Nutrition and Health Series

Adrianne Bendich, PhD, FACN, FASN, Series Editor

For further volumes:
http://www.springer.com/series/7659

Caroline J. Hollins Martin • Ronald Ross Watson
Victor R. Preedy
Editors

Nutrition and Diet in Menopause

Humana Press

Editors
Caroline J. Hollins Martin, PhD, MPhil, BSc
ADM, PGCE, RMT, RM
Department of Midwifery
School of Nursing, Midwifery and Social Work
College of Health and Social Care
University of Salford
Salford, Greater Manchester, UK

Ronald Ross Watson, BS, PhD
Mel and Enid Zuckerman College of Public
Health, and School of Medicine
Arizona Health Sciences Center
University of Arizona
Tucson, AZ, USA

Victor R. Preedy, PhD
Departments of Nutritional Biochemistry
Diabetes and Nutritional Sciences
King's College London
School of Medicine
London, UK

ISBN 978-1-4939-5984-6 ISBN 978-1-62703-373-2 (eBook)
DOI 10.1007/978-1-62703-373-2
Springer New York Heidelberg Dordrecht London

Printed on acid-free paper

Humana Press is a brand of Springer
Springer is part of Springer Science+Business Media (www.springer.com)

Preface

Marked decreases in estrogen production and other endocrine changes are hallmarks of the menopause and affect physiological and psychological function in women. Indeed, it has been reported that the menopause affects most, if not every, organ system in one way or another. The degree of these changes is determined by a number of modulators such as lifestyle, genetics, and dietary factors. However, some of the adverse changes in menopause are considerable, and impose disadvantaged measures of mortality and morbidity. The family unit and communities are also affected. Thus, there is a considerable cost burden to health care providers and services. As a consequence there is a drive to understand, from a scientific point of view, what menopause entails from the cellular level to lifestyle factors. The ultimate objective of such investigations is the formulation of coherent strategies to prevent or cure the adverse effects of menopause. Thus, to achieve an understanding of menopause a holistic approach is needed. However, obtaining this information in a single comprehensive source is currently problematical. This volume, *Nutrition and Diet in Menopause,* aims to achieve this. It is conveniently divided into five parts as follows:

1. *Overviews and general aspects*
2. *Bone and muscle*
3. *Cardiovascular system, metabolism, and cancer*
4. *Psychological aspects and cognitive function*
5. *Preclinical studies: Implications for human health*

There is wide coverage in *Nutrition and Diet in Menopause* including, for example, overviews, body composition, physiological changes, polyphenols, calcium absorption, fortified soy milk, homocysteine, vitamin B12, folate levels, antioxidant vitamins and carotenoids, isoflavones, soy daidzein, tofu, osteoporosis, curcumin, sarcopenia, flaxseed, cardiovascular risk, magnesium, folic acid supplementation, myoinositol, leptin and obesity, fat distribution, cancers including gynecological and breast cancers, vitamin D and cancer, psychology, cognitive decline, black cohosh, and dietary supplements and cognition. Studies on animal models cover α-zearalanol, flaxseed, herba epimedii, and maslinic acid. Finally there is a chapter on supplemental reading and resources.

The contributors are authors of international and national standing, leaders in the field, and trendsetters. Emerging fields of science and important discoveries relating to the menopause are also incorporated in *Nutrition and Diet in Menopause.* The book will be essential reading for nutritionists, dieticians, endocrinologists, cardiologists, health care professionals, research scientists, molecular or cellular biochemists, general practitioners, as well as those interested in women's health in general.

Salford, UK — Caroline J. Hollins Martin
Tucson, AZ, USA — Ronald Ross Watson
London, UK — Victor R. Preedy

Preface

Series Editor Page

The great success of the Nutrition and Health Series is the result of the consistent overriding mission of providing health professionals with texts that are essential because each includes (1) a synthesis of the state of the science and relevant clinical applications; (2) timely, in-depth reviews by the leading researchers in their respective fields; (3) extensive, up-to-date fully annotated reference lists; (4) a detailed index; (5) relevant tables and figures; (6) identification of paradigm shifts and the consequences; (7) virtually no overt overlap of information between chapters, but targeted, inter-chapter referrals; (8) suggestions of areas for future research; and (9) balanced, data-driven answers to patient as well as health professional questions which are based upon the totality of evidence rather than the findings of any single study.

The Series volumes are not the outcome of a symposium. Rather, each editor has the potential to examine a chosen area with a broad perspective, both in subject matter as well as in the choice of chapter authors. The editor(s), whose training(s) is (are) both research and practice oriented, has the opportunity to develop a primary objective for their book, define the scope and focus, and then invite the leading authorities to be part of their initiative. The authors are encouraged to provide an overview of the field, discuss their own research, and relate the research findings to potential human health consequences. Because each book is developed de novo, the chapters are coordinated so that the resulting volume imparts greater knowledge than the sum of the information contained in the individual chapters.

Handbook of Nutrition and Diet in Menopause, edited by Professor Caroline J. Hollins Martin, Ph.D., M.Phil., B.Sc., A.D.M., P.G.C.E., R.M.T., R.M., R.G.N., M.B.Ps.S.; Professor Ronald Ross Watson, Ph.D.; and Professor Victor R. Preedy, Ph.D., D.Sc., F.B.S., F.R.S.P.H., F.R.C.Path., F.R.S.C., clearly exemplifies the goals of the Nutrition and Health Series. The major objective of this comprehensive text is to review the growing evidence that the nutrition provided during adulthood directly affects the changes seen during the menopausal transition. This volume includes 34 up-to-date informative reviews of the current major dietary and health-related issues associated with menopause. Practicing health professionals, researchers, and academicians can rely on the chapters in this volume for objective data-driven sources about essential vitamins and minerals, proteins, fats, and carbohydrates; gynecological cancers; obesity; metabolic syndrome; and osteoporosis. This new comprehensive review of the science behind the nutritional strategies to assure the health of the menopausal woman is of great importance to the nutrition community as well as for health professionals who have to answer patient, client, or graduate student questions about the newest clinical research on nutrition and women's midlife health.

Handbook of Nutrition and Diet in Menopause contains in-depth chapters that review the potential long-term consequences of menopause on the overall health of women, not only at the physical level, including hot flushes (flashes), alterations to the genitourinary system, skin changes, decreased cardiovascular functions, hypertension, headache, back pain, and constipation, as examples. Also examined in relevant chapters are effects on the psychological responses including increased mental tension, irritability, anxiety, sadness, and concentration and memory problems; lack of self-confidence; sleep changes; and libido changes. It is to the credit of Profs. Martin, Watson, and Preedy that they have organized this volume so that it provides an in-depth overview of the critical issues involved in the determination of the best nutrition for middle-aged women, including those with medical conditions that require specific dietary interventions.

The volume contains five related parts. The first part includes chapters containing excellent tables and figures that provide an overview of the physiological changes seen during the menopausal transition. The four chapters include reviews of the endocrine changes and their resulting effects on areas including, but not limited to, loss of fertility, vasomotor symptoms, psychological alterations, body composition, lipid metabolism, increased blood pressure, and the critical role of diet and exercise on maintaining mental as well as physical health during the transition. Perimenopausal changes and postmenopausal health risks are reviewed in detail. Specific physiological areas discussed include the decline of estrogen, thyroid hormone, and growth hormone levels and decreases in the estrogen/androgen ratio. The consequences of these hormonal changes are discussed with regard to body composition changes and weight gain. It is well documented that menopause results in weight gain and fat accumulation, especially visceral fat accumulation, which accelerates as estrogen levels decline. Recent studies are reviewed and point to the potential beneficial effects of moderate exercise and maintenance of body weight as two tactics for reducing certain of the adverse health effects seen in menopausal women. The last chapter in this part reviews the data on the associations between diets rich in polyphenols, especially flavonoids in soy and tea, and reductions in some of the physiological consequences and symptoms of menopause.

The second part on bone and muscle contains ten chapters. Calcium intake is critical to bone health as this essential nutrient is not well absorbed and usual diets do not contain sufficient bioavailable calcium sources. The major food group that contains bioavailable calcium is the dairy group. Several chapters review the effects of reduced estrogen on calcium absorption and transport to bone. This complex biochemical process involves numerous hormones, vitamin D, calcium transport and binding proteins, cell membrane pumps, and other cellular components. Additionally, the type of calcium and the matrix, either from animals or plants, or from supplements, can affect absorption.

Several epidemiological studies have shown that Japanese women have fewer menopausal symptoms based on their soy intake. Soy milk can be used as a calcium source and the bioavailability of the calcium which is fortified in soy milk is dependent upon the type of calcium salt added as well as the acidity of the milk. Soybeans and soy-derived foods, such as tofu, also contain phytoestrogens which are plant derived, phenolic compounds (genistein and daidzein) that are similar in structure to estrogen, although these are not as biologically active. However, a review of randomized control trials that studied the effect of soy isoflavones on bone density reported no significant benefit at major fracture sites in 11 out of 14 trials involving 2,971 postmenopausal women. In contrast, a major study in Japanese women who consumed high levels of soy protein found a decrease in bone fractures. Currently there is an S-equol soy supplement clinical trial under way that may provide a new approach for treatment of menopausal symptoms and osteoporosis.

Oxidative stress adversely affects osteocyte functions. Naturally occurring antioxidants, such as vitamin C and vitamin E are found in diets containing high intakes of nuts, fruits, and vegetables that also contain carotenoids including β-cryptoxanthin and β-carotene. Japanese women, whose diets have included long-term consumption of the β-cryptoxanthin-rich Japanese mandarin orange, have seen benefits to their bone health. The evidence is reviewed in Chap. 8. There is a separate chapter that objectively examines the data linking low intakes of the flavonoid curcumin to osteoporotic risk in menopausal women and concludes that clinical data are needed as animal study findings have been inconsistent.

Homocysteine is an endogenous amino acid, and higher than average serum concentrations have been associated with lower than normal intakes of folic acid, vitamin B6, and vitamin B12. With regard to menopausal women, data suggest that loss of estrogen is associated with increased homocysteine levels. Higher than average homocysteine levels have been associated with several cardiovascular and cerebrovascular risks. Additionally, homocysteine is known to interfere with a key enzyme involved in collagen cross-linking. Cross-link formation is critical for normal collagen structure and bone mechanical properties. Thus, higher homocysteine levels may be associated with damage to the bone's mechanical stability and may increase the risk of fractures.

The final chapter in Part 2 reviews the research on the effects of menopause on skeletal muscle structure, strength, and other functions. There is a linear decline in lean mass (that includes muscle) along with an increase in fat mass in postmenopausal women. Moreover, postmenopausal women have twice the concentration of non-contractile muscle tissue, such as intramuscular fat, compared to younger women. This is primarily due to an imbalance between muscle protein synthesis and muscle protein breakdown, and the increase in oxidative stress and inflammation. Additionally, there are declines in estrogen levels, decreased resting metabolic rate, and a loss of neuromuscular function and apoptosis of muscle cells. Increased physical activity and improvements in diet, including optimal intake of vitamin D, are of some help; however, there is an overall increase in the risk of sarcopenia with menopause and advancing age in women.

The ten chapters in the third part examine the role of nutrition and dietary components on the cardiovascular, metabolic, and cancer risks seen in postmenopausal women. The part includes reviews of the nutritional status of women around the world and contrasts unique dietary habits as well as points out common findings that are associated with the physiological changes seen during estrogen depletion. Increased weight gain and obesity as well as increased metabolic syndrome, cardiovascular, and cancer risks are reviewed in unique chapters. For instance, a detailed chapter describes the adverse health consequences associated with higher than average consumption of red meat in Uruguay. There are also chapters from certain European and Asian communities that confirm that eating fried fish increases, while non-fried fish decreases, cardiovascular risks. The metabolic syndrome is reviewed in several chapters that provide an overview of the endocrine effects of estrogen depletion including significantly increased leptin secretion and insulin resistance, and the potential roles of myoinositol and folic acid, vitamin D, and whole flaxseed. The link between lowered estrogen and reduced serum magnesium levels, altered parathyroid hormone, and vitamin D levels is discussed with regard to consequences to the cardiovascular system as well as bone remodeling. The chapter devoted to gynecological cancers examines the potential for phytoestrogens and other flavonoids from fruits, vegetables, teas, and coffee to affect the risk of endometrial, ovarian, and breast cancers. Several chapters discuss the importance of physical activity and maintenance of ideal body weight with the goal of reducing adverse health effects associated with menopause.

The fourth part contains four informative chapters that examine psychological aspects and cognitive changes that may result from lowered estrogen production during menopause. Acute vasomotor responses to fluctuations in estrogen levels are associated with increased physical as well as emotional stress. However, several epidemiological studies document that physical responses, including hot flushes (flashes) and night sweats, are reported more frequently by women living in North America and Europe, and less so by women from Africa and Latin America. Globally, there are consistent reports of menopause-related psychological symptoms including moodiness, irritability, depression, and impairment of cognitive functions such as memory and concentration. The cultural differences in women's responses to menopausal changes are extensively reviewed. The chapters consistently indicate that further research is needed to determine the role of estrogen in brain functions of menopausal women especially during the expected 20+years of postmenopausal estrogen depletion. There is an extensive review of the many dietary supplements that are purported to reduce menopausal symptoms, including memory loss and cognitive decline. These include soy, red clover, black cohosh, evening primrose oil, dong quai, ginseng, and ginkgo. The 12 placebo-controlled studies that examined the effects of these supplements on cognitive function are carefully reviewed and current data suggest inconsistent and often nonsignificant effects. The detailed review chapter of the clinical data involving studies with black cohosh also suggests the potential for certain adverse effects.

The fifth part contains six chapters that examine preclinical studies of animal models of menopause. Several animal models have been developed specifically for the major chronic diseases seen in postmenopausal women as well as aging men. For example, with regard to Alzheimer's disease, there are transgenic mouse models with selective single or multiple mutations. Models for cardiovascular disease include knockout mouse models, rabbit, and large animal models. The ovarectomized rodent, large animal models, and specific knockout mice are used to study prevention of as well as treatments for osteoporosis. The metabolic syndrome has been studied using pancreatectomy models, transgenic and knockout mouse models, dietary interventions, and spontaneous mutant rodents. All of these models are described and the findings reviewed in the chapters within this part. Certain animal models are relevant as a model of menopausal estrogen changes. The follicle-stimulating hormone receptor knockout mice exhibit changes in the central nervous system and also develop aspects of the metabolic syndrome. These and other relevant animal models are presented in comprehensive tables in Chap. 29. Animal models are important in the development of new drugs and supplements that may be of benefit during menopause and in the postmenopause period. The results of studies with a plant-derived phytoestrogen, α-zearalanol (α-ZAL), a potential replacement for estrogen, are described in the next chapter. The third chapter in this part reviews the numerous animal studies using flaxseed alone and in combination with soy and certain drugs in models of menopausal bone loss and cardiovascular disease. Traditional Chinese medicine (TCM) herbs and plant extracts have been tested for potential anti-osteoporotic effects in ovarectomized mouse models; extracts of the herbs also appear to have some promising activities in these models. Two chapters describe compounds that have TCM substances and specific chemical compounds that have been synthesized from these extracts and tested for efficacy in bone and other models. It may be that the specific compounds will be developed as drugs whereas the extracts will remain classified as dietary components. The final chapter in this part provides valuable information concerning relevant literature and electronic resources available to health professionals interested in nutrition and health for menopausal women.

The logical sequence of the parts as well as the chapters within each part enhance the understanding of the latest information on the current standards of gynecological practice in menopause for clinicians, and related health professionals including the dietician, nurse, pharmacist, physical therapist, behaviorist, psychologist, and others involved in the team effort required for successful treatment of symptoms as well as chronic diseases associated with estrogen loss. This comprehensive volume also has great value for academicians involved in the education of graduate students and postdoctoral fellows, medical students, and allied health professionals who plan to interact with menopausal patients with disorders that may be beneficially affected by nutritional support including the treatment of obesity and the metabolic syndrome.

Cutting-edge discussions of the roles of signaling molecules, growth factors, hormones, cellular and nuclear receptors, and all of the cells and tissues directly involved or affected by the loss of estrogen are included in well-organized chapters that put the molecular aspects into clinical perspective. Of great importance, the editors have provided chapters that balance the most technical information with discussions of its importance for clients and patients.

The volume contains over 150 detailed tables and figures that assist the reader in comprehending the complexities of changes associated with menopause as well as the nutritional factors that can be of benefit during this transition. The overriding goal of this volume is to provide the health professional with balanced documentation and awareness of the newest research and therapeutic approaches including an appreciation of the complexity of the interactions between women's health, diet, and hormonal changes and its consequences on cells and tissues throughout the body. Hallmarks of the 33 chapters include key words and bulleted key points at the beginning of each chapter, complete definitions of terms with the abbreviations fully defined for the reader, and consistent use of terms between chapters. There are over 1,600 up-to-date references; all chapters include a conclusion to highlight major findings. The volume also contains a highly annotated index.

This unique text provides practical, data-driven resources based upon the totality of the evidence to help the reader understand the basics, treatments, and preventive strategies that are involved in the understanding of the role dietary components may play in the prevention of certain chronic conditions associated with menopause. Of equal importance, critical issues that involve cultural preferences seen in countries around the globe are reviewed in well-referenced, informative chapters. The overarching goal of the editors is to provide fully referenced information to health professionals so that they may have a balanced perspective on the value of various preventive and treatment options that are available today as well as in the foreseeable future.

In conclusion, *Handbook of Nutrition and Diet in Menopause*, edited by Professor Caroline J. Hollins Martin, Ph.D., M.Phil., B.Sc., A.D.M., P.G.C.E., R.M.T., R.M., R.G.N., M.B.Ps.S.; Professor Ronald Ross Watson, Ph.D.; and Professor Victor R. Preedy, Ph.D., D.Sc., F.B.S., F.R.S.P.H., F.R.C.Path., F.R.S.C., provides health professionals in many areas of research and practice with the most up-to-date, well-referenced, and comprehensive volume on the current state of the science and medical practice guidelines with regard to maintaining the optimal nutritional and health status of the menopausal woman. This volume will serve the reader as the most authoritative resource in the field to date and is a very welcome addition to the Nutrition and Health Series.

Adrianne Bendich, Ph.D., F.A.C.N., F.A.S.N.
Series Editor

About Series Editor

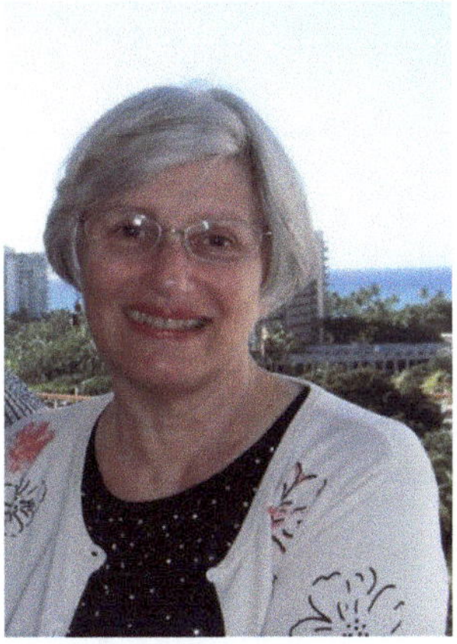

Adrianne Bendich, Ph.D., F.A.C.N., F.A.S.N. Dr. Bendich has successfully served as Series Editor for the Nutrition and Health book series for 15 years and continues to identify key areas of clinical nutrition research that can benefit from the development of targeted, objective volumes edited by the leading researchers in their fields of investigation.

Prior to retiring in September 2010, Dr. Bendich held the position of Director of Medical Affairs at GlaxoSmithKline Consumer Healthcare, where she was responsible for the Medical leadership for the Venture Group, and provided Medical support for well-known brands including TUMS, FiberChoice, Os-Cal, Geritol, and Citrucel. Additionally, she served as a member of GSK's successful Advisory Committee team in support of FDA's Rx to OTC switch of alli®.

Dr. Bendich is internationally recognized as an expert in Women's Health, calcium and vitamin D in bone health, folic acid and pregnancy outcomes, and antioxidants and carotenoid effects on immune functions. She served as the GSK corporate representative to the Women's Health Initiative (WHI) for 9 years as GSK Consumer Healthcare provided all calcium and vitamin D supplements for the WHI study.

She has held memberships and professional positions (ongoing and former): Editorial Board, *Journal of Nutrition in Gerontology and Geriatrics, Antioxidants*, an e-journal, *Journal of Women's Health and Gender-based Medicine*; Associate Editor for *Nutrition*, the International Journal; Chair, Corporate Advisory Committee, Society for Women's Health Research; Member of the Program Advisory Committee for Helen Keller International; Advisor to the Nutrition Department, Montclair State University; Member: Advisory Board, *Current Topics in Nutraceutical Research*; and member ASN's Industry Board and several RIS groups.

Dr. Bendich was a recipient of the Burroughs-Wellcome Fund Professorship and Roche Research Award; she is listed in Who's Who of American Women Scientists and many other Who's Who volumes; she is a recipient of the CRN Apple Award for contributions to the science of vitamin and mineral supplements. In 2012, Dr. Bendich was elected a Fellow of the American Society for Nutrition, the highest honor of the Society.

Dr. Bendich is the author of more than 100 peer-reviewed publications, and Series Editor of "Nutrition and Health" for Springer/Humana Press which includes 48 volumes such as *Preventive Nutrition*, *Handbook of Clinical Nutrition and Aging*, *Diet and Human Immune Functions*, *Handbook of Drug–Nutrient Interactions*, and other reference volumes for health professionals as outlined at http://www.springer.com/series/7659.

About Volume Editors

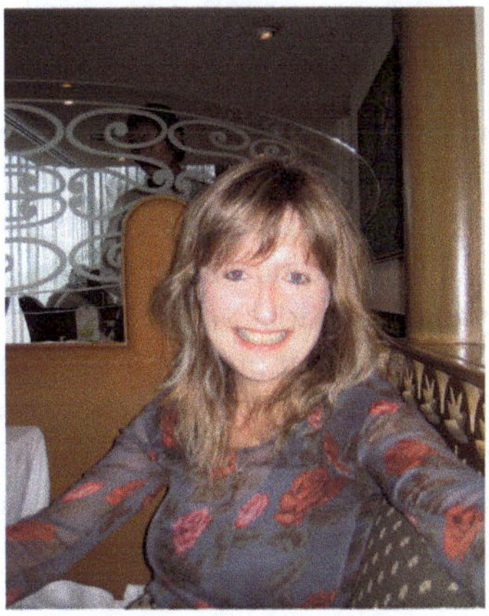

Caroline J. Hollins Martin, Ph.D., M.Phil., B.Sc., A.D.M., P.G.C.E., R.M.T., R.M., R.G.N., M.B.Ps.S., is a Professor in Midwifery in the College of Health and Social Care at the University of Salford. Her background has encompassed a career in women's reproductive health that spans 26 years; the first 11 of these were spent as a clinical midwife in Ayrshire (Scotland) and 15 teaching and researching women's reproductive health within universities. She is an NMC Registered Midwife and Lecturer/Practice Educator. She is also a graduate and postgraduate in psychology and a Member of the British Psychological Society (M.B.Ps.S.). Her research interests lie in social psychology that relates to women's reproductive health, with much of her work relating to obstructing autonomy, evidence-based practice, and providing choice and control to childbearing women. More recently, her focus has shifted to developing useful tools for maternal health practitioners to use in clinical practice, for example, the Birth Participation Scale (BPS) to assess fathers' fears and needs in relation to childbirth and the Birth Satisfaction Scale (BSS) to assess mothers' perceptions of their birth experience. Current research interests lie in shaping perinatal bereavement care, outcomes of maternal activity during labor, and the effects of music upon women's stress levels. To date, she has published 31 peer-reviewed papers, presented 32 conference papers, and written 4 book chapters and is the associate editor for women's reproductive health papers submitted to the *Journal of Nurse Education in Practice*.

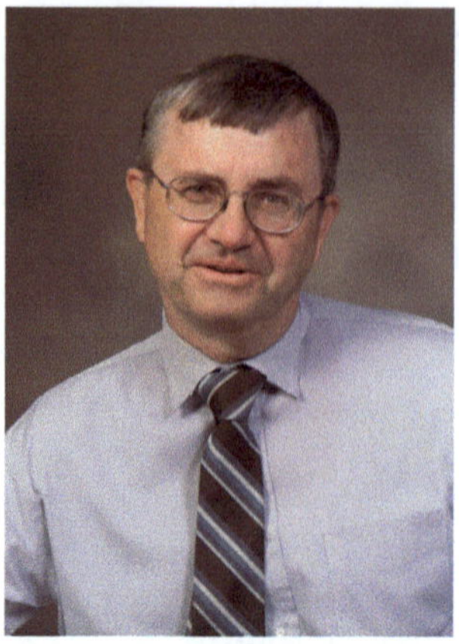

Ronald Ross Watson, Ph.D., attended the University of Idaho but graduated from Brigham Young University in Provo, Utah, with a degree in chemistry in 1966. He earned his Ph.D. in biochemistry from Michigan State University in 1971. His postdoctoral schooling in nutrition and microbiology was completed at the Harvard School of Public Health, where he gained 2 years of postdoctoral research experience in immunology and nutrition.

From 1973 to 1974, Dr. Watson was assistant professor of immunology and performed research at the University of Mississippi Medical Center in Jackson. He was assistant professor of microbiology and immunology at the Indiana University Medical School from 1974 to 1978, and associate professor at Purdue University in the Department of Food and Nutrition from 1978 to 1982. In 1982, Dr. Watson joined the faculty at the University of Arizona Health Sciences Center in the Department of Family and Community Medicine of the School of Medicine. He is currently professor of health promotion sciences in the Mel and Enid Zuckerman Arizona College of Public Health.

Dr. Watson is a member of several national and international nutrition, immunology, cancer, and alcoholism research societies. Among his patents he has one on a dietary supplement passion fruit peel extract, with more pending. He had done DHEA research on its effects on mouse AIDS and immune function for 20 years. He edited a previous book on melatonin (Watson RR. *Health Promotion and Aging: The Role of Dehydroepiandrosterone (DHEA)*. Harwood Academic Publishers, 1999, 164 pages). For 30 years he was funded by Wallace Research Foundation to study dietary supplements in health promotion. Dr. Watson has edited more than 100 books on nutrition, dietary supplements and over-the-counter agents, and drugs of abuse, as scientific reference books. He has published more than 500 research and review articles.

Victor R. Preedy, B.Sc., Ph.D., D.Sc., F.S.B., F.R.C.Path., F.R.S.P.H., F.R.S.C., is a senior member of King's College London (Professor of Nutritional Biochemistry) and King's College Hospital (Professor of Clinical Biochemistry). He is attached to both the Diabetes and Nutritional Sciences Division and the Department of Nutrition and Dietetics. He is also Director of the Genomics Centre and a member of the School of Medicine. Professor Preedy graduated in 1974 with an Honors Degree in Biology and Physiology with Pharmacology. He gained his University of London Ph.D. in 1981. In 1992, he received his Membership of the Royal College of Pathologists and in 1993 he gained his second doctoral degree, for his outstanding contribution to protein metabolism in health and disease. Professor Preedy was elected as a Fellow to the Institute of Biology in 1995 and to the Royal College of Pathologists in 2000. Since then he has been elected as a Fellow to the Royal Society for the Promotion of Health (2004) and The Royal Institute of Public Health (2004). In 2009, Professor Preedy became a Fellow of the Royal Society for Public Health and in 2012 a Fellow of the Royal Society of Chemistry. In his career Professor Preedy has carried out research at the National Heart

Hospital (part of Imperial College London) and the MRC Centre at Northwick Park Hospital. He has collaborated with research groups in Finland, Japan, Australia, the USA, and Germany. He is a leading expert on the science of health. He has lectured nationally and internationally. To his credit, Professor Preedy has published over 570 articles, which include 165 peer-reviewed manuscripts based on original research, 100 reviews, and over 50 books and volumes.

Contents

Contributors

Krasimira Aleksandrova, M.P.H., Ph.D. Department of Epidemiology, German Institute of Human Nutrition Potsdam–Rehbruecke, Nuthetal, Germany

John Aloia, M.D. Winthrop University Hospital, Mineola, NY, USA

Bahram H. Arjmandi, Ph.D. Department of Nutrition, Food and Exercise, Florida State University, Tallahassee, FL, USA

Mylène Aubertin-Leuheure, Ph.D. Groupe de Recherche en Activité Physique Adaptée, Université du Québec à Montréal, Pavillon des Sciences Biologiques, Montréal, QC, Canada

S.S. Avinash, M.B.B.S., M.D. Department of Biochemistry, Father Muller Medical College, Mangalore, Karnataka, India

Isabel Baeza, Ph.D. San Rafael-Nebrija Health Sciences Centre, Nebrija University, Madrid, Spain

Jameela Banu, M.Sc., Ph.D. Coordinated Program in Dietetics and Department of Biology, University of Texas - Pan American, Division of Clinical Immunology and Rheumatology, Department of Medicine, Edinburg Regional Academic Health Center, University of Texas Health Science Center at San Antonio, Edinburg, TX, USA

Medical Research Division, Edinburg Regional Academic Health Center, University of Texas Health Science Center at San Antonio, Edinburg, TX, USA

Sébastien Barbat-Artigas, Ph.D. Groupe de Recherche en Activité Physique Adaptée, Université du Québec à Montréal, Pavillon des Sciences Biologiques, Montréal, QC, Canada

Francesca Basile, M.D. Department of Obstetrics and Gynecology, Catholic University of Sacred Heart, Rome, Italy

Eleonora Bielawska-Batorowicz, M.Sc., Ph.D. Institute of Psychology, University of Łódź, Łódź, Poland

Alessandro Caruso, M.D. Department of Obstetrics and Gynecology, Catholic University of Sacred Hearth, Rome, Italy

Luigi Mario Chiechi, M.D. Department of Bioethics, University of Bari, Bari, Italy

Yuri N. Clement, B.Sc., Ph.D. Faculty of Medical Sciences, Pharmacology Unit, The University of the West Indies, St. Augustine, Trinidad and Tobago

Rosario D'Anna, M.D. Department of Obstetrics and Gynecology, University Hospital, Messina, Italy

Eduardo De Stéfani, M.D. Grupo de Epidemiología, Departamento de Patología, Facultad de Medicina, Universidad de la República, Montevideo, Uruguay

Mónica De la Fuente, M.Sc., Ph.D. Department of Physiology (Animal Physiology II), Faculty of Biology, Complutense University of Madrid, Madrid, Spain

Cristina Di Cesare, M.D. Department of Obstetrics and Gynecology, Catholic University of Sacred Hearth, Rome, Italy

Patrick Rene Diel, Ph.D. Department of Cellular and Molecular Sports Medicine, Institute of Cardiovascular Research and Sports Medicine, German Sports University Cologne, Cologne, Germany

Laura Donati, M.D. Department of Obstetrics and Gynecology, Catholic University of Sacred Hearth, Rome, Italy

Gabriel Fernandes, M.Sc., Ph.D. Division of Clinical Immunology and Rheumatology, Department of Medicine, University of Texas Health Science Center at San Antonio, San Antonio, TX, USA

Joanna Folwarczna, Pharm.D., Ph.D. Department of Pharmacology, School of Pharmacy with Division of Laboratory Medicine, Medical University of Silesia, Katowice, Sosnowiec, Poland

Henk R. Franke, M.D., Ph.D. Department of Obstetrics and Gynecology, Medisch Spectrum Twente Hospital Group, Enschede, The Netherlands

J. Christopher Gallagher, M.D. Bone Metabolism Unit, Department of Endocrinology, Creighton University Medical Center, Omaha, NE, USA

B.K. Manjunatha Goud, M.B.B.S., M.D. Department of Biochemistry, RAK College of Medical Sciences, RAK Medical and Health Sciences University, Ras Al Khaimah, United Arab Emirates

Ted Greiner, Ph.D. Department of Food and Nutrition, College of Human Ecology, Hanyang University, Seoul, South Korea

Jeffrey S. Greiwe, Ph.D. Ausio Pharmaceuticals, LLC, Cincinnati, OH, USA

Berna Haliloglu, M.D. Department of Obstetrics and Gynecology, School of Medicine, University of Maltepe, Istanbul, Turkey

Wei He, M.D. Obesity and Body Composition Research Center, Chronic Disease Research Institute, Zhejiang University School of Public Health, Hangzhou, Zhejiang, China

Francesca Ianniello, M.D. Department of Obstetrics and Gynecology, Catholic University of Sacred Hearth, Rome, Italy

Maria Lieta Interdonato Department of Obstetrics and Gynecology, Policlinico Universitario "G. Martino", Messina, Italy

Kiyoshi Ito, M.D., Ph.D. Department of Disaster Obstetrics and Gynecology, International Research Institute of Disaster Science (IRIDeS), Tohoku University, Sendai, Japan

Richard L. Jackson, Ph.D. Ausio Pharmaceuticals, LLC, Cincinnati, OH, USA

Wangjing Ke, M.D. Arizona Health Sciences Center, Mel and Enid Zuckerman College of Public Health and School of Medicine, University of Arizona, Tucson, AZ, USA

Sylvia Kirchengast, M.A., Ph.D. Department of Anthropology, University of Vienna, Vienna, Austria

Cristina Larroy, Ph.D. Faculty of Psychology, Department of Clinical Psychology, Universidad Complutense de Madrid, Madrid, Spain

Departmento de Psicología Clínica, Facultad de Psicología, Madrid, Spain

Mingyao Liu, Ph.D. The Institute of Biomedical Sciences, East China Normal University, Shanghai, China

Edralin A. Lucas, Ph.D. Nutritional Sciences Department, Oklahoma State University, Stillwater, OK, USA

Jian Luo, Ph.D. The Institute of Biomedical Sciences, East China Normal University, Shanghai, China

Xiaoguang Ma, M.D., M.Phil., Ph.D. Department of Epidemiology and Biostatistics, Arnold School of Public Health, University of South Carolina, Columbia, SC, USA

Gail B. Mahady, Ph.C., Ph.D. Department of Pharmacy Practice, PAHO/WHO Collaborating Centre for Traditional Medicine, College of Pharmacy, University of Illinois, Chicago, IL, USA

Caroline J. Hollins Martin, Ph.D., M.Phil., B.Sc., A.D.M., P.G.C.E., R.M.T., R.M., R.G.N., M.B.Ps.S. Department of Midwifery, School of Nursing, Midwifery and Social Work, College of Health and Social Care, University of Salford, Salford, Greater Manchester, UK

Maureen Meister, B.S. Nutritional Sciences Department, Oklahoma State University, Stillwater, OK, USA

Giancarlo Paradisi, M.D. Department of Obstetrics and Gynecology, Catholic University of Sacred Heart, Rome, Italy

Vinood B. Patel, B.Sc. (Hons), Ph.D. Department of Biomedical Sciences, School of Life Sciences, University of Westminster, London, UK

Hakan Peker, M.D. Department of Obstetrics and Gynecology, Memorial Hizmet Hospital, Istanbul, Turkey

Victor R. Preedy, Ph.D. Division of Diabetes and Nutritional Sciences, School of Medicine, Kings College London, London, UK

Lorena Quagliozzi, M.D. Department of Obstetrics and Gynecology, Catholic University of Sacred Heart, Rome, Italy

Rajkumar Rajendram, A.K.C., B.Sc. (hons), M.B.B.S. (dist), M.R.C.P. (UK), F.R.C.A. Departments of General Medicine and Intensive Care, John Radcliffe Hospital, Oxford, UK

Diabetes and Nutritional Sciences Research Division, King's College London School of Medicine, London, UK

Roshanna Rajendram, B.Sc. (hons) School of Medical and Dental Sciences, University of Birmingham, Birmingham, UK

Alvaro L. Ronco, M.D. Oncology and Radiotherapy Unit, Department of Epidemiology and Scientific Methods, School of Medicine IUCLAEH, Pereira Rossell Women's Hospital, Montevideo, Uruguay

Hironobu Sasano, M.D., Ph.D. Department of Pathology, Tohoku University Graduate School of Medicine, Sendai, Japan

Richard J. Schwen, Ph.D. Ausio Pharmaceuticals, LLC, Cincinnati, OH, USA

Albert Shieh, M.D. Winthrop University Hospital, Mineola, NY, USA

Brenda J. Smith, Ph.D. Nutritional Sciences Department, Oklahoma State University, Stillwater, OK, USA

Sreekantha, M.B.B.S., M.D. Department of Biochemistry, Navodaya Medical College, Raichur, Karnataka, India

Lily Stojanovska, Ph.D. College of Health and Biomedicine, Victoria University, Melbourne, VIC, Australia

Minoru Sugiura, Ph.D. Citrus Research Division, National Institute of Fruit Tree Science, Shizuoka City, Shizuoka, Japan

Anne Lise Tang, Ph.D. College of Health and Biomedicine, Victoria University, Melbourne, VIC, Australia

Lilian U. Thompson, Ph.D. Faculty of Medicine, Department of Nutritional Sciences, Faculty of Medicine, University of Toronto, Toronto, ON, Canada

Yvonne T. van der Schouw, Ph.D. Julius Center for Health Sciences and Primary Care, University Medical Center Utrecht, Utrecht, The Netherlands

Rosa Vera Legal and Forensic Psychology, Vertices Psicólogos, Madrid, Spain

Wen Wang, M.D., Ph.D. Department of Pathophysiology, School of Basic Medical Sciences, Capital Medical University, Beijing, China

Wendy Elizabeth Ward, B. Arts & Sci., M.Sc., Ph.D. Department of Kinesiology and Center for Bone and Muscle Health, Brock University, St. Catharines, ON, Canada

Ronald Ross Watson, B.S., Ph.D. Arizona Health Sciences Center, Mel and Enid Zuckerman College of Public Health and School of Medicine, University of Arizona, Tucson, AZ, USA

Carmen Weigt, Dipl. Biol. German Sports University Cologne, Cologne, Germany

Magdalena Wiacek, Ph.D. Jędrzej Śniadecki Academy of Physical Education and Sports, Gdańskt, Poland

Man-Sau Wong, Ph.D. Department of Applied Biology and Chemical Technology, The Hong Kong Polytechnic University, Kowloon, Hong Kong, China

Nobuo Yaegashi, M.D., Ph.D. Department of Obstetrics and Gynecology, Tohoku University Graduate School of Medicine, Sendai, Japan

Vinod Yalamanchili, M.B.B.S. Bone Metabolism Unit, Department of Endocrinology, Creighton University Medical Center, Omaha, NE, USA

Yan Zhang, Ph.D. University of Shanghai for Science and Technology, Shanghai, China

Shankuan Zhu, M.D., Ph.D. Obesity and Body Composition Research Center, Chronic Disease Research Institute, Zhejiang University School of Public Health, Hangzhou, Zhejiang, China

Igor Z. Zubrzycki, Ph.D., D.Sc. Department of Life Science, Jędrzej Śniadecki Academy of Physical Education and Sports, Gdańskt, Poland

Part I
Overview and General Aspects

Chapter 1
An Overview of the Extent and Nature of Menopause and Its Physiological Basis

Yvonne T. van der Schouw

Keypoints

- Menopause is defined as the permanent cessation of menstruation due to depletion of the follicle pool.
- The menstrual cycle and changes in the cyclic pattern until a complete stop are orchestrated by gonadotrophins, steroids, and inhibins.
- The median age at natural menopause is around 50–51, for centuries and across populations.
- Menopause is associated with vasomotor menopausal symptoms; of other symptoms such as incontinence, depressed feelings, and vaginal dryness it is not clear whether it is the menopause per se that causes these symptoms and complaints, or whether aging also plays a major role.
- Early menopause is associated with increased risk of cardiovascular disease and osteoporosis and a decreased risk of breast cancer.
- These effects are generally ascribed to estrogens, but for osteoporosis and breast cancer this is much more clear than for cardiovascular disease.

Keywords Menopause • Endocrinology • Epidemiology • Physiology • Vasomotor menopausal symptoms

Abbreviations

FMP	Final menstrual period
STRAW	Stages of reproductive aging workshop
LH	Luteinizing hormone
FSH	Follicle-stimulating hormone
GnRH	Gonadotrophin-releasing hormone
VMS	Vasomotor menopausal symptoms
CVD	Cardiovascular diseases
CHD	Coronary heart disease
HT	Hormone therapy
HERS	Heart and estrogen/progestin replacement study
WHI	Women's Health Initiative trial
BMD	Bone mineral density

Y.T. van der Schouw, Ph.D. (✉)
Julius Center for Health Sciences and Primary Care, University Medical Center Utrecht, STR 6.131, P.O. Box 85500, Utrecht, 3508 GA, The Netherlands
e-mail: y.t.vanderschouw@umcutrecht.nl

C.J.H. Martin et al. (eds.), *Nutrition and Diet in Menopause*, Nutrition and Health,
DOI 10.1007/978-1-62703-373-2_1, © Springer Science+Business Media New York 2013

Introduction

The word "menopause" is derived from the Greek word παυσις (pausis, cessation) and the root μεν- (men-, month). Menopause is defined as the permanent cessation of menstruation [1]. Most animals do not have a post-reproductive life, and menopause has been considered as something unique to human [2]. There is a lively debate among evolutionary biologists and anthropologists why human females have menopause. The grandmother theory proposes that natural selection increased the length of the human postmenopausal period—and, thus, extended longevity—as a result of the inclusive fitness benefits of grandmothering [3]. The other theory, also known as the disposable soma theory, states that longevity requires investments in somatic maintenance that reduce the resources available for reproduction [4]. Recently it was shown that menopause is not unique for humans, but is also experienced by nonhuman primates [5, 6].

Menopause occurs with the final menstrual period (FMP), which is known with certainty only in retrospect after 12 consecutive months of amenorrhea. There is no biological marker of menopause [1]. Perimenopause is the time immediately before menopause, when the endocrinological, biological, and clinical features of approaching menopause commence, and the first year after menopause [1].

Treloar was among the first to observe a group of female students in Minnesota starting in 1934 until the 1960s of the previous century, in order to describe menstrual cyclicity during women's lives [7, 8]. The Stages of Reproductive Aging Workshop (STRAW) group have proposed definitions for staging female reproductive aging (Fig. 1.1) [9]. According to STRAW, the menopausal transition is

Menarche (at stage -5) FMP (0) (between stages -1 and +1a)

Stage	-5	-4	-3b	-3a	-2	-1	+1 a	+1b	+1c	+2
Terminology	REPRODUCTIVE				MENOPAUSAL TRANSITION		POSTMENOPAUSE			
	Early	Peak	Late		Early	Late	Early			Late
					Perimenopause					
Duration	*variable*				*variable*	1-3 years	2 years (1+1)		3-6 years	*Remaining lifespan*
PRINCIPAL CRITERIA										
Menstrual Cycle	Variable to regular	Regular	Regular	Subtle changes in Flow/ Length	*Variable Length* Persistent ≥7- day difference in length of consecutive cycles	Interval of amenorrhea of >=60 days				
SUPPORTIVE CRITERIA										
Endocrine FSH AMH Inhibin B			Low Low	Variable Low Low	↑ Variable Low Low	↑ >25 IU/L** Low Low	↑ Variable Low Low		Stabilizes Very Low Very Low	
Antral Follicle Count			Low	Low	Low	Low	Very Low		Very Low	
DESCRIPTIVE CHARACTERISTICS										
Symptoms						Vasomotor symptoms *Likely*	Vasomotor symptoms *Most Likely*			*Increasing* symptoms of urogenital atrophy

* Blood draw on cycle days 2-5 ↑ = elevated
**Approximate expected level based on assays using current international pituitary standard[67-69]

Fig. 1.1 The stages of reproductive aging workshop + 10 staging system (STRAW) for reproductive aging in women. Reproduced from [9] with permission from Wolters Kluwer Health

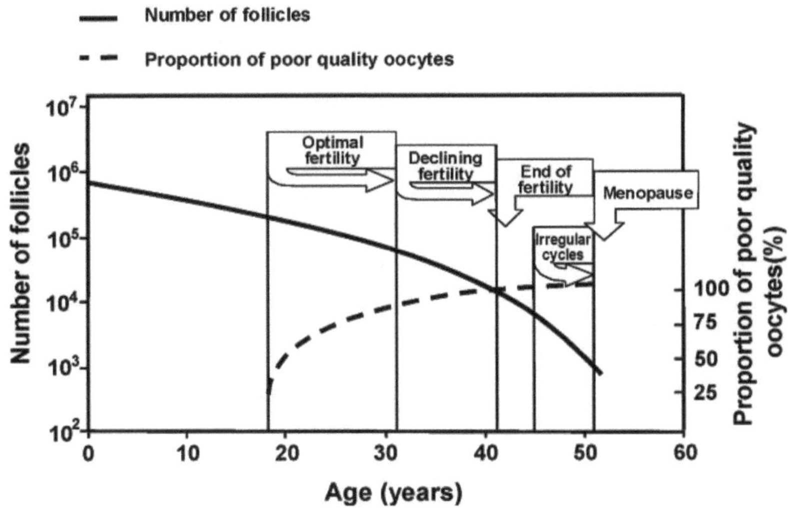

Fig. 1.2 The decline in follicle number and the increase in the proportion of poor-quality oocytes in relation to reproductive events with increasing female age. Redrawn after de Bruin JP 2004 and [106]. Reproduced from [107] with permission from Elsevier

the time before the FMP, when variability in the menstrual cycle is usually increased. It may be subdivided into the early transition, marked by a 7 or more days' persistent difference in cycle lengths from the woman's previous normal range, and late transition, marked by 60 or more days of amenorrhea, observed on at least one occasion.

Menopause is the ultimate result of ovarian aging and the consequence of a decrease in the number of remaining follicles with increasing female age. Women are born with the full stock of primordial follicles, containing six to seven millions [10], to serve the needs of reproduction for the rest of a woman's life. From birth onwards, the follicle pool decreases; a process called atresia makes the follicles deteriorate before or after they have initiated follicle growth [11]. At puberty, only ~300,000 follicles are left, and subsequently with every menstrual cycle hundreds vanish. This also occurs during periods when no ovulation takes place, such as pregnancy, breastfeeding, or oral contraceptive use. The rate of disappearance increases markedly from age 37 to 38 onwards. At 45–46 years, the stock has diminished to several thousands, a critical number, and menstrual bleeding starts to become irregular [12]. When reduced to a thousand or less, the number is too small to maintain the cyclic hormonal process needed for menstruation, and menopause occurs [13]. There is substantial interindividual variation in the onset of menopause, varying roughly between 40 and 60 years, with a mean age of 51 which is rather constant over time and populations worldwide [14]. In parallel to the *quantitative* decline in the number of oocytes also the *quality* of the oocytes held in the follicles declines with increasing female age. This results in a decrease in female fecundity after the age of 31, which may accelerate after age 37, leading to sterility at a mean age of 41 (Fig. 1.2) [15].

Endocrinology

The decrease of the follicle pool appears to be caused by endocrine changes [16]. Gonadotrophins, steroids, and inhibins play a crucial role in the endocrinology of the menopausal transition (Fig. 1.3) [16]. The pituitary is stimulated by gonadotrophin-releasing hormone (GnRH) from the hypothalamus

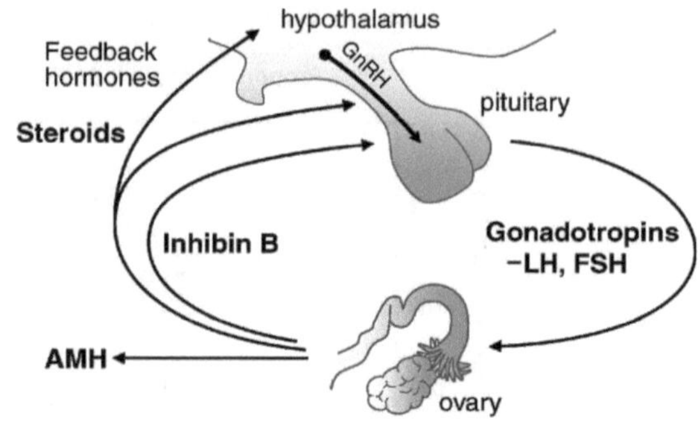

Fig. 1.3 Schematic of hypothalamopituitary-ovarian axis. Antimüllerian hormone (AMH) is also a product of antral follicles, but does not appear to participate in the closed-loop feedback system. Reprinted from [16] with permission from Wolters Kluwer Health

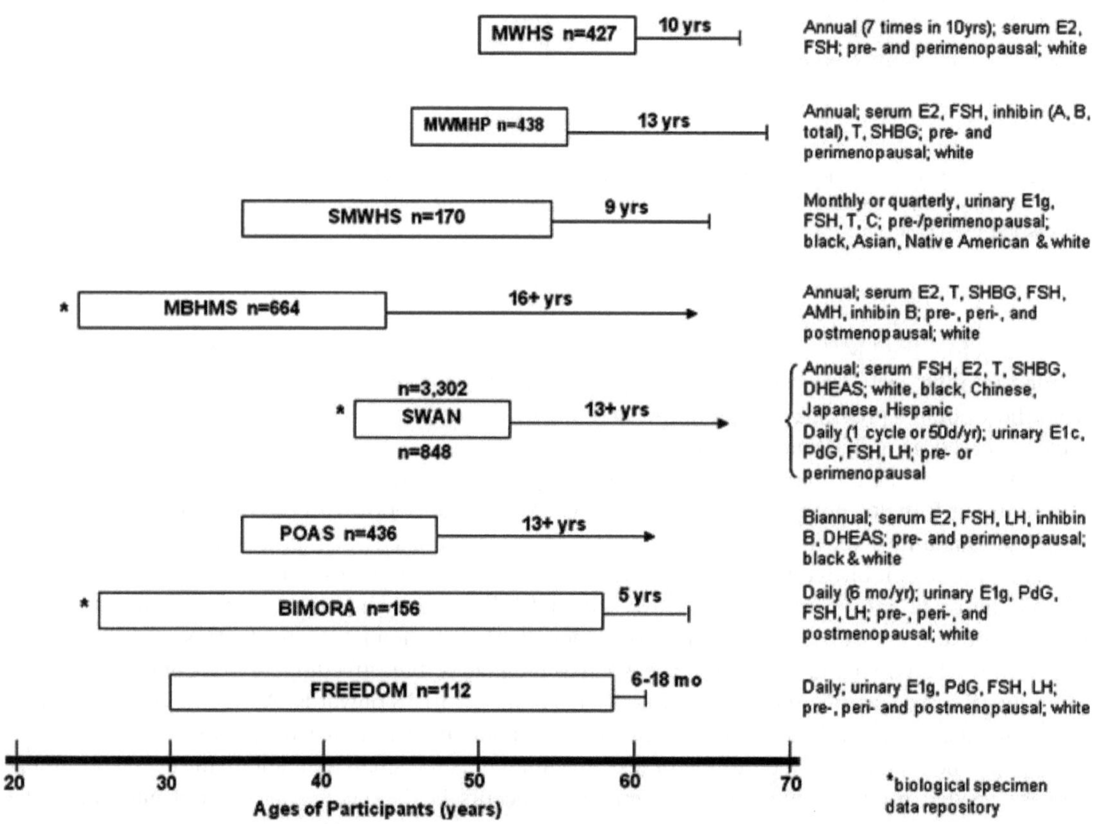

Fig. 1.4 Longitudinal, epidemiologic studies of female reproductive aging that include substantial endocrine data. Studies are in order from least to most recent start date (*top* to *bottom*). Box width depicts the baseline age range of participants for each study. Number of years listed on line to the *right* of each box is the maximum number of years during which endocrine data were/are collected; *arrow* indicates that a study is ongoing. Information to the right includes sampling strategy, hormones measured, allowable menopausal stages at baseline, and ethnicity. All annual or monthly samples were taken during the early follicular phase of the menstrual cycle. Across all studies, women were excluded if they did not have at least one ovary, were pregnant or breastfeeding, or were taking exogenous hormones or other medications known to affect reproductive hormone values. *MWHS* Massachusetts Women's Health Study, *MWMHP* Melbourne Women's Midlife Health Project, *SMWHS* Seattle Midlife Women's Health Study, *MBHMS* Michigan Bone Health and Metabolism Study, *SWAN* Study of Women's Health Across the Nation, *POAS* Penn Ovarian Aging Study, *BIMORA* Biodemographic Models of Reproductive Aging Project, *FREEDOM* Fertility Recognition Enabling Early Detection of Menopause Study. *Hormones*: *C* cortisol, *AMH* anti-Müllerian hormone, *E2* estradiol, *E1c/E1g* estrogen conjugates, *FSH* follicle-stimulating hormone, *LH* luteinizing hormone, *PdG* pregnanediol glucuronide, *T* testosterone, *SHBG* sex hormone-binding globulin, *DHEAS* dehydroepiandrosterone sulfate. Reprinted from [108] with permission from John Wiley and Sons

to produce luteinizing hormone (LH) and follicle-stimulating hormone (FSH). LH and FSH are the regulators of follicle development and hormone secretion by the follicle. In the follicular phase of the menstrual cycle, the granulosa cells of the antral follicle produce estradiol and inhibin B. Estradiol exerts feedback actions on the pituitary and the hypothalamus, whereas inhibin B mainly acts on the pituitary to reduce FSH secretion [17].

Several epidemiological studies have yielded important information on the hormonal changes throughout female reproductive life; they are summarized in Fig. 1.4. When follicles decrease in number, the number of fully functioning granulosa cells also decreases. This initially leads to differentially decreased secretion of inhibin B, as a result of which FSH secretion increases [18, 19]. As a consequence, follicle development will be initiated earlier, and the follicular phase of the still regular menstrual cycles will become shorter. In older women, at least some of their cycles are characterized by elevated follicular phase FSH levels, corresponding to STRAW stage 3.

It is yet unknown what the causes are for cycle irregularity; several mechanisms have been postulated, which are well summarized by Burger et al. [16]. It has been suggested that at the initiation of a cycle, there may be no follicles responsive to the FSH increase between cycles. As a result, the ovarian negative feedback is lacking, inhibin B and estradiol levels remain low, and FSH increases until responsive follicles appear, with the subsequent initiation of the events leading up to ovulation [16, 20]. An alternative theory is that decreasing follicle production might lead to high levels of estrogen secretion around the time of menstrual bleeding, which appear to be associated with shortened cycles. If FSH levels are sufficiently high and sustained, it is possible that other antral follicles may be stimulated to grow and develop in other parts of the cycle, with high estradiol levels, which may explain the wide range of estradiol levels seen in women in the transition [18]. Such elevations may lead to delayed menses or to breakthrough bleeding. Further follicle depletion may then result in failure to ovulate and the progressively increasing frequency of anovulatory cycles in the late menopausal transition. However, occasionally it may be possible to respond normally to gonadotrophin stimulation, with the development of a normal ovulatory cycle as a result. The changes in follicle production may lead to a diminished function of the corpus luteum. Rapid declines in estrogen levels occur during late perimenopause, the last 2 years before the FMP, so mainly in STRAW stage 1 [21, 22].

Epidemiology

The mean age at which natural menopause occurs is generally considered to be 50–51 years. Since the report of age at menopause in different European countries by Backman in 1948 [23] there has been discussion whether there is a secular trend in age at menopause, just as has been observed for age at menarche [24]. A secular trend is defined as an increasing or a decreasing age at which an event occurs.

Backman observed an increasing trend for age at menopause, using reports of menopause to begin at age 40 in ancient times, and increasing from a little bit lower than 46 in 1840 to a little bit over 48 in 1940, as displayed in Fig. 1.5. However, a later more extensive review of ancient Greek and Roman literature concludes that the most cited age at menopause is 50 years [25]. The same investigators also studied European medieval sources from the sixth to the fifteenth century, and conclude that again the most frequently cited age of menopause is 50 years, just like what is currently reported [26]. These reports cast doubt on the existence of a secular trend in age at menopause.

Treloar asked single female students attending the University of Minnesota in the fall of 1934 and the freshmen of the next 3 consecutive years to keep a menstrual diary, basically for the rest of their reproductive life. In 1970, for 324 from the 2,700 enrolled who had reached natural menopause, the mean age at menopause was estimated to be 49.5 years [27]. In 1981, this information was updated and again, the estimate for the mean age at menopause was 49.5 years.

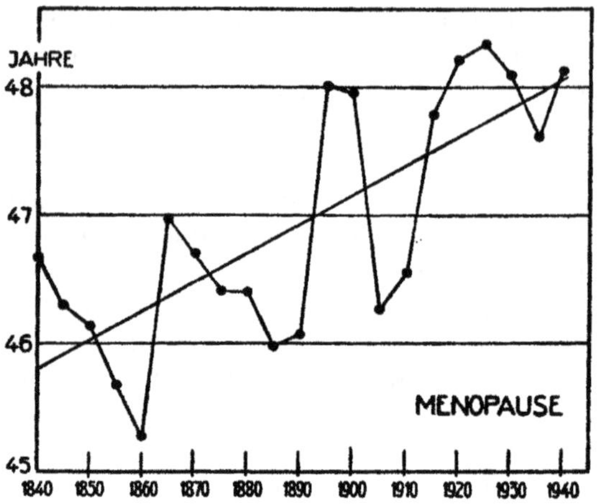

Fig. 1.5 Course of the mean age at menopause per 10 years and for every 5 years in Europe, 1840–1940. Reproduced from [23] with permission from S. Karger AG, Basel

Assessment of mean age at menopause sounds easy, but is in fact difficult. In the oldest reports, ages are often just listed as "between 45 and 50 years." In populations where not all women have become postmenopausal, means and medians are not accurate reflections of the true population means or medians, as they just take into account the menopausal ages of the still premenopausal women, and will therefore be an underestimation [28, 29]. It is well known that women tend to round off their age at menopause to the nearest 5 or 0; therefore, clusters occur at age 40, 45, 50, and 55 [30–32].

Besides these more methodological problems, there are also factors affecting age at menopause, which hamper comparison of mean ages at menopause in different time periods in different populations. Women who had surgical menopause usually have this at younger ages than natural menopause would have occurred. Also smoking advances age at menopause with a year [33]. This may lead to a lower estimated mean age at menopause in populations with a large proportion of smoking or surgically menopausal women. In addition, it has been suggested that nutritional status, geographical altitude, and genetics may affect the age at menopause [29].

In 1985, McKinlay summarized 13 studies covering a period between 1960 and 1985 that provided information on median age at menopause in a more reliable manner using appropriate statistics. A median age at menopause between 50 and 51 years was consistently reported [34]. In 1998, the results were published of a large study on the variability in reproductive factors among 18,997 women in Europe, the Americas, Asia, Australia, and Africa. The median age at natural menopause was estimated to be 50 years overall, and the median ages at menopause ranged moderately between 49 and 52 years among the centers [14]. The authors concluded that there is not much international variation in age at menopause.

Later studies from Sweden, the USA, and The Republic of Chuvasia, Russian Federation, have suggested that there is a secular trend visible in age at menopause [35–39], but also in these studies a median age of 50 was observed, with some variation around that age; and not all studies used proper methods, and sometimes no secular trend was seen after adjustment for education, smoking, and physical activity.

In conclusion, most studies observe a median age at menopause somewhere between 49 and 51, already since ancient Greek and Roman times. Because of influences of external factors on age at menopause, such as surgery, smoking, and oral contraceptive or hormone use, it is questionable whether more precise estimates can be reliably made. The fact that estimates are around the age of 50 for centuries argues against the existence of a secular trend in age at menopause.

Physiology

Vasomotor Menopausal Symptoms

Menopause is associated with many physiological changes, one of the most distinct being vasomotor menopausal symptoms (VMS), i.e., hot flushes or hot flashes and night sweats. VMS are defined as subjective sensations of heat that are associated with objective signs of cutaneous vasodilatation and a subsequent drop in core body temperature [40]. Intensity of VMS widely varies, between women, but also within individual women. Mild VMS can be experienced as a transient warming sensation. With severe VMS, women report abrupt and very intense heat that spreads over the face and the upper body, together with reddening of the face and severe perspiration. These symptoms are objectified by measurement of skin temperature and skin conductance, an electrical measure of sweating [41]. Very frequently these symptoms are followed by chills and shivering. The duration of a hot flush is in general quite short, around 5 min, but can also be up to 15 min [42].

VMS seem to result from a reduced thermoneutral zone [43]. The core body temperature is regulated between an upper threshold for sweating and a lower threshold for shivering. Between these thresholds is a neutral zone within which thermoregulatory responses such as sweating and shivering do not occur [44]. In women without VMS, the null zone is about 0.4 °C. This means that temperature fluctuations of as much as + 0.4 °C do not cause sweating or shivering in women without VMS. However, in women with VMS, the thermoneutral zone disappears and temperature fluctuations quickly lead to sweating or shivering as explained in Fig. 1.6 [45].

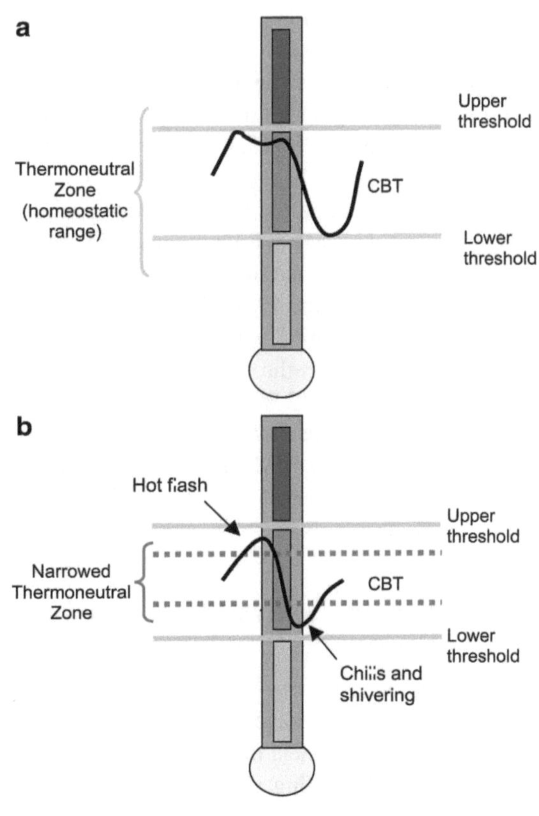

Fig. 1.6 Maintenance of core body temperature (CBT). CBT is critical to organ integrity and optimal function [48]. (**a**) Normal temperature regulation. (**b**) Dysfunctional temperature regulation. Reprinted from [48] with permission from Springer

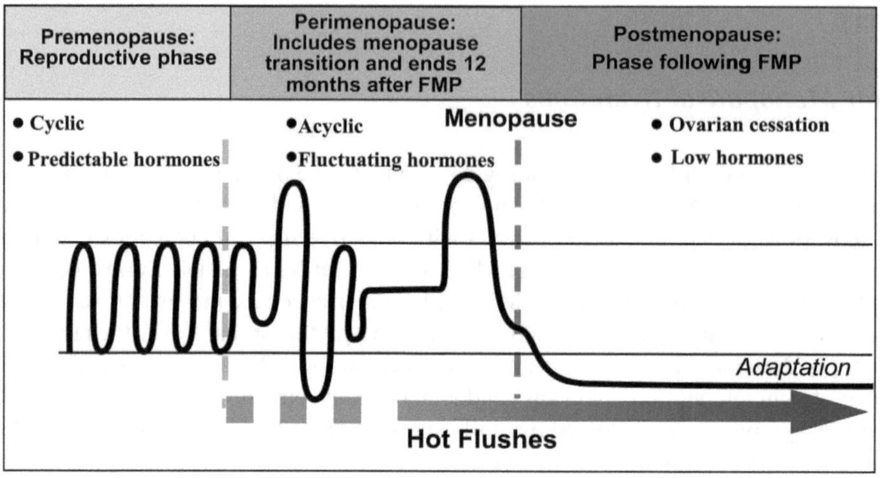

Fig. 1.7 Relationship between estrogen and a woman's reproductive phases and the occurrence of hot flushes. Reprinted from [48] with permission from Springer

Given the observation that VMS occur in most women experiencing dramatic lowering of estrogen levels due to natural or surgical menopause, it is very likely that estrogens do play a role in the initiation of VMS [41]. Strong support for this observation is the fact that estrogen administration practically eliminates VMS [46]. However, studies investigating plasma, urinary, or vaginal levels of estrogens have not been able to find an association with the presence of VMS. Furthermore, estrogen concentrations remain low throughout menopause while VMS usually subside with time after menopause. Therefore, it is not very likely that estrogen deficiency as such is a sufficient risk factor for symptoms, although estrogen deficiency seems to be necessary to explain the occurrence of VMS [41, 47]. It has been suggested that the fluctuations in estrogen levels during perimenopause play a role in the occurrence of VMS [48, 49], as outlined in Fig. 1.7.

Prevalence of VMS in women varies over the lifetime. From approximately 2 years before the FMP, prevalence starts to increase from around 10 % of women reporting VMS to a peak around the first year after the FMP with a mean of 55 % of women [50]. In some studies percentages of women experiencing VMS in the first year after the FMP of as high as 70–80 have been reported [51, 52]. Six to seven years after the FMP, the prevalence of VMS falls to approximately half of the peak prevalence, and it takes until 8 years after the FMP before VMS prevalence has returned to premenopausal levels [50]. Data from the Multiple Outcomes of Raloxifene Evaluation trial show that 10–19 years after menopause still 12 % of women report VMS that were symptoms that were bothersome "some," "most," or "all" of the time, while this was reported by 8 % of women who were 20 years or longer after menopause [53]. VMS seem to be more common in 90 % of women reporting this in the first year, and more abrupt and more severe in women who underwent surgical menopause [54].

Other Menopausal Symptoms and Complaints

Several other symptoms and complaints, i.e., urinary complaints, vaginal dryness, sleep disturbance, and mood symptoms, have been reported to be associated with menopause, although the literature is not completely consistent on whether it is the menopause per se that causes these symptoms and complaints, or whether aging also plays a major role [55]. Studies using factor analysis have shown that menopausal status is more consistently associated with VMS than with psychological or physical symptoms [56], which argues against the existence of a universal menopausal syndrome that includes them all [55].

Urinary incontinence may occur more frequently as a result of atrophy of the bladder trigone, decreased sensitivity of alpha-adrenergic receptors of the bladder and urethral sphincter, or thinning of the urethral mucosa [57]. Urinary tract infections may be a result of increased vaginal pH and vaginal microflora changes to gram-negative organisms [57].

Vaginal atrophy is associated with menopause [58] and may lead to symptoms of dyspareunia, vaginal dryness, itching, and irritation, and the estrogen withdrawal after menopause seems to play a role in its occurrence, as systemic or vaginal estrogen therapy can be used as a relief [57].

The literature on mood changes, development of mental disorders, and depression as a result of menopause is conflicting with several studies that were unable to find such associations, where some were [55]. It has been reported that the increased rate of perimenopausal depression was primarily found in women with a history of depression, suggestive of increased vulnerability in women who are known to have affective disorders [59, 60].

Cardiovascular Disease

Cardiovascular diseases (CVD) are the major cause of disease and death in Western countries, accounting for 30 % of deaths. Morbidity and mortality graphs by sex suggest that women are relatively protected against coronary heart disease until around the age of 50, the age at which menopause occurs [61].

Protection by endogenous estrogens has long been considered a likely explanation for this risk difference. Circulating estrogen levels decline to about 20 % of premenopausal levels around menopause. Early menopause, caused by bilateral oophorectomy, increases the risk of CVD in younger women, but not when estrogen supplementation therapy is given [62–65]. Observational studies support the hypothesis that a later age at menopause decreases CVD risk [66–69]. Whether endogenous estrogens are the key driver of cardiovascular protection is unclear up to now. The Women's Ischemia Syndrome Evaluation study showed that premenopausal women with angiographic coronary artery disease suffered more often from hypoestrogenemia in combination with low FSH and LH levels, as is present in menopause [70]. The few studies that are available on postmenopausal estrogen levels and CVD risk generally do not support an association [71–73], but postmenopausal estrogen levels do not necessarily reflect premenopausal levels.

A logical consequence of increased coronary risk due to ceased estradiol production would be that this risk be reversed by increasing estradiol levels in postmenopausal women through supplementing estrogens after menopause, with the so-called postmenopausal hormone therapy (HT). Extensive data from observational studies support a beneficial effect of HT on the occurrence of CVD in postmenopausal women, amounting to a risk reduction of 35–50 % [74–76]. Moreover, observational data in women who have experienced a cardiac event or a coronary intervention agree with the data from healthy women on HT [77]. This led to the paradigm that estrogen deficit causes CHD and supplying hormone therapy is good for postmenopausal women. However, randomized trials on hormone therapy and clinically manifest CVD did not confirm the findings of the observational studies. None of the large trials observed clear coronary risk reduction in the hormone therapy arms (summarized in [78]). These findings raise serious questions on the validity of the paradigm.

The randomized trials on HT typically targeted older women 10–15 years after menopause and showed no overall benefit. Yet, women randomized to hormone therapy closer to menopause did experience CHD protection, whereas women starting further from menopause did not [79]. These findings suggest that estrogen benefits are not the same across all postmenopausal women at large.

The most critical difference between women using HT in trials and in real life is that outside trials women tend to receive HT because of a reason, e.g., for an indication. The typical indication for HT is suffering from VMS, because HT is the most effective treatment to reduce VMS, and after cessation of HT VMS often recur [80]. In the randomized trials, women with severe VMS were largely excluded as these symptoms could reduce adherence to placebo treatment or giving placebo was considered unethical. In contrast, women enrolled in the observational studies will usually have started HT because they experienced VMS [81].

We have hypothesized that women with VMS are different from women without such symptoms [82]. This difference may lie in their cardiovascular risk profile, or their response to exogenous hormone therapy. Indeed women with VMS have an adverse cardiovascular risk profile [83], which could not be explained by the absolute estradiol level [47], and have increased arterial calcification and a 1.33-fold increased risk of incident CHD [84]. The findings support the view that VMS are associated with increased cardiovascular risk. However, there is no consensus in the literature [85–87].

Whether VMS are a marker of sensitivity to beneficial effects of estrogens on CVD is also currently unclear. The two post hoc analyses of HT trials suggest that in women with baseline VMS HT *increased* the risk of CHD events. However, these findings should be interpreted cautiously. In both trials the mean age of participants was in the mid to late 60s, and the percentage of women reporting VMS was small, in particular in HERS (16 %). Therefore, these women seem to be a selected group and not a reflection of the average group of women experiencing VMS when going through the menopausal transition. Moreover, effect estimates are based on small number of cases, and in HERS the difference in HT risk between women with and without VMS was significant in the first year only, suggesting that a chance finding cannot be excluded [88]. Data from our own group in an observational setting suggest exactly the opposite; among women with intense VMS, ever HT use significantly decreased CHD risk compared with never HT use (HR 0.39 [95 % CI 0.18–0.87]). On the other hand, among women without intense VMS, ever HT use was associated with a borderline significantly increased CHD risk (HR 1.29 [95 % CI 0.97–1.72]) ($P=0.03$ for interaction) [89].

Osteoporosis

Early menopause is consistently associated with lower bone mineral density (BMD); whereas the premenopausal loss in BMD is small, after menopause studies have reported 3–5 % annual decreases [90–92], which is a factor 5–10 higher than the premenopausal loss in BMD. Oophorectomy leads to rapid bone loss from the trabecular and cortical compartments of the skeleton; although longitudinal studies are scarce, the average loss of trabecular bone from the spine has been estimated to be between 12 and 19 % in the first year after bilateral oophorectomy [93, 94]. Evidence for a role of menopause in osteoporosis is strengthened by many observational studies reporting that early menopause increases the risk of fractures, which are nicely summarized by Gallagher in 2007 [95].

There is compelling evidence that in the case of osteoporosis, the effect of early menopause can be attributed to the decrease in estrogen levels. Several observational studies pointed to a 50 % reduction in fracture risk in women using estrogen therapy versus women who do not [96–98], whereas meta-analyses clearly pointed in the same direction [99–101]. A systematic review and meta-analysis including data from the Women's Health Initiative study, the largest randomized trial on postmenopausal hormone therapy, estimated that estrogen therapy for 6.2 years is associated with 52 % reduction in incident fractures [78]. Discontinuation of estrogen therapy leads to rapid bone loss in the first year of 3–6 %, and a loss of fracture protection [102].

Breast Cancer

There is wide consensus that a late menopause increases the risk of breast cancer. Every 1-year increment in age at menopause confers an increase of breast cancer by approximately 3 % [103, 104]. Noteworthy is the marked protective effect from a premature oophorectomy performed before age 40, the risk of breast cancer being reduced by about 50 %. This effect is ascribed to the longer exposure to endogenous estrogens if menopause occurs later. In fact, for breast cancer all available evidence, be it on reproductive factors, endogenous estrogen levels, or exogenous estrogen supplementation, points to an important harmful role of estrogen exposure [105].

Conclusion

Menopause is defined as the permanent cessation of menstruation, and defined present 1 year after the last menstrual cycle. Menopause is due to depletion of the follicle pool. The menstrual cycle and changes in the cyclic pattern until a complete stop are orchestrated by gonadotrophins, steroids, and inhibins.

The median age at natural menopause is around 50–51, for centuries and across populations.

Onset of menopause is associated with VMS, the so-called hot flushes and night sweats, the prevalence of which around the FMP is as high as 80 %. Of other symptoms, such as incontinence, depressed feelings, and vaginal dryness, it is not clear whether it is the menopause per se that causes these symptoms and complaints, or whether aging also plays a major role.

Early menopause is associated with increased risk of CVD and osteoporosis and a decreased risk of breast cancer. These effects are generally ascribed to estrogens, but for osteoporosis and breast cancer this is much more clear than for CVD.

References

1. WHO Scientific Group on Research on the Menopause in the 1990s. Geneva, WHO: WHO Technical report series, Research on the menopause in the 1990s; 1996. Ref Type: Report. 866.
2. Peccei JS. A critique of the grandmother hypotheses: old and new. Am J Hum Biol. 2001;13:434–52.
3. Hawkes K, O'Connell JF, Jones NG, Alvarez H, Charnov EL. Grandmothering, menopause, and the evolution of human life histories. Proc Natl Acad Sci USA. 1998;95:1336–9.
4. Kirkwood TB. Evolution of ageing. Nature. 1977;270:301–4.
5. Walker ML, Herndon JG. Menopause in nonhuman primates? Biol Reprod. 2008;79:398–406.
6. Walker ML, Anderson DC, Herndon JG, Walker LC. Ovarian aging in squirrel monkeys (Saimiri sciureus). Reproduction. 2009;138:793–9.
7. Treloar AE, Boynton RE, Behn BG. Variation of the human menstrual cycle through reproductive life. Int J Fertil. 1967;12:77–126.
8. Treloar AE. Menstrual cyclicity and the pre-menopause. Maturitas. 1981;3:249–64.
9. Harlow SD, Gass M, Hall JE, Lobo R, Maki P, Rebar RW, et al. Executive summary of the stages of reproductive aging workshop+10: addressing the unfinished agenda of staging reproductive aging. Menopause. 2012;19(4):387–95.
10. Baker TG. A quantitative and cytological study of germ cells in human ovaries. Proc R Soc Lond B Biol Sci. 1963;158:417–33.
11. Block E. Quantitative morphological investigations of the follicular system in women; variations at different ages. Acta Anat (Basel). 1952;14:108–23.
12. Richardson SJ, Senikas V, Nelson JF. Follicular depletion during the menopausal transition: evidence for accelerated loss and ultimate exhaustion. J Clin Endocrinol Metab. 1987;65:1231–7.
13. Faddy MJ, Gosden RG, Gougeon A, Richardson SJ, Nelson JF. Accelerated disappearance of ovarian follicles in mid-life: implications for forecasting menopause. Hum Reprod. 1992;7:1342–6.

14. Morabia A, Costanza MC. International variability in ages at menarche, first livebirth, and menopause. World Health Organization Collaborative Study of Neoplasia and Steroid Contraceptives. Am J Epidemiol. 1998;148:1195–205.
15. Noord-Zaadstra BM, Looman CW, Alsbach H, Habbema JD, te Velde ER, Karbaat J. Delaying childbearing: effect of age on fecundity and outcome of pregnancy. BMJ. 1991;302:1361–5.
16. Burger HG, Hale GE, Dennerstein L, Robertson DM. Cycle and hormone changes during perimenopause: the key role of ovarian function. Menopause. 2008;15:603–12.
17. Burger H. The menopausal transition—endocrinology. J Sex Med. 2008;5:2266–73.
18. Burger HG, Dudley EC, Hopper JL, Shelley JM, Green A, Smith A, et al. The endocrinology of the menopausal transition: a cross-sectional study of a population-based sample. J Clin Endocrinol Metab. 1995;80:3537–45.
19. Burger HG, Cahir N, Robertson DM, Groome NP, Dudley E, Green A, et al. Serum inhibins A and B fall differentially as FSH rises in perimenopausal women. Clin Endocrinol (Oxf). 1998;48:809–13.
20. Welt CK, Adams JM, Sluss PM, Hall JE. Inhibin A and inhibin B responses to gonadotropin withdrawal depends on stage of follicle development. J Clin Endocrinol Metab. 1999;84:2163–9.
21. Burger HG, Hale GE, Robertson DM, Dennerstein L. A review of hormonal changes during the menopausal transition: focus on findings from the Melbourne Women's Midlife Health Project. Hum Reprod Update. 2007;13:559–65.
22. Sowers MR, Zheng H, McConnell D, Nan B, Harlow SD, Randolph Jr JF. Estradiol rates of change in relation to the final menstrual period in a population-based cohort of women. J Clin Endocrinol Metab. 2008;93:3847–52.
23. Backman G. Die beschleunigte Entwicklung der Jugend. Verfrühte Menarche, verspätete Menopause, verlängerte Lebensdauer. Acta Anat (Basel). 1947;4:421–80.
24. Tanner JM. Growth at adolescence: with a general consideration of the effects of hereditary and environmental factors upon growth and maturation from birth to maturity. Oxford: Blackwell Scientific Publications; 1962.
25. Amundsen DW, Diers CJ. The age of menopause in classical Greece and Rome. Hum Biol. 1970;42:79–86.
26. Amundsen DW, Diers CJ. The age of menopause in medieval Europe. Hum Biol. 1973;45:605–12.
27. Treloar AE. Menarche, menopause, and intervening fecundability. Hum Biol. 1974;46:89–107.
28. Flint M. Is there a secular trend in age of menopause? Maturitas. 1978;1:133–9.
29. Flint MP. Secular trends in menopause age. J Psychosom Obstet Gynaecol. 1997;18:65–72.
30. Frommer J. Changing age of the menopause. Br Med J. 1964;2:349–51.
31. MacMahon B, Worcester J. Age at menopause, United States 1960–62. US Dept of Health, Education and Welfare, Public Health Service, National Center for Health Statistics, Series 11, Number 19. Washington, DC: US Government Printing Office; 1966.
32. McKinlay S, Jefferys M, Thompson B. An investigation of the age at menopause. J Biosoc Sci. 1972;4:161–73.
33. van Asselt KM, Kok HS, van der Schouw YT, Grobbee DE, te Velde ER, Pearson PL, et al. Current smoking at menopause rather than duration determines the onset of natural menopause. Epidemiology. 2004;15:634–9.
34. McKinlay SM, Bifano NL, McKinlay JB. Smoking and age at menopause in women. Ann Intern Med. 1985;103:350–6.
35. Rodstrom K, Bengtsson C, Milsom I, Lissner L, Sundh V, Bjourkelund C. Evidence for a secular trend in menopausal age: a population study of women in Gothenburg. Menopause. 2003;10:538–43.
36. Nichols HB, Trentham-Dietz A, Hampton JM, et al. From menarche to menopause: trends among US Women born from 1912 to 1969. Am J Epidemiol. 2006;164:1003–11.
37. Kalichman L, Malkin I, Kobyliansky E. Time-related trends of age at menopause and reproductive period of women in a Chuvashian rural population. Menopause. 2007;14:135–40.
38. Dratva J, Gomez Real F, Schindler C, Ackermann-Liebrich U, Gerbase MW, Probst-Hensch NM, et al. Is age at menopause increasing across Europe? Results on age at menopause and determinants from two population-based studies. Menopause. 2009;16:385–94.
39. Pakarinen M, Raitanen J, Kaaja R, Luoto R. Secular trend in the menopausal age in Finland 1997–2007 and correlation with socioeconomic, reproductive and lifestyle factors. Maturitas. 2010;66:417–22.
40. Stearns V, Ullmer L, Lopez JF, Smith Y, Isaacs C, Hayes D. Hot flushes. Lancet. 2002;360:1851–61.
41. Freedman RR. Pathophysiology and treatment of menopausal hot flashes. Semin Reprod Med. 2005;23:117–25.
42. Kronenberg F. Hot flashes: epidemiology and physiology. Ann N Y Acad Sci. 1990;592:52–86.
43. Freedman RR, Krell W. Reduced thermoregulatory null zone in postmenopausal women with hot flashes. Am J Obstet Gynecol. 1999;181:66–70.
44. Savage MV, Brengelmann GL. Control of skin blood flow in the neutral zone of human body temperature regulation. J Appl Physiol. 1996;80:1249–57.
45. Freedman RR. Physiology of hot flashes. Am J Hum Biol. 2001;13:453–64.
46. Nelson HD. Commonly used types of postmenopausal estrogen for treatment of hot flashes: scientific review. JAMA. 2004;291:1610–20.
47. Gast GC, Samsioe G, Grobbee DE, Nilsson PM, van der Schouw YT. Vasomotor symptoms, estradiol levels and cardiovascular risk profile in women. Maturitas. 2010;66:285–90.

48. Deecher DC, Dorries K. Understanding the pathophysiology of vasomotor symptoms (hot flushes and night sweats) that occur in perimenopause, menopause, and postmenopause life stages. Arch Womens Ment Health. 2007;10:247–57.
49. Freeman EW, Sammel MD, Lin H, et al. Symptoms associated with menopausal transition and reproductive hormones in midlife women. Obstet Gynecol. 2007;110:230–40.
50. Politi MC, Schleinitz MD, Col NF. Revisiting the duration of vasomotor symptoms of menopause: a meta-analysis. J Gen Intern Med. 2008;23:1507–13.
51. McKinlay SM, Jefferys M. The menopausal syndrome. Br J Prev Soc Med. 1974;28:108–15.
52. Freeman EW, Sherif K. Prevalence of hot flushes and night sweats around the world: a systematic review. Climacteric. 2007;10:197–214.
53. Huang AJ, Grady D, Jacoby VL, Blackwell TL, Bauer DC, Sawaya GF. Persistent hot flushes in older postmenopausal women. Arch Intern Med. 2008;168:840–6.
54. Bachmann GA. Vasomotor flushes in menopausal women. Am J Obstet Gynecol. 1999;180:S312–6.
55. Nelson HD. Menopause. Lancet. 2008;371:760–70.
56. Avis NE, Brockwell S, Colvin A. A universal menopausal syndrome? Am J Med. 2005;118(Suppl 12B):37–46.
57. Greendale GA, Lee NP, Arriola ER. The menopause. Lancet. 1999;353:571–80.
58. Dennerstein L, Dudley EC, Hopper JL, Guthrie JR, Burger HG. A prospective population-based study of menopausal symptoms. Obstet Gynecol. 2000;96:351–8.
59. Avis NE, Brambilla D, McKinlay SM, Vass K. A longitudinal analysis of the association between menopause and depression. Results from the Massachusetts Women's Health Study. Ann Epidemiol. 1994;4:214–20.
60. Hunter MS. Psychological and somatic experience of the menopause: a prospective study [corrected]. Psychosom Med. 1990;52:357–67.
61. Witteman JC, Moerman CJ, Westendorp IC. Myth of the menopause paradox. Lancet. 1998;352:407.
62. Kannel WB, Hjortland MC, McNamara PM, Gordon T. Menopause and the risk of cardiovascular disease: the Framingham study. Ann Intern Med. 1976;85:447–52.
63. Colditz GA, Willett WC, Stampfer MJ, Rosner B, Speizer FE, Hennekens CH. Menopause and the risk of coronary heart disease in women. N Engl J Med. 1987;316:1105–10.
64. Rivera CM, Grossardt BR, Rhodes DJ, et al. Increased cardiovascular mortality after early bilateral oophorectomy. Menopause. 2009;16:15–23.
65. Parker WH, Jacoby V, Shoupe D, Rocca W. Effect of bilateral oophorectomy on women's long-term health. Womens Health (Lond Engl). 2009;5:565–76.
66. van der Schouw YT, van der Graaf Y, Steyerberg EW, Eijkemans JC, Banga JD. Age at menopause as a risk factor for cardiovascular mortality. Lancet. 1996;347:714–8.
67. de Kleijn MJ, van der Schouw YT, Verbeek AL, Peeters PH, Banga JD, van der Graaf Y. Endogenous estrogen exposure and cardiovascular mortality risk in postmenopausal women. Am J Epidemiol. 2002;155:339–45.
68. Atsma F, Bartelink ML, Grobbee DE, van der Schouw YT. Postmenopausal status and early menopause as independent risk factors for cardiovascular disease: a meta-analysis. Menopause. 2006;13:265–79.
69. Baer HJ, Glynn RJ, Hu FB, Hankinson SE, Willett WC, Colditz GA, et al. Risk factors for mortality in the nurses' health study: a competing risks analysis. Am J Epidemiol. 2011;173:319–29.
70. Bairey Merz CN, Johnson BD, Sharaf BL, Bittner V, Berga SL, Braunstein GD, et al. Hypoestrogenemia of hypothalamic origin and coronary artery disease in premenopausal women: a report from the NHLBI-sponsored WISE study. J Am Coll Cardiol. 2003;41:413–9.
71. Barrett-Connor E, Goodman-Gruen D. Prospective study of endogenous sex hormones and fatal cardiovascular disease in postmenopausal women. BMJ. 1995;311:1193–6.
72. Rexrode KM, Manson JE, Lee IM, et al. Sex hormone levels and risk of cardiovascular events in postmenopausal women. Circulation. 2003;108(14):1688–93.
73. Chen Y, Zeleniuch-Jacquotte A, Arslan AA, Wojcik O, Toniolo P, Shore RE, et al. Endogenous hormones and coronary heart disease in postmenopausal women. Atherosclerosis. 2011;216:414–9.
74. Stampfer MJ, Colditz GA. Estrogen replacement therapy and coronary heart disease: a quantitative assessment of the epidemiologic evidence. Prev Med. 1991;20:47–63.
75. Grodstein F, Stampfer M. The epidemiology of coronary heart disease and estrogen replacement in postmenopausal women. Prog Cardiovasc Dis. 1995;38:199–210.
76. Grodstein F, Manson JE, Colditz GA, Willett WC, Speizer FE, Stampfer MJ. A prospective, observational study of postmenopausal hormone therapy and primary prevention of cardiovascular disease. Ann Intern Med. 2000;133:933–41.
77. Grodstein F, Manson JE, Stampfer MJ. Postmenopausal hormone use and secondary prevention of coronary events in the nurses' health study. a prospective, observational study. Ann Intern Med. 2001;135:1–8.
78. Farquhar C, Marjoribanks J, Lethaby A, Suckling JA, Lamberts Q. Long term hormone therapy for perimenopausal and postmenopausal women. Cochrane Database Syst Rev. 2009;CD004143.
79. Rossouw JE, Prentice RL, Manson JE, Wu L, Barad D, Barnabei VM, et al. Postmenopausal hormone therapy and risk of cardiovascular disease by age and years since menopause. JAMA. 2007;297:1465–77.

80. Lindh-Astrand L, Brynhildsen J, Hoffman M, Hammar M. Vasomotor symptoms usually reappear after cessation of postmenopausal hormone therapy: a Swedish population-based study. Menopause. 2009;16(6):1213–7.
81. Burger HG. WHI risks: any relevance to menopause management? Maturitas. 2007;57:6–10.
82. van der Schouw YT, Grobbee DE. Menopausal complaints, oestrogens, and heart disease risk: an explanation for discrepant findings on the benefits of post-menopausal hormone therapy. Eur Heart J. 2005;26:1358–61.
83. Gast GC, Grobbee DE, Pop VJ, Keyzer JJ, Wijnands-van Gent CJ, Samsioe GN, et al. Menopausal complaints are associated with cardiovascular risk factors. Hypertension. 2008;51:1492–8.
84. Gast GC, Pop VJ, Samsioe G, Grobbee DE, Nilsson PM, Keyzer JJ, et al. Vasomotor menopausal symptoms are associated with increased risk of coronary heart disease. Menopause. 2011;18:51.
85. Tuomikoski P, Mikkola TS, Hamalainen E, Tikkanen MJ, Turpeinen U, Ylikorkala O. Biochemical markers for cardiovascular disease in recently postmenopausal women with or without hot flashes. Menopause. 2010;17:151.
86. Svartberg J, von MD, Kritz-Silverstein D, Barrett-Connor E. Vasomotor symptoms and mortality: the Rancho Bernardo Study. Menopause. 2009;16:888–91.
87. Allison MA, Manson JE, Aragaki A, et al. Vasomotor symptoms and coronary artery calcium in postmenopausal women. Menopause. 2010;17:1145.
88. Allison MA, Manson JE. The complex interplay of vasomotor symptoms, hormone therapy, and cardiovascular risk. Menopause. 2009;16:619–20.
89. Gast GC, Pop VJ, Samsioe GN, Grobbee DE, Nilsson PM, Keyzer JJ, et al. Hormone therapy and coronary heart disease risk by vasomotor menopausal symptoms. Maturitas. 2011;70:373–8.
90. Block JE, Smith R, Glueer CC, Steiger P, Ettinger B, Genant HK. Models of spinal trabecular bone loss as determined by quantitative computed tomography. J Bone Miner Res. 1989;4:249–57.
91. Gudmundsdottir H, Jonsdottir B, Kristinsson S, Johannesson A, Goodenough D, Sigurdsson G. Vertebral bone density in Icelandic women using quantitative computed tomography without an external reference phantom. Osteoporos Int. 1993;3:84–9.
92. Seifert-Klauss V, Link T, Heumann C, Luppa P, Haseitl M, Laakmann J, et al. Influence of pattern of menopausal transition on the amount of trabecular bone loss. Results from a 6-year prospective longitudinal study. Maturitas. 2006;55:317–24.
93. Prior JC, Vigna YM, Wark JD, Eyre DR, Lentle BC, Li DK, et al. Premenopausal ovariectomy-related bone loss: a randomized, double-blind, one-year trial of conjugated estrogen or medroxyprogesterone acetate. J Bone Miner Res. 1997;12:1851–63.
94. Genant HK, Cann CE, Ettinger B, Gordan GS. Quantitative computed tomography of vertebral spongiosa: a sensitive method for detecting early bone loss after oophorectomy. Ann Intern Med. 1982;97:699–705.
95. Gallagher JC. Effect of early menopause on bone mineral density and fractures. Menopause. 2007;14:567–71.
96. Weiss NS, Ure CL, Ballard JH, Williams AR, Daling JR. Decreased risk of fractures of the hip and lower forearm with postmenopausal use of estrogen. N Engl J Med. 1980;303:1195–8.
97. Grady D, Rubin SM, Petitti DB, et al. Hormone therapy to prevent disease and prolong life in postmenopausal women. Ann Intern Med. 1992;117:1016–37.
98. Cauley JA, Seeley DG, Ensrud K, Ettinger B, Black D, Cummings SR. Estrogen replacement therapy and fractures in older women. Study of Osteoporotic Fractures Research Group. Ann Intern Med. 1995;122:9–16.
99. Wells G, Tugwell P, Shea B, Guyatt G, Peterson J, Zytaruk N, et al. Meta-analyses of therapies for postmenopausal osteoporosis. V. Meta-analysis of the efficacy of hormone replacement therapy in treating and preventing osteoporosis in postmenopausal women. Endocr Rev. 2002;23:529–39.
100. Torgerson DJ, Bell-Syer SE. Hormone replacement therapy and prevention of nonvertebral fractures: a meta-analysis of randomized trials. JAMA. 2001;285:2891–7.
101. Nelson HD, Humphrey LL, Nygren P, Teutsch SM, Allan JD. Postmenopausal hormone replacement therapy: scientific review. JAMA. 2002;288:872–81.
102. Heiss G, Wallace R, Anderson GL, Aragaki A, Beresford SA, Brzyski R, et al. Health risks and benefits 3 years after stopping randomized treatment with estrogen and progestin. JAMA. 2008;299:1036–45.
103. Pike MC, Krailo MD, Henderson BE, Casagrande JT, Hoel DG. "Hormonal" risk factors, "breast tissue age" and the age-incidence of breast cancer. Nature. 1983;303:767–70.
104. Breast cancer and hormone replacement therapy: collaborative reanalysis of data from 51 epidemiological studies of 52,705 women with breast cancer and 108,411 women without breast cancer. Collaborative Group on Hormonal Factors in Breast Cancer. Lancet. 1997;350:1047–59.
105. Persson I. Estrogens in the causation of breast, endometrial and ovarian cancers—evidence and hypotheses from epidemiological findings. J Steroid Biochem Mol Biol. 2000;74:357–64.
106. Klinkert ER. Clinical significance and management of poor response in IVF. Ref Type: Thesis/Dissertation: Utrecht University; 2005.
107. Lambalk CB, van Disseldorp J, de Koning CH, Broekmans FJ. Testing ovarian reserve to predict age at menopause. Maturitas. 2009;63:280–91.
108. Ferrell RJ, Sowers M. Longitudinal, epidemiologic studies of female reproductive aging. Ann N Y Acad Sci. 2010;1204:188–97.

Chapter 2
Body Composition and Menopausal Transition: A Bioanthropological Perspective

Sylvia Kirchengast

Key Points

- Menopause is defined as the permanent cessation of menstruation due to depletion of the follicle pool.
- The menstrual cycle and changes in the cyclic pattern until a complete stop are orchestrated by gonadotrophins, steroids, and inhibins.
- The median age at natural menopause is around 50–51, for centuries and across populations.
- Menopause is associated with vasomotor menopausal symptoms; of other symptoms such as incontinence, depressed feelings, and vaginal dryness it is not clear whether it is the menopause per se that causes these symptoms and complaints, or whether aging also plays a major role.
- Early menopause is associated with increased risk of cardiovascular disease and osteoporosis and a decreased risk of breast cancer.
- These effects are generally ascribed to estrogens, but for osteoporosis and breast cancer this is much more clear than for cardiovascular disease.

Keywords Age at menopause • Body composition • Lean mass • Fat mass • Fat distribution • Bone mass • Menopausal transition • Evolution

Introduction

Menopause, the cessation of menstrual function and the irreversible termination of female reproductive capability, is an event experienced by all human females who live beyond 55 years of life [1]. Understanding and interpretation of menopause differs between scientific disciplines. In Western societies menopause is mainly seen as visible sign of female ageing and it is often interpreted as a kind endocrine disease, which can be treated effectively with hormone replacement therapy. As a consequence the medical viewpoint dominates menopause research since a long time. Changes in hormone secretion and menstrual cycle patterns but first of all the occurrence of climacteric complaints were recorded and efficient treatments were tested. Nevertheless, menopause is not a disease per se it is a common experience of all human females who live beyond 55 years of life. Although all menopausal women lost reproductive capability and menstrual cycle stops irreversible, menopause is experienced quite different under

S. Kirchengast, M.A., Ph.D. (✉)
Department of Anthropology, University of Vienna, Althanstrasse 14, 1090 Vienna, Austria
e-mail: sylvia.kirchengast@univie.ac.at

C.J.H. Martin et al. (eds.), *Nutrition and Diet in Menopause*, Nutrition and Health,
DOI 10.1007/978-1-62703-373-2_2, © Springer Science+Business Media New York 2013

different sociocultural conditions. As a consequence from a biocultural viewpoint menopause is not a common disease it reflects simply reproductive ageing and the end of childbearing phase in female life. Numerous studies carried out among menopausal women of different sociocultural background and among women in traditional societies demonstrated that menopause is the product of decades of physiological responses to an environment composed of cultural and biological factors [2].

Menopause from a Bioanthropological Viewpoint

Menopause is not only of medical and biocultural interest, it is also a main focus of bioanthropological research. From an evolutionary life history perspective, menopause is a universal one-time life event which marks the transition from reproductive to postreproductive life; consequently menopause is a marker of reproductive ageing patterns typical of female *Homo sapiens*. Reproductive ageing characterized by a decline of sex steroid levels and a reduced probability of successful reproduction is found among several free living social mammals such as cetaceans, elephants, lions, or first of all primates and captive animals, an obligatory postreproductive life stage of 30 years and more, however, is exclusively found among human females [1]. The majority of women in developed countries experience menopause between 47 and 55 year of life. This seems quite early because the average life expectancy of females in these countries is about 80 years. Consequently postreproductive phase of the human female lasts on the average 30 years in industrialized countries. The maximum life span of recent *Homo sapiens* is even longer and is thought to be about 120 years. Thus human females can spend more than half of their maximum life span potential in postreproductive life. This extremely long postreproductive phase of life among human females is unique in the animal kingdom and makes menopause to an extremely interesting event from an evolutionary point of view [3]. If maximization of reproductive success is the ultimate goal of life, how can such a long postreproductive period be explained in evolutionary terms? Since the 1970s several evolutionary scenarios of human menopause were provided. On the one hand, menopause ensures that old or abnormal eggs are not fertilized. Furthermore, the termination of reproductive capability ensures that mothers have a real chance to be young enough at their last birth to survive until their last offspring is able to survive without a biological mother [1]. These arguments, however, are not able to explain the extreme length of postreproductive phase in human females. Another possibility of an evolutionary benefit of menopause is grandparenting [4]. This point of view resulted in the introduction of the so-called grandmother hypothesis, which suggested increased fitness of women who stops reproduction and invest in their grandchildren. Seeking explanations for a long postreproductive life span resulted in publication of numerous evolutionary explanations of the menopause up to now; however, there is no consensus which scenario is the most likely one. The development of evolutionary scenarios of human menopause is therefore still a main focus of bioanthropological menopause research (see Fig. 2.1).

Additionally to an evolutionary viewpoint, bioanthropological menopause research focus on somatic changes which occur during menopausal transition. These changes, however, have also to be interpreted in an evolutionary sense. The aim of this review is to discuss somatic in particular body composition changes during menopause and to provide beside physiological explanations of these somatic alterations an evolutionary one.

Biological Basis of Menopause

The World Health Organization (WHO) has defined menopause as the permanent cessation of menstruation resulting from loss of ovarian follicular activity [5]. The phase of irregular cycles and starting hormonal changes, which precede menopause, is commonly called perimenopause. From a

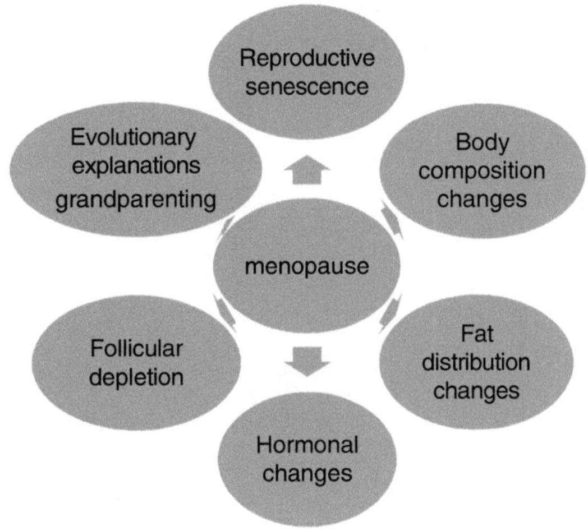

Fig. 2.1 Menopause from a bioanthropological viewpoint

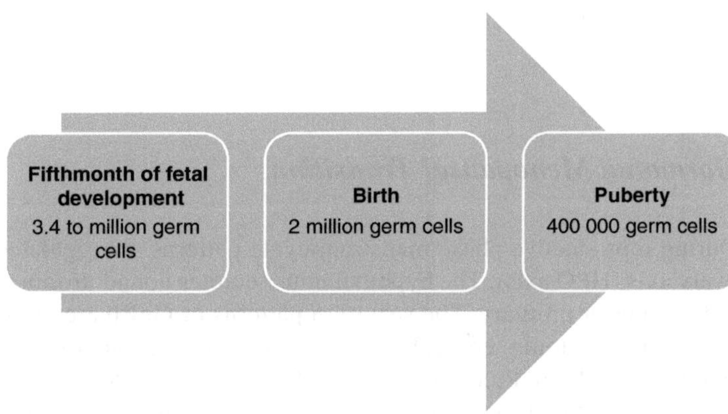

Fig. 2.2 The number of female germ cells decreases dramatically

biomedical viewpoint menopause is widely defined as the last spontaneous menstrual bleeding; however, no human female knows exactly that the actual bleeding is really the last one. Therefore, postmenopause is reached when a woman had no menstrual periods over 12 months.

On cellular level menopause is seen as a result from life long process of follicular atresia that starts during intrauterine phase and continues until menopause [1]. In the female embryo primordial germ cells originating from the yolk sac, develop into oogonia, immature sex cells. Approximately seven million oogonia are formed by the 5th month of fetal development. Oogonia develop to oocytes, almost fully developed sex cells. Oocyte formation, however, ceases by the time a female fetus is 5 months old. Human females are unable to continue to produce oocytes past their fifth month in utero. At this time the process of follicular degeneration and resorption from 3.4 to 7 million germ cells at their peak to less than 1,000 remaining follicles at the time when menopausal transition starts. The exorbitantly high number of seven million oogonia declines to about two million oocytes at the time of birth and to about 400,000 at pubertal onset. Oocytes are embedded in follicular cells, the vast majority of follicles are non-proliferating, produce steroids, and succumb to atresia by apoptosis [1]. Only few follicles develop to preovulatory follicles with a thick layer of granulosa and theca cells, consequently only few oocytes undergo ovulation. The majority of follicles and oocytes, which are developmental units degenerates before ovulation. Oocyte or follicular depletion accelerates as menopause got closer. At the time of menopause the activity of the few remaining follicles decline drastically [1]. This follicular decline results in the hormonal transition typical of menopause (see Fig. 2.2).

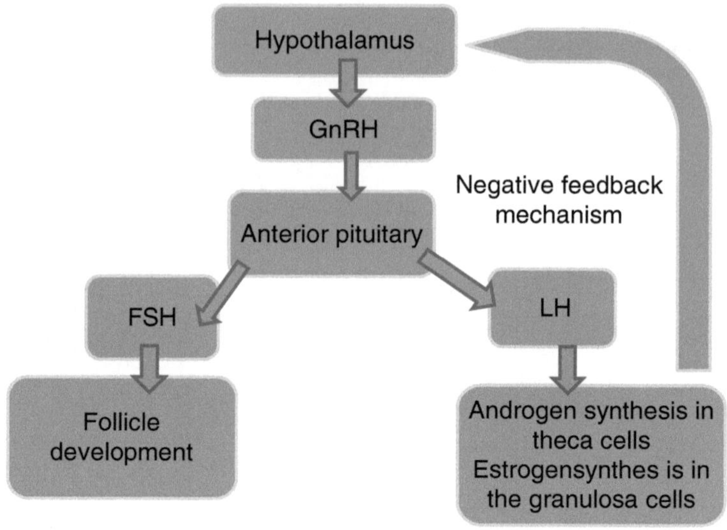

Fig. 2.3 Hypothalamus–pituitary–gonad (HPG) axis

Hormonal Menopausal Transition

During reproductive phase menstrual cycle patterns are regulated by the hypothalamus–pituitary–ovary axis (HPO axis). The hypothalamus secretes gonadotropin releasing hormone (GnRh) directly to the anterior pituitary. The secretion patterns of GnRh are modified by neurotransmitters such as dopamine, serotonin, epinephrine or endorphin. Receptors in the anterior pituitary sense the pulse frequency and amplitude of GnRh and direct the production of the gonadotropins, FSH and LH, which are essential for reproduction. FSH stimulates follicle development, LH the estrogen synthesis in the ovaries. Both stimulate ovulation and LH induces corpus luteum development and in this way progesterone synthesis. FSH binds to specific hormone receptors on the membrane of the granulosa cells LH binds to receptors of the granulose and theca cells. Androgens are secreted under LH stimulation from the theca cells, in the granulosa cells these androgens are converted to estradiol. The hormone secretion of the HPO axis is regulated by a negative feedback mechanism (see Fig. 2.3). During reproductive phase female sex hormone secretion underlies dramatic cyclic fluctuations.

Menopausal transition is characterized by marked endocrine changes which are mainly induced by central neuroendocrine changes and changes within the ovary. The reduction of ovarian follicles during perimenopause results in declining levels of inhibin B, a dimeric protein, and a rise of FSH and LH levels. During perimenopause estradiol levels remain relatively unchanged presumably in response to the elevated FSH levels [6, 7]. As the follicular supply is exhausted estradiol (E_2) and estrone (E) decrease dramatically; FSH and LH, however, remain elevated. Estradiol the most physiologically active estrogen declines most markedly, while estrone continues to be produced through the conversion of androstenedione to estrone in muscle, adipose and other tissues. Consequently the hypothalamus–pituitary–gonad axis (HPG axis) is irreversible disturbed. Beside the decline in estrogens and progesterone (P) a decrease of testosterone (T), androstendione (A), dehydroepiandrosterone (DHEA), dehydroepiandrosterone sulfate (DHEA-S), and sex hormone binding globulin (SHBG) levels after menopausal transition was observed [6, 7]. Additionally

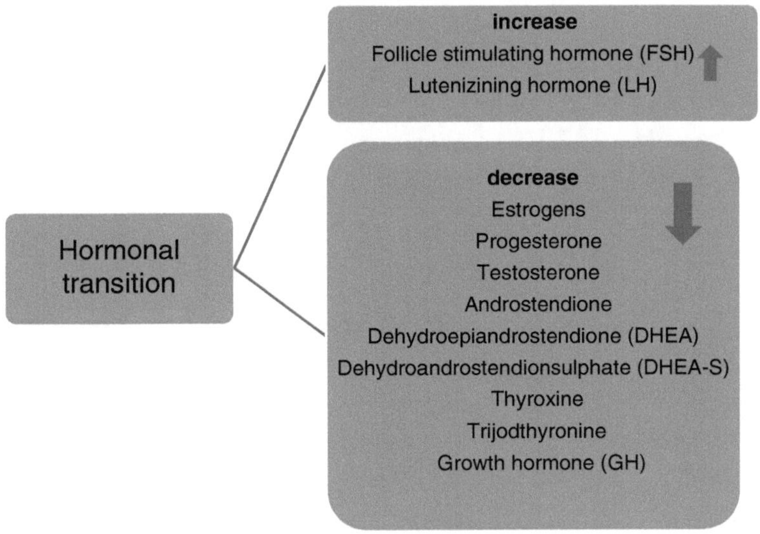

Fig. 2.4 Menopausal transition is characterized by specific hormonal changes

thyroxine (t_4) and triiodothyronine (t_3) levels as well as growth hormone (GH) decrease as results of the general ageing process (see Fig. 2.4).

Menopausal Transition and Body Composition

As pointed out above from a bioanthropological viewpoint menopause is not a disease it is a typical event of biological ageing of human females and ageing per se is not a disease. Biological ageing in general and in both sexes is associated with various changes in body build, body weight, and body composition.

Stature, Body Weight, and Weight Status

With increasing chronological age stature height decreases, on the other hand, body weight increases. Decreasing stature height is mainly due to the age related compression of intervertebral disks, microfractures of vertebral bodies, and an increased curvature of the spine [8]. Contrary to stature height body weight increases with age. Body weight starts to increase slightly since early adulthood (averaging 250 g per year) because of a decrease in lean body mass and metabolic rate. This increase of body weight accelerates during middle adulthood [9]. It is well documented that menopause is associated with weight gain and women exhibited a sharp increase in obesity rates between the ages 45 and 55 [10]. At the onset of menopause a woman's body weight reaches its maximum [11], caused mainly by the increase of fat tissue. Decreasing stature height and increasing body weight results in increased weight status determined by means of body mass index (BMI) (kg/m^2). Consequently the prevalence of overweight and obesity is higher among postmenopausal women compared to premenopausal ones

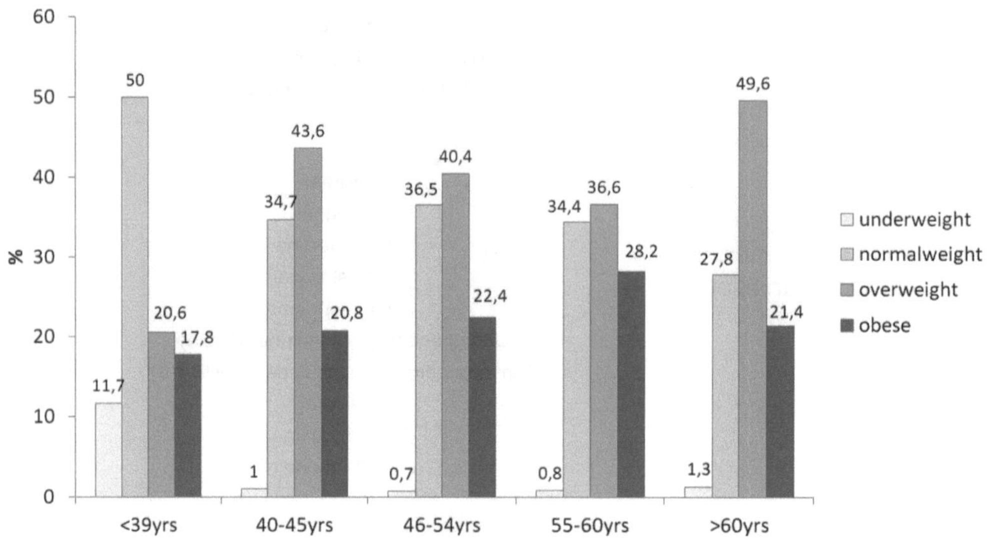

Fig. 2.5 Weight status changes with increasing age (sample of 940 Austrian women). Data source: Viennese body composition project by S. Kirchengast

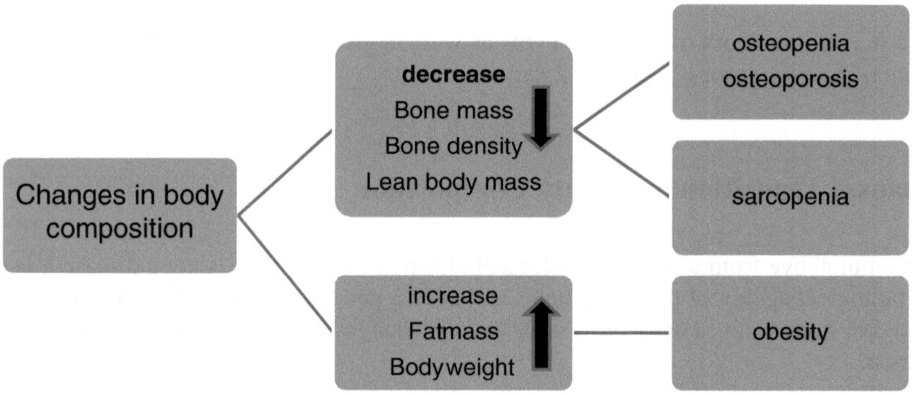

Fig. 2.6 Menopausal transition is characterized by marked changes in body composition

[12]. Women who have never suffered from weight problems experience an undesirable increase of body weight and body mass index [13] and marked alterations in body proportions. During the seventh decade of life (>60 years) body weight begins to decline and this decline accelerates during eighth decade of life (see Fig. 2.5).

Body Composition

Independent of general ageing and weight changes, during menopausal transition dramatic modifications in body composition occur [12, 14–16]. Body composition is mainly constituted by three components: lean soft tissue mass, i.e., muscle mass, bone mass, and fat mass [17]. All three components of body composition undergo certain changes in course of general ageing process and menopausal transition in particular (see Fig. 2.6).

Bone Mass and Bone Density

Age related changes in body composition include a progressive depletion of bone mass and bone density. Adult bone mass is equal to the peak bone mass achieved during early adulthood minus the amount of bone loss afterwards. Bone mass and bone density decline with increasing age, in women an accelerated rate bone loss occurs during menopausal transition and postmenopause. This menopause associated decline in bone mass has deleterious effects and may lead to the development of osteopenia or osteoporosis, which is clinically defined as areal bone mineral density (g/m^2) more than 2.5 SD below the young adult average [18].

Lean Body Mass and Sarcopenia

Ageing is generally associated with a reduction of lean body mass in particular muscle mass. Beside general ageing, menopause induces lean body mass loss, independent of ageing and stature height [16, 19]. This decrease in skeletal muscle mass has dramatic consequences. Skeletal muscle represents the largest component at the tissue-organ level of body composition in healthy adults and it is essential for locomotion and mobility. The state of pathologically reduced skeletal muscle mass is commonly called sarcopenia, from the Greek "poverty of flesh" [20, 21]. Sarcopenia, caused by reduced physical activity and hormonal factors is frequently found among postmenopausal women [22].

Body Fat and Fat Distribution Patterns

Similar to body weight the total amount of body fat as well as the fat percentage increase during middle adulthood and decreases during old age [9]. In course of menopausal transition the increase of fat mass accelerates; however, not only absolute and relative fat mass increase, fat distribution patterns change during menopausal transition too.

Body fat distribution is a typical sign of secondary sexual dimorphism in humans [23]. 65 years ago Vague [24] described differences in fat distribution patterns between men and women. During infancy and childhood fat distribution patterns are quite similar in girls and boys; during pubertal transition, however, marked differences in fat distribution patterns develop. While healthy normal weight boys develop the typical masculine or kind of fat distribution with extremely less subcutaneous fat tissue at the lower body region, i.e., buttocks, thighs, and hips, girls develop the typical gynoid kind of fat patterning with increased fat deposits at the lower body region. With the onset of reproductive maturation these sex specific fat distribution patterns are clearly visible. During adulthood and reproductive phase striking sex differences in body fat distribution intensify. Female waist to hip ratio is significantly lower than the waist to hip ratio of males. While the amount subcutaneous fat tissue is much higher in even slender women compared with weight status and age matched men, men show higher amounts of visceral fat tissue. This is mainly due to the fact that men tend to accumulate adipose tissue in the abdominal region, while healthy women tend to accumulate fat tissue in the gluteal–femoral region. For a similar fat mass, men have on average a twofold higher visceral adipose tissue accumulation compared to women [23]. Android and gynoid fat distribution patterns allow observers to distinguish between male and female body shapes which are commonly called apple shape or pear shape. Additionally in men abdominal fat tissue tends to accumulate in the visceral area to a greater extent than in women [25, 26]. While in men this kind of fat distribution pattern remain stabile through adult life and senescence, in women marked changes in fat distribution occur associated with the end of reproductive phase of life. Menopausal transition is associated with a body fat redistribution towards a dramatic increase in the accumulation of abdominal adipose tissue. Abdominal fat comprises three distinct fat stores: a superficial subcutaneous a deep subcutaneous and a visceral compartment. All three compartments, in particular visceral fat mass increase through menopausal transition [12, 27, 28]. Changes in fat patterning start during late premenopausal phase.

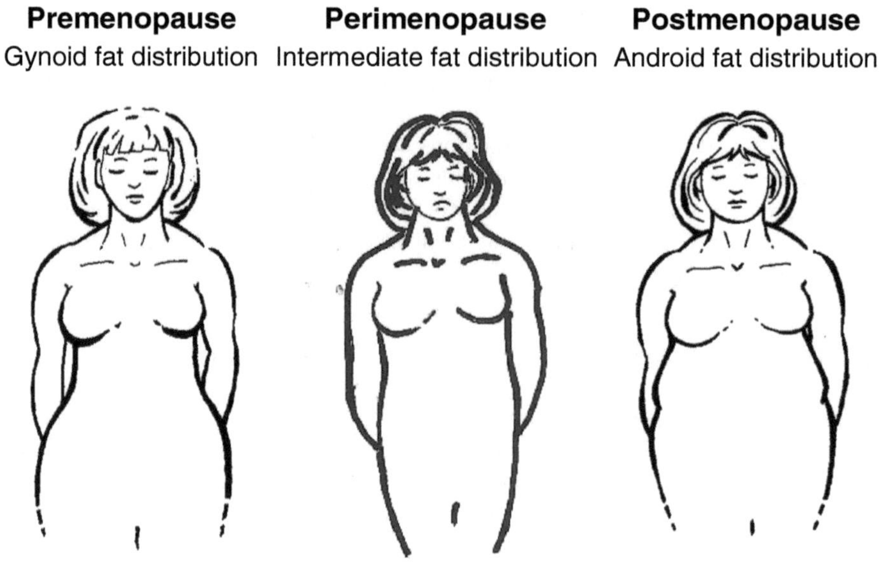

Fig. 2.7 Changes in fat distribution patterns during menopausal transition

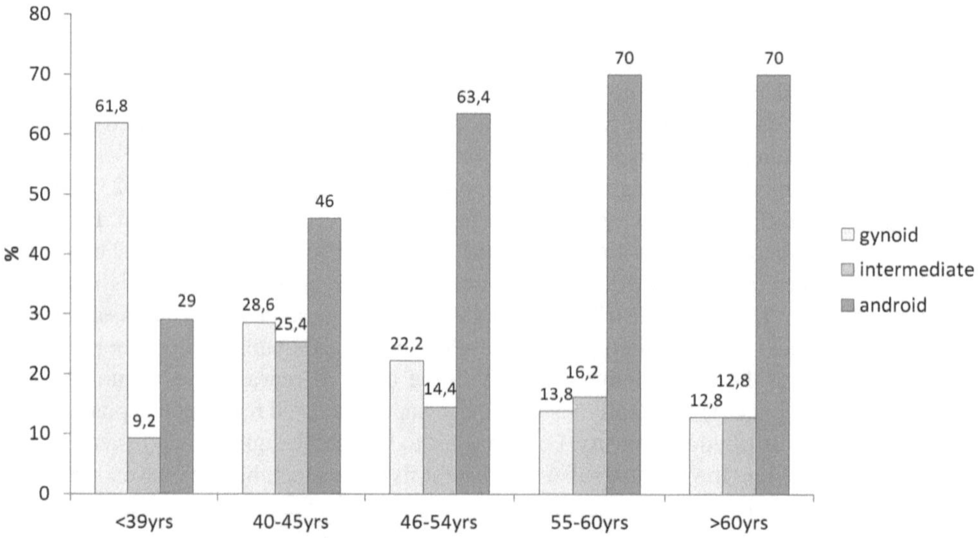

Fig. 2.8 Fat distribution with increasing age (sample of 940 Austrian women). Data source: Viennese body composition project by S. Kirchengast

At the late phase of premenopause and during perimenopause the gynoid fat patterning changes independent of age and weight status to an intermediate stadium of fat distribution between the gynoid and the android type. The amounts of abdominal fat tissue and lower body fat tissue are more or less equal during perimenopause. During the postmenopausal phase of life the intermediate type of fat patterning changes into the typical android fat patterning in the majority of women [28] (Figs. 2.7 and 2.8). With other words, menopausal transition results in a masculinization of female body shape.

Body Composition and Age at Menopause

Age at menopause is determined by the number of oocytes that the woman is born with and the rate at which those oocytes and their follicles are lost through the process of atresia [1]. Consequently age at menopause appears to be highly heritable, although it is also influenced by environmental factors. On important factor seems to be nutritional status. Elias et al. [29] analyzed the impact of Dutch famine during World War II on age at menopause. It could be demonstrated that women who were severely exposed to famine conditions experienced age at menopause on average 0.37 years earlier than women who were not exposed. The influence of famine on age at menopause was much higher when the famine was experienced between the ages 2 and 6. Those women who had suffered from malnutrition at this age reached menopause 1.83 years earlier than women who were not exposed to famine. Inconsistent results exist concerning the association between adult body mass index or body composition and age at menopause [30]. While several studies found no significant relation between adult body composition and menopausal age, others demonstrated a significant positive association between weight status as well as the amount of fat tissue and age at menopause (see Figs. 2.9 and 2.10). Body size and fat distribution have been considered in relation to age at menopause as it is hypothesized that increased peripheral conversion of androgens to estrogens might contribute to a delay of age at menopause. Consequently it was hypothesized that the higher the amount of subcutaneous fat tissue the later menopause occurs [31, 32]. On the other hand, menopause transition promotes somatic changes—as mentioned above—and therefore, a significant association between age at menopause and postmenopausal body composition may be assumed. It could be shown that age at menopause was positively associated with absolute and relative fat mass as well as lean body mass during postmenopause. Additionally a late menopause was associated with a significantly higher bone mass and bone density during postmenopause [33].

Beside natural menopause, artificial menopause as a consequence of hysterectomy is significantly associated with postmenopausal body composition characteristics. Hysterectomy due to nonma-

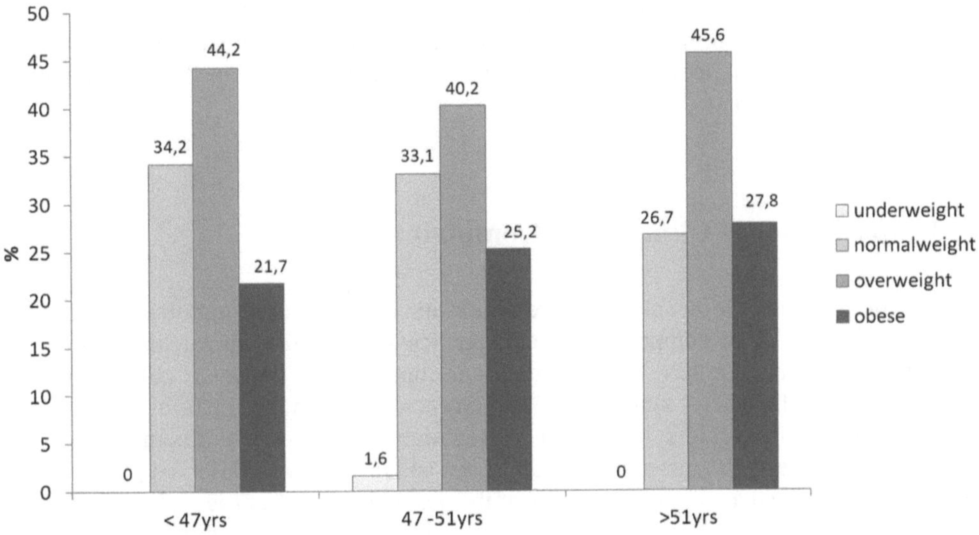

Fig. 2.9 Weight status and age at menopause (sample of 940 Austrian women). Data source: Viennese body composition project by S. Kirchengast

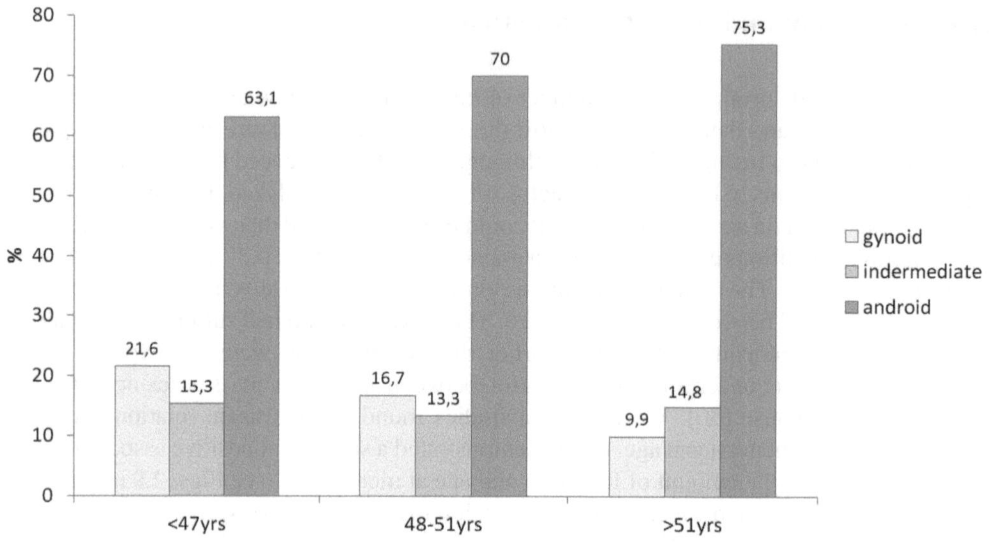

Fig. 2.10 Fat distribution and age at menopause (sample of 940 Austrian women). Data source: Viennese body composition project by S. Kirchengast

lignant cause is among the most common surgical procedures in women aged 40–60 years worldwide, although marked differences in the frequency of hysterectomies are observable between different countries and also within a population. Hysterectomy performed during pre- or perimenopause represents not only an artificial end of reproductive function, it also has an impact on weight status and body composition. Carlson et al. [34] reported a significant weight gain in 12 % of women after hysterectomy, according to Ravn et al. [35] hysterectomized women exhibited 2–11 % more body fat than women who experienced natural menopause. A Viennese study documented a significantly higher weight gain after menopause in hysterectomized women than in those who had a spontaneous menopause (9.1 kg vs. 6.0 kg). Furthermore, the percentage of obese women (BMI < 30.00) was significantly higher among hysterectomized women (34.0 % vs. 17.7 %) [36]. Furthermore, hysterectomized women showed a significantly higher amount of abdominal fat mass. Consequently hysterectomy was associated with a higher risk for the development of the centralized or android fat distribution.

Body Composition and Climacteric Complaints

Menopausal transition is accompanied by several somatic and psychic symptoms commonly called climacteric syndrome. Body composition characteristics and changes in fat distribution patterns through menopausal transition have also an important impact on the course of climacteric or on the degree of severity of climacteric symptoms. With an increasing amount of fat tissue the degree of severity of somatic and psychic symptoms increased significantly [37]. Furthermore, a significant decrease of sexual interest with increasing weight status and fat mass was observed [38]. The majority of symptoms are explained as somatic reactions of the postmenopausal estrogen deficiency. However, during climacteric the subcutaneous fat tissue has a positive impact on the endogenous estrogen levels because the extraovarian estrogen synthesis by aromatization of androgens to weak estrogens is taking place there. Therefore, the increased climacteric symptomatology and the reduced sexual interest associated with increased fat mass may be explained by the adverse effects of psychosocial stress to which women are exposed in our society if their bodies do not correspond to our culture specific beauty ideal [37, 38]. In Western industrialized societies many women interpret weight gain and changes fat distribution patterns as visible signs of ageing and every sign of ageing is interpreted exclusively negatively in the youth-oriented culture of Western societies.

Reasons for Body Composition Changes During Menopausal Transition

But what are the reasons for body composition changes during menopausal transition and postmenopause? From a bioanthropological viewpoint we have to distinguish between proximate or physiological causes and ultimate or evolutionary reasons.

Physiological or Proximate Reasons

Hormonal Factors

Hormonal factors contribute mainly to somatic changes taking place during menopausal transition and postmenopause [39–44]. First of all the decline of estrogen levels, thyroid hormone levels, GH level, and the estrogen–androgen ratio, typical of menopausal transition and postmenopause, are discussed as responsible factors for body composition changes and weight gain. It is well documented weight gain and fat accumulation, especially visceral fat accumulation in women accelerates when estrogen levels decline. This is possibly due to direct effects of estrogen on adipose tissue estrogen, progesterone and androgen receptors which are expressed in adipose tissues [23]. Furthermore, beside the decline in estrogen levels the changes in levels of certain energy homeostasis peptides that also occur with menopause are discussed to be promoters of weight gain during menopausal transition [45]. Furthermore, the weight gain during middle age may be enhanced by the decrease of the lipolytic acting thyroid hormones and GH indicating the decrease of the basal metabolic rate (BMR) [46]. Especially GH and its mediator insulin-like growth factors I (IGF-I) decrease in as a result of estrogen deficiency. The reduction of GH levels is typical of menopausal women and may enhance visceral fat accumulation and weight gain. Hormonal factors are not only responsible for the general weight gain, they are also essential for fat redistribution through menopausal transition. Centralized fat patterning characterized by increased visceral fat mass is in men associated with low testosterone levels [26, 42]. On the other hand, the reduction of dehydroepiandrosterone (DHEA) and its sulfated prohormone dehydroepiandrosterone-sulfate (DHEA-S) have been discussed to be responsible for weight gain and increased visceral fat mass among menopausal women [46]. Beside androgens the decline in estrogen levels is discussed to be responsible for redistribution of body fat through menopausal transition. Gonadal steroid hormones have been proposed to be associated with the increase of the waist to hip ratio in menopausal women and the development of android fat patterning [46]. During reproductive phase in the lower body adipocytes at the gluteal–femoral region an increased lipoprotein lipase activity and a blunted lipolytic response can be observed in comparison with the upper body (abdominal) adipocytes. In the abdominal region the lipolysis is induced by estradiol [47, 48]. The decrease of estrogen levels during the menopausal transition induces marked metabolic changes: the lower body adipocytes no longer show an increased lipoprotein lipase activity and a further increase of lower body fat mass does not take place. On the other hand, the diminished estrogen levels reduce the lipolytic metabolism at the abdominal region and result in an increase of adipose tissue at this region.

Therefore, the menopausal hormonal transition with reduced estrogen secretion may enhance changes in fat patterning, the conversion from more gynoid to more android fat patterning.

Lifestyle Factors

Other proximate causes for body composition changes during menopausal transition are lifestyle factors. The most important component of total daily energy expenditure, the resting metabolic rate, is reduced by ageing and also by menopause independent of the effects of the normal ageing process [12]. Unfortunately at the same time marked behavioral changes occur. The energy expenditure decreases dramatically and a more sedentary lifestyle is typical of middle age, while no changes in eating habits take place. One of the most important somatic consequences of these metabolic alterations and behavioral factors is the increase of body weight, especially an increase of adipose tissue, as a result of a long term positive energy balance. On the other hand, lean body mass, especially muscle mass reduces dramatically as a result of an increased sedentary lifestyle, may be resulting in a pathological state of sarcopenia.

Reproductive History Patterns

Menstrual and reproductive history is considered to be of special importance in explaining somatic changes at the end of the reproductive phase of life [49]. Several studies plead for significant associations between age at menarche and postmenopausal body composition [50, 51]. Other studies yielded significant associations between weight status, body composition as well as fat patterning and parameters of reproductive history, while no menstrual history factors were significantly related to somatic characteristics [52]. Of special importance appear to be the amount of weight gain during pregnancies and the number of births: Obese postmenopausal women reported the significantly highest average weight gain during their pregnancies while normal weight postmenopausal women reported the significantly lowest average pregnancy weight gain. Pregnancy weight gain can in retrospect be identified as the most important triggering life event for the development of obesity and a high amount of body weight. Furthermore, postmenopausal weight status was significantly negatively associated with the age at first birth. Regarding fat distribution, only the number of births seems to be associated significantly with the fat distribution patterns. A gynoid fat patterning seems to be associated significantly positively with the number of births [52]. Concerning body composition, a significant increase of lean soft tissue mass and fat mass during postmenopause with increasing pregnancy weight gain was described [52]. Bone mineral content (BMC) and bone mineral density (BMD) increased significantly with increasing number of births (see Fig. 2.11).

Body Composition Changes During Menopausal Transition from an Evolutionary Point of View

According to Theodosius Dobhansky "Nothing in Biology Makes Sense Except in the Light of Evolution". As pointed out in the introduction section several theories have been formulated to find an evolutionary explanation for the phenomenon of human menopause [4]. But what about the body composition alterations? As mentioned above the main characteristics of somatic changes during menopausal transition are the increase of body fat mass and the visible changes in fat dis-

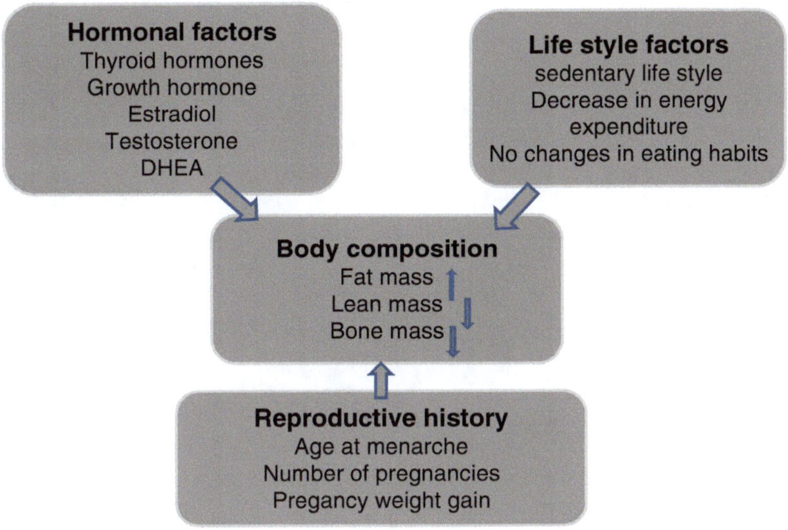

Fig. 2.11 Proximate factors influencing body composition during menopausal transition

tribution patterns. The typical fat distribution of fertile phase of life is the gynoid kind of fat patterning with a quantitatively higher amount of lower body fat, i.e., fat at the hips, buttocks, and thighs, than at the upper body. Cross-cultural analyses using the Human relation area files as data source reveal that in 90 % of investigated cultures a gynoid fat distribution is associated with female attractiveness [53] presumably because gynoid fat patterning is interpreted as an indicator for potential fertility and reproductive success of a female [54, 55]. Body fat at the lower body region is an excellent energy store for phases of increased energetic requirements [23]. The capacity to store lipids within subcutaneous fat depots especially at the lower body region is the key to facing famine and limited caloric supply especially among females. Human females are able to mobilize these energy stores to augment the caloric demands placed on the body during phases of gestation, and lactation. It is no problem for recent female *Homo sapiens* in developed countries to meet the increased energetic requirements of successful reproduction; however, our ancestors did not live in the garden of Eden. They were frequently faced with the problems of malnutrition and starvation. During pregnancy and lactation longer phases food shortages and a lack of sufficient energy had deleterious effects on reproductive outcome [49]. Sufficient energy stores in subcutaneous fat depots were visible indicators that reproductive success is possible even under worse energetic conditions (see Fig. 2.12). Lower body fat stores remain stable even during phases of starvation and malnutrition indicating the potential fertility of young women [55]. In contrast, an android fat patterning, typical for males throughout adult life, is found only among obese young females and among young females suffering from Polycystic Ovary Syndrome (PCOS), the most common endocrine cause of female infertility [56]. An android fat patterning or an android body silhouette is also found during pregnancy when a new conception is impossible. After menopausal transition nearly all postmenopausal women exhibit an android kind of fat patterning independent of their weight status (see Fig. 2.13). Android fat distribution patterns seem therefore to be excellent indicators of infertility or physiological sterility as in case of postmenopause. Therefore, a suggestion for an ultimate or evolutionary explanation of the body composition and fat distribution changes taking place during menopausal transition may be that android fat patterning could serve as an indicator for the irreversible end of female reproductive capability; however, several other evolutionary explanations are possible.

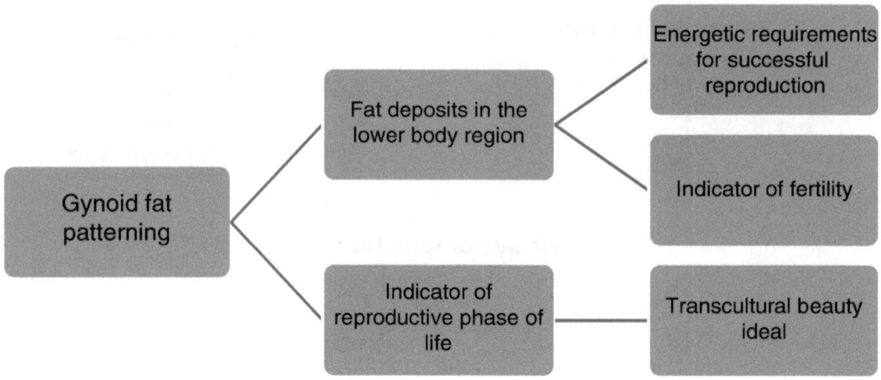

Fig. 2.12 Gynoid fat patterning as an indicator of reproductive phase

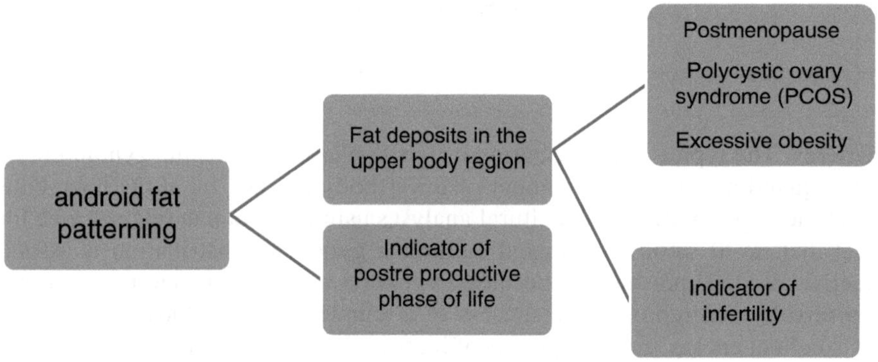

Fig. 2.13 Android fat patterning as an indicator of reduced fertility and sterility

Conclusion

Menopausal transition is associated with weight gain and dramatic changes in body composition. Although these alterations in body composition may increase the risk of various diseases such as metabolic syndrome or osteoporosis, menopause per se is not a disease, it is a natural part of female life history. The redistribution of fat tissue from a gynoid kind of fat distribution, typical of reproductive phase of life towards android fat patterning typical of postmenopause but also hyperandrogenemia in females may be interpreted as a visible marker of physiological sterility of postmenopausal women.

References

1. Leidy Sievert L. Menopause: a biocultural perspective. Rutgers University Press, New Brunswick, New Jersey; 2006.
2. Melby MK, Lampl M. Menopause: a biocultural perspective. Ann Rev Anthropol. 2011;40:43–70.
3. Austad NS. Menopause: an evolutionary perspective. Exp Gerontol. 1994;29:253–66.
4. Hawkes K, O'Connell JF, Jones NG, Alvarez H, Charnov AL. Grandmothering, menopause and the evolution of human life histories. Proc Natl Acad Sci USA. 1998;95:1336–9.

5. World Health Organization (WHO). Research on menopause in the 1990s. WHO technical reports series no.866. Geneva; 1996.
6. Burger HG, Dudley EC, Robertson DM, Dennerstein L. Hormonal changes in the menopause transition. Recent Prog Horm Res. 2002;57:257–75.
7. Burger HG, Hale GE, Robertson DM, Dennerstein L. A review of hormonal changes during the menopausal transition: focus on findings from the Melbourne Women's Midlife Health project. Hum Reprod Update. 2007;13:559–65.
8. Sorkin DJ, Muller DC, Andres R. Longitudinal change in height of men and women: implications for interpretation of the body mass index. Am J Epidemiol. 1999;150:969–77.
9. Kuk JL, Saunders TJ, Davidson LE, Ross R. Age related changes in total and regional fat distribution. Ageing Res Rev. 2009;8:339–48.
10. Dubov G, Brzezinski A, Berry EM. Weight control and the management of obesity after menopause: the role of physical activity. Maturitas. 2003;44:89–101.
11. Astrup A. Physical activity and weight gain and fat distribution changes with menopause: current evidence and research issues. Med Sci Sports Exerc. 1999;31:S564–7.
12. Tchernof A, Poehlmann ET. Effects of the menopause transition on body fatness and body fat distribution. Obes Res. 1998;6:246–54.
13. Kirchengast S, Gruber D, Sator M. Gewichtsproblematik in der Perimenopause. Speculum. 1995;13:19–21.
14. Panotopoulus G, Ruiz JC, Raison J, Guy-Grand B, Basdevant A. Menopause, fat and lean distribution in obese women. Maturitas. 1996;25:11–9.
15. Douchi T, Yamamoto S, Yoshimitsu N, Andoh T, Matsuo T, Nagata Y. Relative contribution of ageing and menopause to changes in lean and fat mass in segmental regions. Maturitas. 2002;42:301–6.
16. Douchi T, Yamamoto S, Nakamura S, Ijuin T, Oki T, Maruta K, et al. The effect of menopause on regional and total body lean mass. Maturitas. 1998;29:247–52.
17. Liu SP, Li JW, Sheng ZF, Wu XP, Liao EY. Relationship between body composition and age, menopause and its effects on bone mineral density at segmental regions in Central Southern Chinese postmenopausal elderly women with and without osteoporosis. Arch Gerontol Geriatr. 2011;53:192–7.
18. Hernandez CJ, Beaupre GS, Carter DR. A theoretical analysis of the relative influences of peak BMD, age related bone loss and menopause on the development of osteoporosis. Osteoporos Int. 2003;14:843–7.
19. Baumgartner RN, Waters DL, Gallagher D, Morley JE, Garry PJ. Predictors of skeletal muscle mass in elderly men and women. Mech Ageing Dev. 1999;107:123–36.
20. Rosenberg IH. Summary comments. Am J Clin Nutr. 1989;50:1231–3.
21. Kyle UG, Genton L, Hans D, Karsegard L, Slosman DO, Pichard C. Age-related differences in fat free mass, skeletal muscle, body cell mass and fat mass between 18 and 94 years. Eur J Clin Nutr. 2001;55:663–72.
22. Messier V, Rabasa-Lhoret R, Barat-Artigar S, Elisha B, Karelis AD, Aubertin-Leheudre M. Menopause and sarcopenia: a potential role for sex hormones. Maturitas. 2011;68:331–6.
23. Shi H, Seeey RJ, Clegg DJ. Sexual differences in the control of energy homeostasis. Front Neuroendocrinol. 2009;30:396–404.
24. Vague J. La differenciation sexuelle facteur determinant des forms da l'obesite. Presse Med. 1947;30:339–40.
25. Blouin K, Veilleux A, Luu-The V, Tchernof A. Androgen metabolism in adipose tissue: recent advances. Mol Cell Endocrinol. 2009;301:97–102.
26. Blouin K, Boivin A, Tchernof A. Androgens and body fat distribution. J Steroid Biochem Mol Biol. 2008;108:272–80.
27. Piche ME, Lapointe A, Weisnagel SJ, Corneau L, Nadeau A, Bergeron J, et al. Regional body fat distribution and metabolic profile in postmenopausal women. J Metab Clin Exp. 2008;57:1101–7.
28. Kirchengast S, Gruber D, Sator M, Hartmann B, Knogler W, Huber J. Menopause associated differences in female fat patterning estimated by dual-energy-x-ray absorptiometry. Ann Hum Biol. 1997;24:45–54.
29. Elias SG, van Noord PA, Peeters PH, den Tonkelaar I, Grobbee DE. Caloric restriction reduces age at menopause: the effect of the 1944–1945 Dutch famine. Menopause. 2003;10:399–405.
30. Hardy R, Mishra GD, Kuh D. Body mass index trajectories and age at menopause in a British birth cohort. Maturitas. 2008;59:304–14.
31. Akahoshi M, Soda M, Nakashima E, et al. The effects of body mass index on age at menopause. Int J Obes Relat Metab Disord. 2002;26:961–8.
32. Kirchengast S. Anthropological aspects of the age at menopause. Homo. 1993;44:263–77.
33. Kirchengast S, Gruber D, Sator M, Huber J. The individual age at menopause—an appropriate indicator of postmenopausal body composition? Int J Anthropol. 1999;14:243–53.
34. Carlson KJ, Miller BA, Fowler F. The main women's health study I: outcomes of hysterectomy. Obstet Gynecol. 1994;83:556–65.
35. Ravn P, Lind C, Nilas L. Lack of influence of simple premenopausal hysterectomy on bone mass and bone metabolism. Am J Obstet Gynecol. 1995;172:891–5.
36. Kirchengast S, Gruber D, Sator M, Huber J. Hysterectomy is associated with postmenopausal body composition characteristics. J Biosoc Sci. 2000;32:37–46.

37. Kirchengast S. Relations between anthropometric characteristics and the degree of severity of the climacteric syndrome in Austrian women. Maturitas. 1993;17:167–80.
38. Kirchengast S, Hartmann B, Gruber D, Huber J. Decreased sexual interest and its relationship to body build in postmenopausal women. Maturitas. 1996;23:63–71.
39. Björntorp P. The regulation of adipose tissue distribution. Int J Obes Relat Metab Disord. 1996;20:291–302.
40. Björntorp P. Hormonal control of regional fat distribution. Hum Reprod. 1997;12:21–5.
41. Brown LM, Clegg DJ. Central effects of estradiol in the regulation of adiposity. J Steroid Biochem Mol Biol. 2010;122:65–73.
42. Janssen I, Powell LH, Kazlauskaite R, Dugan SA. Testosterone and visceral fat in midlife women: the study of women's health across the nation (SWAN) fat patterning study. Obesity. 2010;18:604–10.
43. Yialamas MA, Hayes FJ. Androgens and the ageing male and female. Best Pract Res Clin Endocrinol Metab. 2003;17:223–6.
44. Sowers MR, Wildman RP, Mancuso P, Eyvazzadeh AD, Karvonen-Gutierrez CA, Rillamas-Sun E, et al. Change in adipocytokines and ghrelin with menopause. Maturitas. 2008;59:149–57.
45. Soni AC, Conroy MB, Mackey RH, Kuller LH. Ghrelin, leptin, adiponectin and insulin levels and concurrent and future weight change in overweight postmenopausal women. Menopause. 2012;18:296–301.
46. Milewicz A, Demissie M. Metabolic and endocrine changes in climacteric women. Int Congress Series. 2002; 1229:3–7.
47. Rebuffe-Scrive M, Brönnegard M, Nilson A, Eldh J, Gustafson JA, Björntorp P. Steroid hormone receptors in human adipose tissue. J Endocrinol Metab. 1990;71:1215–9.
48. Rebuffe-Scrive M, Enk L, Crona N. Fat cell metabolism in different regions in women: effects of menstrual cycle, pregnancy and lactation. J Clin Invest. 1985;75:1973–6.
49. Ellison PT. Advances in human reproductive ecology. Ann Rev Anthropol. 1994;23:255–75.
50. Parazzini F, Tavani A, Ricci E, Lavecchia C. Menstrual and reproductive factors and hip fractures in postmenopausal women. Maturitas. 1996;24:191–6.
51. Adams-Campbell LL, Kim KS, Dunston G, Laing AE, Bonney G, Demenais F. The relationship of body mass index to reproductive factors in pre- and postmenopausal African-American women with and without breast cancer. Obes Res. 1996;4:451–6.
52. Kirchengast S, Gruber D, Sator M, Huber J. Postmenopausal weight status, body composition and body fat distribution in relation to parameters of menstrual and reproductive history. Maturitas. 1999;33:117–26.
53. Brown PJ. Culture and evolution of human obesity. Hum Nat. 1991;2:31–57.
54. Singh D. Ideal female body shape: role of body weight and waist-to-hip ratio. Int J Eating Dis. 1994;16:283–8.
55. Kirchengast S, Huber J. Fat distribution patterns in young amenorrhoeic females. Hum Nat. 2001;12:123–40.
56. Kirchengast S, Huber J. Body composition characteristics and body fat distribution in lean women with polycystic ovary syndrome. Hum Rep. 2001;16:1255–60.

Chapter 3
Menopause-Related Physiological Changes and Their Possible Control Through Diet and Exercise

Igor Z. Zubrzycki, Magdalena Wiacek, and Ted Greiner

Key Points

- Menopause is a biological aging associated phenomenon coupled with a reduction in physical fitness, and sometimes combined with emotional disturbance.
- Maintenance of as high level of physical fitness as possible, which has clear links to BMI and lipid profiles, is one of the methods of lessening these detrimental phenomena.
- Walking, its variant Nordic-walking (NW), as well as jogging, and cycling are among the most popular physical activities reducing aging- and/or menopause-associated physical fitness deterioration.
- The same advice as is given to the entire population to consume a moderate diet rich in fruits, vegetables, whole grains, legumes, and low-fat dairy products is likely to reduce some of the negative effects linked to menopause. Increased consumption of soy appears to be justified as one way to alleviate some but by no means all of these.
- Currently, Body Mass Index (BMI), serum levels of total cholesterol (TC), high-density lipoprotein (HDL-C), low-density lipoprotein (LDL-C), triglycerides (TG), blood pressure, follicle-stimulating hormone (FSH), and luteinizing hormone (LH) are often used as factors describing or linked to menopausal transition.
- Changes in systolic blood pressure (SBP) and diastolic blood pressure (DBP) during the menopausal transition are most probably solely due to age increase.
- Much of the commonly seen changes in BMI, and serum concentrations of TC, HDL-C, LDL-C, and TG are likely due to both the menopausal transition and biological age increase. However, culturally mediated changes in diet and exercise patterns at this stage in life may play a role in either worsening or protecting against these changes.
- At present, we are not able to establish clear-cut dependencies between the influence of exercise and/or diet on these specific parameters defining the menopausal transition.

I.Z. Zubrzycki, Ph.D., D.Sc. (✉)
Department of Life Science, Jędrzej Śniadecki Academy of Physical Education and Sports, ul. Kazimierza Górskiego 1, 80-336 Gdańskt, Poland
e-mail: igor@hanyang.ac.kr; igorzubrzycki@yahoo.com

M. Wiacek, Ph.D.
Jędrzej Śniadecki Academy of Physical Education and Sports, ul. Kazimierza Gorskiego 1, 80-336 Gdańskt, Poland
e-mail: magdalenawiacek@yahoo.de

T. Greiner, Ph.D.
Department of Food and Nutrition, College of Human Ecology, Hanyang University, Seongdong-gu, Wangsimni ro 222, Seoul 133-791, South Korea
e-mail: tgreiner@hanyang.ac.kr

C.J.H. Martin et al. (eds.), *Nutrition and Diet in Menopause*, Nutrition and Health,
DOI 10.1007/978-1-62703-373-2_3, © Springer Science+Business Media New York 2013

Keywords Menopausal transition • Physical exercise • Diet • Cardiovascular disease • Blood pressure • Follicle-stimulating hormone • Luteinizing hormone • Aging

Abbreviations

HRQoL	Health related quality of life
NW	Nordic-walking
W	Walking
BMI	Body mass index
TC	Total cholesterol
TG	Triglyceride levels
HDL-C	High-density lipoprotein levels
LDL-C	Low-density lipoprotein levels
BP	Blood pressure
LH	Luteinizing hormone
FSH	Follicle stimulating hormone
CVD	Cardiovascular disease

Introduction

Aging is accompanied by a variety of different factors, such as loss of postural stability, spatial orientation, and strength [1], that induce a decrease in health related quality of life (HRQoL) for both men and women. In women, however, another factor that can affect HRQoL is menopause—defined as the cessation of menstruation due to follicular depletion, resulting in a loss of ovarian sensitivity to gonadotropin stimulation. In other words, the ovaries stop producing an egg each month. During the menopausal transition, aging follicles become more resistant to gonadotropin stimulation, levels of follicle-stimulating hormone (FSH) and luteinizing hormone (LH) increase. The loss of functioning follicles results also in a dramatic decline in circulating estradiol during a period lasting from about 2 years before menopause to 2 years afterwards. The ups and downs of estrogen and, to a lesser extent, progesterone, probably produce most of the symptoms women experience during this transition. Serum testosterone levels do not change. Women's attitudes towards this life transition can influence its apparent impact on their health [2].

The menopausal transition begins at around 45–48 years of age and lasts several years. It is coupled with clinical symptoms and sometimes associated with emotional disturbance—perhaps exacerbated by a perceived loss of attractiveness. In Western culture, menopause has been "medicalized," implying that its symptoms may be reduced via specific preventive means [3]. This point of view has given rise to a variety of "scientifically proven" medical approaches, for example using different types of herbal ingredients all of which have either not undergone or not withstood real scientific scrutiny. However, there is one soy constituent, genistein, which may reduce the frequency and duration of hot flashes [4].

Currently we know that menopause may be accompanied by weight gain in some but not all populations [5] and an increase of vasomotor symptoms [6] resulting in a thermoregulatory imbalance. These in turn may be linked to increased adiposity-driven weight gain [6], in turn often leading to a less favorable serum lipid spectrum. Some studies have shown that total cholesterol (TC) levels, low-density lipoprotein cholesterol (LDL-C), high-density lipoprotein cholesterol (HDL-C), and triglyceride (TG) levels are associated not only with the aging process, per se, but also with the menopausal transition (Fig. 3.1) [7–12]. Adverse lipid profiles may be associated with a detrimentally high body mass index (BMI), which is pronouncedly associated with less increase in FSH during the menopausal transition [12] (Fig. 3.2), and with an earlier cessation of reproductive cycles.

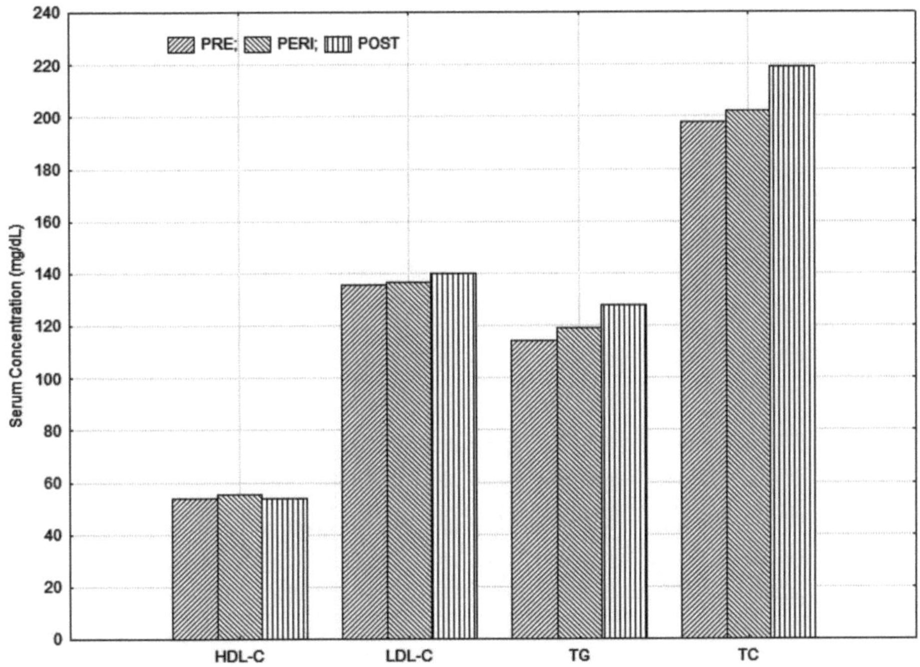

Fig. 3.1 The relationship between lipids profile and menopausal status among untrained women. The bar plot indicates menopause and/or age induced changes in serum concentration of High-density lipoprotein (HDL-C), Low-density lipoprotein (LDL-C), Triglycerides (TG), and Total Cholesterol (TC) among untrained women (after Hagner et al. [11]). For simplicity only the central values of the population are given

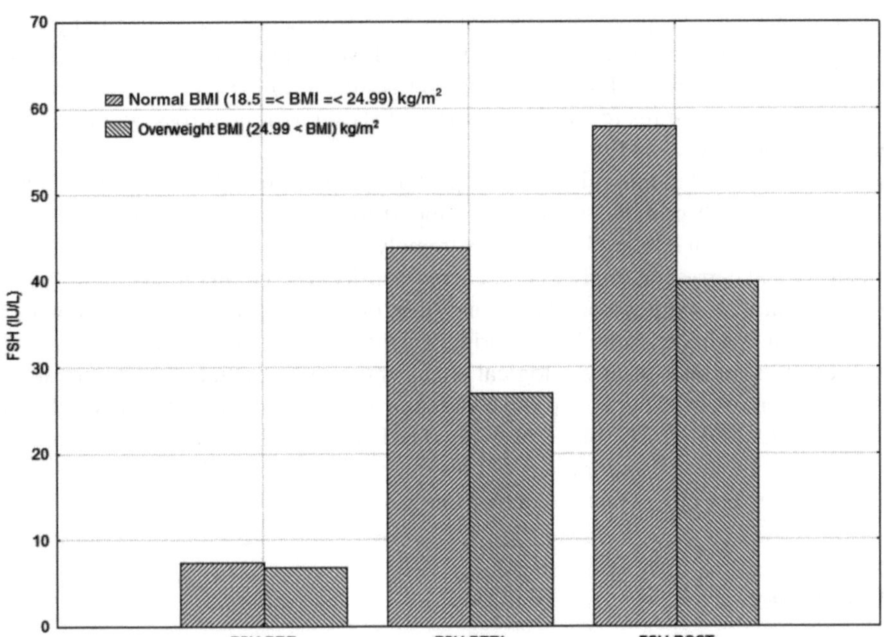

Fig. 3.2 The changes in Body Mass Index and FSH and LH activity as a function of menopausal status. The bar plot indicates relation between Body Mass Index (BMI; kg/m^2) and activity of Follicle Stimulating Hormone (FSH; IU/L) in premenopausal, perimenopausal, and postmenopausal women (after Wiacek et al. [12]). For simplicity only the central values of the population are given

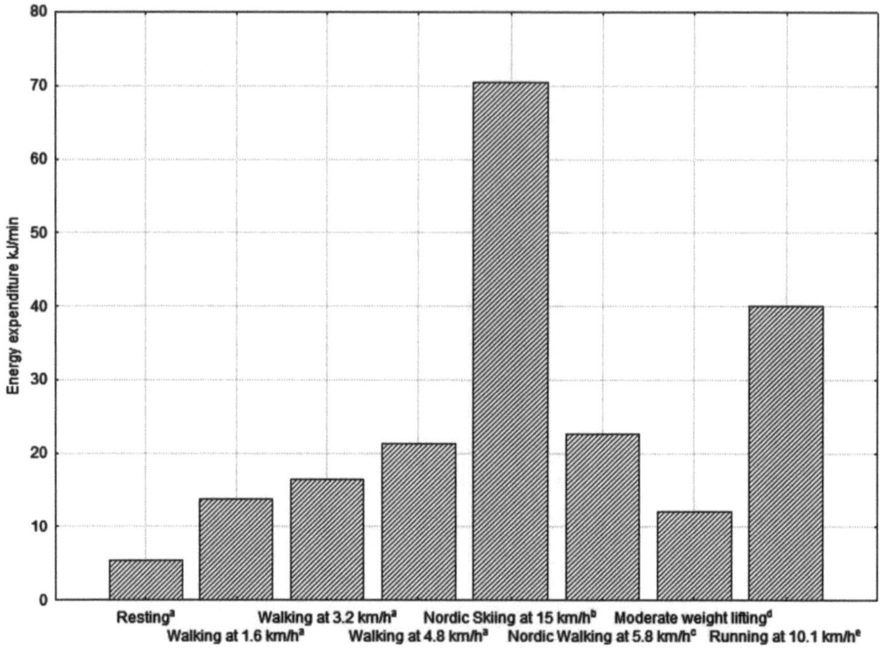

Fig. 3.3 Energy expenditure as a function of specific physical activity. The changes in energy expenditure as a function of physical activity: resting, walking, Nordic skiing, Nordic walking, weight lifting, and running. [a]Levine et al. [92], [b]Niinimaa et al. [93], [c]Church et al. [94], [d]Morgan et al. [95], [e]Hall et al. [96]. For simplicity only the central values of the population are given

One method of reducing the physical deterioration driven by menopause and/or aging is maintaining a high level of physical fitness, which has clear links to BMI and lipid profiles [11]. Among the most popular physical activities are walking and its variant Nordic-walking (NW), as well as jogging, and cycling. The energy expenditures for walking, Nordic walking, Nordic (cross country) skiing, weight lifting, and running are shown in Fig. 3.3.

Clearly diet too is crucial in minimizing the impact of aging on crucial components of physical well-being [13]. While research provides inadequate support to compose a "menopause diet" (other than perhaps recommending high intake of soy), it is extremely important at this time of life to eat a diet high in nutrient density and correspondingly low in energy density. The common pattern of "roller coaster" weight loss and gain that many women have long been on by this time in life can now be especially harmful, as muscle loss is much more likely during weight loss than muscle gain is during weight gain.

Here, we review a number of physiological changes that may be linked to menopause. We have chosen BMI as the most commonly reported indicator related to body fat and weight gain, serum levels of TC, HDL-C, LDL-C, TG, blood pressure, FSH, and LH. These are chosen not only because of their potential public health importance, but also because generally there has been more research on them than on the many others that could be examined.

Body Mass Index

Among many indices correlating height and weight of a human being, BMI expressed as the ratio of weight in kilogram to height squared in meters (W/H^2, Quetelet index) appears to be the most stable and is the one most commonly used as a rough measure of adiposity. The World Health Organization established a classification for underweight, overweight, and obesity according to BMI (Table 3.1).

Table 3.1 WHO classification of obesity accordingly to Body Mass Index

Classification	BMI (kg/m^2)
Underweight	<18.50
Severe thinness	<16.00
Moderate thinness	16.00–16.99
Mild thinness	17.00–18.49
Normal range	18.50–24.99
Overweight	≥25.00
Pre-obese	25.00–29.99
Obese	≥30.00
Obese class I	30.00–34.99
Obese class II	35.00–39.99
Obese class III	≥40.00

However, BMI functions poorly as a measure of adiposity in athletic or heavily muscled subjects. For example, an athletic subject with 15–18 % body fat, common among bodybuilders, may be incorrectly classified as obese. Better alternatives exist such as the fat-free mass index (FFMI) (fat free mass/ht^2) and the body-fat-mass index (BFMI) (body fat mass/ht^2) but these require special equipment and have not been widely enough used in past research to be used in this review.

While a few studies on BMI changes as a function of the menopausal transition indicate that the observed changes are likely due to menopause, per se [14], most find that the commonly seen increase in BMI is probably more related to age increases than menstrual cessation [11], though some argue that declines in levels of exercise are responsible [15]. From a biological perspective, the observed increase in body mass may be driven by a reverse proportional relation between age and resting metabolic rate [16], which may be indirectly influenced by an age-dependent decrease in maximal oxygen uptake capacity (VO_2max).

However, in large surveys in France [5] and Italy [17], there was no significant difference in BMI by menopausal status (and thus not by age either). This may serve to remind us that behavioral factors (and the cultural norms linked to them) rather than biological factors may be responsible for many of the differences we report here, especially any that may be linked to weight gain.

Control through exercise. While exercise clearly plays an important role in weight and BMI changes in menopausal and postmenopausal women [18], it is not a one-off activity, but must be continued if these benefits are to be realized.

Regarding the question of which type of exercise best controls BMI, in studies on the impact of Nordic-walking in premenopausal, perimenopausal, and postmenopausal women [11], a clear positive role of moderate endurance training on BMI values was seen across all menopausal groups. Stationary bicycle exercises (6 weeks; three times per week; 30 min per session) also resulted in significant changes in BMI [19]. Similarly, treadmill walking/jogging, stationary cycling, and rowing at least 3–4 days per week for 8 weeks resulted in a significant decrease in BMI in both Caucasian and African American women [20]. Although in all three studies [11, 19, 20] an increase in VO_2max was also observed, the latter [20] does not report a statistically significant increase in resting metabolic rate (RMR). This observation is rather puzzling in light of other studies clearly pointing to a positive correlation between RMR and VO_2max [21] in premenopausal and postmenopausal women, but the authors claim that the loss of weight during the training program could compensate for the lack of increase in RMR.

Control through diet. Frequency of eating correlates positively with energy intake in both premenopausal and postmenopausal women; however, only in premenopausal women does it correlate with energy expenditure. Thus, it is not surprising that only in postmenopausal women does frequency of eating correlate with percentage body fat [22]. While age appears more important than menopause per se, there may be a detrimental interaction between menopause, diet, and exercise, leading to further weight gain during the menopausal period.

In midlife, women tend to make positive behavioral changes, including dietary improvements [23]. Menopausal Spanish women consume more dairy products [24] and Malaysian postmenopausal women were found to consume 6 % less fat than premenopausal women [25].

However, achieving weight loss or even avoiding gain during the midlife period when menopause typically occurs is challenging. In one group of women 47–52 years old, a 2-year follow-up study showed that only those who decreased food quantity, cut down on fats/sugars, used a commercial weight loss program, and exercised avoided weight gain [26], while others (the majority of whom were attempting to control their weight), gained an average of 1.2 kg. Nevertheless, dietary interventions can be effective in reducing weight and BMI and improving blood lipids in postmenopausal women [27]. In the Women's Healthy Lifestyle Project, among women at an average age of 47 at baseline, behavior change efforts over a 5-year period (during which 35 % became postmenopausal) focused on decreasing intakes of calories and cholesterol and increasing exercise in an attempt to reduce the unfavorable changes typically occurring during menopause [28]. Weight was decreased by 0.1 kg compared to an increase of 2.4 kg in the control group.

There has been speculation that consumption of soy, in addition to other benefits, might assist with weight control. One study providing supplementation with 99 mg isoflavones daily for 1 year had no impact on BMI compared with provision of an equal amount of milk protein [29] but another 3-month trial in postmenopausal Caucasian and African American women providing 20 g soy plus 160 mg of isoflavones daily reduced total and subcutaneous abdominal fat [30]. A 6-month trial in postmenopausal Italian women of a diet very high in soy (referred to below as the "high soy study") resulted in a non-significant decrease in BMI, but adherence to such a profoundly changed diet was not high [31].

Total Cholesterol

Progress in the medical sciences has allowed us to realize that excess cholesterol in the bloodstream may result in a plaque causing atherosclerosis, a thickening and reduction in flexibility of the arteries, often leading to obstruction in blood flow and hypertension. Although current popular and scientific literature portrays cholesterol as the "bad guy," it plays a vital role in homeostasis (i.e. stable internal environment of an organism). For example, cholesterol moderates cell membrane stability making them less temperature dependent. It is also a crucial factor in steroid hormone production and a major participant in vitamin D biosynthesis which in turn is associated with bone mineral density i.e., it is necessary in the maintenance of strong bones. It also regulates function of neurotransmitters. Thus, the use of drugs that inhibit liver cholesterol production has a detrimental influence on our mental capabilities, including memory function. It has to be stressed that the level of TC in our body does not depend on the amount of cholesterol in the diet but is a function of the types of fat consumed; for example saturated fatty acids stimulate cholesterol synthesis.

Analysis of a variety of epidemiological studies led to the Adult Treatment Panel (ATP) III classification [32], consisting of TC, LDL-C and HDL-C, each with a link to CHD risk (Table 3.2).

An analysis of the current literature reveals slight inconsistencies regarding changes in TC level as a function of the menopausal transition. The vast majority of reports [33, 34] indicate that the transition between perimenopause and postmenopause is associated with an increase in TC levels. However, Franklin et al. [33] reported a lack of menopause-induced changes in TC level. This phenomenon may be due to a different analytical approach; in contrast to previous reports, in the latter no adjustment for body mass was made. Since many studies found an increase in fat and body mass, one may assume that these two parameters in turn influence the level of TC.

Table 3.2 Classification of total cholesterol, LDL cholesterol, and HDL cholesterol accordingly to Adult Treatment Panel III

Total cholesterol (mg/dL)		LDL cholesterol (mg/dL)		HDL cholesterol (mg/dL)	
		<100	Optimal	<40	Low
<200	Desirable	100–129	Near optimal/above optimal	40–60	Normal
200–239	Borderline-high	130–159	Borderline-high		
≥240	High	160–189	High	≥60	High
		≥190	Very high		

Control through exercise. TC levels are lower among subjects with higher aerobic fitness in premenopausal, perimenopausal, and postmenopausal women [11]. Some research suggests that a moderate to significant amount of exercise may be required [11], but the minimal amount of exercise required to induce a decrease in TC levels is at present unknown. In studies performed on 28 subjects on a stationary bicycle, the administration of exercise for 14 min at 55 % of each participant's maximal oxygen consumption resulted in an acute decrease in TC levels among all the participants [35]. Not only endurance but also resistance training appears to be beneficial in lowering TC levels [36]. Given that the menopausal increase in TC levels is linked to both the menopausal transition and the aging process, we assume that the administration of almost any exercise program will decrease TC levels throughout the menopausal transition.

Control through diet. Providing a diet high in monounsaturated fats reduces TC levels irrespective of menopausal status [37]. Dietary interventions to improve cardiac health used to focus on fat intake but there is increasing doubt that this is adequate. For example, in one study of Japanese women in midlife (referred to below as "the Japanese study"), diets with a high glycemic load, although lower in TC, even after controlling for menopausal status and several other variables, were associated with no reduction in total serum cholesterol concentrations [38]. Thus, the focus of dietary recommendations has shifted in recent years to increasing intakes of fruits, vegetables, low-fat dairy products, *n*-3 fatty acids, and dietary fiber [39].

In general, diets rich in isoflavones (found largely in soy beans) are found to improve cardiovascular profiles, reducing TC and LDL-C levels, while having no known adverse effects. A recent systematic review [40] estimates that consumption of soy protein was on average associated with a 5.34 mg/dL, or 2.4 %, decrease in TC. This increased to 6.56 mg/dL with consumption of at least 40 mg/day, possibly important in east Asian diets where 50 mg/day is commonly consumed [41]. However, in a review of six randomized trials with at least 2 years of follow-up in postmenopausal women, Howard et al. [42] concluded that a reduction in the risk of coronary heart disease occurs when diets achieve at least a 12 % decrease in serum TC. The differences in intake seen in modified Western diets (often less than 1 mg/day) are probably not large enough to make any difference [43]. The high soy study resulted in a non-significant decrease in TC [31].

High Density Lipoprotein Cholesterol

HDL is synthesized in the liver and small intestine. HDL is composed of different apolipoproteins, including apoA-I, apoC-I, apoC-II, and the enzyme lecithin-cholesterol acyl transferase (LCAT). LCAT converts cholesterol to cholesteryl esters, forming a spherical HDL particle. This cholesterol-rich lipoprotein (*HDL-C*) returns to the liver, where the cholesterol is unloaded. HDL cholesterol (HDL-C) normally makes up 20–30 % of the total serum cholesterol. HDL-C is often referred to as the "good cholesterol" because epidemiological studies have shown that the level of serum HDL-C is reversely proportional to CHD morbidity and mortality, but this protective effect may be lost after menopause. The ATP III panel adjusted the cut-off point for HDL-C cholesterol to 40 mg/dL for both men and women, indicating that subjects having a cholesterol concentration less than 40 mg/dL were at higher risk of CHD [44] (Table 3.2).

Some studies have found a significant [12, 34] and progressive [45] increase in levels of the protective serum high-density lipoprotein cholesterol during the menopausal process, though one study [46] found a decrease during the 2 years preceding menopause and some [5] have found no change. After the final menstrual period, the level of HDL-C usually begins to decline, often reaching the perimenopausal level [11]. One study found a significant decrease in serum HDL-C level from pre-menopause to postmenopause [47], but hormonal levels, age group and BMI levels had not been adequately controlled for. In particular, it is well known that there is a reverse proportional association between BMI and HDL-C levels [48]. Thus, given the typical menopause-related changes in BMI [49], it is likely that the observed changes in HDL-C levels are menopause-driven.

Control through exercise. Some studies report an increase in HDL-C levels in spite of a lack of exercise [50] in women around perimenopause. Later studies indicated that irrespective of baseline levels [11] and regardless of exercise intensity, HDL-C levels increase in women just before and during menopause [51]. Kemmler et al. [52] found that exercise induced only a non-significant positive change in serum HDL-C levels among postmenopausal women. Similarly, Hagner et al. [11] found that exercise induced significant increases in HDL-C levels in pre-menopause and perimenopause but not in the postmenopause. Cauley et al. [53] also found that 2 years of exercise failed to have an impact on HDL-C levels among postmenopausal women.

Control through diet. Neither a low-fat diet, an exercise program, nor a combination of the two increased HDL-C in one study of middle aged men and postmenopausal women with low baseline HDL-C [54]. The Women's Healthy Lifestyle Project also failed to change HDL-C levels [28]. In Japanese women in midlife, diets with a high glycemic load, though lower in TC were associated with lower serum HDL-C cholesterol concentrations after controlling for menopausal status and other variables [38]. Providing a diet high in monounsaturated fats tends to increase HDL-C irrespective of menopausal status [37]. A recent systematic review [40] concluded that consumption of soy protein is not associated with changes in HDL-C. Similarly, the high soy study resulted in no change in HDL-C [31].

Low-Density Lipoprotein Cholesterol

LDL-C particles are synthesized in the liver and transport cholesterol molecules to extra-hepatic tissues that require cholesterol, for example for biosynthesis of the steroid hormones. After fusion of LDL-cholesterol with a cell, through a specific binding mechanism LDL-C particles are catabolised and cholesterol is used by the cell.

LDL-C is the main source of artery-clogging plaque. LDL-C concentration in human blood serum has been divided into five specific ranges as a function of health related quality of life (Table 3.2).

Some studies have found a continuous increase in LDL-C levels across pre-menopause, perimenopause [55], and postmenopause [12]. The Chin-Shan Community Cardiovascular Cohort study [56] found an increase in LDL-C in premenopausal and perimenopausal women but a decrease in postmenopausal women. The French study [5] found a significant increase in the prevalence of high LDL and high TC combined during menopause.

Control through exercise. Prabhakaran et al. [57] found that resistance training may improve lipid profiles among premenopausal women but applicability to perimenopausal and postmenopausal women is to date unknown. Moderate endurance training does appear to influence lipid profiles, reducing LDL-C levels among premenopausal, perimenopausal, and postmenopausal women [11].

Control through diet. Providing a diet high in monounsaturated fats reduces LDL-C levels irrespective of menopausal status [37]. In the Japanese study, diets with a high glycemic load were associated with higher serum LDL-C concentrations in postmenopausal but not premenopausal women [38].

In a study on the influence of an 8 year low-fat diet in postmenopausal women, a 2.7 mg/dL reduction in LDL-C levels was observed [42]. However, after 5 years of implementation, The Women's Healthy Lifestyle Project was unable to reduce LDL-C. Nevertheless, the 3.5 mg/dL increase was significantly less than the 8.9 mg/dL increase in the control group [28]. Prediger et al. [40] found little evidence that consumption of soy protein was associated with changes in LDL-C. The high soy study resulted in a non-significant reduction in LDL-C [31]. However, it may be that even though diet and exercise each alone have only a minor impact, together they seem able to reduce LDL-C in perimenopausal [58] and postmenopausal women [54].

Serum Triglyceride

A TG (triacylglycerol) is a molecular comprising one molecule of glycerol and three molecules of fatty acids. TG are the main components of animal fats and vegetable oils. Analogous to cholesterol TG play an important role in elasticity of cell membranes and their depots serve as insulation against cold. The correlations found between serum TG levels and CHD rendered these parameters as risk markers for CHD. For example, TG level ≥200 mg/dL is consonant with an elevated level of atherogenic factors that increase the risk for CHD significantly more than TG alone. These observations were included in ATPIII [32] proposed TG classification, Table 3.3.

Elevation in blood TG levels is a derivative of a variety of factors, which can be divided into two groups. The first group comprises factors related to quality of life i.e., obesity, physical inactivity, tobacco smoking, excess alcohol intake, and high-carbohydrate diet and the second to diseases inducing elevation of TG level, i.e., type 2 diabetes, chronic renal failure, nephrotic syndrome, and genetic factors.

Two studies [33, 59] report fairly constant TG levels across the menopausal transition. However, other have found a consistent increase in TG levels along with increases in BMI in women during this period [60]. A large French survey found no increase in obesity with menopause but a significant increase in TG [5]. Aging rather than menopause per se appears to be the main factor involved [12].

Control through exercise. Exercise appears to reduce TG levels, even in postmenopausal women; one study found significant decreases after 2 years of exercise (four sessions per week, 60–70 min per session + two 25-min home training sessions) [52]. Another study obtained decreases after only 10 weeks of aerobic and resistance training [61] and a third after 12 weeks of endurance training [11]. A recent study in young women found that, unlike for young men, they had significant decreases in TG in the immediate post-exercise period (3 h) independent of exercise intensity [62]. The minimum

Table 3.3 Triglyceride categories accordingly to Adult Treatment Panel III

Triglyceride category	ATP III levels (mg/dL)
Normal triglycerides	<150
Borderline-high triglycerides	150–199
High triglycerides	200–499
Very high triglycerides	≥500

required exercise level to decrease TG levels, especially during the menopausal transition, is at present unknown.

Control through diet. The Women's Healthy Lifestyle Project was unable to reduce TG but the 18.2 mg/dL increase was significantly less than the 29.9 mg/dL increase in the control group over the 5-year intervention period [28]. In the Japanese study, diets with a high glycemic load, though lower in fat, were associated with higher serum TG concentrations [38]. This effect was more pronounced in postmenopausal than premenopausal women.

The high soy study resulted in a nonsignificant decrease in serum TG [31]. A recent systematic review [40] concluded that consumption of soy protein is not associated with changes in TG.

Blood Pressure

The last few decades of study on hypertension related health risk indicated that the specific attention should be given to systolic blood pressure (SBP) changes, since these are the main risk factors for cardiovascular diseases. Extensive analysis of the assonant changes in SBP and diastolic blood pressure (DPB) has revealed specific age dependent correlations between the SPB, DPB, and the mean arterial pressure (MAP). SPB rises continuously to the ninth decade of life. This phenomenon is associated with a congruent two-phase increase in the pulse pressure (PP). In the first phase, DBP rises until the age of about 50 when it may level off for the rest of life or fall later in life.

The Joint National Committee on Prevention, Detection, Evaluation, and Treatment of High Blood Pressure (JNC) report [63] introduced a classification of blood pressure in regards to human health status (Table 3.4).

The French study [5], comparing postmenopausal with perimenopausal women within a relatively narrow age range (average 4 years difference in age), found 14.5 % hypertension in the former compared to 7.4 % in the latter group. Zanchetti et al. [64] also found an increase after controlling for age, BMI, and other factors, but only among women undergoing menopause at a younger age. Another study of 671 women referred for coronary angiography [65] found no statistically significant increase in SBP as a function of the menopausal transition when data were adjusted for age. Similarly, a recent analysis of NHANES data [34] concluded that changes in SBP during the menopausal transition were solely due to age increases (Fig. 3.4). DBP also does not appear to change across the premenopausal, perimenopausal, and postmenopausal transition [56].

Control through exercise. In the French study [5], 46 % of postmenopausal women were sedentary compared to 43 % of perimenopausal women and thus a decline in levels of exercise was unlikely to explain the higher level of hypertension in the former group. An early meta-analysis of the literature on SBP among adult women [66] failed to find any clear impact of aerobic exercise on resting SBP. Bond et al. [67] had similar findings in premenopausal African-American women. However, some

Table 3.4 Blood pressure, systolic blood pressure (SBP) and diastolic blood pressure (DBP) classification according to JNC 7

SBP/DBP	JNC 7 category
<120/80	Normal
120–139/80–89	Prehypertension
≥140/90	Hypertension
140–159/90–99	Stage 1 hypertension
≥160/100	Stage 2 hypertension

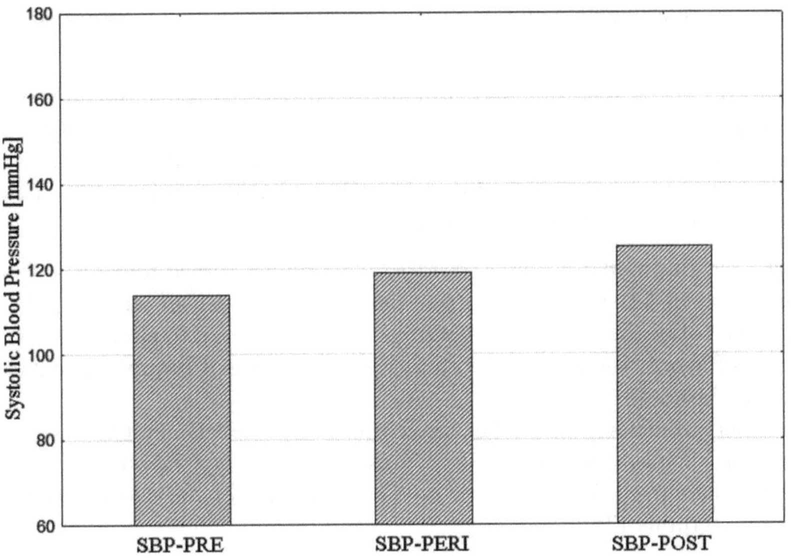

Fig. 3.4 Changes in systolic blood pressure as a function of menopausal status [34]. Relation between Systolic Blood Pressure (SBP) as a function of menopausal status—unpublished results (Wiacek and Zubrzycki). For simplicity only the central values of the population are given. *SBP-PRE* median value of systolic blood in premenopausal group, *SBP-PERI* median value of systolic blood pressure in perimenopausal group, *SBP-POST* median value of systolic blood pressure in postmenopausal group

recent studies do find an impact. For example, Figueroa et al. [68] achieved a reduction in both systolic and diastolic blood pressure in postmenopausal women with 12 weeks of moderate-intensity combined resistance and endurance training. Among women with hypertension, exercise has also proven to have a positive effect in decreasing SBP [69].

Control through diet. In a study by Wing et al. [55], weight increase was positively associated with an increase in SBP. In a 5-year follow-up of perimenopausal women (defined as women aged 47–56), Juntunen et al. [70] similarly concluded that avoiding weight gain via exercise and diet was necessary to prevent postmenopausal hypertension. However, the Women's Healthy Lifestyle Project failed to achieve changes in systolic blood pressure [28]. The high soy study among postmenopausal women also resulted in no change in blood pressure [31].

Luteinizing Hormone

LH is produced by the anterior pituitary, stimulating in females development of the *corpus luteum*, a structure formed from tissues of ruptured ovarian follicles. Along with other hormones, including FSH, it takes part in the regulation of the menstrual cycle. Its highest concentration is apparently during the ovulatory phase.

One study reported that only age seemed to be involved [71] and another [72] concluded that menopause alone was responsible for changes in LH levels. However, over the past decade, most studies have suggested that both age and menopause cause an increase in LH levels [12], the study performed on women aged 35–60 encompassed in NHANES III and NHANES 1999–2002 [34] found that LH increased in a similar fashion in perimenopausal as in postmenopausal women. Thus, more research is needed to determine whether the LH increase is driven by a menopause per se, the aging process, or both.

Control through exercise. It has been shown that LH pulsatility-driven amenorrhea occurs among female subjects engaging in a variety of intensive sports, including running and cycling, or in ballet [73]. This phenomenon may be linked with exercise-driven energy depletion-induced amenorrhea congruent with the level of physical fitness leading to metabolic stress manifested by lower SBP, higher VO_2max, lower TC and LDL-C levels, and higher HDL-C levels [23].

Control through diet. During the last two decades, attention has turned towards soy isoflavones as a means of suppression of LH mid-cycle surges among premenopausal women [74]. Though some research did not find soy per se to be very effective [75], a recent trial found that genistein, making up about half of the isoflavones found in soy, with a single daily dose of 30 mg, did reduce the frequency and duration of hot flashes [4].

Among the variety of dietary approaches for controlling LH levels in menopausal women, the use of herbal ingredients such as dandelion, ginkgo, ginseng, raspberry, wild yam, black cohosh, phytoestrogens from soy, red clover, flax, and dong quai has become popular. However, none of these has withstood scientific scrutiny [76].

Follicle Stimulating Hormone

FSH is a glycoprotein gonadotropin secreted by the anterior pituitary in response to gonadotropin-releasing hormone. FSH is primarily responsible for stimulating growth of the ovarian follicle.

In French women 45–55 years of age, serum FSH was 7 IU/L in early perimenopause, 35.9 IU/L in late perimenopause, and 47.8 IU/L in postmenopause [5]. The Melbourne Women's MidLife Health Project study found that the level of FSH begins to rise around 2 years before the final menstrual period [77]. An extensive study comprising four cohorts in TERMIN [78], the Melbourne Women's Midlife Health Project (MWMHP) [79], the Seattle Midlife Women's Health Study (SMWHS) [80], and the Study of Women's Health Across the Nation (SWAN) [81] all reported stronger coupling between FSH concentration and the late menopausal transition than the early menopausal transition. They also revealed a continuous increase in FSH levels across postmenopause up to the level of about 40 IU/L. Notwithstanding the clear-cut changes in FSH levels as a function of the menopause, FSH level is of negligible diagnostic value i [82].

Control through exercise. At present, only a handful of studies have reported on changes in FSH levels as a function of exercise in premenopausal and postmenopausal women and none of them have focused on perimenopause. A study of exercise and FSH levels in premenopausal women of about 26 years of age found an exercise-induced decrease in FSH levels, but only at the 90 % confidence interval [83]. A study on 50 sedentary Brazilian postmenopausal women had a similar finding [84]; 16-week resistance training resulted in a statistically significant decrease in FSH levels at $P<0.001$. No significant changes were seen in BMI, muscle mass or fat percentage. However, Trevisan et al. [85] found no impact of resistance training on FSH levels in postmenopausal women. Aerobic training also proved to be an inefficient means of decreasing FSH levels in postmenopausal women, *vide* the study by Cardoso et al. [86].

Control through diet. Among the handful of studies on this subject is a report [87] indicating no change in FSH activity as a function of a galactose-rich diet in perimenopausal women. A study on supplementation with soy and wheat in postmenopausal women found a decrease in serum FSH in the wheat flour group compared with the soy group [88].

Table 3.5 Literature-derived relationships between menopausal-transition driven changes in Body Mass Index (BMI), Total Cholesterol (TC), Triglyceride levels (TG), High-density lipoprotein levels (HDL-C), Low-density lipoprotein levels (LDL-C), Blood Pressure (BP), Luteinizing Hormone activity (LH), and Follicle Stimulating Hormone activity (FSH), and the potential for controlling such changes through physical exercise or diet

Parameter	Menopausal transition	Control through exercise	Control through diet
BMI	Often increased	Aerobic endurance	Likely/uncertain
TC	Increase	Aerobic endurance/resistance	Likely
TG	Increase	Aerobic endurance	Uncertain
HDL-C	Fluctuation	Aerobic endurance	Uncertain
LDL-C	Uncertain	Aerobic endurance	Likely
BP	Uncertain	Uncertain	Uncertain
LH	Increase	Uncertain	Likely/uncertain
FSH	Increase	Likely/uncertain	Uncertain

Conclusions

This analysis of current knowledge on the associations between the menopausal transition and anthropometric and physiological parameters, including BMI, TC, HDL-C, LDL-C, TG, LH, FSH, and blood pressure, focused on evidence regarding the extent to which diet and exercise can modify these associations. In Table 3.5 we summarize our conclusions based on current knowledge of these associations. One may clearly see that in many cases the influence of exercise or diet on the specific parameter, if not unknown, is uncertain. Though it was pointed out many years ago that research on these issues needed to be done, including psychosocial factors, and examining effects in heterogeneous populations, little research of this kind has been done [89]. As a result, there are still serious shortcomings in our knowledge of these relationships, hindering attempts to improve HQoL through specific or tailored diet and/or exercise regimes.

However, we believe that the evidence so far available suggests that an increase in weight and the appearance of obesity should not be viewed as tightly linked either to menopause or aging. Most of the observations suggesting such a link have so far been reported from North America and other societies where diet and exercise behaviors, in turn influenced by cultural, commercial food industry, and other factors amenable to change, are at least partially involved. Thus, many of the negative changes often seen during menopause should not be viewed as inevitable. The maintenance and even strengthening of healthy dietary and exercise habits before, through and even after menopause is feasible [90] and will likely pay off in a healthier and longer-lasting [91] old age among women.

References

1. Wiacek M, Hagner W, Hagner-Derengowska M, et al. Correlations between postural stability and strength of lower body extremities of women population living in long-term care facilities. Arch Gerontol Geriatr. 2009;48:346–9.
2. Ayers B, Forshaw M, Hunter MS. The impact of attitudes towards the menopause on women's symptom experience: a systematic review. Maturitas. 2010;65:28–36.
3. Rogers A. Human behavior in the social environment. McGraw-Hill Humanities/Social Sciences/Languages. United States; 2005.
4. Evans M, Elliott JG, Sharma P, Berman R, Guthrie N. The effect of synthetic genistein on menopause symptom management in healthy postmenopausal women: a multi-center, randomized, placebo-controlled study. Maturitas. 2011;68:189–96.
5. Tremollieres FA, Pouilles JM, Cauneille C, Ribot C. Coronary heart disease risk factors and menopause: a study in 1684 French women. Atherosclerosis. 1999;142:415–23.

6. van Poppel MN, Brown WJ. "It's my hormones, doctor"—does physical activity help with menopausal symptoms? Menopause. 2008;15:78–85.
7. Davis CE, Pajak A, Rywik S, Williams DH, Broda G, Pazucha T, et al. Natural menopause and cardiovascular disease risk factors. The Poland and US Collaborative Study on Cardiovascular Disease Epidemiology. Ann Epidemiol. 1994;4:445–8.
8. Akahoshi M, Soda M, Nakashima E, Shimaoka K, Seto S, Yano K. Effects of menopause on trends of serum cholesterol, blood pressure, and body mass index. Circulation. 1996;94:61–6.
9. Bonithon-Kopp C, Scarabin PY, Darne B, Malmejac A, Guize L. Menopause-related changes in lipoproteins and some other cardiovascular risk factors. Int J Epidemiol. 1990;19:42–8.
10. Matthews KA, Wing RR, Kuller LH, Meilahn EN, Plantinga P. Influence of the perimenopause on cardiovascular risk factors and symptoms of middle-aged healthy women. Arch Intern Med. 1994;154:2349–55.
11. Hagner W, Hagner-Derengowska M, Wiacek M, Zubrzycki IZ. Changes in level of VO2max, blood lipids, and waist circumference in the response to moderate endurance training as a function of ovarian aging. Menopause. 2009;16:1009–13.
12. Wiacek M, Hagner W, Zubrzycki IZ. Measures of menopause driven differences in levels of blood lipids, follicle-stimulating hormone, and luteinizing hormone in women aged 35 to 60 years: National Health and Nutrition Examination Survey III and National Health and Nutrition Examination Survey 1999–2002 study. Menopause. 2011;18:60–6.
13. Cuzick J, Glasier A, La Vecchia C, Maraganore DM, Negri E, Rossi M, et al. Perimenopausal risk factors and future health. Hum Reprod Update. 2011;17:706–17.
14. Svendsen OL, Hassager C, Christiansen C. Age- and menopause-associated variations in body composition and fat distribution in healthy women as measured by dual-energy X-ray absorptiometry. Metabolism. 1995;44:369–73.
15. Sternfeld B, Wang H, Quesenberry CP, Abrams B, Everson-Rose SA, Greendale GA, et al. Physical activity and changes in weight and waist circumference in midlife women: findings from the study of women's health across the nation. Am J Epidemiol. 2004;160:912–22.
16. Luhrmann PM, Edelmann-Schafer B, Neuhauser-Berthold M. Changes in resting metabolic rate in an elderly German population: cross-sectional and longitudinal data. J Nutr Health Aging. 2010;14:232–6.
17. Pasquali R, Casimirri F, Pascal G, Tortelli O, Labate AMM, Bertazzo D, et al. Influence of menopause on blood cholesterol levels in women: the role of body composition, fat distribution and hormonal milieu. J Intern Med. 1997;241:195–203.
18. Choquette S, Riesco E, Cormier E, Dion T, Aubertin-Leheudre M, Dionne IJ. Effects of soya isoflavones and exercise on body composition and clinical risk factors of cardiovascular diseases in overweight postmenopausal women: a 6-month double-blind controlled trial. Br J Nutr. 2011;105:1199–209.
19. Dunai A, Novak M, Chung SA, Kayumov L, Keszei A, Levitan R, et al. Moderate exercise and bright light treatment in overweight and obese individuals. Obesity (Silver Spring). 2007;15:1749–57.
20. Santa-Clara H, Szymanski L, Ordille T, Fernhall B. Effects of exercise training on resting metabolic rate in postmenopausal African American and Caucasian women. Metabolism. 2006;55:1358–64.
21. Van Pelt RE, Jones PP, Davy KP, Desouza CA, Tanaka H, Davy BM, et al. Regular exercise and the age-related decline in resting metabolic rate in women. J Clin Endocrinol Metab. 1997;82:3208–12.
22. Yannakoulia M, Melistas L, Solomou E, Yiannakouris N. Association of eating frequency with body fatness in pre- and postmenopausal women. Obesity (Silver Spring). 2007;15:100–6.
23. De Cree C. Comment on health issues for women athletes: exercise-induced amenorrhea. J Clin Endocrinol Metab. 1999;84:4750–1.
24. Ubeda N, Basagoiti M, Alonso-Aperte E, Varela-Moreiras G. Dietary food habits, nutritional status and lifestyle in menopausal women in Spain. Nutr Hosp. 2007;22:313–21.
25. Pon LW, Noor-Aini MY, Ong FB, Adeeb N, Seri SS, Shamsuddin K, et al. Diet, nutritional knowledge and health status of urban middle-aged Malaysian women. Asia Pac J Clin Nutr. 2006;15:388–99.
26. Williams L, Germov J, Young A. Preventing weight gain: a population cohort study of the nature and effectiveness of mid-age women's weight control practices. Int J Obes (Lond). 2007;31:978–86.
27. Abedi P, Lee MHS, Kandiah M, Yassin Z, Shojaeezade D, Hosseini M, et al. Diet intervention to improve cardiovascular risk factors among Iranian postmenopausal women. Nutr Res Pract. 2010;4:522–7.
28. Loucks AB. Energy balance and body composition in sports and exercise. J Sports Sci. 2004;22:1–14.
29. Kok L, Kreijkamp-Kaspers S, Grobbee DE, Lampe JW, van der Schouw YT. Soy isoflavones, body composition, and physical performance. Maturitas. 2005;52:102–10.
30. Christie DR, Grant J, Darnell BE, Chapman VR, Gastaldelli A, Sites CK. Metabolic effects of soy supplementation in postmenopausal Caucasian and African American women: a randomized, placebo-controlled trial. Am J Obstet Gynecol. 2010;203:153.e151–9.
31. Chiechi LM, Secreto G, Vimercati A, Greco P, Venturelli E, Pansini F, et al. The effects of a soy rich diet on serum lipids: the Menfis randomized trial. Maturitas. 2002;41:97–104.
32. Third Report of the National Cholesterol Education Program (NCEP) Expert Panel on Detection, Evaluation, and Treatment of High Blood Cholesterol in Adults (Adult Treatment Panel III). Third Report of the National

Cholesterol Education Program (NCEP) Expert Panel on detection, evaluation, and treatment of high blood cholesterol in adults (Adult Treatment Panel III) final report. Circulation. 2002;106:3143–421.
33. Franklin RM, Ploutz-Snyder L, Kanaley JA. Longitudinal changes in abdominal fat distribution with menopause. Metabolism. 2009;58:311–5.
34. Wiacek M, Jegal BS, Hagner W, Hagner-Derengowska M, Zubrzycki IZ. Age- and menopause-related differences in physiological factors of health quality in women aged 35–60. Arch Gerontol Geriatr. 2012;54(2):385–90.
35. Lennon DL, Stratman FW, Shrago E, Nagle FJ, Hanson PG, Madden M, et al. Total cholesterol and HDL-cholesterol changes during acute, moderate-intensity exercise in men and women. Metabolism. 1983;32:244–9.
36. Boyden TW, Pamenter RW, Going SB, Lohman TG, Hall MC, Houtkooper LB, et al. Resistance exercise training is associated with decreases in serum low-density lipoprotein cholesterol levels in premenopausal women. Arch Intern Med. 1993;153:97–100.
37. Mata P, Garrido JA, Ordovas JM, Blazquez E, Alvarezsala LA, Rubio MJ, et al. Effect of dietary monounsaturated fatty acids on plasma lipoproteins and apolipoproteins in women. Am J Clin Nutr. 1992;56:77–83.
38. Montoye HJ, Mikkelsen WM, Block WD, Gayle R. Relationship of oxygen uptake capacity, serum uric acid and glucose tolerance in males and females, age 10–69. Am J Epidemiol. 1978;108:274–82.
39. Tobita Y, Otaki H, Kusaka Y, Iki M, Kajita E, Sato K. [A cross-sectional analysis on relationships between maximum oxygen uptake and risk factors for cardiovascular diseases]. Sangyo Eiseigaku Zasshi. 1995;37:409–15.
40. Prediger CCD, Olinto MTA, Nacul LC, Ziegler DR, Pattussi MP. Effects of soy protein containing isoflavones on women's lipid profile: a meta-analysis. Rev Nutr. 2011;24:161–72.
41. Somekawa Y, Chiguchi M, Ishibashi T, Aso T. Soy intake related to menopausal symptoms, serum lipids, and bone mineral density in postmenopausal Japanese women. Obstet Gynecol. 2001;97:109–15.
42. Howard BV, Van Horn L, Hsia J, Manson JE, Stefanick ML, Wassertheil-Smoller S, et al. Low-fat dietary pattern and risk of cardiovascular disease: the Women's Health Initiative Randomized Controlled Dietary Modification Trial. JAMA. 2006;295:655–66.
43. Kreijkamp-Kaspers S, Kok L, Bots ML, Grobbee DE, van der Schouw YT. Dietary phytoestrogens and plasma lipids in Dutch postmenopausal women; a cross-sectional study. Atherosclerosis. 2005;178:95–100.
44. National Cholesterol Education Program. Third Report of the Expert Panel on detection, evaluation, and treatment of high blood cholesterol in adults (ATP III Final Report). Bethesda, MD; 2002.
45. Kim CJ, Kim TH, Ryu WS, Ryoo UH. Influence of menopause on high density lipoprotein-cholesterol and lipids. J Korean Med Sci. 2000;15:380–6.
46. Jensen J, Nilas L, Christiansen C. Influence of menopause on serum lipids and lipoproteins. Maturitas. 1990;12:321–31.
47. Nerbrand C, Lidfeldt J, Nyberg P, Schersten B, Samsioe G. Serum lipids and lipoproteins in relation to endogenous and exogenous female sex steroids and age. The women's health in the lund area (WHILA) study. Maturitas. 2004;48:161–9.
48. Ernst ND, Obarzanek E, Clark MB, Briefel RR, Brown CD, Donato K. Cardiovascular health risks related to overweight. J Am Diet Assoc. 1997;97:S47–51.
49. McNeil CJ, Vandervoort AA, Rice CL. Peripheral impairments cause a progressive age-related loss of strength and velocity-dependent power in the dorsiflexors. J Appl Physiol. 2007;102:1962–8.
50. Brownell KD, Bachorik PS, Ayerle RS. Changes in plasma lipid and lipoprotein levels in men and women after a program of moderate exercise. Circulation. 1982;65:477–84.
51. Spate-Douglas T, Keyser RE. Exercise intensity: its effect on the high-density lipoprotein profile. Arch Phys Med Rehabil. 1999;80:691–5.
52. Kemmler W, Lauber D, Weineck J, Hensen J, Kalender W, Engelke K. Benefits of 2 years of intense exercise on bone density, physical fitness, and blood lipids in early postmenopausal osteopenic women: results of the Erlangen Fitness Osteoporosis Prevention Study (EFOPS). Arch Intern Med. 2004;164:1084–91.
53. Cauley JA, Kriska AM, LaPorte RE, Sandler RB, Pambianco G. A two year randomized exercise trial in older women: effects on HDL-cholesterol. Atherosclerosis. 1987;66:247–58.
54. Stefanick ML, Mackey S, Sheehan M, Ellsworth N, Haskell WL, Wood PD. Effects of diet and exercise in men and postmenopausal women with low levels of HDL cholesterol and high levels of LDL cholesterol. N Engl J Med. 1998;339:12–20.
55. Wing RR, Matthews KA, Kuller LH, Meilahn EN, Plantinga PL. Weight gain at the time of menopause. Arch Intern Med. 1991;151:97–102.
56. Torng PL, Su TC, Sung FC, Chien KL, Huang SC, Chow SN, et al. Effects of menopause on intraindividual changes in serum lipids, blood pressure, and body weight—the Chin-Shan Community Cardiovascular Cohort study. Atherosclerosis. 2002;161:409–15.
57. Prabhakaran B, Dowling EA, Branch JD, Swain DP, Leutholtz BC. Effect of 14 weeks of resistance training on lipid profile and body fat percentage in premenopausal women. Br J Sports Med. 1999;33:190–5.
58. Wildman RP, Schott LL, Brockwell S, Kuller LH, Sutton-Tyrrell K. A dietary and exercise intervention slows menopause-associated progression of subclinical atherosclerosis as measured by intima-media thickness of the carotid arteries. J Am Coll Cardiol. 2004;44:579–85.

59. Cho EJ, Min YJ, Oh MS, Kwon JE, Kim JE, Lee WS, et al. Effects of the transition from premenopause to postmenopause on lipids and lipoproteins: quantification and related parameters. Korean J Intern Med. 2011;26:47–53.
60. Sundquist J, Winkleby MA, Pudaric S. Cardiovascular disease risk factors among older black, Mexican-American, and white women and men: an analysis of NHANES III, 1988–1994. Third National Health and Nutrition Examination Survey. J Am Geriatr Soc. 2001;49:109–16.
61. Fahlman MM, Boardley D, Lambert CP, Flynn MG. Effects of endurance training and resistance training on plasma lipoprotein profiles in elderly women. J Gerontol A Biol Sci Med Sci. 2002;57:B54–60.
62. Henderson GC, Krauss RM, Fattor JA, Faghihnia N, Luke-Zeitoun M, Brooks GA. Plasma triglyceride concentrations are rapidly reduced following individual bouts of endurance exercise in women. Eur J Appl Physiol. 2010;109:721–30.
63. Chobanian AV, Bakris GL, Black HR, Cushman WC, Green LA, Izzo JL, Jr., et al. The Seventh Report of the Joint National Committee on prevention, detection, evaluation, and treatment of high blood pressure: the JNC 7 report. JAMA. 2003;289:2560–72.
64. Zanchetti A, Facchetti R, Cesana GC, Modena MG, Pirrelli A, Sega R, et al. Menopause-related blood pressure increase and its relationship to age and body mass index: the SIMONA epidemiological study. J Hypertens. 2005;23:2269–76.
65. Gierach GL, Johnson BD, Merz CNB, Kelsey SF, Bittner V, Olson MB, et al. Hypertension, menopause, artery disease risk in the and coronary women's ischemia syndrome evaluation (WISE) study. J Am Coll Cardiol. 2006;47:50s–8.
66. Kelley GA, Kelley KS. Aerobic exercise and resting blood pressure in women: a meta-analytic review of controlled clinical trials. J Womens Health Gend Based Med. 1999;8:787–803.
67. Bond V, Millis RM, Adams RG, Oke LM, Enweze L, Blakely R, et al. Attenuation of exaggerated exercise blood pressure response in African-American women by regular aerobic physical activity. Ethn Dis. 2005;15:S5-10–3.
68. Figueroa A, Park SY, Seo DY, Sanchez-Gonzalez MA, Baek YH. Combined resistance and endurance exercise training improves arterial stiffness, blood pressure, and muscle strength in postmenopausal women. Menopause. 2011;18:980–4.
69. Hagberg JM, Brown MD. Does exercise training play a role in the treatment of essential hypertension? J Cardiovasc Risk. 1995;2:296–302.
70. Juntunen M, Niskanen L, Saarelainen J, Tuppurainen M, Saarikoski S, Honkanen R. Changes in body weight and onset of hypertension in perimenopausal women. J Hum Hypertens. 2003;17:775–9.
71. MacNaughton J, Banah M, McCloud P, Hee J, Burger H. Age related changes in follicle stimulating hormone, luteinizing hormone, oestradiol and immunoreactive inhibin in women of reproductive age. Clin Endocrinol (Oxf). 1992;36:339–45.
72. Klein NA, Battaglia DE, Fujimoto VY, Davis GS, Bremner WJ, Soules MR. Reproductive aging: accelerated ovarian follicular development associated with a monotropic follicle-stimulating hormone rise in normal older women. J Clin Endocrinol Metab. 1996;81:1038–45.
73. Warren MP. Health issues for women athletes: exercise-induced amenorrhea. J Clin Endocrinol Metab. 1999;84:1892–6.
74. Cassidy A, Bingham S, Setchell KD. Biological effects of a diet of soy protein rich in isoflavones on the menstrual cycle of premenopausal women. Am J Clin Nutr. 1994;60:333–40.
75. Duncan AM, Merz BE, Xu X, Nagel TC, Phipps WR, Kurzer MS. Soy isoflavones exert modest hormonal effects in premenopausal women. J Clin Endocrinol Metab. 1999;84:192–7.
76. Wylie-Rosett J. Menopause, micronutrients, and hormone therapy. Am J Clin Nutr. 2005;81:1223S–31.
77. Burger HG, Cahir N, Robertson DM, Groome NP, Dudley E, Green A, et al. Serum inhibins A and B fall differentially as FSH rises in perimenopausal women. Clin Endocrinol (Oxf). 1998;48:809–13.
78. Treloar AE, Boynton RE, Behn BG, Brown BW. Variation of the human menstrual cycle through reproductive life. Int J Fertil. 1967;12:77–126.
79. Dennerstein L, Dudley EC, Hopper JL, Guthrie JR, Burger HG. A prospective population-based study of menopausal symptoms. Obstet Gynecol. 2000;96:351–8.
80. Mitchell ES, Woods NF, Mariella A. Three stages of the menopausal transition from the Seattle midlife women's health study: toward a more precise definition. Menopause. 2000;7:334–49.
81. Sowers M, Crawford S, Sternfeld B, Morgenstein D, Gold E, Greendale G, et al. SWAN: a multicenter, multiethnic, community-based cohort study of women and the menopausal transition. In: Lobo R, Kelsey J, Marcus R, editors. Menopause: biology and pathobiology. San Diego, CA: Academic; 2000. p. 175–88.
82. Burger HG. Diagnostic role of follicle-stimulating hormone (FSH) measurements during the menopausal transition—an analysis of FSH, oestradiol and inhibin. Eur J Endocrinol. 1994;130:38–42.
83. Bonen A, Ling WY, MacIntyre KP, Neil R, McGrail JC, Belcastro AN. Effects of exercise on the serum concentrations of FSH, LH, progesterone, and estradiol. Eur J Appl Physiol Occup Physiol. 1979;42:15–23.

84. Orsatti FL, Nahas EA, Maesta N, Nahas-Neto J, Burini RC. Plasma hormones, muscle mass and strength in resistance-trained postmenopausal women. Maturitas. 2008;59:394–404.
85. Trevisan M, Burini R. Resting metabolism of post-menopause women submitted to a training program with weights (hypertrophy). Rev Bras Med Esporte. 2007;13:116–9.
86. Ardoso CG, Jr., Rosas FC, Oneda B, Labes E, Tinucci T, Abrahao SB, et al. Aerobic training abolishes ambulatory blood pressure increase induced by estrogen therapy: a double blind randomized clinical trial. Maturitas. 2011;69:189–94.
87. Cooper GS, Baird DD, Darden FR. Measures of menopausal status in relation to demographic, reproductive, and behavioral characteristics in a population-based study of women aged 35–49 years. Am J Epidemiol. 2001;153:1159–65.
88. Murkies AL, Lombard C, Strauss BJ, Wilcox G, Burger HG, Morton MS. Dietary flour supplementation decreases post-menopausal hot flushes: effect of soy and wheat. Maturitas. 1995;21:189–95.
89. Kuller LH, Meilahn EN, Cauley JA, Gutai JP, Matthews KA. Epidemiologic studies of menopause: changes in risk factors and disease. Exp Gerontol. 1994;29:495–509.
90. Beasley JM, Schenk JM, Ludman E, Lampe JW, Reed SD, Grothaus L, et al. Brief telephone intervention increases soy intake in peri- and postmenopausal US women: the herbal alternatives trial (HALT). J Am Diet Assoc. 2010;110:1189–97.
91. van den Brandt PA. The impact of a Mediterranean diet and healthy lifestyle on premature mortality in men and women. Am J Clin Nutr. 2011;94:913–20.
92. Levine JA, Schleusner SJ, Jensen MD. Energy expenditure of nonexercise activity. Am J Clin Nutr. 2000;72:1451–4.
93. Niinimaa V, Shephard RJ, Dyon M. Determinations of performance and mechanical efficiency in nordic skiing. Br J Sports Med. 1979;13:62–5.
94. Church TS, Earnest CP, Morss GM. Field testing of physiological responses associated with nordic walking. Res Q Exerc Sport. 2002;73:296–300.
95. Morgan B, Woodruff SJ, Tiidus MP. Aerobic energy expenditure during recreational weight training in females and males. J Sport Sci Med. 2003;2:117–22.
96. Hall C, Figueroa A, Fernhall B, Kanaley JA. Energy expenditure of walking and running: comparison with prediction equations. Med Sci Sports Exerc. 2004;36:2128–34.

Chapter 4
The Role of Polyphenols in Menopause

Isabel Baeza and Mónica De la Fuente

Key Points

- Menopause gives rise to an increase in the rate of the ageing process, thus causing premature ageing.
- Oxidative stress occurs with menopause-related loss of oestrogens, this being responsible for premature ageing and much their of its associated physiological deterioration.
- Polyphenols are a group of pigments widely distributed in plants and are responsible for colouring. Besides, they play a protective role due to their antioxidant activity.
- Antioxidants, concretely polyphenols, can decrease the oxidative stress situation during menopause.
- Diets rich in polyphenols, especially flavonoids such as soy food and tea, can decrease the physiological consequences and symptoms of menopause, improving the state of health.
- Diets and supplements containing flavonoids such as isoflavones (phytoestrogens) could be an alternative to the pharmacological treatments frequently prescribed for menopausal and postmenopausal women.
- Since polyphenols improve immune system function, which is a marker of health, biological age and a predictor of longevity, the ingestion of these antioxidants could aid in slowing down the ageing process during menopause.

Keywords Polyphenols • Ageing • Menopause • Oxidative stress • Antioxidants • Immunosenescence

Abbreviations

ER	Estrogen receptor
CAT	Catalase
GPx	Glutathione peroxidase
GSH	Reduced glutathione

I. Baeza, Ph.D.
San Rafael-Nebrija Health Sciences Centre, Nebrija University, Madrid 28036, Spain
e-mail: isabelbaezamonedero@yahoo.es

M. De la Fuente, Ph.D. (✉)
Department of Physiology (Animal Physiology II), Complutense University of Madrid,
José Antonio Novais 2 Street Madrid, 28040, Spain
e-mail: mondelaf@bio.ucm.es

C.J.H. Martin et al. (eds.), *Nutrition and Diet in Menopause*, Nutrition and Health,
DOI 10.1007/978-1-62703-373-2_4, © Springer Science+Business Media New York 2013

GSSG	Oxidized glutathione
HRT	Hormonal replacement therapy
Mn-SOD	Mn-Superoxide dismutase
ROS	Reactive oxygen species
TNFα	Tumor necrosis factor alpha

Introduction

The role of polyphenols in menopause can be understood in the context of the ageing process and its characteristics. Ageing may be defined as a progressive and general impairment of the functions of an organism that leads to a lower ability to adaptively react to changes and preserve homeostasis. This difficulty in preserving the homeostasis is the basis of the increase of age-related morbidity and mortality. Thus, although with ageing all the physiological systems are affected, the regulatory systems, namely, nervous, endocrine and immune systems, are those in which the age-related deleterious effects are most clearly shown [1, 2]. Moreover, these systems are intimately linked, the communication between these regulatory systems being mediated by cytokines, hormones and neurotransmitters through the presence of their receptors on the cells of the three systems. Because of this, it is currently recognised that there is a "neuro-endocrine-immune" system, which allows the preservation of homeostasis and therefore of health [3]. This system also suffers an age-related deterioration [2, 4]. In addition, the above mentioned age-related impairment of physiological functions is linked to a chronic oxidative and inflammatory stress (a progressive imbalance between endogenous antioxidant/anti-inflammatory and oxidant/pro-inflammatory compounds, with higher levels of the latter) affecting all cells and especially those of the regulatory systems [2, 5]. Moreover, we have proposed the theory of oxidation-inflammation in ageing, in which the deterioration of the immune system with ageing, which is termed immunosenescence, can be involved in the "oxi-inflamm-ageing" situation of the organism and thus modify its rate of ageing [2, 6, 7].

Ageing is also a very heterogeneous process and thus there are different rates of age-related physiological changes in each system or tissue of the organism and in the diverse members of a population of the same chronological age. This fact justified the introduction of the concept of "biological age", which determines the rate of ageing experienced by each individual and therefore its life expectancy, having a better predictive value for longevity than chronological age [2]. Thus, the biological age is related to the mean longevity, which can be defined as the mean of the time that the members of a population that have been born on the same date live. Subjects of a population with a higher rate of ageing show an older biological age and a shorter lifespan. Although currently it is impossible to increase the maximum longevity (the maximum time that a subject belonging to a determined species can live), which is fixed in each species, the mean lifespan of individual organisms shows marked variability and can be increased by determined environmental factors. These allow the maintenance of good health and the approach to the maximum lifespan in good condition, this being in humans presently about 75–85 years in developed countries. In order to determine the "biological age" the parameters that change with age and show the tendency to a premature death should be analysed [8]. Since a positive relation has been shown between the good function of immune cells and longevity [9, 10], we have proposed several immune function parameters as adequate markers of "biological age" and therefore as predictors of longevity [2]. Moreover, the redox situation and inflammatory state of the immune cells are related to their functional capacity and to the lifespan of a subject. Subjects with a higher oxidative and inflammatory state in their immune cells show a worse function of these cells and die before their counterparts [2]. In addition, a confirmation of the central role of the immune system in oxi-inflamm-ageing is that several lifestyle strategies such as the administration of adequate amounts of antioxidants in the diet and physical and mental activity, improve the functions of immune cells, decreasing their oxidative and inflammatory stress, and consequently increasing the longevity of individuals [7].

If the ageing process has as its base an oxidative stress situation, an imbalance with higher amounts of oxidants and lower amounts of antioxidants [2, 11], it is logical that the incorporation of antioxidant compounds would recuperate the balance of oxidants/antioxidants needed for an appropriate cell function [1, 2, 7]. In fact, antioxidants are compounds that protect cells against the damaging effects of reactive oxygen species (ROS). These oxidant molecules, although necessary for many cell functions, can cause, if they are present in excess, damage to proteins, lipids and DNA [2, 11]. The antioxidant compounds and antioxidant enzymes are mainly responsible for the neutralisation of this excess of ROS avoiding their noxious effects on cells [1, 2, 7, 12].

In the context of the above, menopause, which is a depletion of a finite ovarian follicle supply [13] and therefore resultins in a complete failure of the ovary to produce hormones such as oestrogens, represents a situation of premature ageing. In fact, the cessation of the ovarian function at the time of menopause and the resulting hormonal changes are associated with many physiopathological reactions that are somehow related to those typically attributed to ageing, making women more prone to experience disease and disability [12]. Furthermore, many of the menopausal symptoms are linked to oestrogen loss and to high levels of oxidative stress [12]. Since oestrogens are antioxidant compounds and they also increase the expression of antioxidant defences of the organism [14], their loss in menopause could be the principal reason for the oxidative stress situation that accelerates the ageing process (Fig. 4.1).

Menopause marks the start of a new phase in the life of women. Although during the last decades of the twentieth century human life expectancy in developed countries has increased, the age at which women encounter their major age related hormonal change, that is, menopause, has remained essentially constant at about 50 years. Therefore, women spend nearly a third of their lives in an oestrogen-deficient state [12]. Due to this, research on menopause and especially on possible treatments to decrease its physiological consequences and symptoms, is very useful. Many of these studies have to be carried out in experimental animals such as mice and rats. Since rodents become anovulatory at a mature age (10–12 months old) but maintain a basal gonadal steroid secretion, in contrast to what happens in women [15], ovariectomy in these animals becomes the best tool to mimic human ovarian hormone loss, this being a "model of menopause".

Oestrogen Replacement Therapies and Plant-Derived Oestrogens

Since oestrogens have a regulatory role in many organs, the rapid decline in their circulating levels associated with menopause has many implications in a wide range of non-reproductive functions. They play a major role in the onset of menopausal hot flushes, bone loss, vaginal epithelium atrophy, acceleration of arteriosclerosis, skin ageing, immune dysfunctions, altered subcutaneous fat distribution, etc. [12]. Moreover, the psycho-emotional symptoms associated with menopause overlap depressive symptoms and include disturbed sleep, concentration, anxiety, irritability, frustration, mood lability, depression and fatigue.

Until recently, it had been generally accepted that the most effective treatment of menopausal symptoms was hormonal replacement therapy (HRT) with female sex hormones. Therefore, the fight against menopausal effects has been traditionally approached with HRT using exogenous oestrogens, whose administration causes rapid alleviation of menopausal symptoms and reduces the risk of heart disease and osteoporosis. Nevertheless, most women are still reluctant to use HRT mainly due to the possible increased risk of breast and endometrial cancer, vaginal haemorrhage, cardiovascular diseases, etc. [12]. Therefore, in view of these concerns about the safety of HTR, there has been a recent growing demand for alternative treatments that are able to protect against climacteric symptoms and minimise

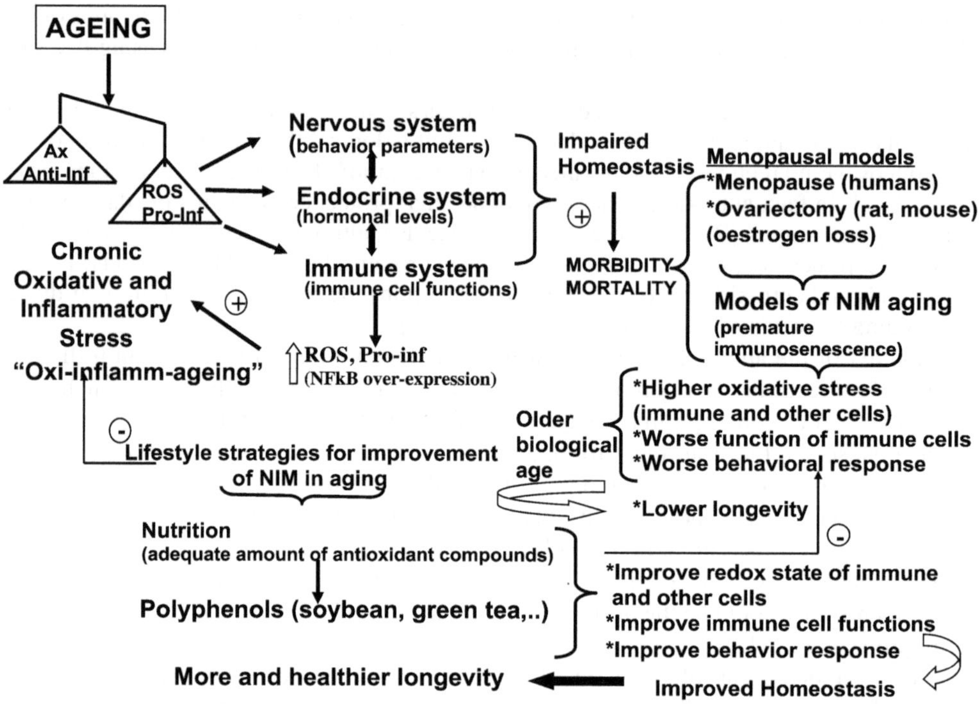

Fig. 4.1 Role of polyphenols in the ageing process. Ageing is a chronic oxidative stress condition affecting all cells, especially those of the regulatory systems, i.e. the nervous, endocrine and immune system and the communication among them. This explains the impaired homeostasis and the increased morbidity and mortality found in old age. In addition, we have proposed an "oxi-inflamm-ageing" situation in which the immune system is involved. Thus, this system, in its communication with the other homeostatic systems, can modulate the ageing process of the organism, concretely the rate of ageing. Menopause in humans and ovariectomy in rodents, as a consequence of oestrogen loss are useful models for the study of ageing of neuroimmunomodulation (NIM) since these subjects show high oxidative stress in the immune and other cells, impaired immune cell functions and behavioural responses. Thus, they show an older biological age and therefore more physiological deteriorations. An adequate nutrition, with ingestion of appropriate amounts of antioxidant compounds, such as plant-derived polyphenols, could be a good strategy of lifestyle to improve the immune functions, the redox state and the behavioural responses. Thus, these kind of diets could retard the ageing process, improving homeostasis and possibly increasing the longevity of the individuals. *Ax* antioxidant compounds, *Anti-inf* anti-inflammatory compounds, *ROS* reactive oxygen species, *Pro-Inf* pro-inflammatory compounds

at the same time the undesirable side-effects mentioned above. In this context, plant-derived oestrogens such as phytoestrogens, which are also antioxidants, seems to be a feasible alternative to the pharmacological treatments usually prescribed for menopausal and postmenopausal women [14].

Polyphenolic Antioxidants: Soybean and Green Tea Flavonoids

Polyphenols are a group of substances widely distributed in the plant kingdom. They are pigments and thus responsible for the colouring of plants, in which they play a protective role. They have many physiological actions, the best known being their antioxidant activity. Although their role in human health has been widely suggested this subject is very complex and needs much more research [16]. The functional activities of polyphenols are determined by their chemical structure. In this respect, they are characterised

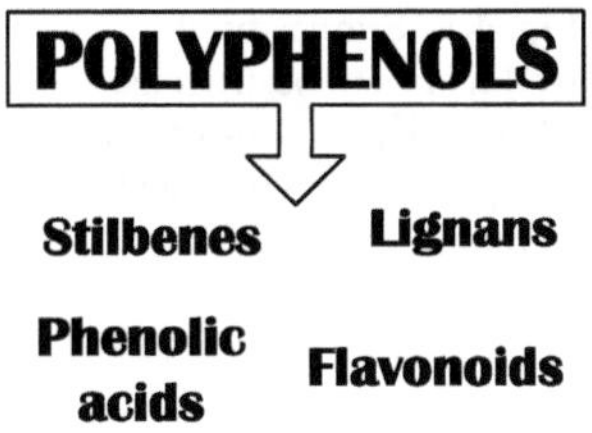

Fig. 4.2 Classification of the four main types of polyphenols

Table 4.1 The most important polyphenol compounds present in different foods

Group of polyphenols	Polyphenol	Food
Stilbenoids	Resveratrol	Grape skins and seeds, wine, nuts, peanuts
	Pterostilbene	Grapes; blueberries
Lignans		Seeds (sesame, sunflower, …); fruits (berries) whole grains (rye, oats, …); bran (wheat, oats, …)
Phenolic acids	Gallic acid	Tea; mango; strawberry; rhubarb
	Vanillin	Vanilla beans; cloves
	Curcumin	Mustard; curry
Flavonoids		
Anthocyanins	Pelargonidin	Raspberry; strawberry
	Cyanidin	Red apple; pear; cherry; plum; cocoa
Flavonols	Quercetin	Onions; tea; wine; apples; beans; cranberries
	Rutin	Citrus fruits; apricot; tomato; parsley; tea
Flavanols	Catechins	Tea; grapes; apple; cocoa; lentils
Flavanones	Naringenin	Citrus fruits
Isoflavones	Daidzein	Soy; peanuts; legumes
	Genistein	Soy; peanuts; legumes

by the presence of one or more phenol groups per molecule. Currently more than 8,000 polyphenols are known, but few plants containing an abundance of these compounds are common sources of food in the human diet [17]. These include the skin of red grapes, several fruits, vegetables, cereal grains, nuts and beverages such as tea, fruit juice, wine, coffee and chocolate [18]. Polyphenols have been classified into 16 groups according to their chemical structure, the most important being: stilbenes, lignans, phenolic acids and flavonoids (Fig. 4.2). The main stilbene is resveratrol, found primarily in grape skin, blackberry and peanuts. "Lignans" is a general term for a large family of compounds, whose main dietary source is linseed, but they are present also in whole-wheat flour, vegetables, fruits, coffee and tea. In the group of phenolic acids there are many polyphenols, which are derived from benzoic acid or cinnamic acid, the main sources of these compounds being cereals, vegetables, aromatic herbs, prunes and coffee. The group of flavonoids, which can be classified in several subgroups of compounds such as anthocyanins, flavonols, flavanols, flavanones and isoflavones, amongst others, are essential components of diet (Table 4.1). They have many biological properties, which contribute to gene and metabolism regulation as well as the scavenging of free radicals and thus they modulate cell cycle, proliferation and the redox state of cells. These compounds show antioxidant, anti-inflammatory, antithrombotic, antiviral, anticancerogenic and antiallergic properties as well as modulating immune system response [18]. Nowadays, many researchers focus on flavonoids, which appear to have played a major role in the successful medical treatments of ancient times, and their use has persevered up to now.

Isoflavones, one of the groups of flavonoids, are considered widespread in the plant kingdom, and they have been classically defined as phytoestrogens, for being compounds that exert oestrogenic effects. These isoflavones share structural features with oestrogens, and therefore they are able to evoke biological responses (Fig. 4.3). The presence of the phenolic ring enables isoflavones to bind

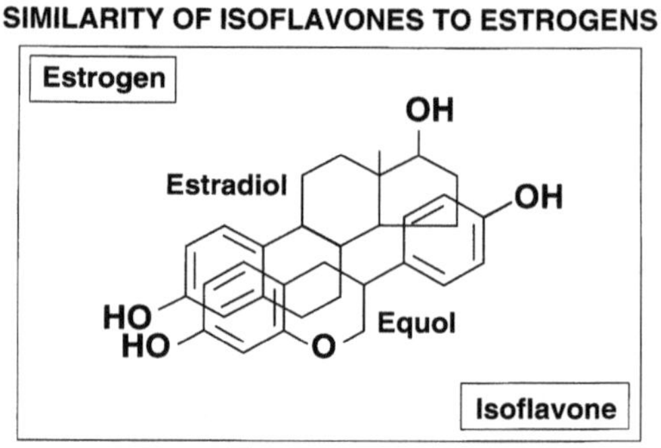

Fig. 4.3 Similarity of isoflavones to oestrogens. Chemical structures of equol (a type of isoflavone) and estradiol (an oestrogen)

both types of oestrogen receptors: ERα and ERβ. Unlike endogenous oestrogen, however, isoflavones bind with a much higher affinity to ERβ, which suggests that they may be more accurately defined as selective oestrogen receptor modulators capable of both pro-oestrogenic and anti-oestrogenic effects. However, they are much weaker than human oestrogens, with 10^2 to 10^5 times less activity [19].

Soy bean flavonoids: Isoflavones are mainly found in "*Leguminosae*" and are especially abundant in soybean (*Glycine max.*). Soybeans and their proteins have long been staples in the diets of the people of China and Japan, but their incorporation into the Western diet is minimal [20]. The number of foods sold in the West that have ingredients derived from soybeans has been increasing. Many of these have soybean oil, soy protein, or other ingredients serving functional roles in the food. Therefore, with increasing interest among consumers in dietary choices that help to improve health and reduce risk of disease, products in which soy is featured are quite readily available [20]. They have been found to have a wide range of hormonal and non-hormonal activities that provide plausible mechanisms for the potential health benefits of diets rich in these compounds. Among the soy food isoflavones, the best known and widely available are genistein, daidzein and glycitein [19].

Tea flavonoids: The most significant components of the tea plant are also polyphenols. The history of tea began over 5,000 years ago in ancient China. Currently, tea is the most popular beverage consumed by two-third of the world's population, well ahead of coffee, beer, wine and carbonated soft drinks [21]. Green, black and oolong tea are all derived from the *Camellia sinensis* plant, and the differences between these three varieties of tea lie in the differences in the manufacturing process. While green tea does not undergo fermentation, black tea is completely fermented, and oolong tea contains a mixture of both fermented and non-fermented leaves [21]. Green tea is favoured in Japan and China, and it has been considered a medicine and a healthy beverage since ancient times. Initial research on the benefits of green tea was carried out in these countries because of local customs, and traditional Chinese medicine has recommended this plant for headaches, body aches and pains, digestion, depression, detoxification, as an energizer and, in general, to prolong life. Although tea has been consumed for centuries, it has only recently been studied extensively as a health-promoting beverage that may act to prevent a number of chronic diseases and cancers [21–23].

Green tea leaves contain three main components, which act upon human health: xanthic bases (caffeine and theophylline), essential oils and, especially, polyphenolic compounds. The main green tea polyphenols are catechins, which constitute approximately 30 % of the dry leaf weight of the *Camellia sinensis* plant. Catechins contain a benzopyran skeleton with a phenyl group substituted at the 2-position and a hydroxyl (or ester) function at the 3-position. They consist of (−)-epicatechin, (−)-epicatechin-3-gallate, (−)-epigallocatechin and (−)-epigallocatechin-3-gallate [22, 23]. Its polyphenol content has made green tea attract a great deal of attention, as these compounds are strong antioxidants and present important biological properties, including chemopreventive efficacy, the induction of apoptotic cell death and cell cycle arrest in tumour cells, the reduction of plasma cholesterol levels, and, subsequently, the prevention of cardiovascular diseases and cancer [21, 22, 24].

Role of Polyphenolic Antioxidants in Menopause Effects

Organic polyphenols found in plants are the most abundant antioxidants in our diet. Many effects of flavonoids, which will be mentioned, are due to their antioxidant properties. They show the ability to scavenge ROS and they can neutralise free radicals since they are one-electron donors. Thus, they are capable of protecting unsaturated fatty acids in membranes against oxidation by ROS [19, 25]. Moreover, soybean isoflavones share with oestradiol the ability to up-regulate the expression of antioxidant defence genes such as glutathione peroxidase (GPx) and Mn-superoxide dismutase (Mn-SOD) [26]. In addition, tea catechins also display in the organism a crucial role as radical and oxidant scavengers, protecting the human body from oxidative stress [21, 22, 24]. Catechins are hypothesised to contribute, along with antioxidant vitamins (e.g. vitamins C and E) and enzymes (e.g. superoxide dismutase (SOD) and catalase), to the local antioxidant defence system [27].

Cardiovascular Diseases

The incidence of cardiovascular diseases rapidly increases in women after menopause thus resulting in an increased risk of heart disease [28]. Therefore, it could be suggested that endogenous oestrogens in premenopausal women provide protection against cardiovascular disease. Soybean isoflavones have been described as preventing atherosclerosis and reducing risk markers of cardiovascular disease [19, 25, 29]. Certain types of green tea cathechins may have the same preventive role when administered to postmenopausal women, as some studies suggest that their consumption is inversely related to the risk of coronary heart disease [21, 22, 27].

Regarding the most commonly described vasomotor symptoms during the menopausal transition, which are mainly hot flushes and night sweats, some authors have described soy phytoestrogens as good candidates for decreasing these symptoms [30], while others have found no effects [31].

Bone Health and Osteoporosis

Osteoporosis is a worldwide problem that affects mostly women, and it is clear that hormonal changes after menopause increase the rate of bone resorption, leading to greater risk of suffering this disease [28]. In this respect, it has already been described that soybean isoflavones improve bone mineral density in postmenopausal women, thus preventing such oestrogen-related bone loss [29]. Green tea consumption has also been associated with increased bone mineral density, one positive effect being the proliferation and improved activity of bone cells [27]. In fact, tea consumption has been described as protecting against the risk of hip fractures in people over 50 and as increasing bone mineral density in menopausal women. The same results have been obtained in ovariectomized rats, where bone mineral density increased after green tea polyphenol supplementation [22, 32].

Cancer Incidence

Disregulated proliferation appears to be a hallmark of increased susceptibility to neoplasia. Cancer prevention is generally associated with inhibition, reversion or retardation of cellular hyper-proliferation. Since advanced metastasised cancers are mostly incurable, an effort to control the process of carcinogenesis through chemoprevention has become an important, feasible strategy for cancer treatment. It is generally agreed that dietary flavonoids behave as general cell growth inhibitors. They have been demonstrated to inhibit proliferation in many kinds of cultured human cancer cell lines, and this mainly occurs through anti-aromatase, anti-proliferative and anti-angiogenic mechanisms [19, 29].

Numerous studies have also demonstrated that green tea and tea polyphenols possess a chemopreventive potential. Many of these effects are mediated by catechins, and this has been demonstrated in many different animal models of lung, skin, breast, oesophagus, prostate, rectal and liver cancers [21]. The results from all the above experiments indicate that tea offers a broad inhibitory role in the initiation, promotion and progression of carcinogenesis. However, the molecular mechanisms for these inhibitory actions are not fully understood. Possibly, these are most likely related to the antioxidant effects of the tea polyphenols, which protect DNA from damage and/or methylation, inhibit proteasome activity in tumour cells, induct apoptosis and inhibit tumour promotion-related events as well as angiogenesis.

Body Weight Control

Obesity has increased at an alarming rate in recent years and is now a worldwide health problem. Adipose tissue distribution is regulated by female sex hormones, so metabolic changes due to menopause lead to increased obesity in postmenopausal women [28]. In this respect, the effects of long-term feeding with tea catechins have been widely studied, suggesting a potential role of green tea in body weight control. Thus, green tea extracts may display thermogenic properties and promote fat oxidation, reducing or preventing body weight gain, together with visceral and liver fat accumulation [22, 27]. Furthermore, epidemiological observations and laboratory studies have shown that green tea has an effect on glucose tolerance and insulin sensitivity, increasing the activity of this hormone through an enhanced glucose uptake of adipocytes [27].

Cognition and Psycho-Emotional Symptoms

Oestrogens have been associated with cognitive and emotional processing since their receptors are present on neurons (on both dendrites and presynaptic terminals) and glial cells. These hormones have been reported to have beneficial effects on the nervous system, and it has been described that they can promote cognitive function when administered after the menopausal transition [33]. In addition, research using isoflavone supplementation in postmenopausal women, yields controversial results, with some studies suggesting that soybean isoflavones displayed a favourable effect on cognitive function, particularly verbal memory [34], whilst others describe no improvements or appreciable effects [35]. There are also reports that indicate that tea can improve neurologic and psychologic functions. Tea catechins possess divalent metal chelating, antioxidant and anti-inflammatory activities, penetrating the brain barrier and protecting against neuronal death in a wide array of cellular and animal models of neurological diseases [22]. Other components of tea, such as theanine, act as neurotransmitters in the brain and decrease blood pressure in animal models of hypertension. Moreover, this compound modulates brain serotonin and dopamine levels, thus improving memory, learning ability and affecting emotions [22]. Among age-associated pathologies and neurodegenerative diseases, green tea has been shown to afford significant protection against Parkinson's disease, Alzheimer's disease and ischemic damage [36].

Immune Function

The available data show that female sex hormones stimulate immune function, this being responsible of the usually better immune response of females than males in the mammalian species [2, 37–39]. As mentioned above, a great deal of research has shown that the ageing process is associated with a general impairment of immune function, commonly known as "immunosenescence", which has as its basis an oxidative stress situation [2, 6, 7]. Thus, we can understand how the oestrogen loss associated with menopause or ovariectomy accelerates immunosenescence in women and experimental animals, respectively. The consequences include impaired cellular and humoral immune responses and an altered oxidant/antioxidant balance, resulting in a pro-oxidative state [37–41]. Monocyte and macrophage functions such as the chemotaxis, phagocytosis and microbicidal capacities result dramatically altered as a consequence of ovariectomy (in experimental animals) or either premature ovarian failure (in women) [40, 42]. Lymphocytes are important effector cells whose activation is essential for the immune response, and among their key functions we can cite the chemotaxis and proliferative capacities and the NK activity, all three being severely impaired after menopause/ovariectomy [37–40, 43, 44]. In addition, it has been postulated that the oestrogen loss associated with the menopausal transition is directly linked to the higher levels of pro-inflammatory cytokines found in postmenopausal women [44]. Moreover, a marked overproduction of pro-inflammatory cytokines leads to immunosuppression [2]. In postmenopausal women and ovariectomised animals an increase in the oxidative imbalance has also been observed. In fact, these subjects show increased levels of oxidant such as oxidised glutathione (GSSG) and decreased levels of antioxidant such as reduced glutathione (GSH), which is the most abundant endogenous antioxidant, and constituting one of the first lines of defence against oxidation. As a consequence of this oxidative stress situation an increase in the oxidation damage to lipids, proteins and nucleic acids occurs [39, 41, 43]. Based on all the above, we suggested that menopause/ovariectomy is a situation of premature immunosenescence, and since ovariectomised animals also show senescence behavioural responses [40], they are prematurely ageing [39, 40] (Table 4.2).

In this respect, the administration of antioxidants, and concretely soybean isoflavones, to postmenopausal women and ovariectomised animals improves macrophage and lymphocyte functions such as those mentioned above (chemotaxis, phagocytosis, T-cell proliferation, NK activity, etc.) [38, 41, 43, 45, 46]. Moreover, in ovariectomised animals it has been recently described that the oral administration of a combined treatment of soybean isoflavones with green tea results in a stimulating effect of macrophage and lymphocyte activities [47] (Table 4.2). As previously mentioned, the structure of isoflavones resembles the steroid hormone 17β-oestradiol, being able to bind to the oestrogen receptors and acting though the same intracellular signalling pathways [19]. This could be the mechanism through which isoflavones exert their stimulatory effects on the immune cells, in a similar manner to oestrogens, due to the presence of their receptors in certain immune cells including T cells, monocytes and macrophages, natural killer cells and dendritic cells [48].

Green tea polyphenols (mainly catechins) have also been reported to play an immunomodulatory role in the organism. They inhibit endothelial exocytosis by limiting leucocyte adherence to the endothelial cells of the vessel walls increasing the synthesis of NO [49]. Regarding this, catechins present in green tea have been described as decreasing inflammation in a variety of animal models, including endotoxemia, asthma, autoimmune encephalitis and cystitis. They even limit infiltration of leucocytes into the skin of humans exposed to UV light. Regarding the molecular mechanisms that are responsible for such effects, it seems that they inhibit the activation of transcription factors (as NF-kB and AP-1) through the partial inhibition of the mitogen-activated MAP-Kinase (MAPK) cascade. This leads to a decrease in the expression of inflammatory gene products including lipoxygenase, cyclooxygenase, nitric oxide synthase and TNF-alpha. Catechins also induce apoptosis of several immune cells, which is another possible mechanism of its anti-inflammatory effects [49].

Table 4.2 Changes in function and oxidative-inflammatory stress parameters in immune cells from old and ovariectomised female experimental animals (mice and rats) versus adults and sham animals, as well as effects of a diet supplemented with antioxidants in old and ovariectomised animals

	Old animals	Ovariectomized animals	Antioxidant supplementation
Immune functions			
Mobility (chemotaxis) of macrophages	Decrease	Decrease	Increase
Phagocytosis capacity of macrophages	Decrease	Decrease	Increase
Digestion capacity (intracellular ROS)	Decrease	Decrease	Increase
Mobility (chemotaxis) of lymphocytes	Decrease	Decrease	Increase
Lymphoproliferative response to mitogens	Decrease	Decrease	Increase
Natural Killer (NK) activity	Decrease	Decrease	Increase
IL-2 release	Decrease	Decrease	Increase
Oxidant and pro-inflammatory compounds			
Extra-cellular superoxide anion	Increase	Increase	Decrease
Oxidised glutathione (GSSG)	Increase	Increase	Decrease
Oxidised/reduced glutathione (GSSG/GSH)	Increase	Increase	Decrease
Pro-inflammatory cytokines (TNFα; IL-6)	Increase	Increase	Decrease
Antioxidant and anti-inflammatory defences			
Reduced glutathione (GSH) levels	Decrease	Decrease	Increase
Superoxide dismutase (SOD) activity	Decrease	Decrease	Increase
Catalase (CAT) activity	Decrease	Decrease	Increase
Glutathione peroxidase (GPx)	Decrease	Decrease	Increase
Glutathione reductase (Gr)	Decrease	Decrease	Increase
Anti-inflammatory cytokines (IL-10)	Decrease	Decrease	Increase
Oxidative damage			
Malondialdehyde (MDA) (lipid peroxidation)	Increase	Increase	Decrease

In addition, it is of great relevance to notice that nutritional treatments with plant-derived polyphenols restore the oxidative balance with a decrease in the GSSG levels [41] and improve the redox status by trapping ROS and protecting against oxidative damage to lipid membranes, proteins and nucleic acids [22].

We have recently proposed an involvement of the immune system in the ageing process of the organism, concretely in the rate of ageing [2, 6, 7]. Thus, a worse immune function such as that accelerates occurs in a menopause/ovariectomy situation accelerates the ageing process. Nevertheless, the treatment with antioxidant polyphenols can be a good strategy to restore and even improve the rate of ageing.

Longevity

Longevity studies have been carried out on the Japanese population, which consumes green tea and soybean on a daily basis, and the results have shown a significant decrease in cancer as well as age-related conditions causing death. This has been found to be associated with the increased consumption of these products, especially in people over 79 years of age [22]. These results indicate that daily consumption of green tea in sufficient amounts would help to prolong life by avoiding premature death, particularly that caused by cancer [22].

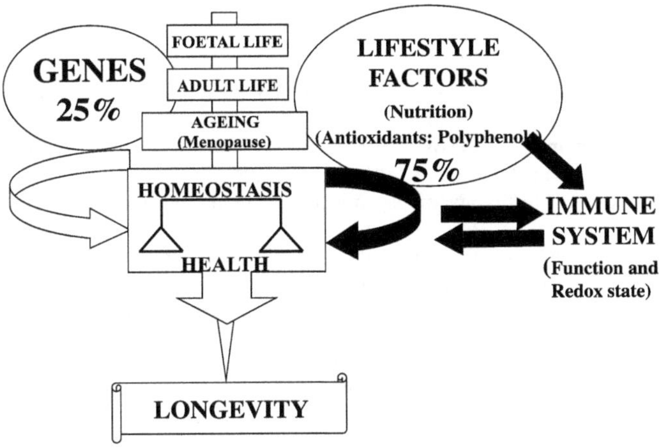

Fig. 4.4 How diet with appropriate amount of antioxidants, such as polyphenols, improves the ageing process and enabling a long and healthy mean longevity to be reached? The base of a functional longevity is the health maintenance, and this depends on preservation of homeostasis (the balance at all physiological levels). This health preservation depends approximately in a proportion of 25 % of the genes, but in a 75 % of the style of life and environmental factors. One of these factors of lifestyle is the nutrition and concretely the antioxidant compounds that we can take through diet. With ageing it is more difficult to maintain the homeostasis as consequence of deterioration of the regulatory systems. This loss of homeostasis is established at different rate in each subject, and this rate is the result of individual epigenetic mechanisms acting on genes from foetal life throughout the life of the subject. With the loss of oestrogens (menopause) females can accelerate the ageing process. Since the functions and redox states of the immune system are good markers of health and predictors of longevity, we have proposed their study in order to determine each particular rate of ageing and its response to changes in the style of life and environmental factors. Moreover, a younger immune system can be obtained with the ingestion of appropriate amounts of antioxidants and since the immune system is involved in the rate of ageing, this strategy of lifestyle can help achieve healthy longevity

Conclusions

Since it has been demonstrated that the immune system is an excellent marker of health, rate of ageing and predictor of longevity [2, 50], the impairment of this system in subjects with menopause/ovariectomy-related oestrogen loss shows with their accelerated ageing. In addition, the base of a functional longevity is health maintenance and this depends on the genes (approximately in a proportion of 25 %) and on the style of life and environmental factors (in a 75 %). The administration to aged subjects of adequate amounts of antioxidants in the diet improves several functions of immune cells, decreasing their oxidative stress, and consequently increasing the longevity of individuals [2, 6, 7] (Fig. 4.4). Thus, the replacement therapies in postmenopausal women with plant-derived polyphenols such as the ones present in soybean or green tea, constitute a promising tool to be applied. Despite all the results on these antioxidants described in the present chapter, more interventional trials are still required to reach definitive conclusions with respect their efficacy and safety in menopause transition. The next challenges to be faced will be to investigate on several physiological systems, especially the homeostatic systems, the effects of a wider number of possible diet-polyphenols, a wider range of doses as well as of the best design of administration, in order to optimise the beneficial effects of these compounds on health and longevity.

Acknowledgements This work was supported by grants of the MCINN (BFU2008-04336; BFU2011-30336), Research Group of UCM (910379ENEROINN) and RETICEF (RD06/0013/0003) (RD12/0043/0018) (ISCIII).

References

1. De la Fuente M, Hernanz A, Vallejo MC. The immune system in the oxidative stress conditions of aging and hypertension: favorable effects of antioxidants and physical exercise. Antioxid Redox Signal. 2005;7(9–10):1356–66.
2. De la Fuente M, Miquel J. An update of the oxidation-inflammation theory of aging: the involvement of the immune system in oxi-inflamm-aging. Curr Pharm Des. 2009;15:3003–26.
3. Besedovsky HO, Del Rey A. Physiology of psychoneuroimmunology: a personal view. Brain Behav Immun. 2007;21:34–44.
4. De la Fuente M. Role of neuroimmunomodulation in aging. Neuroimmunomodulation. 2008;15:213–23.
5. Harman D. Aging: a theory based on free radical and radiation chemistry. J Gerontol. 1956;2:298–300.
6. Alonso-Fernandez P, De la Fuente M. Role of the immune sytem in aging and longevity. Curr Aging Sci. 2011;4(1):78–100.
7. De la Fuente M, Cruces J, Hernandez O, et al. Strategies to improve the functions and redox state of the immune system in aged subjects. Curr Pharm Des. 2011;17:3966–93.
8. Bulpitt CJ, Antikainen RL, Markowe HL, et al. Mortality according to a prior assessment of biological age. Curr Aging Sci. 2009;2:193–9.
9. Guayerbas N, Puerto M, Victor VM, et al. Leukocyte function and life span in a murine model of premature immunosenescence. Exp Gerontol. 2002;37:249–56.
10. Guayerbas N, De La Fuente M. An impairment of phagocytic function is linked to a shorter life span in two strains of prematurely aging mice. Dev Comp Immunol. 2003;27:339–50.
11. Dowling DK, Simmons LW. Reactive oxygen species as universal constraints in life-history evolution. Proc Biol Sci. 2009;276:1737–45.
12. Miquel J, Ramirez-Bosca A, Ramirez-Bosca JV, et al. Menopause: a review on the role of oxygen stress and favorable effects of dietary antioxidants. Arch Gerontol Geriatr. 2006;42(3):289–306.
13. Richardson SJ, Nelson JF. Follicular depletion during the menopausal transition. Ann N Y Acad Sci. 1990;592:13–20.
14. Viña J, Gambini J, Lopez-Grueso R, et al. Females live longer than males: role of oxidative stress. Curr Pharm Des. 2011;17(36):3959–65.
15. Nelson HD. Menopause. Lancet. 2008;371:760–70.
16. Visioloi F, De la Lastra CA, Andres-Lacueva C, et al. Polyphenols and human health: a prospectus. Crit Rev Food Sci Nutr. 2011;51(6):524–46.
17. Queen BL, Tollefsbol TO. Polyphenols and aging. Curr Aging Sci. 2010;3:34–42.
18. Manach C, Scalbert A, Morand C, et al. Polyphenols: food sources and bioavailability. Am J Clin Nutr. 2004;79:727–47.
19. Dijsselbloem N, Vanden Berghe W, De Naeyer A, et al. Soy isoflavone phyto-pharmaceuticals in interleukin-6 affections. Multi-purpose nutraceuticals at the crossroad of hormone replacement, anti-cancer and anti-inflammatory therapy. Biochem Pharmacol. 2004;68(6):1171–85.
20. Lee M. Phytoestrogens as bioactive agents in functional foods: Canadian regulatory update. J AOAC Int. 2006;89(4):1135–7.
21. Chen D, Milacic V, Chen MS, et al. Tea polyphenols, their biological effects and potential molecular targets. Histol Histopathol. 2008;23(4):487–96.
22. Khan N, Mukhtar H. Tea polyphenols for health promotion. Life Sci. 2007;81(7):519–33.
23. Ellinger S, Muller N, Stehle P, et al. Consumption of gree tea or green tea products: is there an evidence for antioxidant effects from controlled interventional studies? Phytomedicine. 2011;18(11):903–15.
24. Singh BN, Shankar S, Srivastava RK. Green tea catechin, epigallocatechin-3-gallate (EGCG): mechanisms, perspectives and clinical applications. Biochem Pharmacol. 2011;82(12):1807–21.
25. Havsteen BH. The biochemistry and medical significance of the flavonoids. Pharmacol Ther. 2002; 96(2–3):67–202.
26. Borras C, Gambini J, Gomez-Cabrera MC, et al. Genistein, a soy isoflavone, up-regulates expression of antioxidant genes: involvement of estrogen receptors, ERK1/2, and NFkappaB. FASEB J. 2006;20(12):2136–8.
27. Cabrera C, Artacho R, Gimenez R. Beneficial effects of green tea—a review. J Am Coll Nutr. 2006;25(2):79–99.
28. Jung BH, Jeon MJ, Bai SW. Hormone-dependent aging problems in women. Yonsei Med J. 2008;49(3):345–51.
29. Sirtori CR, Arnoldi A, Johnson SK. Phytoestrogens: end of a tale? Ann Med. 2005;37(6):423–38.
30. Maclennan AH, Broadbent JL, Lester S, Moore V. Oral oestrogen and combined oestrogen/progestogen therapy versus placebo for hot flushes. Cochrane Database Syst Rev. 2004; (4):CD002978.
31. Lethaby AE, Brown J, Marjoribanks J, Kronenberg F, Roberts H, Eden J. Phytoestrogens for vasomotor menopausal symptoms. Cochrane Database Syst Rev. 2007; (4):CD001395.
32. Shen CL, Wang P, Guerrieri J, Yeh JK, Wang JS. Protective effect of green tea polyphenols on bone loss in middle-aged female rats. Osteoporos Int. 2008;19(7):979–90.

33. Rettberg JR, Hamilton RT, Mao Z, To J, Zhao L, Appt SE, et al. The effect of dietary soy isoflavones before and after ovariectomy on hippocampal protein markers of mitochondrial bioenergetics and antioxidant activity in female monkeys. Brain Res. 2011;1379:23–33.
34. Kritz-Silverstein D, Von Muhlen D, Barrett-Connor E, Bressel MA. Isoflavones and cognitive function in older women: the SOy and Postmenopausal Health In Aging (SOPHIA) study. Menopause. 2003;10(3):196–202.
35. Fournier LR, Ryan Borchers TA, Robison LM, et al. The effects of soy milk and isoflavone supplements on cognitive performance in healthy, postmenopausal women. J Nutr Health Aging. 2007;11(2):155–64.
36. Mandel S, Youdim MB. Catechin polyphenols: neurodegeneration and neuroprotection in neurodegenerative diseases. Free Radic Biol Med. 2004;37(3):304–17.
37. Gameiro CM, Romao F, Castelo-Branco C. Menopause and aging: changes in the immune system—a review. Maturitas. 2010;67(4):316–20.
38. Baeza I, Alvarado C, Alvarez P, et al. Improvement of leukocyte functions in ovariectomised aged rats after treatment with growth hormone, melatonin, oestrogens or phyto-oestrogens. J Reprod Immunol. 2009;80:70–9.
39. Baeza I, De Castro NM, Arranz L, et al. Ovariectomy causes immunosenescence and oxi-inflamm-ageing in peritoneal leukocytes of aged female mice similar to that in aged males. Biogerontology. 2011;12(3):227–38.
40. Baeza I, De Castro NM, Gimenez-Llort L, et al. Ovariectomy, a model of menopause in rodents, causes a premature aging of the nervous and immune systems. J Neuroimmunol. 2010;219:90–9.
41. Baeza I, Fdez-Tresguerres J, Ariznavarreta C, et al. Effects of growth hormone, melatonin, oestrogens and phytoestrogens on the oxidized glutathione (GSSG)/reduced glutathione (GSH) ratio and lipid peroxidation in aged ovariectomized rats. Biogerontology. 2010;11(6):687–701.
42. Hoek A, van Kasteren Y, de Haan-Meulman M, et al. Dysfunction of monocytes and dendritic cells in patients with premature ovarian failure. Am J Reprod Immunol. 1993;30(4):207–17.
43. Arranz L, Fernandez C, Rodriguez A, et al. The glutathione precursor N-acetylcysteine improves immune function in postmenopausal women. Free Rad Biol Med. 2008;45:1252–62.
44. Gameiro C, Romao F. Changes in the immune system during menopause and aging. Front Biosci (Elite Ed). 2010;2:1299–303.
45. Ryan-Borchers TA, Park JS, Chew BP, et al. Soy isoflavones modulate immune function in healthy postmenopausal women. Am J Clin Nutr. 2006;83(5):1118–25.
46. Baeza I, de Castro NM, Alvarado C, et al. Improvement of immune cell functions in aged mice treated for five weeks with soybean isoflavones. Ann N Y Acad Sci. 2007;1100:497–504.
47. Baeza I, De Castro NM, Arranz L, et al. Soybean and green tea polyphenols improve immune function and redox status in very old ovariectomized mice. Rejuvenation Res. 2010;13(6):665–74.
48. Bird MD, Karavitis J, Kovacs EJ. Sex differences and estrogen modulation of the cellular immune response after injury. Cell Immunol. 2008;252(1–2):57–67.
49. Yamakuchi M, Bao C, Ferlito M, et al. Epigallocatechin gallate inhibits endothelial exocytosis. Biol Chem. 2008;389(7):935–41.
50. Wayne SJ, Rhyne RL, Garry PJ, Goodwin JS. Cell-mediated immunity as a predictor of morbidity and mortality in subjects over 60. J Gerontol. 1990;45(2):M45–8.

Part II
Bone and Muscle

Chapter 5
Intestinal Calcium Absorption Efficiency in Women and the Influence of Menopause

John Aloia and Albert Shieh

Key Points

- Intestinal calcium absorption efficiency is the percentage of a given amount of consumed calcium that is absorbed.
- Estrogen deficiency secondary to menopause is associated with decreased intestinal calcium absorption efficiency.
- One possible mechanism by which menopause causes decreased calcium absorption is that estrogen deficiency leads to a down-regulation of key calcium transport molecules within intestinal cells.
- A second possible mechanism by which menopause causes decreased calcium absorption is that estrogen deficiency leads to decreased synthesis of calcitriol.
- A third possible mechanism by which menopause causes decreased calcium absorption is that estrogen deficiency leads to intestinal resistance to calcitriol.
- Efforts to elucidate the effect of menopause on serum calcitriol, calcium, and parathyroid hormone have been inconclusive.
- Decreased calcium absorption following menopause is associated with a negative change in calcium balance, decreased bone mineral density, and increased fracture risk.
- Optimization of calcium intake following menopause is important for maintaining skeletal health.

Keywords Calcium absorption • Estrogen • Calcitriol • Estrogen deficiency • Efficiency

Abbreviations

TRPV6	Transient receptor potential vanilloid type 6
VDR	Vitamin D receptor
ERa	Estrogen receptor alpha
KO	Knockout
FSH	Follicular stimulating hormone
mRNA	Messenger ribonucleic acid
PTH	Parathyroid hormone
EAR	Estimated average requirement
RDA	Recommended daily allowance

J. Aloia, M.D. (✉) • A. Shieh, M.D.
Winthrop University Hospital, 222 Station Plaza North, Suite 510, Mineola, NY 11501, USA
e-mail: jaloia@winthrop.org; shiehalbert@gmail.com

C.J.H. Martin et al. (eds.), *Nutrition and Diet in Menopause*, Nutrition and Health,
DOI 10.1007/978-1-62703-373-2_5, © Springer Science+Business Media New York 2013

Introduction

Intestinal calcium absorption efficiency is the percentage of a given amount of consumed calcium that is absorbed. Estrogen has been proposed to have direct and indirect effects on calcium absorption, and its deficiency as a consequence of menopause is associated with a decline in fractional calcium absorption. This chapter begins with a summary of calcium absorption physiology, continues with a review of mechanisms by which estrogen deficiency across menopause may effect a decline in fractional calcium absorption, and concludes with a discussion of the clinical consequences of this phenomenon with respect to calcium balance, bone mineral density, and fracture risk.

Physiology of Intestinal Calcium Transport

Intestinal calcium absorption occurs through two pathways: the transcellular route, and paracellular transfer. The active saturable transcellular process is dependent on calcitriol, and occurs primarily in the duodenum. The paracellular process refers to calcium diffusion between enterocytes across the transepithelial electrochemical gradient, and occurs throughout the length of the intestine.

Transcellular Calcium Absorption

The transcellular calcium transport pathway involves three steps: (1) calcium entry into the enterocyte via the apical calcium channel, transient receptor potential vanilloid type 6 (TRPV6); (2) transport across the cell via the calcium binding protein, calbindin-D_{9k}; and (3) extrusion across the basolateral membrane via the plasma membrane calcium pump, PMCA1b (Fig. 5.1).

Calcitriol is classically described as the principal mediator of transcellular calcium transport. In vitamin D receptor (VDR) knockout mice, a rachitic phenotype secondary to impaired calcium absorption is observed [1]. Indeed, calcitriol has been shown to induce expression of TRPV6, calbindin-D_{9k}, and PMCA1b [1]. Interestingly, mice missing either TRPV6 or calbindin-D_{9k} retain some responsiveness of intestinal calcium transport to calcitriol, emphasizing our still incomplete understanding of vitamin D-mediated transcellular calcium absorption [1].

In addition to calcitriol, estrogen is increasingly recognized as an independent mediator of the transcellular pathway. Estrogen receptor α (ERα) knockout mice express lower levels of the apical calcium channel TRPV6 in the duodenum [2]. Intestinal cells also express receptors for estrogen, and respond to estradiol-17β with increased calcium transport [3]. When given to VDR knockout mice following ovariectomy, estradiol increases duodenal TRPV6 expression, and enhances calcium absorption [2, 4] (Fig. 5.2).

Paracellular Calcium Absorption

Paracellular calcium absorption involves the diffusion of calcium across the luminal–serosal electrochemical gradient. While recognized more classically for its role in the transcellular pathway, calcitriol is now also recognized as a potential regulator of paracellular transport. Claudins are the major transmembrane components of tight junctions, and VDR KO mice express decreased levels of claudin-2 and claudin-12 [5]. Importantly, the in vitro administration of calcitriol induces expression of claudin-2 and claudin-12 in intestinal epithelial cell lines, resulting in increased paracellular calcium conductance [5].

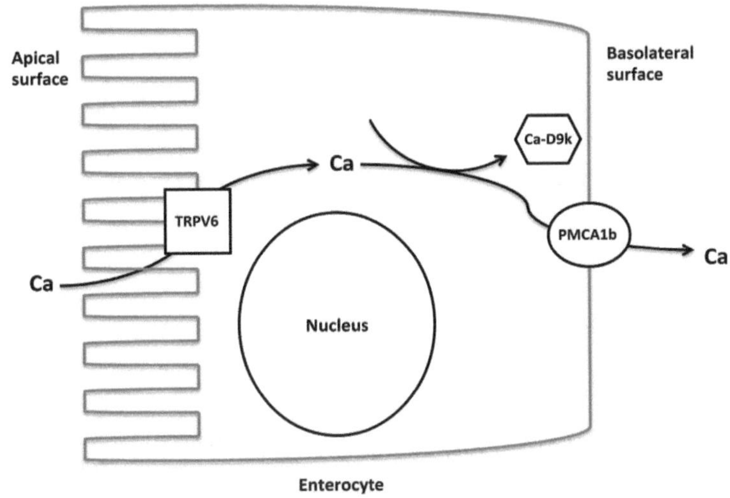

Fig. 5.1 Transcellular intestinal calcium absorption. In order for ingested calcium to be utilized by the body, it must first be absorbed by intestinal cells (enterocytes), and subsequently enter the bloodstream. One mechanism by which enterocytes absorb calcium is through a process called transcellular transport. As depicted in this schematic, transcellular calcium absorption occurs through the following steps: (1) Ingested calcium enters the enterocyte through the apical surface of the cell via a calcium channel called TRPV6; (2) Once the calcium is inside the enterocyte, it is carried across the width of the cell from the apical surface to the basolateral surface possibly via the transport protein Ca-D9k; (3) Once the calcium arrives at the basolateral surface, it exits the cell through another transmembrane protein called PMCA1b, allowing the calcium to enter the bloodstream [1]. *Ca* calcium, *TRPV6* transient receptor potential vanilloid type 6, *Ca-D*$_{9k}$ calbindin-D$_{9k}$

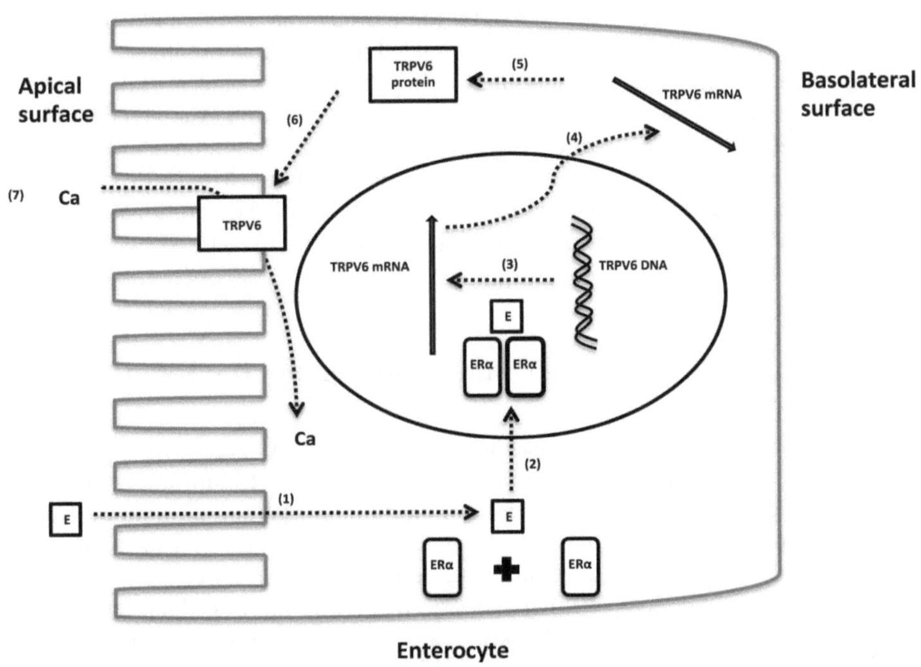

Fig. 5.2 A potential mechanism for estrogen-mediated calcium absorption. While vitamin D has classically been characterized as the primary mediator of intestinal calcium absorption, estrogen also appears to play an important role in promoting transcellular calcium absorption independently of the actions of calcitriol and the vitamin D receptor. As depicted in this schematic, estrogen may promote calcium absorption through the following steps: (1–2) Estrogen enters the intestinal cell (enterocyte), binds to the estrogen receptor, and enters the nucleus. (3–6) Estrogen induces the production of the calcium channel TRPV6. (7) Increased production of TRPV6 increases the ability of the enterocyte to absorb more calcium [2–4]. *Ca* calcium, *E* estrogen, *ERα* estrogen receptor α, *TRPV6* transient receptor potential vanilloid type 6

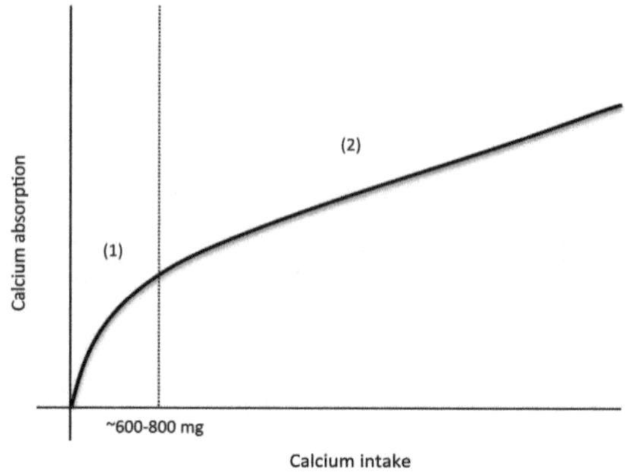

Fig. 5.3 Relationship between dietary calcium intake and net calcium absorption. This schematic depicts the relationship between dietary calcium intake and calcium absorption. (1) At calcium intake levels below 600–800 mg per day, calcium absorption occurs through active transcellular transport (a process mediated by calcium channels and calcium transport proteins), with net calcium absorption rising rapidly with increased calcium intake. (2) At calcium intake levels above 600–800 mg per day, the active transport molecules becomes saturated, and passive diffusion of calcium between intestinal cells predominates, with net calcium absorption rising more slowly, in a linear fashion with increased calcium intake [6, 7]

Calcium Absorption Efficiency

Calcium absorption efficiency is the percentage of a given amount of consumed calcium that is absorbed. At calcium intake levels below 600–800 mg per day, the transcellular pathway predominates, with calcium absorption efficiency inversely related to the size of the ingested load [6, 7]. For example, when calcium absorption was measured in healthy premenopausal adult women to whom calcium loads ranging from 15 to 500 mg were administered, absorption averaged 64.0 % at the lowest load (9.6 mg), and 28.6 % at the highest (143.0 mg) [8]. As calcium intake levels increase above 600–800 mg, the nonsaturable paracellular mechanism predominates, with diffusion increasing linearly with the luminal calcium concentration such that 5–10 % of the additional intake above the quantity that saturates the transcellular mechanism is absorbed (Fig. 5.3) [6, 7].

Calcium Absorption Efficiency in Women Throughout the Life Cycle

Calcium absorption efficiency has been measured using various techniques [9]. Metabolic balance studies measure apparent absorption by determining the difference between calcium intake and fecal calcium [8]. With the advent of radioactive and stable calcium isotopes, single- and dual-isotope techniques have been used. There are two types of single-isotope assays: (1) a low-carrier method in which serum radiocalcium is measured serially after administration of a radioactive calcium isotope with a 20–50 mg calcium carrier load [10–12], and (2) a high-carrier test in which serum radiocalcium is measured 5 h after administration of a radioactive calcium isotope with a 200 mg calcium load [13]. The dual-isotope method involves the co-administration of different oral and intravenous calcium isotopes [14]. The ratio of oral to intravenous isotope content in the urine is then used to calculate calcium absorption [14]. These various techniques have been utilized to elucidate the changes in calcium absorption efficiency throughout the female life cycle in both cross-sectional and longitudinal analyses [15–20].

Calcium Absorption in Childhood, Adolescence, and Adulthood Before Menopause

When 51 girls between 4.9 and 16.7 years of age were enrolled in a cross-sectional study, and calcium absorption measured by a dual-isotope assay, calcium absorption efficiency was 27.7 % before puberty (defined as Tanner stage 1), 34.4 % during early puberty (defined as Tanner stage 2 or 3), and 25.9 % 2 years after early puberty (defined as Tanner stage 4 or 5) [17]. In young adult women, fractional calcium absorption remained at approximately 25–30 % based on a series of controlled metabolic studies [21].

Calcium Absorption Across the Menopause Transition

Menopause, defined as the cessation of menstruation, occurs at a mean age of 51 years [22], and is associated with a decline in calcium absorption efficiency [16, 19, 20]. This decline was delineated in cross-sectional comparisons of premenopausal and postmenopausal women, as well as longitudinal studies of middle-aged women across the menopause transition [16, 19, 20, 23]. Intestinal calcium absorption begins to decline as menstruation becomes irregular [22]. A prospective longitudinal analysis of 72 premenopausal women (defined as having regular menses and normal serum FSH) with a mean age of 47.3 reported that 18 months after enrollment, the majority of patients continued to have regular menses, with very few having undergone menopause (defined as lacking menses and having an elevated FSH) [23]. In 24 subjects who began to report irregular menses, however, calcium absorption as determined by a single-isotope technique declined significantly from baseline, whereas no change was observed in those maintaining regular menstrual cycles [23]. In addition to this study reporting a decline in fractional calcium absorption during the perimenopause window, various cross-sectional and longitudinal studies have examined the changes in calcium absorption associated with completion of the menopause transition [16, 19, 20]. When calcium absorption was measured by a single-isotope assay in 492 women between the ages of 20–80, menopausal status and serum estradiol concentrations were major determinants of calcium absorption [20]. Analysis of 526 absorption studies obtained by dual-isotope and balanced-based methods over a 17-year period from middle-aged women revealed a one-time decrease in fractional calcium absorption from 30.6 % to 27.3 % associated with the completion of menopause [16]. More recently, in 34 women enrolled before menopause and followed longitudinally for eight years across the menopause transition, the hourly fractional calcium absorption rate as determined by a single-isotope assay decreased from 0.78 to 0.64 [19].

Calcium Absorption After Menopause

Beyond its decline associated with the onset of menopause, calcium absorption efficiency decreases further as postmenopausal women continue to age [15, 16, 19]. For example, in the previously cited longitudinal study of healthy women between ages 35 and 62, fractional calcium absorption decreased by 0.21 percent per year starting at age 40 in addition to the one-time decrease associated with the menopause transition [16]. After the seventh decade of life, absorption efficiency appears to drop yet again by approximately 30 % as suggested by two separate cross-sectional analyses, both using the single-isotope method to measure calcium absorption [15, 19].

Estrogen Deficiency and Impaired Calcium Absorption in Postmenopausal Women

The role that decreased ovarian estrogen production plays in the observed decline in calcium absorption efficiency across the menopause transition is underscored by studies in which estrogen replacement in postmenopausal women restored fractional calcium absorption [24, 25]. The question remains of whether estrogen deficiency has a direct or indirect effect on the gut to impair intestinal calcium absorption efficiency across the menopause transition (Fig. 5.4).

Evidence for a Direct Effect of Estrogen Deficiency on the Gut

There is increasing evidence in animal models that estrogen can directly modulate intestinal calcium absorption through the estrogen receptor [2, 3]. For example, estrogen receptor mRNA was detected in rat intestinal cells by Northern blot analysis, with functional estrogen receptors (confirmed by receptor binding techniques) that responded directly to in vitro administration of 17β-estradiol with enhanced calcium transport [3]. In estrogen receptor α (ERα) knockout mice, the expression of the apical calcium channel TRPV6 was reduced [2]. In VDR KO mice that underwent ovariectomy, estrogen therapy induced TRPV6 expression in the duodenum [4]. Taken together, the above data suggests that estrogen may promote calcium absorption through the transcellular pathway by regulating TRPV6 expression independently of calcitriol and the VDR.

Indeed, in multiple human trials of postmenopausal women with osteoporosis, estrogen therapy improves calcium absorption [24, 25]. It is difficult to discern from these studies, however, the extent to which the increase in calcium absorption is attributable to a direct and/or indirect effect of estrogen on the intestinal epithelium.

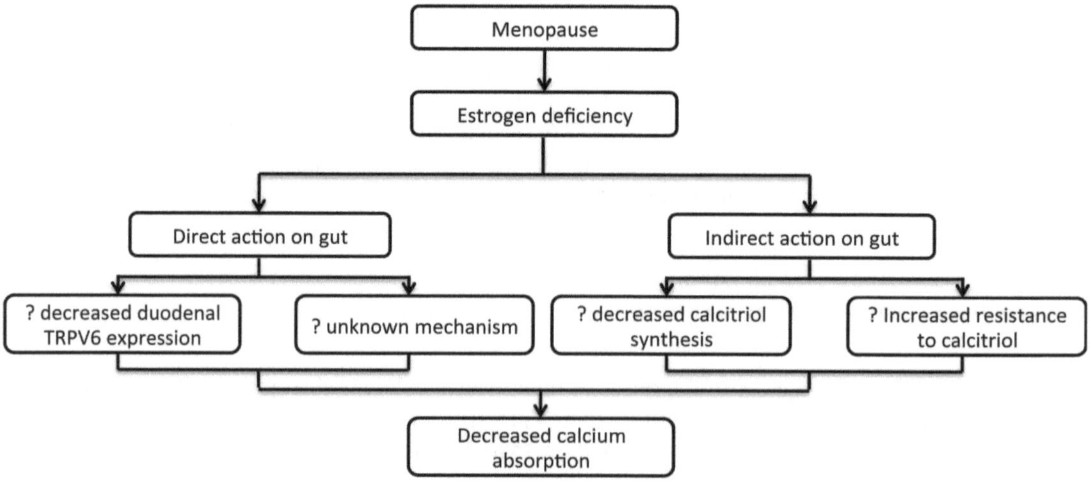

Fig. 5.4 Effects of menopause on calcium absorption. Menopause is associated with a decrease in intestinal calcium absorption. One possible mechanism by which this occurs is that estrogen deficiency secondary to menopause leads to decreased expression of the calcium channel TRPV6 by the intestinal cell, and therefore decreased calcium absorption. A second potential mechanism is that estrogen deficiency leads to decreased production of calcitriol and/or increased intestinal resistance to the actions of calcitriol, resulting in diminished calcium absorption [2, 3, 24, 25, 27, 28]. *TRPV6* transient receptor potential vanilloid type 6

Evidence for an Indirect Effect of Estrogen Deficiency on the Gut

In trials of women with postmenopausal osteoporosis, administration of estrogen therapy was associated with an increase in serum calcitriol and a restoration of calcium absorption efficiency to premenopausal levels [24–26]. For example, in a trial of 71 postmenopausal women, calcitriol levels increased significantly from baseline after administration of estrogen-progestin in combination with 1,700 mg per day of calcium, whereas calcitriol levels did not change in those who received calcium only [26]. Another study reported that postmenopausal osteoporotics randomized to receive 1.25–2.5 mg per day of conjugated equine estrogen experienced a significant increase in serum calcitriol concentrations (23.6–33.2 pg/ml; $p<0.005$), as well as a significant increase in fractional calcium absorption [24]. Similarly, when 21 postmenopausal women received 1.25 mg/day of conjugated equine estrogen, calcitriol levels and calcium absorption also rose significantly from baseline [25].

These findings led to the proposal that decreased ovarian estrogen production associated with menopause leads to decreased calcitriol synthesis and therefore reduced calcium absorption [27, 28]. Based on this paradigm, two potential mechanisms for impaired calcium absorption following menopause were suggested [26–28]. The first assumes that the primary disturbance is an increase in bone resorption secondary to estrogen deficiency, which leads to increased serum ionized calcium, decreased parathyroid hormone (PTH) secretion, decreased calcitriol synthesis, and decreased intestinal calcium absorption [27, 28]. The second presumes that the primary disturbance is decreased calcitriol synthesis secondary to estrogen deficiency, which leads to decreased intestinal calcium absorption, decreased serum ionized calcium, increased PTH secretion, and a restoration of calcitriol synthesis [27, 28]. Both pathways share in common decreased calcitriol synthesis and decreased intestinal calcium absorption efficiency, but differ in potential changes in serum calcium and PTH levels (Fig. 5.5). To that end, various studies have attempted to confirm a decline in circulating calcitriol levels and elucidate the precise change in serum calcium and PTH concentrations across the menopause transition [28–32].

With respect to calcitriol, a decline in serum levels across the menopause transition has not been definitively proven [21, 28–30]. A cross-sectional comparison of age-matched premenopausal and postmenopausal women reported higher total serum calcitriol levels among postmenopausal subjects, but the calculated free calcitriol index was no different between the two groups when corrected for vitamin D-binding protein [31]. In 19 premenopausal women followed for 8 years prospectively, serum estrogen levels began to decline before menopause, but no significant change in either total or free calcitriol was observed before or after cessation of menstruation [29]. Several subsequent longitudinal observational studies involving 10 and 34 participants also demonstrated no change in circulating calcitriol across menopause [28, 30].

In terms of whether serum PTH concentration increases or decreases with menopause, results have been similarly inconclusive [28, 31–33]. Historically, estrogen has been proposed to have the ability to decrease total serum calcium because of its antiresorptive properties [33]. In fact, estrogen therapy has been evaluated as a potential treatment modality for hypercalcemia secondary to primary hyperparathyroidism [33]. A recent review of relevant clinical trials concluded that hormone therapy indeed suppresses total serum calcium, but does not affect serum ionized calcium or intact PTH [33]. Based on its ability to suppress serum calcium concentrations, one could postulate that estrogen deficiency associated with menopause would lead to higher serum calcium levels and subsequent suppression of PTH secretion. This, however, has not been confirmed in studies of changes in calcium and PTH across the menopause transition [28, 31, 32]. For example, an early cross-sectional study of 22 age-matched premenopausal and postmenopausal women found that serum calcium was significantly higher in the postmenopausal group, but no difference between the two groups existed with respect to serum PTH [31]. A subsequent large-scale cross-sectional analysis of 655 women between the ages of 35 and 90 also found that serum calcium increased significantly, but serum PTH remained constant across the menopause transition [32]. The difference in serum calcium between the premenopausal

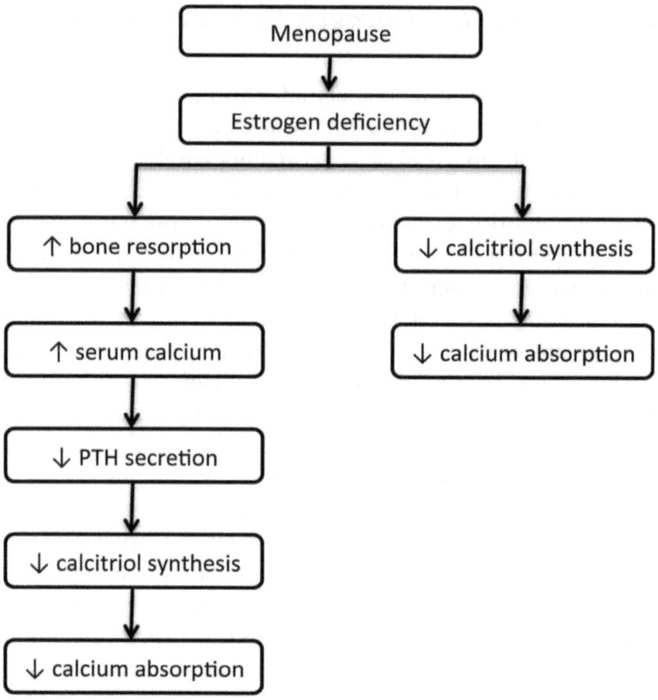

Fig. 5.5 Potential effects of menopause on calcitriol synthesis and calcium absorption. Estrogen deficiency resulting from menopause has been proposed to cause decreased calcitriol synthesis, and therefore decreased calcium absorption. One possible mechanism by which this occurs is that decreased estrogen leads to increased bone resorption (breakdown), increased serum calcium, decreased parathyroid hormone (PTH) secretion, decreased calcitriol synthesis, and therefore decreased calcium absorption. A second potential mechanism is that decreased estrogen leads to decreased calcitriol synthesis, decreased calcium absorption, decreased calcium, and increased PTH secretion. Various studies have attempted to elucidate the changes in serum calcitriol, calcium, and PTH that occur across the menopause transition, but results are inconclusive [27–32]

and postmenopausal subjects became insignificant, however, once calcium levels were adjusted for differences in serum albumin [32]. More recently, when 104 premenopausal women were followed over an 8-year period, 34 participants underwent menopause. In these subjects, calcium absorption decreased significantly and was associated with an increase in total and ionized calcium, but no change in serum PTH [28]. Other studies have attempted to explicitly determine if there exists a correlation between calcium absorption and serum PTH across the menopause transition [28, 34]. Among 262 postmenopausal women aged 40–87 years in whom calcium absorption was measured by a single-isotope assay, no correlation between calcium absorption and serum PTH was found [28]. In an even larger analysis of 482 postmenopausal women, similar findings were reported [34]. To summarize, the inconclusive evidence regarding changes in serum calcitriol, calcium, and PTH levels across the menopause transition, and the lack of correlation between calcium absorption and PTH secretion in postmenopausal subjects underscores our still incomplete understanding of how—and even whether—decreased estrogen production leads to decreased calcitriol synthesis and reduced intestinal calcium absorption.

Another proposed mechanism by which estrogen deficiency may decrease calcium absorption efficiency is that it limits intestinal responsiveness to calcitriol [35, 36]. In female rats that underwent oophorectomy, the number of calcitriol receptors in jejunal villous cells was reduced by 37 % [33]. In humans, a study involving 44 healthy ambulatory women between 20 and 87 years of age who underwent duodenal biopsy during gastroduodenoscopy revealed that vitamin D receptor concentration when measured by an immunoradiometric assay decreased significantly with age [37]. However, whether this change is a consequence of menopause, advancing age, or both cannot be concluded from this study. When 14 premenopausal women who underwent oophorectomy were placed on calcitriol, and then randomized to estrogen therapy or placebo, serum calcitriol levels between the estrogen and placebo arms were not different, but intestinal calcium absorption was significantly higher in the estrogen group indicating a possible component of intestinal resistance related to estrogen deficiency [36]. More recently, calcium absorption data from 492 women was used to build a predictive model to relate calcium absorption to various covariates. The resulting predictive models revealed calcium absorption to be a function of serum calcitriol in both premenopausal and postmenopausal women, but had a lower intercept in postmenopausal subjects, suggesting intestinal resistance to calcitriol in the setting of decreased ovarian estrogen production [20].

Clinical Significance of Decreased Calcium Absorption Efficiency in Postmenopausal Women

Calcium Balance

It is generally accepted that after menopause, there is a negative change in calcium balance [21, 27, 38, 39]. For example, a calcium balance analysis of postmenopausal women reported negative balance by 50–70 mg per day in the majority of subjects [38]. In a subsequent calcium balance study of 207 women with an average calcium intake of 650 mg per day, balance was −20 mg per day in 42-year-old (premenopausal) women compared to −43 mg per day in 47-year-old (postmenopausal) women [39]. This change was attributed equally to decreased intestinal calcium absorption and increased urinary calcium loss [39]. This study also established that calcium balance was a function of calcium intake before and after menopause, but that the parameters of the relationship were different in estrogen-replete versus deficient states [27, 39]. More specifically, for any given intake, absorption was about 14 mg less in postmenopausal women [27, 39]. Of note, hormone replacement therapy in postmenopausal subjects restored calcium balance to levels identical to those observed in premenopausal participants [27, 39].

The precise calcium intake quantity necessary to achieve neutral calcium balance in postmenopausal women has not been definitively established. In the above cited report, an intake of 990 mg per day in premenopausal and estrogen-treated postmenopausal women was calculated [39]. In contrast, postmenopausal women who did not receive hormone replacement therapy required 1,504 mg per day [39]. Most recently, a series of controlled metabolic studies undertaken by the USDA was reviewed, and calcium balance data from 155 subjects (73 female, 82 male) with calcium intake ranging from 415 to 1,740 mg per day were reported [21]. When the relation between daily calcium intake and output was examined by fitting random coefficient models, neutral calcium balance was predicted at a calcium intake of 741 mg per day [21]. While this study included both males and females across a wide age range, the authors found that neither age nor gender were significant determinants of the relation between calcium intake and output [21]. The predicted calcium intake requirement of 741 mg per day should therefore be applicable to postmenopausal women.

Osteoporosis

Changes in the handling of calcium by the gut across the menopause transition likely contribute to bone loss in postmenopausal women [40, 41]. In healthy elderly subjects with normal bone density, calcium absorption was decreased, and adaptation to low dietary calcium impaired when compared to

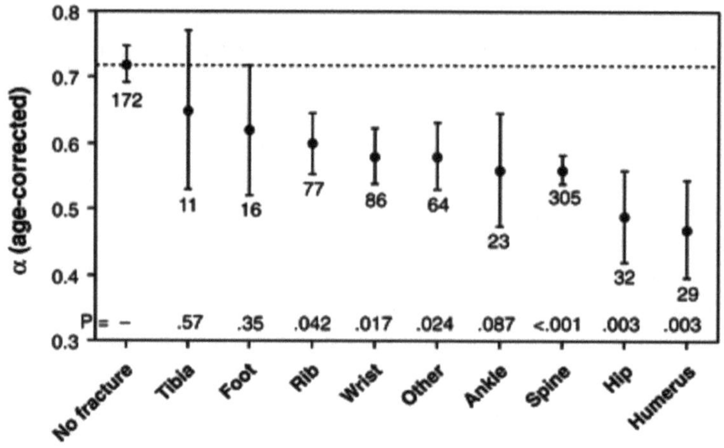

Fig. 5.6 Calcium absorption in postmenopausal women with and without peripheral fractures The decline in intestinal calcium absorption that occurs following the menopause transition is clinically significant. As demonstrated in this figure (reprinted with kind permission from Springer Science+Business Media: Osteoporosis International; Radiocalcium absorption is reduced in postmenopausal women with vertebral and most types of peripheral fractures; Volume 15; 2004; Page 29; B.E. Christopher Nordin, O'Loughlin, PD, et al.; Fig. 2), calcium absorption in postmenopausal women with spine, hip, humeral, wrist, and rib fractures is significantly lower than that in postmenopausal women without fractures [44]

non-elderly subjects. In elderly subjects with osteoporosis, these abnormalities were even more pronounced [40]. When 49 postmenopausal women with osteoporosis were compared to age-matched controls without osteoporosis, the hourly fractional calcium absorption rate as measured by a single-isotope assay was 0.57 in those with osteoporosis versus 0.81 in those without [41]. Further, in osteoporotic patients, fractional calcium absorption positively correlated with vertebral bone density [41]. Beyond its relation to bone density, decreased calcium absorption in postmenopausal women was also associated with vertebral, hip, humeral, wrist, and rib fractures [42–45] (Fig. 5.6).

Recommended Daily Calcium Intake

The 2011 Institute of Medicine report on dietary reference intakes for calcium recommends an estimated average requirement (EAR) and recommended daily allowance (RDA) of 1,000 and 1,200 mg per day, respectively, for women between 51 and 70 years of age [46]. As vitamin D and calcium are known to interact physiologically, these calcium recommendations assume a vitamin D-replete state [46]. In terms of vitamin D, the IOM recommends an EAR and RDA of 400 and 600 IU per day, respectively, for women 51–70 years of age [46]. For women over 70, the EAR and RDA are 400 and 800 IU per day [46]. These vitamin D recommendations were based on a review of the relation between vitamin D status and integrated bone health outcomes (calcium absorption, bone accretion, bone maintenance, bone loss, and fractures), as well as simulated dose–response curves [46].

With respect to calcium, the EAR and RDA intake quantities were derived from an analysis of randomized clinical trials pertaining to the effect of calcium supplementation on bone mineral density (which the IOM considered to be a surrogate of fracture risk), as well as calcium balance data [46]. The IOM acknowledged that available studies on the relation between calcium supplementation and BMD were limited by inconsistent reporting of background diet, and therefore total estimated calcium intake [46]. There was, however, general evidence that suggested a benefit to taking an average of

1,100 mg per day of calcium among women over the age of 60 with respect to BMD [46]. Recognizing the limitations of existing data, the fact that women over age 51 represent a spectrum of physiological conditions, and a desire to err on the side of caution to ensure public health protection, the IOM arrived at an EAR of 1,000 mg per day by adding 200 mg per day to the aforementioned 741 mg per day intake that was calculated to achieve neutral calcium balance [21, 46].

Conclusion

Intestinal calcium absorption consists of the active transcellular and passive paracellular transport of calcium across the transepithelial barrier. The decreased ovarian production of estrogen as a consequence of the menopause transition is associated with impaired intestinal calcium absorption. Mechanisms by which estrogen deficiency either directly or indirectly acts on the gut to alter calcium transport physiology have been suggested, but not definitively elucidated by currently available evidence. The reduced calcium absorption efficiency observed across menopause manifests clinically as a negative change in calcium balance, an increased association with osteoporosis, and an increased risk of fracture. In postmenopausal women, it is therefore important to optimize calcium intake to ensure maintenance of skeletal health. Based on data suggesting a benefit to calcium supplementation with respect to bone mineral density, and available calcium balance analyses, the Institute of Medicine currently recommends an EAR and RDA of calcium of 1,000 and 1,200 mg per day, respectively, in vitamin D-replete women 51 years and older.

References

1. Christakos S. Vitamin D: molecular mechanism of action. Ann N Y Acad Sci. 2007;1116:340–8.
2. Van Cromphaut SJ. Intestinal calcium transporter genes are upregulated by estrogens and the reproductive cycle through vitamin D receptor-independent mechanisms. J Bone Miner Res. 2003;10:1725–36.
3. Arjmandi BH. Evidence for estrogen receptor-linked calcium transport in the intestine. Bone Miner. 1993;21:63–74.
4. O'Loughlin PD. Oestrogen deficiency impairs intestinal calcium absorption in the rat. J Physiol. 1998;15:313–22.
5. Fujita H. Tight junction proteins claudin-2 and -12 are critical for vitamin D-dependent Ca2+ absorption between enterocytes. Mol Biol Cell. 2008;19:1912–21.
6. Heaney RP. Calcium absorption as a function of calcium intake. J Lab Clin Med. 1975;85:881–90.
7. Nordin BE. Calcium homeostasis. Clin Biochem. 1990;23:3–10.
8. Heaney RP. Influence of calcium load on absorption fraction. J Bone Miner Res. 1990;5:1135–8.
9. Nordin BE. Calcium absorption revisited. Am J Clin Nutr. 2010;92:673–4.
10. Avioli LV. The influence of age on the intestinal absorption of 47-Ca absorption in post-menopausal osteoporosis. J Clin Invest. 1965;44:1960–7.
11. Nordin BE. Calculation of calcium absorption rate from plasma radioactivity. Clin Sci. 1968;35:177–82.
12. Nordin BEC. Modification and validation of a single-isotope radiocalcium absorption test. J Nucl Med. 1998;39:108–13.
13. Heaney RP. Estimation of true calcium absorption. Ann Intern Med. 1985;103:516–21.
14. DeGrazia JA. A double isotope method for measurement of intestinal absorption of calcium in man. J Lab Clin Med. 1965;66:822–9.
15. Bullamore JR. Effect of age on calcium absorption. Lancet. 1970;2:535–7.
16. Heaney RP. Calcium absorption in women: relationships to calcium intake, estrogen status, and age. J Bone Miner Res. 1989;4:469–75.
17. Abrams SA. Calcium metabolism in girls: current dietary intakes lead to low rates of calcium absorption and retention during puberty. Am J Clin Nutr. 1994;60:739–43.
18. Kovacs CS. Calcium and bone metabolism in pregnancy and lactation. J Clin Endocrinol Metab. 2001;86:2344–8.
19. Nordin BE. Effect of age on calcium absorption in postmenopausal women. Am J Clin Nutr. 2004;80:998–1002.

20. Aloia JF. Serum vitamin D metabolites and intestinal calcium absorption efficiency in women. Am J Clin Nutr. 2010;92:835–40.
21. Hunt CD. Calcium requirements: new estimations for men and women by cross-sectional statistical analyses of calcium balance data from metabolic studies. Am J Clin Nutr. 2007;86:1054–63.
22. McKinlay SM. Smoking and age at menopause in women. Ann Intern Med. 1985;103:350–6.
23. Wishart JM. Effect of perimenopause on calcium absorption: a longitudinal study. Climacteric. 2000;3:102–8.
24. Gallagher JC, Riggs BL, DeLuca HF. Effect of estrogen on calcium absorption and serum vitamin D metabolites in postmenopausal osteoporosis. J Clin Endocrinol Metab. 1980;51:1359–64.
25. Civitelli R. Effects of one-year treatment with estrogens on bone mass, intestinal calcium absorption, and 25-hydroxyvitamin D-1 alpha-hydroxylase reserve in postmenopausal osteoporosis. Calcif Tissue Int. 1988;42:77–86.
26. Aloia JF. Biochemical short-term changes produced by hormonal replacement therapy. J Endocrinol Invest. 1991;14:927–34.
27. Heaney RP. Calcium nutrition and bone health in the elderly. Am J Clin Nutr. 1982;36:986–1013.
28. Falch JA. Early postmenopausal bone loss is not associated with a decrease in circulating levels of 25-hydroxyvitamin D, 1,25-dihydroxyvitamin D, or vitamin D-binding protein. J Clin Endocrinol Metab. 1987;64:836–41.
29. Hartwell D. Changes in vitamin D metabolism during natural and medical menopause. J Clin Endocrinol Metab. 1990;71:127–32.
30. Prince RL. The effects of the menopause on calcitriol and parathyroid hormone: responses to a low dietary calcium stress test. J Clin Endocrinol Metab. 1990;70:1119–23.
31. Prince RL. The effects of menopause and age on calcitropic hormones: a cross-sectional study of 655 healthy women aged 35 to 90. J Bone Miner Res. 1995;10:835–42.
32. Nordin BE. A longitudinal study of bone-related biochemical changes at the menopause. Clin Endocrinol (Oxf). 2004;61:123–30.
33. Khan A. Medical management of asymptomatic primary hyperparathyroidism: proceedings of the third international workshop. J Clin Endocrinol Metab. 2009;94:373–81.
34. Nordin BE. Calcium malabsorption does not cause secondary hyperparathyroidism. Calcif Tissue Int. 2009;85:31–6.
35. Chan SD. Oophorectomy leads to a selective decrease in 1,25-dihydroxycholecalciferol receptors in rat jejunal villous cells. Clin Sci (Lond). 1984;66:745–8.
36. Gennari C. Estrogen preserves a normal intestinal responsiveness to 1,25-dihydroxyvitamin D3 in oophorectomized women. J Clin Endocrinol Metab. 1990;71:1288–93.
37. Ebeling PR. Evidence of an age-related decrease in intestinal responsiveness to vitamin D: relationship between serum 1,25-dihydroxyvitamin D3 and intestinal vitamin D receptor concentrations in normal women. J Clin Endocrinol Metab. 1992;75:176–82.
38. Marshall DH. Calcium, phosphorus and magnesium requirement. Proc Nutr Soc. 1976;35:163–73.
39. Heaney RP. Menopausal changes in calcium balance performance. J Lab Clin Med. 1978;92:953–63.
40. Gallagher JC. Intestinal calcium absorption and serum vitamin D metabolites in normal subjects and osteoporotic patients: effect of age and dietary calcium. J Clin Invest. 1979;64:729–36.
41. Nordin BE. The relation between calcium absorption, serum dehydroepiandrosterone, and vertebral mineral density in postmenopausal women. J Clin Endocrinol Metab. 1985;60:651–7.
42. Gallagher JC. The crush fracture syndrome in postmenopausal women. Clin Endocrinol Metab. 1973;2:293–315.
43. Francis RM. Calcium malabsorption in elderly women with vertebral fractures: evidence for resistance to the action of vitamin D metabolites on the bowel. Clin Sci. 1984;66:103–10.
44. Morris HA. Calcium absorption in normal and osteoporotic postmenopausal women. Calcif Tissue Int. 1991;49:240–3.
45. Nordin BE. Radiocalcium absorption is reduced in postmenopausal women with vertebral and most types of peripheral fractures. Osteoporos Int. 2004;15:27–31.
46. IOM (Institute of Medicine). Dietary reference intakes for calcium and vitamin D. Washington, DC: The National Academies Press; 2011.

Chapter 6
Calcium Absorption from Fortified Soymilk in Osteopenic Postmenopausal Women

Lily Stojanovska and Anne Lise Tang

Key Points

- Consumption of soy isoflavones is becoming increasingly popular among postmenopausal women seeking to reduce symptoms associated with menopause and estrogen deficiency.
- Isoflavones might protect against chronic diseases associated with menopause, such as osteoporosis and cardiovascular disease.
- Consumption of soy protein and isoflavones may be associated with attenuation of bone loss, lowering of urinary calcium and increase of bone mineral density in postmenopausal women.
- The biologically active isoflavone isomers are the aglycone configurations of genistein and daidzein. Intestinal microflora reduces daidzein to equol, a highly active metabolite with estrogen-like chemical structure.
- Soymilk fortification might be an effective way to increase calcium intake although calcium bioavailability in soymilk is highly determined by the type of fortificant used.
- Fermentation of soy milk with probiotics with *Lactobacillus* and *Bifidobacterium* has the potential benefit of increasing calcium bioavailability and absorption.
- Reduction in phytic acid content of soy milk can potentially increase absorption not only of calcium but also iron, zinc, copper and magnesium.
- Calcium absorption and bioavailability from calcium fortified soymilk is found to be similar to that of cows' milk in osteopenic postmenopausal women

Keywords Soymilk • Isoflavones • Osteopenic women • Calcium absorption • Isoflavones

Abbreviations

BMC	Bone mineral composition
BMD	Bone mineral density
CFSM	Calcium fortified soymilk
DXA	Dual-energy X-ray absorptiometry
LAB	Lactic acid bacteria

L. Stojanovska, Ph.D. (✉) • A.L. Tang, Ph.D.
College of Health and Biomedicine, Victoria University, St. Albans Campus, PO Box 14428, Melbourne, VIC 8001, Australia
e-mail: lily.stojanovska@vu.edu.au; annelisetang@yahoo.com

C.J.H. Martin et al. (eds.), *Nutrition and Diet in Menopause*, Nutrition and Health,
DOI 10.1007/978-1-62703-373-2_6, © Springer Science+Business Media New York 2013

Introduction

Calcium is a nutrient essential for maintenance of bone health and mineralisation [1]. In women, the loss of bone mineral greatly increases around the time of menopause as circulating estrogen declines, thus increasing the risk of osteoporosis [2]. Prevention of osteoporosis in women depends in part on maintenance of high calcium intake throughout life and particularly after menopause to slow the rate of bone loss [3]. Calcium nutrition not only is important for bone health but also has been implicated in such disorders as hypertension, colon cancer and kidney stones [4].

In Western, well-developed countries, around 60 % of dietary calcium comes from foods, including cows' milk [5]. Calcium found in cows' milk is in the form of calcium phosphate, which binds with the milk protein, casein, to form a complex. Acidification of the complex causes the calcium phosphate to dissolve and the protein to precipitate, thus allowing for optimum calcium bioavailability. Other factors that may affect calcium absorption are phytic acid, phosphorus, oxalic acid and dietary fibres. Phytic acid, also known as phytate, is a storage form of phosphorus in seeds, particularly abundant in cereal grains, oilseeds and legumes such as soybeans [6]. Phytic acid is known to interfere with calcium bioavailability as the human gastrointestinal tract does not possess an endogenous enzyme, phytase, capable of hydrolysing phytic acid [7]. In addition, other dietary nutrients such as proteins and fats as well as biological modulators such as vitamin D, parathyroid hormone and calcitonin also affect calcium bioavailability [8].

There is an increased awareness that diets high in plant-based foods may provide protection from many hormone-dependent diseases due to the high phytochemical content found in plants. Isoflavones are naturally occurring plant chemicals belonging to the phytoestrogen class, thought to have beneficial effects for a range of conditions including menopausal symptoms, although such effects still require substantiation [9]. In particular, isoflavones are hypothesised to provide relief from hot flushes [10, 11] and protect against chronic diseases, such as osteoporosis, breast cancer and cardiovascular disease [12, 13]. Some studies in postmenopausal women have shown that long-term consumption of isoflavones can have bone-sparing effects due to attenuation of bone loss [13, 14], while others [15] have reported no effect. Furthermore, researchers [16] have proposed that the greatest benefits may be in subjects whose intestinal bacteria degrade daidzein, which is a primary soy isoflavone, into equol, a highly active metabolite.

Soy milk is rich in isoflavone content. Many postmenopausal women may choose to consume soymilk rather than cows' milk due to the perceived health benefits of isoflavones. As such, soymilk is being increasingly consumed in developed countries. Consumption of soymilk may lead to reduced calcium intake as native soymilk contains approximately 20 mg Ca/100 ml compared with cows' milk with approximately 120 mg Ca/100 ml [17]. Commercially available soymilk is now fortified to the same level as cows' milk with calcium phosphate or carbonate, although the type of the fortificant and the methods of fortification vary considerably between products [18]. Soymilk fortification appears to be an effective way to increase calcium intake and the total amount of absorbed calcium, although calcium bioavailability will depend considerably on the choice of the fortificant [19]. The bioavailability rather than the total content of calcium in soymilk is thus an important issue.

One way to potentially enhance the biological activity and nutritional value of soymilk is through fermentation with probiotics. Probiotics are a living microbial food supplement which may have beneficial effects on human health. The fermentation of soymilk in vitro with β-probiotic bacterial strains allows isoflavones to undergo enzymatic hydrolysis into biologically available aglycone structures and increase calcium solubility [20]. Little is known on whether fermentation of soy milk will also increase calcium absorption from the small intestine.

To date, few studies have examined the absorption of calcium from different kinds of fortified soymilk available on the market [17, 19]. As postmenopausal women need up to 1,500 mg calcium per day to prevent osteoporosis, it is important to determine whether they can obtain the calcium that they need from the fortified soymilk.

Calcium and Its Requirements

Calcium is a mineral that accounts for 1–2 % of the adult human body weight and plays a vital role in the development and maintenance of a healthy skeleton [21]. The primitive function of the skeleton is to serve as a source and as a sink for calcium and phosphorus, i.e. as a reserve to offset shortage and as a place for safely storing dietary surpluses, at least after periods of depletion [22]. This feature can be observed when animals placed on low calcium intake, show reduced bone mass as calcium is needed to maintain homeostasis in the extracellular fluids. This activity is mediated by parathyroid hormone and involves actual bone destruction, not leaching of calcium from bone [22].

Calcium and bone balance are synonymous; if the bone balance is negative, then external calcium balance must also be negative [23]. Previous reports have shown the calcium requirement was calculated from calcium balances in normal subjects on a range of calcium intakes. In 212 such balances on 85 subjects published in the literature, the mean value was found to be 550 mg/day [23]. This value was based largely on American balance studies conducted on young adults and may not apply to populations where protein and sodium intakes are lower or higher.

Factors Affecting Calcium Absorption and Excretion

Several nutritional factors influence calcium absorption by way of nutrient interactions which tend to have negative impact on the calcium economy. The principal interacting nutrients are fibre, caffeine, sodium and protein [22]. Fibre and caffeine have variable influence on calcium intestinal absorption; from soluble fibre in green, leafy vegetables having no influence at all on absorption to insoluble fibre in wheat bran which reduces absorption of co-ingested calcium [22]. Phytate and oxalate can also reduce the availability of any calcium contained in the same food; unlike bran, phytate and oxalate generally do not affect co-ingested calcium from other foods. Although caffeine is thought to have deleterious effect on the calcium economy, it has the smallest effect of the known interacting nutrients [22]. Sodium and protein have greater influence on urinary excretion of calcium which can be significant for the calcium economy when calcium intakes are low [22]. Sodium, protein and phosphorus can increase urinary calcium loss across the full range of their intakes. Sodium and calcium share the same transport system in the proximal tubule, and every 2,300 mg of sodium excreted by the kidneys pulls 20–60 mg of calcium out with it. Similarly every gram of protein metabolised in adults additionally causes an increment in urine calcium loss of about 1 mg [22]. Differences in protein and sodium intake among national groups are perhaps part of the reason that studies in different countries have shown strikingly different calcium requirements [22]. There is no clear evidence that phosphorus reduces calcium absorption. An analysis of 567 metabolic balances performed in healthy middle-aged women studied on their usual diets, indicate that variation in phosphorus intake over a nearly sixfold range had no detectable effect on calcium absorption efficiency [24]. In adults, variation in the calcium to phosphorus ratio from 0.2 to more than 2.0 are without effect on calcium balance, providing adjustments are made for calcium intake [24].

Calcium Sources

Foods are the calcium sources for humans. Foods that provide more than 100 mg of calcium per serving are limited to dairy products, greens of the mustard family, calcium-set tofu, sardines, and some nuts, especially hazelnut and almonds. Smaller amounts of calcium are found in many leafy vegetables; while with the exception of shellfish, calcium levels are low in most meats, poultry and fish [22]. The calcium present in beans is only about half as that available as the calcium of milk and the calcium of high oxalate vegetables, such as spinach and rhubarb, is almost completely unavailable [22].

In Western countries, diets that are low in dairy products are generally also low in calcium (~300–400 mg). Consequently, there has been an increasing trend of fortification of foods with low levels of calcium. In the USA, fortified foods range from juice to bread to potato chips to rice. Satisfactory bioavailability still needs to be determined for those fortified foods; a soy beverage fortified to the calcium load of cows' milk was shown to deliver only 75 % of the calcium delivered by cows' milk [17]. Recent entries into the soy and rice beverage markets as well as several of the calcium fortified orange juices exhibited even poorer physical characteristics [18].

The main calcium supplement available in the US market is calcium carbonate formulated so that it disintegrates in the gastric juice [22]. Calcium carbonate is well absorbed and generally well tolerated. Calcium citrate and calcium malate fortificants are also good sources but can be more costly [22].

Estimation of True Calcium Absorption

There is a great deal of variability in calcium absorption. In healthy women, gross absorption efficiency spans at least a threefold range from 15 % to 45 %, even after adjustment for differences in intake [25]. The reasons for much of this inter-individual variability are unclear. While it is known that there is a high degree of within-individual consistency in absorptive performance over time, i.e. some individuals are efficient absorbers and others are poor absorbers [25].

The most reliable and sensitive method of measuring true calcium absorption is the tracer method, using either stable or radioactive calcium isotopes. The radioactive tracer method has been most widely used due to its established methodology and low cost [25], while the stable isotope tracer method is increasingly being practised in recent years [26]. It tends to be costly to perform, although it provides an accurate measure of calcium absorption and has minor ethical constraints. The food sources can be labelled with the tracer intrinsically, where by the isotope is incorporated biosynthetically into the food, or extrinsically, where the tracer calcium is added directly to the food source [27] and the tracer is allowed to mix and exchange uniformly with the food. The food source is then consumed and the level of tracer calcium is measured in the blood over a period of time to determine the rate and amount of calcium absorption [26].

Soymilk

Soymilk consists of a water extract of soybeans, resembling dairy milk in both appearance and composition. Based on the method of preparation, soymilk is grouped into "traditional" soymilk and "modern" soymilk [28]. Traditional soymilk for small scale use has a limited shelf life possessing a beany flavour and a bitter or astringent taste. Modern soymilk, however, is produced using the state of the art technology to maximise taste, flavour, nutritional value and convenience. The resulting soymilk has a relatively bland taste with reduced beany flavour, and in most cases it is flavoured, sweetened, and/or fortified for better taste or nutrition, and packaged for longer life [28]. Much of the soymilk available commercially is now prepared from soy protein isolate rather than from whole soybeans as manufacturers often find production from soybean isolate simpler providing a more consistent product.

Commercially available soymilk usually contains 8–10 % total solids with protein constituting about 3.6–4.0 %, fat 0–2 %, and carbohydrates between 3 and 7 % of the solids [28]. Thus, soymilk composition compares favourably with that of cows' milk. Additionally, soymilk is cholesterol and lactose free. Genotypic changes in protein subunit composition can strongly affect the particle size distribution and the stability of soymilk, however, the use of heat treatment and homogenisation improves particle size distribution [28]. Soymilk generally contains most of the active phytochemicals present in soybeans, including high amounts of isoflavones.

Fortification of Soymilk

When compared to cows' milk (~120 mg Ca/100 ml) native soymilk is relatively poor in calcium (~20 mg Ca/100 ml). Manufacturers have addressed this issue by fortifying soymilk with calcium which appears to be an effective way to increase calcium intake and the total amount of absorbed calcium [29].

Most of the calcium in cows' milk is found as a colloidal caseinate-phosphate complex that is readily released during digestion and hence has high bioavailability. Calcium bioavailability in soymilk, is highly determined by the type of fortificant used [19]. Several commercial calcium salts have been used for fortification of soymilk and soy beverages, including calcium carbonate, calcium chloride, calcium phosphate and others [30]. The bioavailability of these salts may depend not just on their nature, but also on the nature of proteins present in the soymilk, which can act as carriers during the absorption process. With some fortificants and some types of soymilk, the calcium may react strongly with soymilk proteins, particularly after heat processing, leading to sedimentation and gelation. Stabilisers and emulsifiers have therefore been used to try to maintain calcium in suspension as well as to improve mouth-feel and appearance [30]. In soymilks, fortification with a type of calcium carbonate appears to yield similar calcium absorption to that of cows' milk.

Many foods apart from soymilk can be fortified with calcium. However, studies in the USA suggest that the quality of calcium fortification in many beverages is uneven at best, so that consumers are likely to be misled with respect to the calcium benefit conferred by the beverage. For example, tracer equilibrium of calcium varied from 25 % to 79 % in a range of soy and rice beverages tested [18].

Soy Isoflavones

Soybeans and soy derived foods contain phytoestrogens which are plant derived, phenolic compounds with a structural resemblance to human estrogen, although they are not as biologically active. The biologically active, estrogen-like isoflavone isomers are the aglycone configurations of genistein and daidzein [48].

Isoflavones and to some extent lignans are two main phytoestrogens of interest in clinical nutrition with isoflavones having been studied most extensively. When ingested, intestinal microflora induces fermentation on these plant compounds hydrolysing the glucosides into bioavailable aglycones, thus reducing daidzein to equol, a highly active metabolite [31] (Fig. 6.1). Daidzein, genistein and equol are therefore the major isoflavones detected in the human blood and urine [32]. The chemical similarity of estrogen to equol is shown in Fig. 6.2.

Soy Isoflavones and Menopause

Soy isoflavones are becoming increasingly popular among women who are looking for health products to modify symptoms associated with menopause and estrogen deficiency. A review of the literature suggests some evidence for the efficacy of soy preparations for menopausal symptoms including hot flushes and mood swings [12]. A significant inverse correlation has been reported between baseline hot flushes and the reduction in hot flushes achieved by isoflavone therapy, suggesting that isoflavone supplementation was more apparent in women experiencing a high number of hot flushes per day [10, 11]. Soy germ isoflavone has also been found to exert favourable effects on vasomotor symptoms and

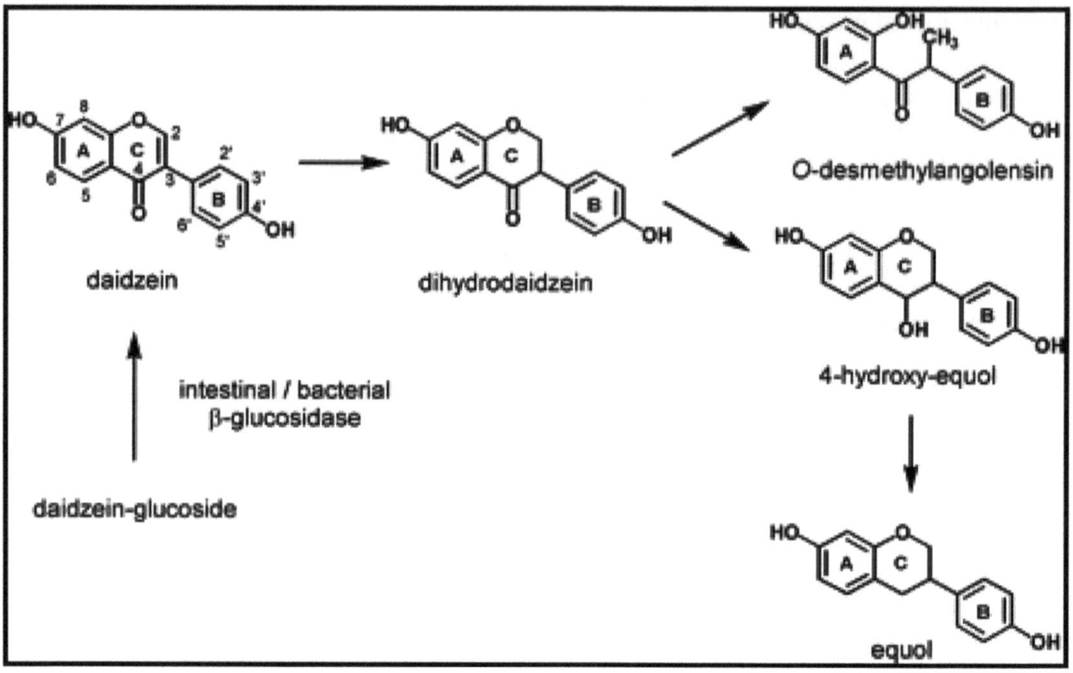

Fig. 6.1 Intestinal bacterial metabolism of the soy isoflavone daidzein to the isoflavone equol (Adapted with permission from Rüfer CE, Glatt H, Kulling SE. Structural elucidation of hydroxylated metabolites of the isoflavan equol by gas chromatography–mass spectrometry and high-performance liquid chromatography–mass spectrometry. Drug Metab Dispos. 2006; 34 (1), 51–60 [31])

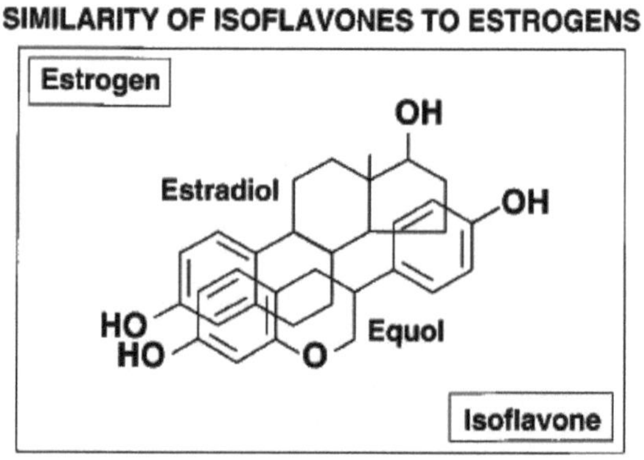

Fig. 6.2 Comparison of the chemical structure of the isoflavone molecule to human estradiol showing similarities of the two molecules (Adapted with permission from Setchell & Cassidy, 1999 [9])

on the lipid profile in postmenopausal women, indicating that it may be useful as an alternative therapy to hormone replacement therapy [33]. Another study in postmenopausal women reported that a soy-rich diet may be efficacious in increasing maturation of vaginal cells. Maturation indices may therefore be a useful marker for examining the efficacy of soy-based dietary interventions against menopausal effects and vaginal atrophy [34]. Isoflavones have been reported to increase nitric oxide breakdown and decrease endothelin-1 levels, thus improving vascular permeability in menopausal women [33].

Soy isoflavones may also have a positive influence on cognitive function, including reception, learning, memory, thinking and expression. As the learning and memory functions are pivotal, many studies on cognitive function focus on these. Soy isoflavones appear to improve cognitive functions by mimicking the effects of estrogen in the brain [35]. Soy isoflavones, however, do not appear to be useful in the treatment of depression [36]. A recent review [37] has questioned recommendations for soy isoflavone consumption since the review found the beneficial effects on climacteric complaints were very weak. In addition there were no clinical endpoint studies with the exclusive aim of investigating the effect of soy or soy isoflavone intake on incidence of mammary cancer and few examining their effects on cardiovascular events [37].

Isoflavones have also been hypothesised to protect against chronic diseases such as osteoporosis, breast cancer and cardiovascular disease. Clinical studies in postmenopausal women have examined the effects of soy food, soy protein isolate or isoflavone tablets on bone mineral content (BMC) and bone mineral density (BMD) or bone turnover markers. Soy isoflavone supplements were shown to moderately decrease levels of the bone resorption marker, urinary deoxypyridinoline (DPD), although they had no effect on bone formation markers, serum bone alkaline phosphatase (BAP) and serum osteocalcin (OC) in menopausal women [38]. In another study, an intake of 100 mg soy isoflavone per day for 1 year was shown to stabilise bone loss in early menopause [39], while a more recent study [15], treatment with two soy isoflavones, 80 and 120 mg/day for 36 months in postmenopausal women did not show a bone-sparing effect, except for a modest effect at the femoral neck [15]. Spence et al. [40] reported consumption of isolated soy protein lowered loss of urinary calcium but was not associated with improved calcium retention, and soy isoflavones did not significantly affect calcium metabolism [40]. While results from another intervention study reported that soy isoflavones had little favourable effect on body composition or physical performance in postmenopausal women [41].

A review of the literature indicates that the results available to date are inconclusive because of the heterogeneity in study designs, treatment dose, duration of treatment, type of soy preparation or subject characteristics, with few studies of sufficient duration to determine the long-term efficacy of isoflavone especially on menopausal symptoms and bone. The estrogen-like effect of soy isoflavone has also given rise to safety concerns [42] with trial data indicating no serious safety concerns with the short term use and low dose of soy isoflavones [15].

Bone Strength and Osteopenia

The bone tissue is in a continual process of breakdown and rebuilding, ensuring that bones are repaired and remain strong [43]. Bone strength is a product of both BMD and bone quality, including bone turnover and mineralisation [43]. Decrease in BMD can lead to osteopenia. Both BMD and BMC can be measured by various methods but bone quality is not readily quantifiable. Various techniques are available to quantify bone mass such as DXA (dual-energy X-ray absorptiometry) and Q-CT (quantitative computed tomography), p-DXA (peripheral dual-energy X-ray absorptiometry) with the most accurate and precise technique being the DXA scan [44]. Bone densitometry can reveal the state of bone health. According to the World Health Organisation criteria, osteopenia is defined by a T-score ranging from −1 to −2.5, compared to normal BMD with a T-score range of −1 to +1.

A strong correlation exists between fracture risk and bone density, and this relationship is even stronger than that between cholesterol and heart disease (Fig. 6.3).

Calcium Bioavailability from Fortified Soymilk in Osteopenic Postmenopausal Women

A clinical study conducted in our laboratory [45] compared the calcium absorption of fortified soymilk (CFSM) to cows' milk in osteopenic postmenopausal women. The soy milk tested, commercially available, was fortified with a phosphate of calcium to achieve similar calcium content to cows' milk. The study, being the first to examine calcium absorption from an Australian fortified soy milk, showed

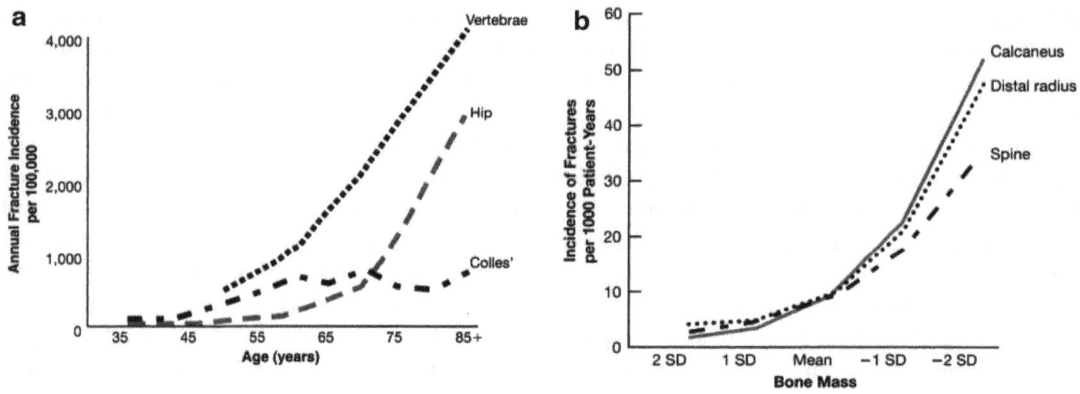

Fig. 6.3 (**a**) Fracture risk with aging in white women. (**b**) Fracture risk versus bone density (Adapted with permission from Camacho & Miller PD, 2007 [43])

the bioavailability of calcium in CFSM is similar to that of cows' milk [45]. Further investigations are needed over a longer term to show whether similar benefit accrues in bone building and maintenance when consuming cows' milk compared to CFSM.

Various factors contribute toward increased calcium absorption and bioavailability. Reducing the phytic acid content of soy milk can potentially increase the absorption not only of calcium but also other minerals such as iron, zinc, copper and magnesium [7]. In addition, fermentation of soy foods with probiotics (*Lactobacillus acidophilus*, *L. casei*, *L. plantarum*, *Bifidobacterium bifidum* and *B. longum*) has also the potential benefit of increasing calcium bioavailability and absorption. Probiotic foods contain live microorganisms, such as lactic acid bacteria (LAB), which promote health by improving the balance of microflora in the intestines as well as improve mineral bioavailability [46, 47]. Studies have shown that during fermentation with certain strains of LAB, the enzyme phytase produced can help catalyse the stepwise hydrolysis of phytic acid [6], while fermentation of dough using certain LAB can produce the enzyme phytase [48], therefore potentially assisting with optimal calcium absorption. However, in a pilot study conducted in our laboratory [49] we compared calcium absorption of fortified soymilk with that of fermented and fortified soymilk in osteopenic postmenopausal women and reported that fermentation has little effect on calcium absorption (Fig. 6.4) [49].

Fermentation of soymilk with LAB may have various potential benefits in enhancing the calcium bioavailability from fortified soymilk and provide a health promoting fermented fortified soy beverage that can be accessible to the general population with the aim of minimising osteoporosis. According to the results obtained in our in vitro study [20], the fermentation of CFSM with probiotics may be a promising way to enhance calcium bioavailability, contribute to bone health and provide the known beneficial effects of probiotic consumption. Longer studies with larger sample size are required to determine beneficial effects in vivo.

Conclusion

Prevention of osteoporosis in women depends in part on maintenance of high calcium intake throughout life and particularly after menopause to slow the rate of bone loss. Calcium nutrition not only is important for bone health but also has been implicated in such disorders as hypertension, colon cancer and kidney stones. Recent studies on calcium absorption and bone metabolism have shown that consumption of soy protein and isoflavones may be associated with attenuation of bone loss, lowering of urinary calcium and increase of bone mineral density in postmenopausal women.

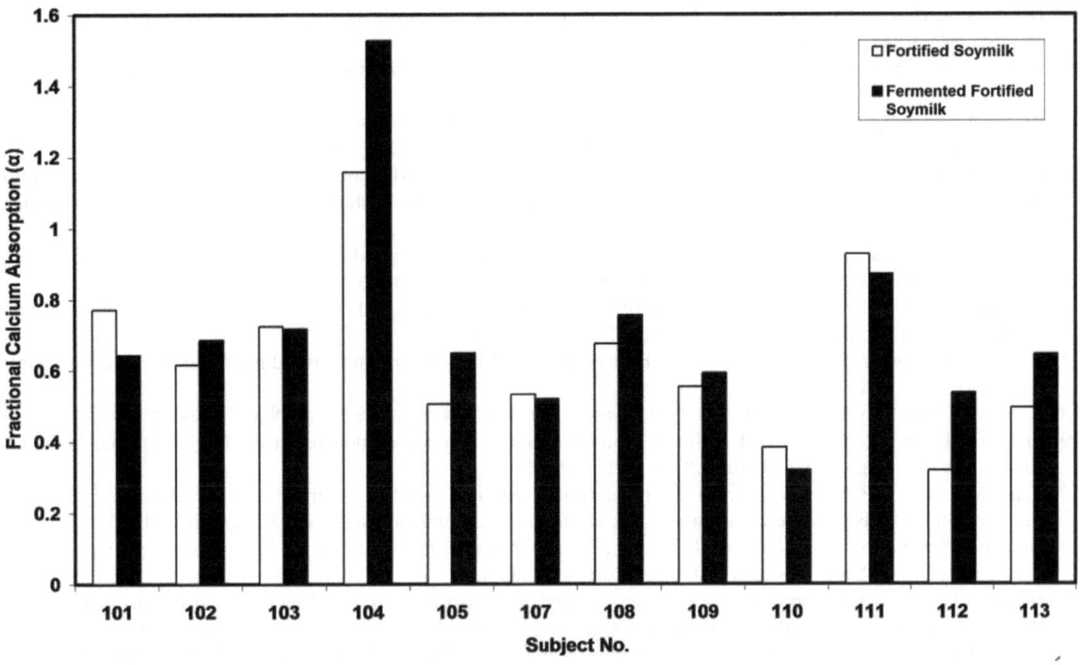

Fig. 6.4 Fractional calcium absorption from calcium fortified soymilk and fermented calcium fortified soya milk (Adapted with permission from Tang et al., 2011 [49])

The calcium absorption from soymilk fortified with calcium is found to be similar to that of cows' milk in osteopenic postmenopausal women. Soymilk can therefore be successfully fortified to deliver the same levels of calcium as cows' milk, and may be used as a substitute for cows' milk in the diets of osteopenic postmenopausal women, vegetarians and individuals with lactose or other forms of intolerance.

References

1. Nordin BEC. Calcium in health and disease. Food Nutr Agricult. 1997;20:13–26.
2. Nordin BEC. Calcif Tissue Int. 2008;83:365–7.
3. The North American Menopause Society. Management of osteoporosis in postmenopausal women: 2010 position statement. Menopause. 2010;17:25–54.
4. McCarron DA, Heaney RP. Estimated healthcare savings associated with adequate dairy food intake. Am J Hypertens. 2004;17:88–97.
5. Calcium, Vitamin D and Osteoporosis - A guide for consumers. Osteoporosis Australia, 4th edition, 2010; 6–10. www.osteoporosis.org.au.
6. Reale A, Mannina L, Tremonte P, et al. Phytate degradation by lactic acid bacteria and yeasts during the wholemeal dough fermentation: a 31P NMR study. J Agric Food Chem. 2004;52:6300–5.
7. Lonnerdal B, Jayawickrama L, Lien LE. Effect of reducing the phytate content and of partially hydrolyzing the protein in soy formula on zinc and copper absorption and status in infant rhesus monkeys and rat pups. Am J Clin Nutr. 1999;69:490–6.
8. Heaney RP. Bone as Calcium nutrient source. In: Weaver CM, Heaney RP, editors, Calcium in human health. New Jersey Humana Press; 2006; 7–12.
9. Setchell KDR, Cassidy A. Dietary isoflavones: biological effects and relevance to human health. Nutr J. 1999;129(3):758s–67.
10. Messina M, Hughes C. Efficacy of soyfoods and soybean isoflavone supplements for alleviating menopausal symptoms is positively related to initial hot flush frequency. J Med Food. 2003;6:1–11.

11. Howes LG, Howes JB, Knight DC. Isoflavone therapy for menopausal flushes: a systematic review and meta-analysis. Maturitas. 2006;55(3):203–11.
12. Huntley AL, Ernst E. Soy for the treatment of perimenopausal symptoms—a systematic review. Maturitas. 2004;47(1):1–9.
13. Atkinson C, Compston JE, Day NE, et al. The effects of phytoestrogen isoflavones on bone density in women: a double blind, randomized, placebo-controlled trial. Am J Clin Nutr. 2004;79:326–33.
14. Chen YM, Ho SC, Lam SSH, et al. Soy isoflavones have a favorable effect on bone loss in chinese postmenopausal women with lower bone mass: a double-blind, randomized, controlled trial. J Clin Endocrinol Metab. 2003;88(10):4740–7.
15. Alekel DL, van Loan MD, Koehler KJ, et al. The soy isiflavone for reducitn bone loss (SIRBL) study: a 3-y randomized controlled trial in postmenopausal women. Am J Clin Nutr. 2010;91:218–30.
16. Vantanparasat H, Chilibeck PD. Does the effect of soy phytoestrogens on bone in postmenopausal women depend on the equol-producing phenotype? Nutr Rev. 2007;65:294–9.
17. Heaney RP, Dowell MS, Rafferty K, et al. Bioavailability of the calcium in fortified milk, with some observations on method. Am J Clin Nutr. 2000;71(5):1166.
18. Heaney RP, Rafferty K, Bierman J. Not all calcium-fortified beverages are equal. Nutr Today. 2005;40(1):39–44.
19. Zhao Y, Martin BR, Weaver CM. Calcium bioavailability of calcium carbonate fortified soymilk is equivalent to cow's milk in young women. J Nutr. 2005;135:2379–82.
20. Tang AL, Shah NP, Wilcox G, et al. Fermentation of calcium-fortified soymilk with lactobacillus: effects on calcium solubility, isoflavone conversion, and production of organic acids. J Food Sci. 2007;72(9):431–6.
21. Gueldner SH, Grabo TN, Newman ED, et al. Osteoporosis: clinical guidelines for prevention, diagnosis and management. New York: Springer Publising Company; 2008.
22. Heaney RP. Osteoporosis: protein, minerals, vitamins and other micronutrients. In: Bendich A, Deckelbaum RJ, editors. Preventive nutrition: the comprehensive guide for health professionals. 3rd ed. Totowa, NJ: Humana Press Inc.; 2005.
23. Nordin BEC, Need AG, Morris HA. Metabolic bone and stone disease. 3rd ed. New York: Churchill Livingston; 1993.
24. Heaney RP. Dietary protein and phosphorus do not affect calcium absorption. Am J Clin Nutr. 2000;72:758–61.
25. Heaney RP. Absorbing calcium. Clin Chem. 1999;45:161–2.
26. Patterson KY, Veillon C. Stable isotopes of minerals as metabolic tracers in human nutrition research. Exp Biol Med. 2001;226:271–82.
27. Fairweather-Tait S, Fox TE, Harvey LJ, Teucher B, Dainty J. Methods for analysis of trace-element absorption. In: Jackson M, editor. Advances in isotope methods for the analysis of trace elements in man: Boca Raton (FL), CRC Press, 2001.
28. Liu K. Soybeans as functional foods and ingredients. Champaign, IL: AOCS Press; 2004.
29. Lopez-Huertas E, Teucher B, Boza JJ, et al. Absorption of calcium from milks enriched with fruto-oligosaccharides, tricalcium phosphate, and milk solids. Am J Clin Nutr. 2006;83:310–6.
30. Singh G, Arora S, Sharma GS, et al. Heat stability and calcium bioavailability of calcium-fortified milk. Lebenson Wiss Technol. 2007;40:625–31.
31. Rüfer CE, Glatt H, Kulling SE. Structural elucidation of hydroxylated metabolites of the isoflavan equol by gas chromatography—mass spectrometry and high-performance liquid chromatography-mass spectrometry. Drug Metab Dispos. 2006;34(1):51–60.
32. Tham D, Gardner C, Haskell W. Potential health benefits of dietary phyto-oestrogens: a review of the clinical, epidemiological, and mechanistic evidence. J Clin Endocrinol Metab. 1998;83:2223–35.
33. Petri Nahas E, Nahás Neto J, De Luca L, et al. Benefits of soy germ isoflavones in postmenopausal women with contraindication for conventional hormone replacement therapy. Maturitas. 2004;48(4):372–80.
34. Chiechi LM, Putignano G, Guerra V, et al. The effect of a soy rich diet on the vaginal epithelium in postmenopause: a randomized double blind trial. Maturitas. 2003;45(4):241–6.
35. Cherma D, Coomarasamt A, El-Toukhy T. Non-hormonal therapy of post-menopausal vasomotor symptoms; a structured evidence-based review. Arch Gynecol Obstet. 2007;276:463–9.
36. de Sousa-Muñoz RL, Filizola RG. Efficacy of soy isoflavones for depressive symptoms of the climacteric syndrome. Maturitas. 2009;63(1):89–93.
37. Wuttke W, Jarry H, Seidlová-Wuttke D. Isoflavones—safe food additives or dangerous drugs? Ageing Res Rev. 2007;6(2):150–88.
38. Taku K, Melby MK, Kurzer MS, et al. Effects of soy isoflavone supplements on bone turnover markers in menopausal women: Systematic review and meta-analysis of randomized controlled trials. Bone. 2010;47(2):413–23.
39. Huang H-Y, Yang H-P, Yang H-T, et al. One-year soy isoflavone supplementation prevents early postmenopausal bone loss but without a dose-dependent effect. J Nutr Biochem. 2006;17(8):509–17.
40. Spence LA, Lipscomb ER, Cadogan J, et al. The effect of soy protein and soy isoflavones on calcium metabolism in postmenopausal women: a randomized crossover study. Am J Clin Nutr. 2005;81(4):916–22.

41. Kok L, Kreijkamp-Kaspers S, Grobbee DE, et al. Soy isoflavones, body composition, and physical performance. Maturitas. 2005;52(2):102–10.
42. Messina MJ, Wood CJ. Soy isoflavones, estrogen theraphy and breast cancer risk: analysis and commentary. Nutr J. 2008;7:17–28.
43. Camacho PM, Miller PD. Osteoporosis: a guide for clinicians. Philadelphia: Wolters Kluwer/Lippincott Williams & Wilkins; 2007.
44. A picture of osteoporosis. Canberra: Australian Institute of Health and Welfare, 2008.
45. Tang AL, Walker KZ, Wilcox G, et al. Calcium absorption in Australian osteopenic postmenopausal women: an acute comparative study of fortified soymilk to cows' milk. Asia Pac J Clin Nutr. 2010;19(2):243–9.
46. Gibson GR, Rastall RA, Fuller R. The health benefits of probiotics and prebiotics. In: Fuller R, Perdigon G, editors. Gut flora, nutrition, immunity and health. Blackwell Publishing Ltd; 2003. p. 52–69.
47. Tsangalis D, Ashton JF, Stojanovska L, et al. Development of an isoflavone aglycone-enriched soymilk using soy germ, soy protein and bifidobacteria. Food Res Int. 2004;37:301–12.
48. Angelis MD, Gallo G, Corbo MR, et al. Phytase activity in sour dough lactic acid bacteria: purification and characterization of a phytase from Lactobacillus sanfranciscensis CB1. Int J Food Microbiol. 2003;87(2003):259–70.
49. Tang AL, Wilcox G, Walker KZ, et al. Fermentation of calcium-fortified soya milk does not appear to enhance acute calcium absorption in osteopenic postmenopasual women. Br J Nutr. 2011;105:282–6.

Chapter 7
Postmenopausal Homocysteine, Vitamin B12, Folate Levels and Bone Metabolism: A Focus on Fractures

Berna Haliloglu and Hakan Peker

Key Points

- Plasma homocysteine concentrations are increased in postmenopausal women in comparison with premenopausal women.
- High homocysteine levels, low folate and vitamin B12 status have been associated with osteoporotic fractures in some, but not all, studies.
- Whether high levels of homocysteine have a direct effect on bone or whether the effect is mediated through folate and/or vitamin B12 deficiencies is uncertain.
- Supplementation with folate and vitamin B12 may also reduce the risk of fractures.
- Whether the risk reduction is due to the lowering of serum homocysteine or an increase in B12/folate is not known.
- Although the evidence is limited, supplemental folic acid or vitamin B12 for the treatment of osteoporosis or primary prevention of fracture is not recommended.

Keywords Menopause • Homocysteine • Vitamin B12 • Folate • Bone

Abbreviations

BMD	Bone mineral density
FSH	Follicle stimulating hormone
Hcy	Homocysteine
SAM	S-Adenosylmethionine
SAH	S-Adenosylhomocysteine
CBS	Cystathionine-ß-synthase

B. Haliloglu, M.D. (✉)
Department of Obstetrics and Gynecology, School of Medicine,
University of Maltepe, Ataturk Cd. Cam Sk. 3/A Istanbul, Turkey
e-mail: bernahaliloglu@yahoo.com; berna.haliloglu@maltepe.edu.tr

H. Peker, M.D.
Department of Obstetrics and Gynecology, Memorial Hizmet Hospital,
Bahcelievler Mah. 34180 Istanbul, Turkey
e-mail: drhakanpeker@hotmail.com

C.J.H. Martin et al. (eds.), *Nutrition and Diet in Menopause*, Nutrition and Health,
DOI 10.1007/978-1-62703-373-2_7, © Springer Science+Business Media New York 2013

MS	Methionine synthase
MTHFR	5,10-Methylenetetrahydrofolate reductase
THF	Tetrahydrofolate
BHMT	Betaine homocysteine methyltransferase
DMG	Dimethylglycine
HRT	Hormone replacement therapy
HHcy	Hyperhomocysteinemia

Introduction

Menopause is the most significant period for bone loss in women, when rapid metabolic and endocrine changes occur. The rate of bone loss is highly dependent upon hormonal, environmental, and genetic factors. Bone loss initiates before the last menstrual period and the percent decrease in BMD in the first 5 years postmenopause can be as high as 9–13 % [1]. In a longitudinal study including healthy premenopausal and perimenopausal women, no bone loss was observed in premenopausal women, while accelerated bone loss was observed in the 2–3 years prior to cessation of menstruation, with a significant correlation between the rate of bone loss and elevation of FSH and bone turnover markers [2].

Several factors are known to affect bone metabolism, and to increase the risk of bone fractures. Recently, elevated Hcy levels have been reported to be responsible for bone fractures [3]. However, confusing data exist regarding the relation between Hcy and bone loss in postmenopausal women because of heterogeneity of studies [4, 5]. The mechanism for increased fracture risk and Hcy is not also clear.

Levels of Hcy are inversely related to the folates and possibly vitamin B12 [6]. While some studies reported that folate deficiency, but not Hcy and vitamin B12, had an important role in the vertebral BMD decline of postmenopausal women, others showed that vitamin B12 was an independent risk factor for osteoporosis and bone fractures [6, 7]. Hence, whether bone is affected by increased Hcy levels or by deficiency of the cofactors necessary for Hcy remethylation to methionine is unclear.

This topic reviews the relationship between postmenopausal bone fracture risk and elevated Hcy levels, vitamin B12 and folate deficiencies, and the evidence evaluating the use of vitamin supplements that lower Hcy levels.

Etiology of Hyperhomocysteinemia

Homocysteine is a thiol amino-acid synthesized during the metabolic conversion of methionine to cysteine. Dietary methionine is converted to the methyl donor SAM and is demethylated to SAH and Hcy. Once generated, Hcy is metabolized by two different pathways: transsulfuration or remethylation [8]. The transsulfuration of Hcy to cysteine is catalyzed by CBS which requires pyridoxal phosphate (vitamin B6) as a cofactor. Hcy can also be remethylated through the folate cycle. This pathway requires the MS and vitamin B12 as well as the MTHFR and folic acid, which enters the cycle as THF. In liver and kidney, Hcy is also remethylated by the enzyme BHMT, which transfers a methyl group to Hcy via demethylation of betaine to DMG (Fig. 7.1).

Elevations in the plasma Hcy concentration may arise from genetic defects in the enzymes involved in Hcy metabolism, nutritional deficiencies in vitamin cofactors, or other factors. Some drugs used in the treatment of hypercholesterolemia may increase Hcy levels by approximately 30 %; however, the clinical significance of this is uncertain. Cigarette smoking and chronic kidney failure may also elevate Hcy levels [9].

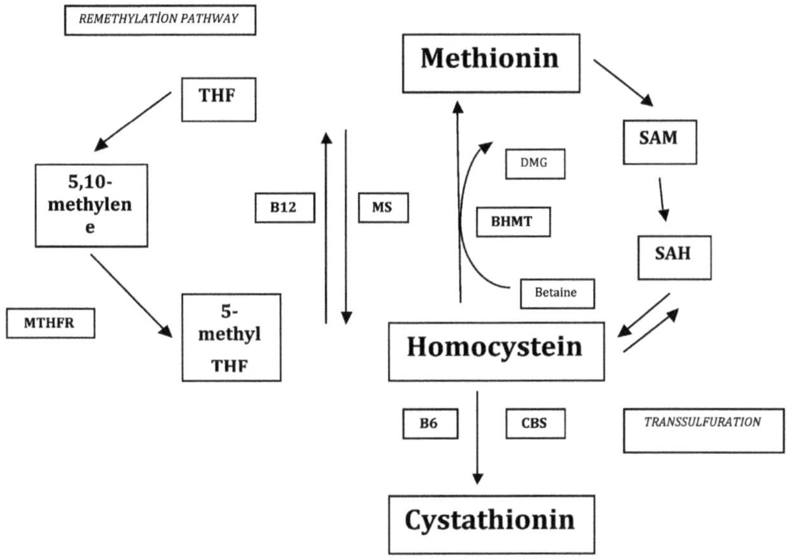

Fig. 7.1 Homocysteine metabolism. Hcy uses two pathways for biotransformation: transsulfuration and remethylation. In transsulfuration, Hcy is transformed into cysteine by two reactions that involve CBS with vitamin B6 as a cofactor. The remethylation pathway involves the MS which uses vitamin B12 as a cofactor and methylenetetrahydrofolate as the substrate. The formation of methylenetetrahydrofolate is catalyzed by MTHFR which uses folic acid as a cofactor

Mutations in genes responsible for the metabolism of Hcy can result in severe forms of HHcy, termed homocystinuria. The most common form of genetic HHcy results from production of a thermolabile variant of MTHFR with reduced enzymatic activity (T mutation). The gene encoding for this variant contains an alanine-to-valine substitution at amino acid 677 (C677T). The prevalence of variant gene is estimated 10 % [10].

On the other hand, increased blood levels of Hcy may reflect deficiency of folate, vitamin B6, and/or vitamin B12. Plasma folate and B12 levels, in particular, are strong determinants of the Hcy concentration. Homocysteine levels are inversely related to folate consumption, reaching a stable baseline level when folate intake exceeds 400 μg/day. Vitamin B6 is a weaker determinant [11].

The etiology of HHcy was summarized in Table 7.1.

Plasma Hcy and Menopausal Status

Menopause is that stage of a woman's life when ovulation ceases and ovarian hormonal activity begins to be insufficient. Menopausal status seems to be an important determining factor for plasma Hcy levels. It is well known that plasma Hcy concentrations are reduced in premenopausal women in comparison with postmenopausal women. In premenopausal women, the higher concentrations of serum 17 β-estradiol may account in part for the lower levels of Hcy [12].

The levels of Hcy vary throughout the menstrual cycle. The mean concentrations of Hcy were found as 7.8 μmol/l in the luteal phase and 8.9 μmol/l in the follicular phase in premenopausal women; however, there has been no correlation between the levels of Hcy and those of estradiol or progesterone [12]. Therefore, when making any determination of Hcy it is important to note what phase of the menstrual cycle that the patient is in at the time of the test.

Table 7.1 Etiology of hyperhomocysteinemia

Genetic mutations	MTHFR polymorphism
Nutritional deficiencies	Folate deficiency
	Cobalamine deficiency
	Pyridoxine deficiency
Disease states	CBS deficiency
	MS deficiency
	Chronic renal disease
	Severe psoriasis
	Pernicious anemia
Drugs	Cholestryamine
	Methotrexate
	Antiepileptics
Caffeinated coffee	
Tobacco	

HHcy is a pathological condition characterized by an increase in plasma concentration of total Hcy. There have been numerous genetic, nutritional and systemic reasons for increased Hcy levels

Studies on endogenous estrogen and Hcy concentrations are scarce. Wouters et al. [13] have reported that plasma Hcy concentration after methionine loading was negatively correlated with serum estradiol concentration. However, a decreased serum estrogen concentration may not necessarily lead to a decrease in Hcy concentration [14]. Numerous studies have confirmed a reduction in the Hcy levels after HRT [12]. It has been suggested that combined estrogen and progesterone therapy would be capable of even greater reductions in the levels of Hcy than the administration of estrogen alone. Nevertheless, other studies showed no change for Hcy levels after estrogen treatment in surgically postmenopausal women [12]. Hence, it is possible that menopause rather than estrogen may modify plasma Hcy levels.

The reduction of Hcy levels in postmenopausal women may also be achieved by administering folic acid. Two studies reported significant inverse correlation between the levels of Hcy and folic acid in postmenopausal women, but neither of them found any correlation between the levels of vitamin B12 [12]. A diet-rich in folic acid provides a reduction in the Hcy concentrations in postmenopausal women, even when the basal concentrations in serum are normal [15]. Additionally, low doses of 400–500 μg per day have resulted sufficient to reduce the levels of Hcy in premenopausal and postmenopausal women [12].

HHcy and Bone Fractures

The relationship between Hcy and skeletal abnormality was first established in studies of homocystinuria, caused by deficiency of CBS. Two population-based studies, from the Netherlands and Framingham, USA, have demonstrated an association between increased levels of Hcy and risk of osteoporotic fracture in both male and female subjects [16].

Clinical studies examining the association between Hcy and fracture show inconsistent results. High Hcy levels in adults have been associated with osteoporotic fractures in some, but not all, studies [4, 5].

Table 7.2 Studies investigating the association of homocysteine, folate, and vitamin B12 with bone mineral density in postmenopausal women

Author	Race	Year	Homocysteine	Folate	Vitamin B12
Cagnacci A	Italian	2003	Not related	Related	Not related
Golbahar J	Iranian	2004	Not related	Related	Not studied
Herrmann M	German	2005	Not related	Not studied	Not studied
Baines M	British	2007	Not related	Related	Not related
Bozkurt N	Turkish	2009	Related	Not related	Related
Haliloglu B	Turkish	2010	Not related	Not related	Not related
Rumbak I	Crotian	2011	Not related	Not related	Not related
Ouzzif Z	Moroccan	2010	Related	Not related	Related

There have been conflicting results about the relationship between BMD and Hcy, vitamin B12 and folate levels. The different findings may be result from the heterogeneity of studies

Table 7.3 The "bone quality" term represents mechanical stability involving numerous factors

Geometry
Bone mass distribution
Interconnection of spongy trabeculae
Cross-linking of collagen molecules
Integration of collagen molecules in bone matrix

The "bone mineral density" cannot provide information about the microstructure of bone matrix which is probably crucial for mechanical stability. The "bone quality" term seems to be more illustrative to define mechanical properties of bone

As previously shown, the levels of Hcy, vitamin B12 and folates are related to each other. One study reported that Hcy at the top fourth quartile is a risk factor for bone fractures and is also characterized by significantly lower levels of folates, and in lesser extent, of vitamin B12 [6]. On the other hand, the first quartile of folates is associated with increased levels of Hcy and decreased levels of vitamin B12. The relation between Hcy, folates and vitamin B12 show that inferences of cause-effect relationship with BMD or bone fractures gained by measuring one single parameter may be misleading.

Even if all these three parameters are considered, conflicting results were reported in literature. While some studies showed that folates but not Hcy or vitamin B12 independently relate to vertebral BMD, others reported no association between vitamin B12, folate and Hcy levels vertebral BMD in postmenopausal women [6, 17, 18]. Vitamin B12 levels, but not folates were found to be related with BMD and osteoporosis in some studies, while low levels of folates, but not vitamin B12 levels were shown associated with low BMD in women in the Hordaland Homocysteine Study [18]. The studies investigating the relationship between BMD and Hcy, vitamin B12 and folate levels were summarized in Table 7.2.

On the other hand, BMD is not the sole predictor of whether an individual will experience a fracture. Bone quality is a broad term involving numerous factors such as geometry, bone mass distribution, trabecular bone architecture and bone mineral and matrix tissue properties (Table 7.3). It is possible that the underlying mechanism of the relation between HHcy and bone fractures might be the mechanistic link which cannot be shown with BMD as mentioned below. In addition, included population, race, age, size of sample, design of study, levels of folate, vitamin B12 and Hcy may all represent differences between studies in the literature (Table 7.4).

Table 7.4 Main causes of different results in studies investigating relationship between BMD and Hcy levels

Age
Population
Vitamin B12 and folate levels
Menopausal status
Dietary habits
Size of sample
Design of study
Site of BMD measurement

BMD measurement could not provide information about the microstructure of bone matrix (e.g., cross-linking of collagen molecules, integration of collagen molecules in bone matrix, interconnection of spongy trabeculae), which is probably crucial for mechanical stability. Therefore, underlying mechanism of increased Hcy levels and osteoporotic fractures may be a mechanistic link which cannot be shown with BMD measurements

Table 7.5 The underlying mechanism of increased Hcy levels and osteoporosis

Protein homocysteinylation
Oxidative damage
Interfering lysyl oxidase action
Collagen posttranslational modifications
Stimulation of osteoclast formation and activity

The reason of different results of studies investigating the relationship between BMD and Hcy levels may be multifactorial as shown below

Role of Hcy Levels

Recent data show a correlation between Hcy levels and fracture risk. Hcy is nonenzymatically added to free cysteinyl residues in proteins and can cleave disulfide bridges with damage to the folding pattern of the proteins [17]. As a result, protein homocysteinylation can lead to changes in the biological functions of proteins such as collagen. Moreover, moderate to high Hcy levels are known to cause oxidative damage which can possibly harm the trabecular structures [17]. Hcy is known to interfere with lysyl oxidase action, thus altering collagen posttranslational modifications and cross-link profiles. Proper cross-link formation is critical for normal collagen structure and bone mechanical properties [18]. Thus, higher Hcy levels may damage bone mechanical stability and cause fractures.

Loss of bone mass, measured by BMD, is considered an important risk factor for bone fragility and fracture. However, there is considerable overlap in BMD between populations that do and do not develop bone fractures [18]. The BMD measurement and none of the existing biochemical turnover markers have been shown to provide information about the microstructure of bone matrix (e.g., cross-linking of collagen molecules, integration of collagen molecules in bone matrix, interconnection of spongy trabeculae), which is probably crucial for mechanical stability.

For this reason, the underlying mechanism of increased Hcy levels and osteoporosis may be a mechanistic link which cannot be shown with BMD and biochemical bone turnover marker measurements. In spite of several studies reported that increased Hcy levels were a risk factor for osteoporotic fractures, most studies levels found no relationship between Hcy levels and BMD/biochemical bone turnover markers [5, 6, 17]. Hence, despite increased Hcy levels reported to be a risk factor for osteoporotic fractures, the lack of correlation between Hcy and BMD or biochemical bone turnover markers in most studies is not surprising. In the light of these findings, relation between Hcy and bone fractures seems to be more complicated (Table 7.5).

Role of Folate and Vitamin B12 Levels

Several studies as well as some recent animal studies have indicated that an alimentary deficiency of folate and vitamin B12 is capable of inducing a moderate HHcy. However, no effect detectable of these metabolic alterations on bone quality was found in mice [8]. In contrast, another study in rats demonstrated that administration of a Hcy-supplemented diet is associated with a significant alteration of cancellous bone structure and bone strength [19]. One explanation for these conflicting results might be due to different bone tissue accumulation of Hcy. The administration of the Hcy-supplemented diet may led to a tissue specific accumulation of Hcy, while tissue concentrations of Hcy in bone were not affected by the folate- and vitamin B12-deficient diet.

Vitamin B12 was advocated as an independent risk factor for osteoporosis and bone fractures and also claimed to show its effects when below a cut-off value of 220 pmol/L [6]. Another study indicates that women those that had vitamin B12 levels below 207 pmol/L had a higher annual rate of reduction in total hip BMD, but not calcaneal BMD, than those with higher levels [7]. In spite of these studies, others reported no association between vitamin B12 levels and BMD [5, 16]. The difference in findings of the association of serum vitamin B12 levels with BMD may be result from population demographic differences and the site of assessment of BMD.

Although low folate levels were shown as a risk factor for osteoporosis in Italian, Iranian and British women [6, 16, 20], other studies reported no relationship between folate and BMD in Crotian and Turkish women [17, 18]. HHcy, due to folate deficiency, was shown to be related with lower BMD values in postmenopausal Iranian women [20]. Folates may exert effects other than the reduction of Hcy levels. Folates are necessary for protein and nucleic acid methylation and for the nitric oxide synthesis pathway [6]. The latter may be related with bone metabolism. Nitric oxide donors have shown to decrease bone resorption and increase bone formation [6]. However, another study [21] reported plasma Hcy, but not folate levels, were associated with osteoporosis in relatively young postmenopausal Turkish women. It seems that dietary habits, racial differences, the site of BMD measurement, and study population differences (gender, age, etc.) may affect the study results investigating the relationship between BMD and folate levels as well as vitamin B12. Additionally, it has been shown that experimental folate and vitamin B 12 deficiencies had no effect on bone quality in rats [22].

The Effect of Vitamin Supplementation on Bone Fractures

Concentrations of Hcy show a strong inverse correlation with folates and much weaker one with vitamin B12. The reduction of Hcy levels in postmenopausal women may also be achieved by administering folic acid. Mineral water fortified with folic acid, vitamins B6, B12, and D, and calcium enhance folate status and reduce plasma Hcy concentration in normohomocysteinemic subjects without folate deficiency [8, 12]. Additionally, a daily vitamin B12 intake of 6 μg was shown to be sufficient to correct Hcy levels in postmenopausal Danish women [23].

Combination folate and vitamin B12 therapy may lower fracture risk in elderly patients with residual hemiplegia after an ischemic stroke [24]. On the other hand, a predefined secondary analysis of the HOPE-2 trial suggests that this approach is not effective in individuals selected on the basis of cardiovascular disease (rather than fracture risk) [25]. In this trial, adults at high risk for cardiovascular disease were randomly assigned to treatment with daily folic acid (2.5 mg), vitamin B12 (1 mg), and vitamin B6 (50 mg) or placebo. Mean baseline Hcy concentration was normal and vitamin supplementation did not reduce the incidence of vertebral or nonvertebral fractures compared with placebo.

Whether the risk reduction is due to the lowering of serum Hcy or an increase in B12/folate is not known. In addition, it is not known whether this therapeutic approach will be effective in patients with normal baseline Hcy, serum B12, and folate concentrations or in other populations. Recommendation of supplemental folic acid or vitamin B12 for the treatment of osteoporosis or primary prevention of fracture is still debated.

Conclusions

Increased Hcy levels are precisely known to be a risk factor for osteoporotic fractures. HHcy may be due to folate and/or vitamin B12 deficiencies. It is not clear, however, whether high levels of Hcy have a direct effect on bone or whether the effect is mediated through another factor, such as folate and/or vitamin B12 deficiencies. Further research is needed to determine how Hcy and vitamin B12/folate influence fracture risk, and whether vitamin supplementation may help maintain bone mass and reduce the risk of fracture in women.

References

1. Ravn P, Hetland ML, Overgaard K, Christiansen C. Premenopausal and postmenopausal changes in bone mineral density of the proximal femur measured by dual-energy X-ray absorptiometry. J Bone Miner Res. 1994;9:1975–80.
2. Chapurlat RD, Garnero P, Sornay-Rendu E, et al. Longitudinal study of bone loss in pre- and perimenopausal women: evidence for bone loss in perimenopausal women. Osteoporos Int. 2000;11:493.
3. Van Meurs JB, Dhonukshe-Rutten RA, Plujim SM, van der Klift M, de Jonge R, Lindemans J, et al. Homocysteine levels and the risk of osteoporotic fracture. N Engl J Med. 2004;350:2033–41.
4. Herrmann M, Kraenzlin M, Pape G, Sand-Hill M, Herrmann W. Relation between homocysteine and biochemical bone turnover markers and bone mineral density in peri- and postmenopausal women. Clin Chem Lab Med. 2005;43:1118–223.
5. Cagnacci A, Baldassari F, Rivolta G, Arangino S, Volpe A. Relation of homocysteine, folate, and vitamin B12 to bone mineral density of postmenopausal women. Bone. 2003;3:956–9.
6. Cagnacci A, Bagni B, Zini A, Cannoletta M, Generali M, Volpe A. Relation of folates, vitamin B12 and homocysteine to vertebral bone mineral density change in postmenopausal women. A five-year longitudinal evaluation. Bone. 2008;42:314–20.
7. Stone KL, Bauer DC, Sellmeyer D, Cummings SR. Low serum B12 levels are associated with increased hip bone loss in older women: a prospective study. J Clin Endocrinol Metab. 2004;89:1217–21.
8. Holstein JH, Herrmann M, Schmalenbach J, Obeid R, Ölkü I, Klein M, et al. Deficiencies of folate and vitamin B12 do not affect fracture healing in mice. Bone. 2010;47:151–5.
9. Bazzano LA, He J, Muntner P, Vupputuri S, Whelton PK. Relationship between cigarette smoking and novel risk factors for cardiovascular disease in the United States. Ann Intern Med. 2003;138:891.
10. Abrahamsen B, Madsen JS, Tofteng CL, Stilgren L, Bladbjerg EM, Kristensen SR, et al. Are effects of MTHFR (C677T) genotype on BMD confined to women with low folate and riboflavin intake? Analysis of food records from the Danish osteoporosis prevention study. Bone. 2005;36:577–83.
11. Ubbink JB, Vermaak WJ, van der Merwe A, Becker PJ. Vitamin B-12, vitamin B-6, and folate nutritional status in men with hyperhomocysteinemia. Am J Clin Nutr. 1993;57:47.
12. Calle M, Usandizaga R, Sancha M, Magdaleno F, Herranz A, Cabrillo E. Homocysteine, folic acid and B-group vitamins in obstetrics and gynaecology. Eur J Obstet Gynecol Reprod Biol. 2003;107:125–37.
13. Wouters MG, Moorrees MT, van der Mooren MJ, Blom HJ, Boers GH, Schellekens LA, et al. Plasma homocysteine and menopausal status. Eur J Clin Invest. 1995;25:801–5.
14. Nagata C, Shimizu H, Takami R, Hayashi M, Takeda N, Yasuda K. Soy product intake is inversely associated with serum homocysteine level in premenopausal Japanese women. J Nutr. 2003;133:797–800.
15. Blouin S, Thaler HW, Korninger C, Schmid R, Hofstaetter JG, Zoehrer R, et al. Bone matrix quality and plasma homocysteine levels. Bone. 2009;44:959–64.
16. Baines M, Kredan MB, Usher J, Davison A, Higgins G, Taylor W, et al. The association of homocysteine and its determinants MTHFR genotype, folate, vitamin B12 and vitamin B6 with bone mineral density in postmenopausal British women. Bone. 2007;40:730–6.

17. Haliloglu B, Aksungar FB, Ilter E, Peker H, Akin FT, Ozekici U. Relationship between bone mineral density, bone turnover markers and homocysteine, folate and vitamin B12 levels in postmenopausal women. Arch Gynecol Obstet. 2010;281:663–8.
18. Rumbak I, Zizic V, Sokolic L, Cvijetic Z, Kajfez R, ColicBaric I. Bone mineral density is not associated with homocysteine level, folate and vitamin B(12) status. Arch Gynecol Obstet. 2012;285(4):991–1000.
19. Herrmann M, Tami A, Wildemann B, Wolny M, Wagner A, Schorr H, et al. Hyperhomocysteinemia induces a tissue specific accumulation of homocysteine in bone by collagen binding and adversely affects bone. Bone. 2009;44:467–75.
20. Golbahar J, Hamidi A, Aminzadeh MA, Omrani GR. Association of plasma folate, plasma total homocysteine, but not methylenetetrahydrofolate reductase C667T polymorphism, with bone mineral density in postmenopausal Iranian women: a cross-sectional study. Bone. 2004;35:760–5.
21. Bozkurt N, Erdem M, Yılmaz E, Erdem A, Biri A, Kubatova A, et al. The relationship of homocysteine, B12 and folic acid with the bone mineral density of the femur and lumbar spine in Turkish postmenopausal women. Arch Gynecol Obstet. 2009;280:381–7.
22. Herrmann M, Wildemann B, Wagner A, Wolny M, Schorr H, Taban-Shomal O, et al. Experimental folate and vitamin B12 deficiency does not alter bone quality in rats. J Bone Miner Res. 2009;24:589–96.
23. Bor MV, Lydeking-Olsen E, Moller J, Nexo E. A daily intake of approximately 6 μg vitamin B-12 appears to saturate all the vitamin B-12-related variables in Danish postmenopausal women. Am J Clin Nutr. 2006;83:52–8.
24. Sato Y, Honda Y, Iwamoto J, et al. Effect of folate and mecobalamin on hip fractures in patients with stroke: a randomized controlled trial. JAMA. 2005;293:1082.
25. Sawka AM, Ray JG, Yi Q, et al. Randomized clinical trial of homocysteine level lowering therapy and fractures. Arch Intern Med. 2007;167:2136.

Chapter 8
Antioxidant Vitamins and Carotenoids Associated with Bone Mineral Density in Postmenopause Female Subjects: Japanese Perspectives

Minoru Sugiura

Key Points

Recent studies show that a high dietary intake of fruit and vegetables rich in antioxidants may reduce the risk of osteoporosis. These findings suggest that antioxidants exert beneficial effects on bone metabolism by suppressing oxidative stress. Carotenoids exist in abundance in these foods and have been known to contribute to the body's defense against reactive oxygen species. Our study showed the association of bone mineral density with antioxidant carotenoids. Our findings suggest that high intakes of fruit and vegetables rich in β-cryptoxanthin and β-carotene might provide benefits to bone health in postmenopausal Japanese females. To determine whether these carotenoids are beneficial micronutrients to bone health, further studies will be required.

Keywords Bone mineral density • Carotenoids • Fruit and vegetables • Postmenopausal Japanese female • Oxidative stress

Abbreviations

BMD Bone mineral density
FFQ Food frequency questionnaire

Introduction

Findings from many of the recent nutritional epidemiological studies [1–4] have demonstrated a significant negative association between fruit and vegetable intake and the risk of lifestyle-related diseases, such as cancer, cardiovascular diseases and diabetes. Fruit and vegetables are an important source of nutrients such as vitamins, minerals, and fiber. Recent studies have called attention to the physiological functions of carotenoids, which exist in abundance in these foods. Oxidative stress has recently been revealed to play a key role in the pathogenesis of cancer, cardiovascular diseases, and diabetes. It has also been observed [5–10] that the powerful antioxidant properties found in all varieties of carotenoids could be effective in preventing these lifestyle-related diseases.

M. Sugiura, Ph.D. (✉)
Citrus Research Division, National Institute of Fruit Tree Science,
485-6 Shimizu-Okitsu-nakachou, Shizuoka City, Shizuoka 424-0292, Japan
e-mail: msugiura@affrc.go.jp

C.J.H. Martin et al. (eds.), *Nutrition and Diet in Menopause*, Nutrition and Health,
DOI 10.1007/978-1-62703-373-2_8, © Springer Science+Business Media New York 2013

Several other recent nutritional epidemiological studies [11–15] have also concluded that high intake of fruit is effective in the formation and maintenance of healthy bone. These beneficial properties are attributed to the rich vitamin C content of fruit that is essential for the synthesis of collagen which is required for bone formation. Excess intake of animal protein has been shown to induce metabolic acidosis due to relatively high sulfur amino acid contents, which activates, in turn, bone resorption and exerts a harmful effect on the bones. The intake of cations, such as potassium, calcium, and magnesium, is believed to be crucial for preventing these problems. Fruits, which are rich in potassium and other minerals, have been suggested to be involved in the prevention of born resorption by correcting metabolic acidosis. The report *Diet, Nutrition and the prevention diseases* [1] published in 2003 by the World Health Organization (WHO) and Food and Agriculture Organization (FAO) states, in fact, that increased fruit and vegetable intake might play an important part in the maintenance and formation of healthy bone as well as in the prevention of osteoporosis-related fractures. In the face of many epidemiological studies pointing to the fact that fruit and vegetable intake is beneficial to bone health, one question arises: are vitamins and minerals the only factors influencing bone metabolism? Several studies have recently been looking into how phytocemicals, including flavonoid and carotenoids that are present in fruit and vegetables in abundance, can affect the bones. This paper therefore aims at describing how carotenoids, especially β-cryptoxanthin found in Japanese mandarin orange in abundance, could be effective in preventing osteoporosis.

Carotenoids and β-Cryptoxanthin

Major Carotenoids in Human Serum

Carotenoids are a widely distributed group of naturally occurring pigments, usually red, orange or yellow in color. As many as 750 types of carotenoids [16] have been isolated and identified. The word "carotenoid" is a general term that refers to a group of compounds that have a basic skeleton consisting of 40 carbons formed by eight linked isoprene units. Carotenoid structure is based on a 22-carbon polyene chain containing nine conjugated double bonds, with hydroxy, carbonyl, carboxyl, and epoxy groups attached on both ends of the molecule. People consume carotenoids from various foods. There are six types of major carotenoids [17] in human serum: lycopene, α-carotene, β-carotene, lutein, zeaxanthin, and β-cryptoxanthin (Fig. 8.1). Three of these carotenoids, namely, α-carotene, β-carotene, and β-cryptoxanthin, are converted to vitamin A in the body.

There has recently been great advancement in the understanding of the physiological functions of carotenoids which have been revealed to exhibit various physiological functions, as evidenced by their provitamin A activity as well as their antioxidant, cancer inhibition, and immunostimulatory effects. Furthermore, recent nutritional epidemiological studies [5–10] have provided evidence of new physiological functions of carotenoids that seem to play a role in the prevention of lifestyle-related diseases, such as cancer, cardiovascular diseases and diabetes. Many studies have, in fact, shown that oxidative stress contributes to the development of a wide range of lifestyle-related diseases, including cancer, myocardial infarction, diabetes, and liver diseases. The chemical structure of carotenoids is characterized by extended conjugated double bonds which make carotenoids a powerful antioxidant that can help prevent various diseases by providing protection against oxidative stress.

Of the six major carotenoids found in human serum, little is known on the physiological functions of β-cryptoxanthin, compared with those of β-carotene or lycopene. This may be due to the fact [18, 19] that the concentrations of β-cryptoxanthin in human serum and breast milk is relatively low in many countries where people do not have a habit of eating the Japanese mandarin orange which contains high concentrations of β-cryptoxanthin. It is therefore conceivable that β-cryptoxanthin has not received much attention compared to other types of carotenoids. Mandarin oranges, which are locally

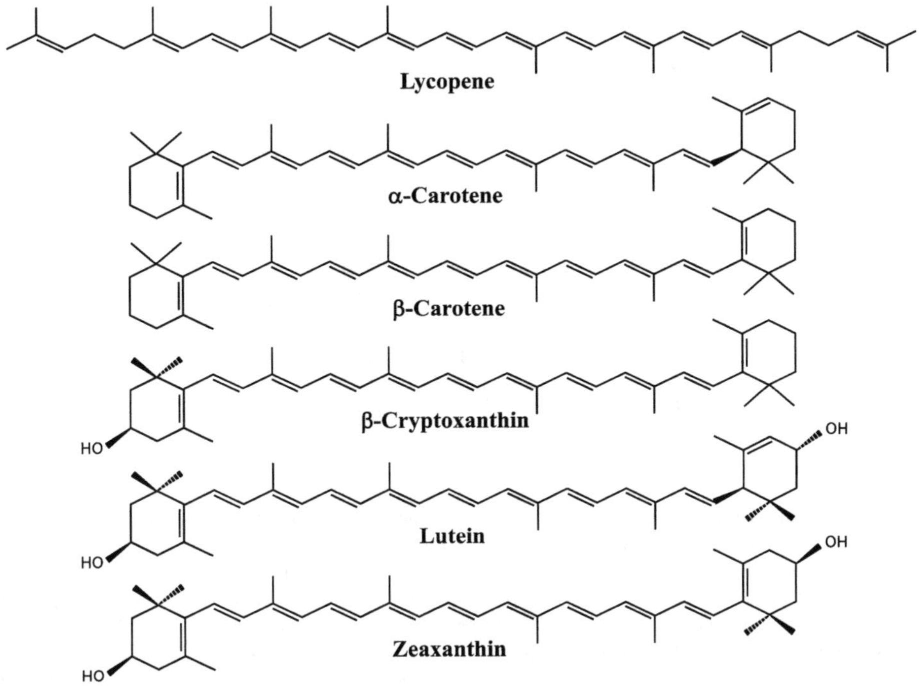

Fig. 8.1 Chemical structure of main six carotenoids

grown in Japan, are the most widely consumed citrus fruit in Japan. In view of this, β-cryptoxanthin intake and its serum level in the Japanese population are probably considerably higher than those in people living in other parts of the world. This leads to the assumption that β-cryptoxanthin greatly contributes to improving the health of Japanese people.

Serum β-Cryptoxanthin Levels

Findings from nutritional epidemiological studies [20, 21] published to date in Europe and the USA show some very interesting trends, namely that serum β-cryptoxanthin is generally maintained at high levels despite the low β-cryptoxanthin intake. For example, according to a report [21] published by a research group in Australia, although the daily β-cryptoxanthin intake in the population studied was 0.2 mg, which was one-tenth of the intakes of β-carotene, lycopene or other carotenoids, the serum concentrations of these substances were found to be at the same levels. This finding leads to assume that β-cryptoxanthin is easily absorbed and that it can also survive relatively long in the body. Our survey [22], on the other hand, has revealed that serum β-cryptoxanthin levels rise dramatically during January, when mandarin oranges are in high season, in a manner dependent on the frequency of mandarin orange intake (Fig. 8.2), and that even during the preharvest month of September, serum β-cryptoxanthin levels are maintained at significantly higher levels in individuals with higher frequency of mandarin orange intake during the winter season. This finding indicates that β-cryptoxanthin accumulates in the body over a relatively long period of time. Furthermore, a detailed follow-up on seasonal changes in serum β-cryptoxanthin levels over a year revealed mandarin oranges to be the only food source affecting the serum concentrations of β-cryptoxanthin [23].

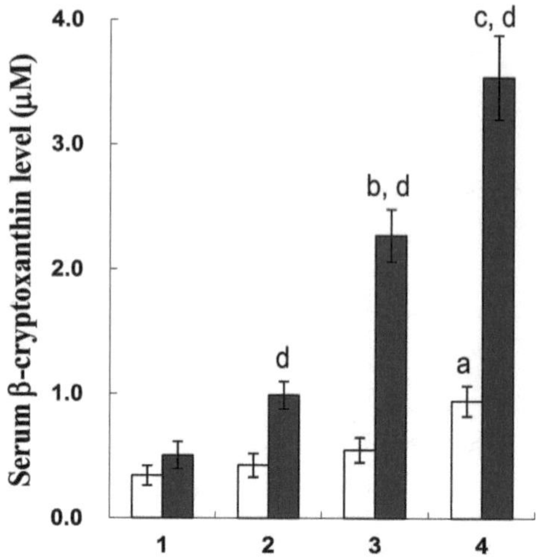

Fig. 8.2 Relationship of serum β-cryptoxanthin level with Japanese mandarin intake. The levels of Satsuma mandarin consumption are as follows: Level 1: "I rarely eat Satsuma mandarin." Level 2: "Although I sometimes eat Satsuma mandarin, I eat fewer than three pieces of this fruit a week." Level 3: "I eat one to three Satsuma mandarins daily." Level 4: "I eat more than four Satsuma mandarins daily." Open columns show the results in September, closed show those in January. All data are represented as means ± S. E. M. Number of observations in group of levels 1, 2, 3, and 4 are 5, 11, 52, and 26, respectively. $^{a}P<0.05$ versus data of September in group of level 1, $^{b}P<0.05$, $^{c}P<0.01$ versus data of January in group of level 1 in Scheffe's test. $^{d}P<0.001$ versus data of September in the same group in paired *t*-test

Characteristics of β-Cryptoxanthin as Identified in Epidemiological Studies

Epidemiological research on the association between fruit and vegetable intake and lifestyle-related diseases has witnessed remarkable progress in recent years, and carotenoids are regarded as one of the factors playing a key role in the prevention of lifestyle-related diseases. Many researchers have in fact focused their attention on carotenoids and have tried to identify and analyze the types of carotenoids that are most effective in preventing these types of diseases. Interestingly, according to the previous epidemiological studies [24–26] on carotenoids, β-cryptoxanthin was found to be the only type of carotenoid that showed an association with lung cancer, diabetes, and rheumatism. It is noteworthy that a statistically significant negative association between β-cryptoxanthin and lung cancer risks in smokers has been reported in several studies [27–29]. These findings suggest that β-cryptoxanthin may be physiologically superior to other carotenoids, but its underlying mechanism of action has not yet been fully elucidated.

β-cryptoxanthin is a type of carotenoid that has a hydroxyl (OH) group attached to one of the rings at the end of the carbon chain. Despite being a xanthophyll, it has pro-vitamin A activity as well as the ability to bind to a carotene binding protein and a retinoic acid receptor [30, 31]. Moreover, due to the presence of the OH group, β-cryptoxanthin has a higher polarity than β-carotene. However, its polarity is not quite as strong as lutein and zeaxanthin, which have an OH group at both ends of their carbon chain. Due to these physicochemical properties specific to β-cryptoxanthin, the localization of β-cryptoxanthin in tissues or cells differs slightly from other types of carotenoids, which may be related to the diverse characteristics of β-cryptoxanthin. Further studies are necessary to provide more detailed information about the characteristics of β-cryptoxanthin.

Recent Findings on Bone Health and Carotenoids

Recent experimental studies [32, 33] have revealed the involvement of oxidative stress in osteoblast apoptosis as well as born resorption mediated by osteoclasts. Several epidemiological studies [34, 35] have in fact demonstrated the association of oxidative stress with BMD and osteoporosis. These findings suggest that antioxidants exert beneficial effects on bone metabolism by suppressing oxidative stress. Furthermore, in recent years, there has been accumulating evidence on the antioxidant potential of carotenoids that are contained in abundance in fruit and vegetables.

Maggio et al. [36] surveyed postmenopausal Italian women and reported for the first time that the serum concentrations of various types of carotenoids including β-carotene are significantly lower in subjects with osteoporosis compared to their healthy counterparts. Yang et al. [37] investigated postmenopausal American women and reported that the serum concentrations of β-cryptoxanthin and lycopene are low in women with osteoporosis. While the above-mentioned results were derived from case–control studies, there have also been numerous cohort studies performed on the benefits of carotenoids. Sahni et al. [38] conducted a 4-year follow-up of elderly men and women in the USA to investigate the association between carotenoid intake and changes in the BMD of the vertebrae, hipbone, and radius, and found that the rate of BMD loss was slower in subjects with a high total intake of carotenoids. Furthermore, a total of 17 years of follow-up revealed that, of all carotenoids, a higher intake of lycopene was especially associated with a reduced risk for hip and nonvertebral fractures [39]. This follow-up, however, failed to reveal any significant effect of β-cryptoxanthin on the reduction of fracture risks. Although varying results from studies targeting different populations likely reflect differences in dietary habits, further epidemiological research is needed to identify the types of carotenoids that are particularly beneficial to bone metabolism.

Findings from an Epidemiological Study (Mikkabi Study) Targeting Residents of Mandarin Orange-Producing Areas

Since 2003, we have been conducting a nutritional epidemiological study (Mikkabi study) targeting the residents of Mikkabi, a town located in the north ward of Hamamatsu City in Shizuoka Prefecture, which is known as the leading mandarin orange producer in Japan. The goal of this study is to find out the types of life-style related diseases that may be prevented by mandarin orange intake. To this end, we have been analyzing how β-cryptoxanthin, which is found in abundance particularly in mandarin oranges, may be associated with various measures of health. In our previous cross-sectional studies [40–45], individuals with high serum β-cryptoxanthin levels (that is, who regularly ate mandarin oranges) were found to be associated with lower risks for liver diseases, arteriosclerosis, insulin resistance, metabolic syndrome, and oxidative stress. As part of Mikkabi study, we have been conducting a BMD survey since 2005 to find out if mandarin oranges are effective in preventing osteoporosis. The findings [46, 47] obtained from Mikkabi study on the association between β-cryptoxanthin and BMD are described in detail in the subsections that follow.

Association Between Serum β-Cryptoxanthin Levels and BMD

Mikkabi residents who participated in a community health checkup and who gave informed consent were included in the survey. A fasting blood sample was taken to measure serum carotenoids levels. BMD was measured at the distal third of the nondominant radius using a dual-energy X-ray absorptiometry scan (see Fig. 8.3).

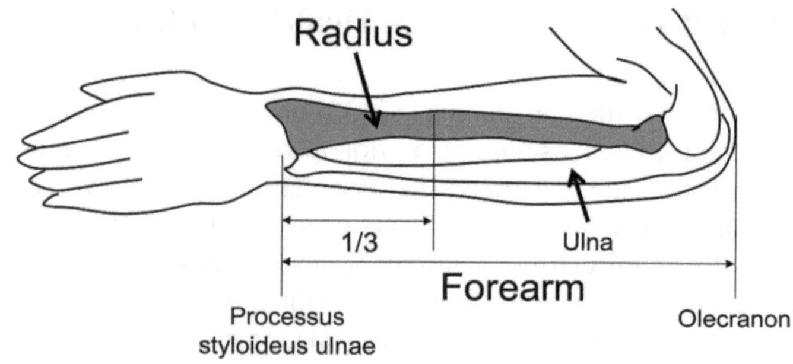

Fig. 8.3 Bone structure of antebrachial region (radius and ulna). Bone mineral density was measured by dual X-ray at *arrowhead*

Table 8.1 Characteristics of the study subject stratified by menopausal status[a]

	Subjects			
	Premenopausal		Postmenopausal	
n	161		293	
Age (years)	44.1	(5.3)	60.2	(6.2)
Body mass index (kg/m^2)	22.4	(3.7)	22.5	(3.0)
Total energy intake (MJ/day)	8.03	(1.83)	8.20	(2.01)
Calcium intake (mg/day)	566	(190)	651	(256)
Vitamin D intake (μg/day)[b]	195	(177–215)	256	(238–276)
Bone mineral density (g/cm^2)	0.677	(0.055)	0.561	(0.084)[c]
Range		0.412–0.817		0.366–0.820
Serum carotenoid (μmol/L)[b]				
Lutein	0.46	(0.44–0.48)	0.54	(0.51–0.56)
Lycopene	0.46	(0.43–0.49)	0.37	(0.35–0.39)
α-Carotene	0.19	(0.17–0.20)	0.21	(0.20–0.23)
β-Carotene	0.84	(0.77–0.91)	1.12	(1.06–1.18)
β-Cryptoxanthin	0.89	(0.79–1.01)	1.75	(1.61–1.90)
Zeaxanthin	0.19	(0.18–0.20)	0.20	(0.20–0.21)
Current tobacco use (%)	3.7		1.7	
Exercise habits (%)[d]	14.9		21.5	
Regular alcohol intake (%)[d]	19.9		11.0	
Current supplement use (%)	9.9		9.6	

[a]Data are mean (standard deviation), geometric mean (95 % confidence interval), range, or percent
[b]These variables were represented as original scale after analysis by log (natural) transformed values
[c]$P < 0.001$ versus premenopausal female
[d]≥1 times/week

A self-administered questionnaire was used to collect information about a subject's history of osteoporosis, medications and/or hormone use, and lifestyle, including tobacco use (current smoker, ex-smoker, or nonsmoker), exercise (1+ times per week), regular alcohol intake (1+ times per week), dietary supplement use (nonuser, occasional-user, current-user), and dietary habits. Diet was assessed with a modified validated simple food-frequency questionnaire (FFQ) developed especially for the Japanese. This study was approved by the ethics committees of the National Institute of Fruit Tree Science and the Hamamatsu University School of Medicine. The total daily calorie intake as well as vitamin and mineral intake was calculated for 454 females who completed the questionnaire and underwent BMD measurement and serum carotenoid analysis. Based on these data, the association between serum carotenoid levels and BMD was analyzed cross-sectionally.

The radial BMD in postmenopausal female subjects was significantly lower than that in premenopausal female subjects (Table 8.1). In multiple linear regression analysis, the radial BMD in postmenopausal female subjects was weakly but significantly correlated with serum β-carotene and

Table 8.2 Multiple linear regression analysis for the association between bone mineral density with serum carotenoid concentrations[a]

	Standard regression coefficients	P-value
Lutein	–0.064	0.209
Lycopene	0.007	0.891
α-Carotene	0.028	0.582
β-Carotene	0.102	0.047
β-Cryptoxanthin	0.105	0.047
Zeaxanthin	–0.051	0.307

[a]Standard regression coefficients of the radial BMD with serum carotenoid concentrations were calculated by multiple linear regression analysis after adjusting for confounding factors

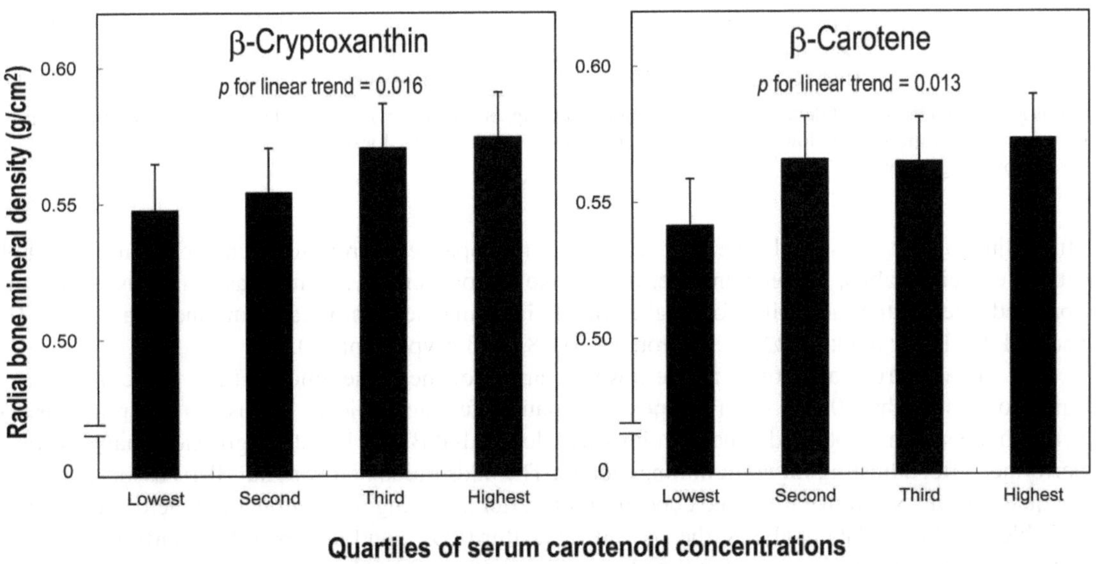

Fig. 8.4 Multivariate-adjusted means of bone mineral density by quartiles of serum β-carotene and β-cryptoxanthin concentrations in postmenopausal female subjects. Multivariate-adjusted means of bone mineral density were calculated after adjusting for age, weight, height, years since menopause, current tobacco use, regular alcohol intake, exercise habits, supplement use, and total energy intake. P-values over the quartiles of serum carotenoids were assessed with a test for linear trends using linear regression

β-cryptoxanthin concentrations after adjusting for age, years since menopause, weight, height, current tobacco use, regular alcohol intake, exercise habits, use of dietary supplements, and total energy intake (Table 8.2). After further adjusting for intakes of calcium, magnesium, potassium, and vitamins C, D, and E, a significant correlation was observed in β-cryptoxanthin (data not shown). No other statistically significant correlations were observed.

Then, 293 postmenopausal women with no history of osteoporosis were divided into quartiles on the basis of serum levels of six types of carotenoids. The multivariate adjusted mean of the radial BMD by the quartiles of the serum carotenoid concentration was calculated after adjusting for confounding factors. In postmenopausal female subjects, although no significant differences among each quartile were observed in all six serum carotenoids, the multivariate adjusted means of the radial BMD showed significant increasing trends under linearity with the quartiles of serum β-cryptoxanthin and β-carotene (Fig. 8.4). The results show the multivariate adjusted means of the radial BMD by quartiles of serum β-carotene and β-cryptoxanthin concentrations in postmenopausal female subjects

Table 8.3 The dds ratios (and 95 % confidence intervals) of high group (upper 3 quartiles) compared with lowest quartile of serum carotenoid concentrations on low bone mineral density in postmenopausal female subjects[a]

Serum carotenoids		n	Mean and range of serum carotenoid (mmol/L)		Odds ratios	95 % CI
Lutein	Lowest (Q1)	71	0.34	(0.21–0.42)	1.00	
	High (Q2–Q4)	222	0.62	(0.44–2.11)	0.59	(0.29–1.22)
Lycopene	Lowest (Q1)	76	0.20	(0.07–0.30)	1.00	
	High (Q2–Q4)	217	0.46	(0.32–1.10)	1.53	(0.77–3.03)
α-Carotene	Lowest (Q1)	81	0.12	(0.06–0.15)	1.00	
	High (Q2–Q4)	212	0.27	(0.17–2.74)	1.19	(0.60–2.36)
β-Carotene	Lowest (Q1)	70	0.60	(0.32–0.82)	1.00	
	High (Q2–Q4)	223	1.36	(0.84–3.37)	0.51	(0.25–1.04)
β-Cryptoxanthin	Lowest (Q1)	73	0.67	(0.22–1.07)	1.00	
	High (Q2–Q4)	220	2.41	(1.10–10.53)	0.45	(0.22–0.95)
Zeaxanthin	Lowest (Q1)	63	0.14	(0.09–0.16)	1.00	
	High (Q2–Q4)	230	0.23	(0.18–0.46)	1.02	(0.49–2.11)

[a]Odds ratios (and 95 % confidence intervals) of high group (upper 3 quartiles) compared with lowest quartile of serum carotenoid concentrations on low bone mineral density were calculated by logistic regression analysis after adjusting for confounding factors

after adjusting for age, weight, height, years since menopause, current tobacco use, regular alcohol intake, exercise habits, supplement use, and intake of total energy. Similar associations were also observed after further adjusting for intakes of calcium, magnesium, potassium, and vitamins D, C, and E (P for linear tend: 0.022 for β-carotene, 0.018 for β-cryptoxanthin).

Low radial BMD was defined as the lowest quartile of the value among study participants; i.e., equal to or less than 0.501 g/cm^2 in postmenopausal female subjects. To assess the relationship between the serum carotenoid concentrations with low radial BMD, logistic regression analyses were performed after adjusting for confounding factors. The odds ratios of low radial BMD associated with the quartiles of six serum carotenoid concentrations after adjusting for confounding factors are shown in Table 8.3. In the data analyses, the second (Q2), third (Q3), and highest (Q4) quartiles of serum carotenoid concentrations were combined as a high group (Q2-Q4). The odds ratios of low radial BMD in the high groups (Q2-Q4) against the lowest quartile (Q1) used for the reference group were calculated. After adjusting for age, weight, and height, significantly lower odds ratio for low radial BMD in postmenopausal female subjects was observed in the group with high serum β-cryptoxanthin. Multivariate adjustment was further conducted to control for potential confounders. After adjusting for age, years since menopause, weight, height, current tobacco use, regular alcohol intake, exercise habits, use of dietary supplements, and total energy intake in postmenopausal female subjects, significantly lower odds ratio for low radial BMD was observed in the group with high serum β-cryptoxanthin compared to the respective lowest quartile used for reference (Table 8.3). However, after further adjusting for intakes of calcium, magnesium, potassium, and vitamins C, D, and E, this significantly lower odds ratio was not observed in the group with high serum β-cryptoxanthin (data not shown). In addition, no significant associations were observed between other types of carotenoids and the risk for low radial BMD.

Interaction Between Other Antioxidants and β-Cryptoxanthin

Based on our finding that β-cryptoxanthin was weakly but significantly associated with BMD measured at the distal third of the nondominant radius of postmenopausal women, we speculated about a possible

Table 8.4 Factor-loading matrix for the three dietary patterns of antioxidant vitamins and carotenoids intakes identified among 293 postmenopausal Japanese female subjects[a]

	Factor 1	Factor 2	Factor 3
	Carotene pattern	Retinol pattern	β-Cryptoxanthin pattern
Retinol[b]		0.825	
Vitamin C	0.435	0.285	0.773
Vitamin E	0.464	0.711	0.258
Lycopene	0.633		
α-Carotene	0.788		
β-Carotene	0.852	0.257	0.369
Lutein	0.740	0.447	0.270
β-Cryptoxanthin			0.920
Zeaxanthin		0.712	
Percentage of variance (%)	30.3	22.8	20.1

[a]Data for 293 subjects from the self-administered food frequency questionnaire. Absolute values <0.25 were excluded from the table for simplicity
[b]Preformed retinol

interaction between β-cryptoxanthin and other antioxidant vitamins and carotenoids. Although analytical data on the serum concentrations of six major types of carotenoids have been collected in Mikkabi study, no measurement has been made of the serum concentrations of vitamins. Thus, the data from FFQ were used to estimate the daily intake of three types of vitamins (retinol, vitamin C, and vitamin E) and six types of carotenoids (lycopene, α-carotene, β-carotene, β-cryptoxanthin, lutein, and zeaxanthin) in each subject to assess how the intake of these vitamins and carotenoids may affect BMD. The daily intake of each type of vitamins and carotenoids was calculated for each subject.

A principal component analysis was used to derive the dietary patterns on the basis of the intakes of nine antioxidant vitamins and carotenoids obtained from the FFQ. To identify the number of factors to be retained, we used the criterion of eigenvalues > 1.0, the most widely used criterion in factor analysis. Finally, we decided to retain three factors for further analysis. We applied a Varimax rotation to the factor-loading matrix to achieve a simpler structure with greater interpretability. After the Varimax rotation, the factor scores for each subject were saved from the principal component analysis. The factor-loading matrix represents correlation coefficients between individual antioxidants and dietary patterns. The percentage of variance explained by each factor was calculated by dividing the sum of the squares of the respective factor loadings by the number of variables.

The factor-loading matrices for the three retained factors are shown in Table 8.4. The high positive loadings indicate strong associations between given antioxidants and dietary patterns. Factor 1 had heavy loadings on β-carotene, α-carotene, lutein, lycopene, and vitamins E and C. This pattern was especially heavily loaded on carotenoids and was labelled the "Carotene" pattern. Factor 2 had heavy loadings on preformed retinol, zeaxanthin, vitamin E, lutein, vitamin C, and β-carotene. This pattern, heavily loaded on preformed retinol, zeaxanthin, and vitamin E, was labelled the "Retinol" pattern. Factor 3 had heavy loadings on β-cryptoxanthin, vitamin C, β-carotene, lutein, and vitamin E. This pattern, heavily loaded on β-cryptoxanthin and vitamin C, was labelled the "β-cryptoxanthin" pattern. Overall, the three dietary patterns accounted for 73.1 % of the variance in antioxidant vitamin and carotenoid intake.

Subjects were divided into three categories according to tertiles of factor scores. To assess the relationship between dietary patterns and low radial BMD, logistic regression analyses were performed. The odds ratios of low radial BMD associated with the tertiles of factor scores of each of the three dietary patterns after adjustments for confounding factors are shown in Table 8.5. The odds ratios for the risk of low radial BMD in the highest tertile of factor scores against the lowest tertile

Table 8.5 The odds ratios (and 95 % confidence intervals) of tertiles of three dietary patterns on low bone mineral density in postmenopausal Japanese female subjects[a]

Dietary patterns	Factor score	*n*	Odds ratios	95 % CI	*P* for trend
Carotene pattern	Lowest	97	1.00		
	Middle	98	0.94	(0.44–2.00)	
	Highest	98	1.38	(0.66–2.89)	0.340
Retinol pattern	Lowest	97	1.00		
	Middle	98	1.35	(0.61–2.98)	
	Highest	98	3.09	(1.28–7.47)	0.009
β-Cryptoxanthin pattern	Lowest	97	1.00		
	Middle	98	0.54	(0.25–1.18)	
	Highest	98	0.22	(0.09–0.54)	0.001

[a]Odds ratios (and 95 % confidence intervals) of highest tertile of factor scores against the lowest tertile used for the reference group were calculated after adjusting for confounding factors

Table 8.6 The odds ratios (and 95 % confidence intervals) of tertiles of antioxidant intakes on low bone mineral density in postmenopausal Japanese female subjects[a]

Dietary intake		*n*	Range (mg/day) or (μg/day)	Odds ratios	95 % CI	*P* for trend
Retinol[b]	Lowest	97	(29–213)	1.00		
	Middle	98	(218–383)	1.65	(0.74–3.69)	
	Highest	98	(386–3531)	3.22	(1.38–7.51)	0.007
Vitamin C	Lowest	96	(47–139)	1.00		
	Middle	99	(140–214)	1.02	(0.47–2.22)	
	Highest	98	(215–625)	0.25	(0.10–0.66)	0.001
β-Cryptoxanthin	Lowest	98	(0.00–0.30)	1.00		
	Middle	101	(0.31–1.21)	0.47	(0.22–1.01)	
	Highest	94	(1.22–7.91)	0.40	(0.17–0.92)	0.068

[a]Odds ratios (and 95 % confidence intervals) of highest tertile compared with lowest group on low bone mineral density were calculated by logistic regression analysis after adjusting for confounding factors
[b]Preformed retinol

used for the reference group were calculated. In the "Carotene" pattern, there was no significant association between the factor score and low radial BMD. In the "Retinol" pattern, a significantly higher odds ratio was observed in the highest tertile of factor score after adjustments for age, years since menopause, weight, height, current tobacco use, regular alcohol intake, exercise habits, use of dietary supplements, and total energy. On the other hand, in the "β-cryptoxanthin" pattern, a significantly lower odds ratio was observed in the highest tertile of factor scores after multivariate adjustment.

The multivariate-adjusted odds ratios for the risk of low BMD values according to the intake of each type of antioxidant vitamins and carotenoids were also calculated. The odds ratios for the risk of low radial BMD associated with the tertiles of daily intakes of each antioxidant vitamin and carotenoid after adjustments for confounding factors are shown in Table 8.6. A significantly higher odds ratio was observed in the highest tertile of preformed retinol intake after multivariate adjustments. In contrast, a significantly lower odds ratio was observed in the highest tertile of vitamin C intake after multivariate adjustments. Also, a significantly lower odds ratio was observed in the highest tertile of β-cryptoxanthin intake after adjustments for age, years since menopause, weight, height, current tobacco use, regular alcohol intake, exercise habits, use of dietary supplements, and total energy. However, these negative associations between vitamin C and β-cryptoxanthin intakes with the risk of low BMD values were no longer significant after further adjusting for β-cryptoxanthin intake and vitamin C intake, respectively.

Table 8.7 The odds ratios (and 95 % confidence intervals) of four groups stratified by dietary intakes of vitamin C and β-cryptoxanthin on low bone mineral density in postmenopausal Japanese female subjects[a]

		Daily intake of β-cryptoxanthin (mg/day)					
		Low intake (0–0.96 mg/day)			High intake (0.97–7.91 mg/day)		
		n	Odd ratios	95 % CI	n	Odd ratios	95 % CI
Daily intake of vitamin C (mg/day)	Low intake (47–169 mg/day)	113	1.00	(Reference)	34	0.73	(0.27–1.99)
	High intake (170–625 mg/day)	36	0.52	(0.18–1.52)	110	0.42	(0.19–0.93)

[a]Age, weight, height, years since menopause, current tobacco use, regular alcohol intake, exercise habits, supplement use, and total energy intake were adjusted

Next, study subjects were divided into two groups by median values of vitamin C and/or β-cryptoxanthin intake. And then, all subjects were ranked into four groups as follow: group 1; lower intake of vitamin C (47–169 mg/day) with lower intake of β-cryptoxanthin (0–0.96 mg/day), group 2; lower intake of vitamin C (47–169 mg/day) with higher intake of β-cryptoxanthin (0.97–7.91 mg/day), group 3; higher intake of vitamin C (170–625 mg/day) with lower intake of β-cryptoxanthin (0–0.96 mg/day), group 4; higher intake of vitamin C (170–625 mg/day) with higher intake of β-cryptoxanthin (0.97–7.91 mg/day). In both groups of higher intake of vitamin C with lower intake of β-cryptoxanthin and/or lower intake of vitamin C with higher intake of β-cryptoxanthin, significantly lower odds ratios were not observed against the lower intake group of both of them used for the reference group. In contrast, a significantly lower odds ratio was observed in the higher intake group of both of them after adjustments for age, years since menopause, weight, height, current tobacco use, regular alcohol intake, exercise habits, use of dietary supplements, and total energy (Table 8.7).

From these results, we concluded that the intakes of vitamin C and β-cryptoxanthin may be significantly but partially associated with radial BMD and these associations may be caused by a combination of vitamin C and β-cryptoxanthin. To our knowledge, there has been no experimental or epidemiological study of the combined effect of vitamin C and carotenoid on bone metabolism. It is conceivable that, rather than vitamin C alone, vitamin C intake combined with the intakes of other antioxidants such as carotenoids may yield an important dietary pattern conducive to the maintenance of bone health. Further studies on the complicated interactions of antioxidants on bone metabolism are required.

Association Between Serum β-Cryptoxanthin Levels and the Risk of Developing Osteoporosis

We conducted a follow-up on subjects from Mikkabi study. Those who participated in previous BMD surveys and completed 4 years of follow-up were examined longitudinally. Here, we provide some of the findings that have emerged so far from our preliminary study.

In Japan, osteoporosis is at present diagnosed based on the criteria presented in the *Guideline on the Management (Medical Treatment) of Osteoporosis* issued by Japan Osteoporosis Society. According to this guideline, a T-score (which shows how a patient's BMD compares with young healthy adults) of 70–80 % indicates low BMD and a T-score lower than 70 % indicates the possibility of osteoporosis. Our follow-up revealed that, although 11.8 % of the postmenopausal women who were past menopause by the time they entered the study were suspected of already having osteoporosis at baseline, this percentage increased significantly to 18.5 % at 4 years. The analysis of the association between serum carotenoid levels at the beginning of the study and changes in BMD over

4 years shows that the groups of subjects with higher serum concentrations of carotenoids, excluding lutein and zeaxanthin, tended to have less decrease in BMD during the 4-year period. In our next analysis, subjects excluding those who were suspected of having osteoporosis at baseline were categorized into the following three groups based on their BMD test results at 4 years: normal group, low BMD group, and osteoporosis group. The serum carotenoid levels at baseline were estimated for each group after statistically adjusting for factors that can affect BMD. This analysis revealed that subjects who developed osteoporosis during the survey period had significant lower serum concentrations of β-cryptoxanthin and β-carotene at baseline, compared to the normal group. In other words, subjects who had had higher serum concentrations of β-cryptoxanthin and β-carotene to begin with were less likely to develop osteoporosis in later years (these study results are currently being submitted for publication).

Possible Preventive Effects of β-Cryptoxanthin on Osteoporosis

Mikkabi study showed that serum β-cryptoxanthin levels in postmenopausal women were weakly but significantly associated with BMD measured at the distal third of the radius, and revealed a strong negative association between β-cryptoxanthin pattern, which loaded heavily on the intake of β-cryptoxanthin and vitamin C, and the risk of low BMD values. These findings suggest that high intake of nutrients such as vitamin C and minerals together with β-cryptoxanthin have additional beneficial effects on the prevention of BMD loss in postmenopausal Japanese women. One normal-size mandarin orange is expected to contain 1.2 mg β-cryptoxanthin and 25 mg vitamin C. In view of this, to prevent menopause-related BMD loss, vitamin C needs to be consumed not only from mandarin oranges but also from other food sources. To date, there have been no reports from experimental studies on the combined effects of vitamin C and β-cryptoxanthin on bone metabolism. Further research is thus needed in this area. On the other hand, our preliminary longitudinal analysis revealed that serum β-cryptoxanthin and β-carotene levels had been significantly lower at baseline in subjects who developed osteoporosis in later years, which suggests that, of all types of carotenoids, β-cryptoxanthin and β-carotene might especially be involved in the prevention of BMD loss.

Recent studies [32–35] have also implicated the possible involvement of oxidative stress in BMD loss and increased risk of fractures. In fact, experimental evidence shows that smokers have increased risk of fractures, that osteoporosis patients have lower concentrations of serum vitamin C and vitamin E and exhibit elevated serum oxidative stress marker levels, and that NF-$_{\kappa}$B proteins that play an important role in bone resorption become activated when exposed to oxidative stress. Although all types of carotenoids are known to have potent antioxidative properties, no association was found between carotenoids other than β-cryptoxanthin and β-carotene and BMD in our study. This finding suggests that mechanisms other than antioxidant activity might be involved in the effect of carotenoids on BMD. Further research is needed in this respect.

Our observation is consistent with experimental results previously reported. Very recently, Yamaguchi et al. [48–50] have reported the beneficial effects of β-cryptoxanthin on bone metabolism in in vitro and in vivo studies. They found [48] that β-cryptoxanthin enhanced the calcium content and alkaline phosphatase activity in the femoral-diaphyseal and femoral-metaphyseal tissues of young rats at physiological low concentrations in vitro, while lycopene and lutein had no effects at the same dose. Furthermore, they found [49] a stimulatory effect on bone formation and an inhibitory effect on bone resorption in a tissue culture. In an in vivo study, they found [50] that the oral administration of β-cryptoxanthin caused a significant increase in the calcium content and alkaline phosphatase activity in the femoral-diaphyseal and femoral-metaphyseal tissues. These previous results support our findings [46, 47] showing that β-cryptoxanthin may have a direct stimulatory effect on bone formation and an inhibitory effect on bone resorption. The development of osteoporosis may be reduced by the dietary intake of β-cryptoxanthin.

Several epidemiological research teams overseas are currently attempting to examine longitudinally how carotenoids might by associated with osteoporosis, changes in BMD, or risks of fractures. Most of the epidemiological studies on the association between carotenoids and bone health have been carried out using either cross-sectional or case control design to examine how carotenoid intake may affect BMD or bone health. Even a few studies that assessed this association using serum carotenoid levels were based on cross-sectional analyses. According to these studies, lycopene, β-carotene, and β-cryptoxanthin have all been reported to be associated with bone health.

It is also important to take into account that dietary habits in populations vary across studies. Thus, studies conducted in Europe or the USA, where lycopene intake is relatively high, tend to implicate lycopene as the type of carotenoid affecting bone metabolism. On the other hand, a few studies [36, 37] targeting Spanish and American populations have reported on the efficacy of β-cryptoxanthin. In recent years, Framingham research group [38, 39], renowned for their accomplishments in epidemiological research, has published results from their longitudinal analysis of the association between carotenoid intake and BMD. This group analyzed how carotenoid intake affects changes in BMD over 4 years and concluded that high intake of lycopene has inhibitory effects on BMD loss. Nonetheless, they found no association between β-cryptoxanthin and bone health.

In general, literature on epidemiological research regarding the association between carotenoids and bone health is poor. No studies have, in fact, been conducted to date to longitudinally analyze the association between serum carotenoid levels and bone health. In this respect, ours is the first study that conducts a longitudinal analysis of the association between serum carotenoid levels and BMD and demonstrates the possible inhibitory effects of β-cryptoxanthin and β-carotene on BMD loss (unpublished data). In general, when the carotenoid intake of each subject is estimated based on data collected from a diet survey administered to them, the estimated intake levels may not necessarily reflect the actual amount of carotenoid ingested or absorbed into the body. On the other hand, data on serum carotenoid levels is a relatively accurate measure of the actual amount of carotenoids present in the body, which therefore gives a more detailed account of the association between carotenoid levels and BMD.

In contrast to findings collected in Europe and the USA, no significant association has been observed between lycopene and bone health in the subjects who participated in our study. This may be partly due the fact that groups of subjects in Mikkabi study have much lower dietary intake and serum levels of lycopene compared to individuals living in other parts of the world. Similarly, although higher serum concentrations of α-carotene has contributed to some extent to decreasing the rate of BMD loss, the association has not been found to be significant. A more extended follow-up may reveal a significant association. On the other hand, our analyses failed to show any association of lutein and zeaxanthin with BMD. Of the carotenoids studied, lutein was found to be consumed in highest amount by the subjects in the Mikkabi study, and the serum concentration of lutein was also found to be higher than those of α-carotene or lycopene. However, no association was found between lutein and bone health. This finding suggests that none of these carotenoids are involved in the maintenance of bone health.

Taken together, our findings lead us to conclude that β-cryptoxanthin and β-carotene are probably the two types of carotenoids that are involved in the prevention of BMD loss in postmenopausal Japanese women. However, further evidence from epidemiological research is needed in order to draw a definitive conclusion on this issue.

Conclusions

In our survey, serum concentrations of β-cryptoxanthin and β-carotene were weakly but positively associated with the radial BMD in postmenopausal Japanese female subjects. Furthermore, a high intake of vitamin C with β-cryptoxanthin is inversely associated with low radial BMD. In our longitudinal analysis, subjects who had had higher serum concentrations of β-cryptoxanthin and β-carotene to begin with were less likely to develop osteoporosis in later years. These associations suggest that high intakes of fruit and vegetables rich in β-cryptoxanthin and β-carotene might provide benefits to bone health in postmenopausal Japanese female. To determine whether these carotenoids are beneficial micronutrients to bone health, further studies will be required.

References

1. World Health Organization. Diet, nutrition and the prevention of chronic diseases. World Health Organ Tech Rep Ser. 2003;916:i–viii. 1–149.
2. Bazzano LA, He J, Ogden LG, Loria CM, Vupputuri S, Myers L, et al. Fruit and vegetable intake and risk of cardiovascular disease in US adults: the first National Health and Nutrition Examination Survey Epidemiologic Follow-up Study. Am J Clin Nutr. 2002;76:93–9.
3. Ford ES, Mokdad AH. Fruit and vegetable consumption and diabetes mellitus incidence among U.S. adults. Prev Med. 2001;32:33–9.
4. Montonen J, Järvinen R, Heliövaara M, Reunanen A, Aromaa A, Knekt P. Food consumption and the incidence of type II diabetes mellitus. Eur J Clin Nutr. 2005;59:441–8.
5. Gutteridge JM. Biological origin of free radicals, and mechanisms of antioxidant protection. Chem Biol Interact. 1994;91:133–40.
6. Rock CL, Jacob RA, Bowen PE. Update on the biological characteristics of the antioxidant micronutrients: vitamin C, vitamin E, and the carotenoids. J Am Diet Assoc. 1996;96:693–702.
7. Stanner SA, Hughes J, Kelly CN, Buttriss J. A review of the epidemiological evidence for the 'antioxidant hypothesis'. Public Health Nutr. 2004;7:407–22.
8. Knekt P, Ritz J, Pereira MA, O'Reilly EJ, Augustsson K, Fraser GE, et al. Antioxidant vitamins and coronary heart disease risk: a pooled analysis of 9 cohorts. Am J Clin Nutr. 2004;80:1508–20.
9. Ford ES, Will JC, Bowman BA, Narayan KM. Diabetes mellitus and serum carotenoids: findings from the Third National Health and Nutrition Examination Survey. Am J Epidemiol. 1999;149:168–76.
10. Comstock GW, Bush TL, Helzlsouer K. Serum retinol, beta-carotene, vitamin E, and selenium as related to subsequent cancer of specific sites. Am J Epidemiol. 1992;135:115–21.
11. Macdonald HM, New SA, Golden MH, Campbell MK, Reid DM. Nutritional associations with bone loss during the menopausal transition: evidence of a beneficial effect of calcium, alcohol, and fruit and vegetable nutrients and of a detrimental effect of fatty acids. Am J Clin Nutr. 2004;79:155–65.
12. New SA, Bolton-Smith C, Grubb DA, Reid DM. Nutritional influences on bone mineral density: a cross-sectional study in premenopausal women. Am J Clin Nutr. 1997;65:1831–9.
13. Prynne CJ, Mishra GD, O'Connell MA, Muniz G, Laskey MA, Yan L, et al. Fruit and vegetable intakes and bone mineral status: a cross-sectional study in 5 age and sex cohorts. Am J Clin Nutr. 2006;83:1420–8.
14. McGartland CP, Robson PJ, Murray LJ, Cran GW, Savage MJ, Watkins DC, et al. Fruit and vegetable consumption and bone mineral density: the Northern Ireland Young Hearts Project. Am J Clin Nutr. 2004;80:1019–23.
15. Tucker KL, Chen H, Hannan MT, Cupples LA, Wilson PW, Felson D, et al. Bone mineral density and dietary patterns in older adults: the Framingham Osteoporosis Study. Am J Clin Nutr. 2002;76:245–52.
16. Britton G, Liaaen-Jensen S, Pfander H. Carotenoids handbook. Basel: Birkhauser Verlag; 2004.
17. Bieri JG, Brown ED, Smith JC. Determination of individual carotenoids in human plasma by high performance liquid chromatography. J Liq Chrom. 1985;8:473–84.
18. Michaud DS, Giovannucci EL, Ascherio A, Rimm EB, Forman MR, Sampson L, et al. Associations of plasma carotenoid concentrations and dietary intake of specific carotenoids in samples of two prospective cohort studies using a new carotenoid database. Cancer Epidemiol Biomarkers Prev. 1998;7:283–90.
19. Canfield LM, Clandinin MT, Davies DP, Fernandez MC, Jackson J, Hawkes J, et al. Multinational study of major breast milk carotenoids of healthy mothers. Eur J Nutr. 2003;42:133–41.
20. Albanes D, Virtamo J, Taylor PR, Rautalahti M, Pietinen P, Heinonen OP. Effects of supplemental beta-carotene, cigarette smoking, and alcohol consumption on serum carotenoids in the Alpha-Tocopherol, Beta-Carotene Cancer Prevention Study. Am J Clin Nutr. 1997;66:366–72.
21. Wahlqvist ML, Wattanapenpaiboon N, Macrae FA, Lambert JR, MacLennan R, Hsu-Hage BH. Changes in serum carotenoids in subjects with colorectal adenomas after 24 mo of beta-carotene supplementation. Australian Polyp Prevention Project Investigators. Am J Clin Nutr. 1994;60:936–43.
22. Sugiura M, Matsumoto H, Kato M, Nagao A, Yano M. Serum concentration of β-Cryptoxanthin in Japan reflects the frequency of satsuma mandarin (Citrus unshiu Marc.) consumption. J Health Sci. 2002;48:350–3.
23. Sugiura M, Matsumoto H, Kato M, Ikoma Y, Yano M, Nagao A. Multiple linear regression analysis of the seasonal changes in the serum concentration of beta-cryptoxanthin. J Nutr Sci Vitaminol. 2004;50:196–202.

24. Männistö S, Smith-Warner SA, Spiegelman D, Albanes D, Anderson K, van den Brandt PA, et al. Dietary carotenoids and risk of lung cancer in a pooled analysis of seven cohort studies. Cancer Epidemiol Biomarkers Prev. 2004;13:40–8.
25. Montonen J, Knekt P, Järvinen R, Reunanen A. Dietary antioxidant intake and risk of type 2 diabetes. Diabetes Care. 2004;27:362–6.
26. Cerhan JR, Saag KG, Merlino LA, Mikuls TR, Criswell LA. Antioxidant micronutrients and risk of rheumatoid arthritis in a cohort of older women. Am J Epidemiol. 2003;157:345–54.
27. Yuan JM, Ross RK, Chu XD, Gao YT, Yu MC. Prediagnostic levels of serum beta-cryptoxanthin and retinol predict smoking-related lung cancer risk in Shanghai, China. Cancer Epidemiol Biomarkers Prev. 2001;10:767–73.
28. Yuan JM, Stram DO, Arakawa K, Lee HP, Yu MC. Dietary cryptoxanthin and reduced risk of lung cancer: the Singapore Chinese Health Study. Cancer Epidemiol Biomarkers Prev. 2003;12:890–8.
29. Voorrips LE, Goldbohm RA, Brants HA, van Poppel GA, Sturmans F, Hermus RJ, et al. A prospective cohort study on antioxidant and folate intake and male lung cancer risk. Cancer Epidemiol Biomarkers Prev. 2000;9:357–65.
30. Matsumoto A, Mizukami H, Mizuno S, Umegaki K, Nishikawa J, Shudo K, et al. beta-Cryptoxanthin a novel natural RAR ligand, induces ATP-binding cassette transporters in macrophages. Biochem Pharmacol. 2007;74:256–64.
31. Rao MN, Ghosh P, Lakshman MR. Purification and partial characterization of a cellular carotenoid-binding protein from ferret liver. J Biol Chem. 1997;272:24455–60.
32. Almeida M, Han L, Martin-Millan M, O'Brien CA, Manolagas SC. Oxidative stress antagonizes Wnt signaling in osteoblast precursors by diverting beta-catenin from T cell factor- to forkhead box O-mediated transcription. J Biol Chem. 2007;282:27298–305.
33. Jilka RL, Weinstein RS, Parfitt AM, Manolagas SC. Quantifying osteoblast and osteocyte apoptosis: challenges and rewards. J Bone Miner Res. 2007;22:1492–501.
34. Basu S, Michaëlsson K, Olofsson H, Johansson S, Melhus H. Association between oxidative stress and bone mineral density. Biochem Biophys Res Commun. 2001;288:275–9.
35. Yalin S, Bagis S, Polat G, Dogruer N, Cenk Aksit S, Hatungil R, et al. Is there a role of free oxygen radicals in primary male osteoporosis? Clin Exp Rheumatol. 2005;23:689–92.
36. Maggio D, Polidori MC, Barabani M, Tufi A, Ruggiero C, Cecchetti R, et al. Low levels of carotenoids and retinol in involutional osteoporosis. Bone. 2006;38:244–8.
37. Yang Z, Zhang Z, Penniston KL, Binkley N, Tanumihardjo SA. Serum carotenoid concentrations in postmenopausal women from the United States with and without osteoporosis. Int J Vitam Nutr Res. 2008;78:105–11.
38. Sahni S, Hannan MT, Blumberg J, Cupples LA, Kiel DP, Tucker KL. Inverse association of carotenoid intakes with 4-y change in bone mineral density in elderly men and women: the Framingham Osteoporosis Study. Am J Clin Nutr. 2009;89:416–24.
39. Sahni S, Hannan MT, Blumberg J, Cupples LA, Kiel DP, Tucker KL. Protective effect of total carotenoid and lycopene intake on the risk of hip fracture: a 17-year follow-up from the Framingham Osteoporosis Study. J Bone Miner Res. 2009;24:1086–94.
40. Sugiura M, Nakamura M, Ikoma Y, Yano M, Ogawa K, Matsumoto H, et al. High serum carotenoids are inversely associated with serum gamma-glutamyltransferase in alcohol drinkers within normal liver function. J Epidemiol. 2005;15:180–6.
41. Sugiura M, Nakamura M, Ikoma Y, Yano M, Ogawa K, Matsumoto H, et al. Serum carotenoid concentrations are inversely associated with serum aminotransferases in hyperglycemic subjects. Diabetes Res Clin Pract. 2006;71:82–91.
42. Nakamura M, Sugiura M, Aoki N. High beta-carotene and beta-cryptoxanthin are associated with low pulse wave velocity. Atherosclerosis. 2006;184:363–9.
43. Sugiura M, Nakamura M, Ikoma Y, Yano M, Ogawa K, Matsumoto H, et al. The homeostasis model assessment-insulin resistance index is inversely associated with serum carotenoids in non-diabetic subjects. J Epidemiol. 2006;16:71–8.
44. Sugiura M, Nakamura M, Ogawa K, Ikoma Y, Matsumoto H, Ando F, et al. Associations of serum carotenoid concentrations with the metabolic syndrome: interaction with smoking. Br J Nutr. 2008;100:1297–306.
45. Sugiura M, Nakamura M, Ogawa K, Ikoma Y, Matsumoto H, Ando F, et al. Synergistic interaction of cigarette smoking and alcohol drinking with serum carotenoid concentrations: findings from a middle-aged Japanese population. Br J Nutr. 2009;102:1211–9.
46. Sugiura M, Nakamura M, Ogawa K, Ikoma Y, Ando F, Yano M. Bone mineral density in post-menopausal female subjects is associated with serum antioxidant carotenoids. Osteoporos Int. 2008;19:211–9.
47. Sugiura M, Nakamura M, Ogawa K, Ikoma Y, Ando F, Shimokata H, et al. Dietary patterns of antioxidant vitamin and carotenoid intake associated with bone mineral density: findings from post-menopausal Japanese female subjects. Osteoporos Int. 2011;22:143–52.
48. Yamaguchi M, Uchiyama S. Effect of carotenoid on calcium content and alkaline phosphatase activity in rat femoral tissues in vitro: the unique anabolic effect of beta-cryptoxanthin. Biol Pharm Bull. 2003;26:1188–91.
49. Yamaguchi M, Uchiyama S. beta-Cryptoxanthin stimulates bone formation and inhibits bone resorption in tissue culture in vitro. Mol Cell Biochem. 2004;258:137–44.
50. Uchiyama S, Yamaguchi M. Oral administration of beta-cryptoxanthin induces anabolic effects on bone components in the femoral tissues of rats in vivo. Biol Pharm Bull. 2004;27:232–5.

Chapter 9
Soy Protein Isoflavones and Their Effect on Bone in Postmenopausal Women

J. Christopher Gallagher and Vinod Yalamanchili

Key Points

- A high intake of soy is thought to be responsible for a lower incidence of osteoporosis in Asian countries compared to the Western countries.
- A review of randomized control trials that studied the effect of soy isoflavones on bone density reported no significant difference from placebo at the spine and hip in 11 out of 14 trials involving 2,971 postmenopausal women.
- The amount of isoflavones studied ranged from 40 to 300 mg/day and the proportion of genistein and daidzein varied amongst studies.
- Meta-analyses reported inconsistent results probably because the included studies varied in each meta-analysis.
- Despite these facts their use in bone health has generally been promoted by nutritional and holistic sources that do not follow the concept of evidence-based studies.

Keywords Soy protein • Isoflavones • Genistein • Daidzein • Equol • Bone • Menopause • Women

Introduction

Soy is the product of soybean, a widely grown plant used in many different types of food either as a primary source of protein or as a supplement for enriching other foods with protein. Use is much higher in Asian communities than Western countries. There has been an increasing interest in nutrition and medicine in the value of soy as a source of isoflavones and their effects on health.

Isoflavones are nonsteroidal compounds that are often described as phytoestrogens or plant estrogens because they have been shown to bind to estrogen receptors in cell systems and act as selective estrogen receptor modulators [1, 2]. The common phytoestrogens include isoflavones, coumestans, and lignans. Genistin and daidzin are the main compounds found in soy along with the minor aglycone forms genistein and daidzein and small amount of the isoflavone glycitin and its aglycone glycitein. Genistein and daidzein are found largely in soybeans and soy products such as tempeh, miso, red clover, kudzu,

J.C. Gallagher, M.D. (✉) • V. Yalamanchili, M.B.B.S.
Bone Metabolism Unit, Department of Endocrinology, Creighton University Medical Center, 601 North 30th Street, Suite 6718, Omaha 68131, NE, USA
e-mail: jcg@creighton.edu; vinod@creighton.edu

C.J.H. Martin et al. (eds.), *Nutrition and Diet in Menopause*, Nutrition and Health,
DOI 10.1007/978-1-62703-373-2_9,

Table 9.1 Estimated soy isoflavone intake in different postmenopausal populations

Country	Mean intake of soy isoflavones mg/day mean (SD)
Caucasians	1.52 (6.02)[a]
China	21.9 (37.5)[b]
Taiwan	24.0 (24.5)[c]
Japanese	54.3 (1.00)[d]
African-Americans	0.42 (2.76)[a]
Korea	7.96 (4.52)[e]
Holland	7.45 (10.55)[f]
Hong Kong	4.50 (5.4)[g]

This table summarizes that Asian populations consume more soy isoflavones when compared to Western population
[a]Greendale (2002)
[b]Mei et al. (2001)
[c]Tai et al. (2011)
[d]Somekawa et al. (2001) [42]
[e]Song et al. (2008)
[f]Kreijkamp et al. (2004)
[g]Ho SC et al. (2008) (soy protein)

tofu, and American groundnut and have been the focus of most in vitro and in vivo experimental studies. The daily intake of soy isoflavones varies with different populations and is summarized in Table 9.1.

The theoretical background for soy having an effect on bone is based on several properties of soy. Isoflavones bind to estrogen receptor beta (ER-β) and their binding is much stronger to ER-β than estrogen receptor alpha (ER-α) [1–3]. Because ER-β is expressed in bone isoflavones might be expected to have an effect on bone [4]. There are other actions of isoflavones on bone; genistein through its action as a tyrosine kinase inhibitor can act as an inhibitor of osteoclastic resorption [5]. Another of the isoflavones—daidzein—is metabolized to equol by intestinal microflora and in animal and human studies equol has about 100-fold stronger binding to estrogen receptors than daidzein. Equol has shown a protective effect on bone loss in mice [6]. Although humans have the ability to convert daidzein to equol, only about 25–30 % of Western people produce equol [7].

In animal models of osteoporosis, studies have demonstrated an effect of isoflavones in rats in preventing bone loss; however, the comparative doses used are severalfold times greater than those used in human studies [8]. A long-term study in postmenopausal monkeys comparing estrogen and isoflavones showed that estrogen but not isoflavones prevented bone loss [9]. Given the composition of soy isoflavones the results in clinical studies will depend on the product used. For example, soy protein is an extract of soybean that contains equal amounts of genistein and daidzein and less glycitein whereas soy germ contains more daidzein and glycitein than genistein. Some nutritional supplements are derived from soy germ and others from the whole bean. Also processing of soy products such as tofu can cause variation in final isoflavone content.

Despite the theoretical and potential value of these products, information is lacking on their physiologic action in humans and their use in health has generally been promoted by nutritional and holistic sources that do not necessarily follow the concepts of evidence-based studies. The subject of this review is the effect of soy products on bone. Our review is based on studies that studied the effects of soy isoflavones on bone metabolism.

Epidemiology

There is minimal epidemiological data on soy intake and bone health. A significant positive relationship between metacarpal BMD and soy protein intake was reported based on food frequency questionnaire from nearly 1,000 Japanese women aged 40–49 years; however whether the association was due to higher protein intake [10] or isoflavones is not known [11].

In a multiethnic study of premenopausal women in the USA, Greendale et al. found that higher genistein intake was associated with 7.7 % higher BMD at the spine and 12 % higher BMD at the femoral neck in premenopausal Japanese women but there was no relationship in Japanese peri- and postmenopausal women, and no relationship between genistein intake and BMD in any Chinese women [12]. Dietary analysis showed soy isoflavone intake to be twice as high in Japanese compared to Chinese women and 1,200 times higher than that in Caucasian women.

In another study of Chinese postmenopausal women marginally higher spine BMD was found in the highest compared to lowest tertile of isoflavone intake but there was no difference in hip BMD; however serum estradiol levels were twice as high in the highest isoflavone tertile compared to the lowest tertile and also could explain the differences in BMD [13].

In a population-based study of 454 health Chinese women, Ho et al. [14] reported that there was statistically significant cross-sectional association between a soy protein intake of 20 mg/day and hip BMD ($p=0.019$) and total body BMD ($p=0.004$) in early postmenopausal women but not in late postmenopause. In 34 young Korean women who consume soy protein as a part of their diet, multiple 24-h recalls were collected over 2 years to estimate average soy intakes and the average daily isoflavone intake was about 8 mg; it was found that soy protein intake was associated positively with BMD at the femoral neck [15].

Intervention Studies of Soy Isoflavones and Bone Mineral Density

In general 2-year studies are preferred for assessing bone efficacy because a positive increase in BMD at 1 year can be due to a transient mild antiresorptive effect that results in the filling in of the remodeling space, i.e., the osteoclastic cavities present at the onset of treatment. This positive change on bone density can become negative in subsequent years. In these studies the type of soy product and the amounts of the bioactive isoflavones genistein, daidzein, and glycitein vary amongst studies; the relative amounts for each study are summarized in Table 9.2 and the BMD results of each study are briefly discussed in the following paragraphs and summarized in Tables 9.2 and 9.3.

Table 9.2 Dose of isoflavones and components used in randomized control trials

Study	Isoflavones (mg/day)	Genistein (mg/day)	Daidzein (mg/day)	Glycitein (mg/day)
Tai et al. (2011)	300	172.5	127.5	–
Levis et al. (2011)	200	91	103	–
Alekel et al. (2010)[a]	80 and 120	31 and 46	40 and 60	9 and 13
Vupadhyayula et al. (2009)	90	47	38	5
Wong et al. (2009)[a]	80 and 120	44 and 66	26 and 39	10 and 15
Kenny et al. (2009)[b]	105	57	45	7
Brink et al. (2008)	110	75	32	3
Marini et al. (2007)	54	54	–	–
Newton et al. (2006)	83	46	32	6
Arjmandi et al. (2005)	60	–	–	–
Lydeking-Olsen et al. (2004)	76	–	–	–
Chen et al. (2004)[a]	40 and 80	18 and 36	16 and 32	6 and 12
Kreijkamp-Kaspers et al. (2004)	99	52	41	6
Morabito et al. (2002)	54	54	–	–

[a]Studies with two treatment groups
[b]Glycoside forms of isoflavones were used instead of aglycone forms
"–" represents either "data not reported" or "not used"

Table 9.3 2-Year randomized clinical trials of the effect of soy isoflavones on bone mineral density (BMD)

Study	Study design and population	Country	Dosage of soy isoflavones	Mean change in BMD over 2 years		BMD rates of bone loss		
				Placebo	Treatment	Spine	Hip	Total body
Tai et al. (2011)	2-Year randomized double blind *N*=431 Postmenopausal osteopenic women Age 45–65 years	Taiwan	*Two groups*: 300 mg/day or placebo	Spine: −1.72 % Total hip: −1.35 %	Spine: −1.09 % Total hip: −0.81 %	NS	NS	NR[a]
Levis et al. (2011)	2-Year randomized double blind *N*=248 Postmenopausal women Age 45–65 years	USA	*Two groups*: 200 mg/day or placebo	Spine: −2.0 % Total hip: −1.2 % Femur neck: −2.2 %	Spine: −2.3 % Total hip: −1.4 % Femur neck: −2.1 %	NS	NS	NR
Alekel et al. (2010)	3-Year randomized and double-blinded study *N*=224 postmenopausal women Age 46–65 years	USA	*Three groups*: 80 mg/day, 120 mg/day, or placebo	Reported no difference between placebo and the two soy treatment groups over time	Spine: −2.08 % Total femur: −1.43 %, Femoral neck: −2.56 % Total body: −1.66 %	NS	ITT NS Complier analysis 120 mg/day better than placebo at femoral neck*	NS
Vupadhyayula et al. (2009)	2-Year randomized double-blinded trial *N*=203 postmenopausal women Age 55–70 years	USA	*Three groups*: Soy protein no isoflavones, milk protein—control, soy protein+90 mg isoflavones	*Soy protein no isoflavones* Spine: −1.94% Total hip: −1.70 % Femur neck: −2.26 % Trochanter: −1.95 % Total body: −2.61 % *Milk protein—control* Spine: −2.11 % Total hip −1.30 % Femur neck: −1.34 % Trochanter: −1.19 % Total body: −2.53 %	*Soy protein +90 mg isoflavones* Spine: −1.55 % Total hip: −1.13 % Femur neck: −1.31 % Trochanter: −0.69 % Total body: −2.82 %	NS	NS	NS

Wong et al. (2009)	2-Year randomized and double-blinded study *N*=403 postmenopausal women Age 45–65 years	USA	*Three groups*: 80 mg isoflavones, 120 mg/day isoflavones, or placebo	Total body: –0.024 g/cm² or –3.1 % over 2 years	Total body: 80 mg/day: –0.037 g/cm² 120 mg/day: –0.038 g/cm²	NS	NS	Treatment (120 mg/day) significantly better than placebo* NS for 80 mg
Marini et al. (2007)	2-Year randomized and double-blinded study *N*=389 postmenopausal osteopenic women Age 49–67 years	Italy	*Two groups*: genistein 54 mg or placebo	Spine: –0.053 g/cm² Femur neck: –0.037 g/cm²	Spine: +0.049 g/cm² Femur neck: +0.035 g/cm² Difference from placebo Spine: +12.0 % Femur neck: +9.2 %	Treatment Significant*	Treatment did better than placebo*	NR
Lydeking-Olsen et al. (2004)	2-Year randomized and double-blinded study *N*=107 Postmenopausal women Age<75 years	Denmark	*Four groups*: Soymilk+76 mg, isoflavones, progesterone, combination, or placebo	Spine: –4.2 % Femur neck: +0.2 %	*Soymilk* Spine: +1.1 % Femur neck: –0.9 % *Combination* Spine: –2.8 % Neck: –1.3 %	Treatment Significant*	NS	NR

NS No significant difference
[a]Not reported
* Should better than placebo *(P < 0.05)*

There have been seven long-term trials lasting 2 or more years of the effect of isoflavones on bone and they include data on 1,987 subjects. There have been two positive studies (478 subjects) and five negative studies (1,509 subjects) on isoflavones and bone. Of the two positive studies, the first evaluated the effect of supplemented soymilk on bone; it was a small trial of 89 postmenopausal women in Denmark (22–23/group) randomized to soymilk supplemented with isoflavones 76 mg, transdermal progesterone, a combination of both soymilk and transdermal progesterone, or placebo [16]. After 2 years there was a significant difference in spine BMD between the placebo and supplemented soymilk groups but no difference between placebo and the combination of soymilk and progesterone. There were no significant treatment effects of isoflavones on hip BMD and no treatment effect on bone markers.

In the second positive 2-year trial, 389 early postmenopausal women from Italy were randomized to either genistein 56 mg/day or placebo [17]. Compared to placebo genistein significantly increased spine density by 10.0 % and femoral neck BMD by 10.5 %. Surprisingly the bone markers (pyridinoline and deoxypyridinoline) only decreased by 11 and 10 % on genistein compared to placebo. Considering the large change in BMD, normally one would expect at least a 50–75 % decrease in bone markers.

There have been five long-term and large studies of isoflavones on bone that produced negative results (Table 9.4). In a controlled randomized trial 200 women from North America, mean age 61 years, were randomized to three dose groups, 25 g of soy protein isolate with 90 mg isoflavones/day containing genistein and daidzein, and glycitein was compared to soy protein with minimal isoflavones 5 mg and control group of milk protein. There was no significant difference amongst the groups in the rate of bone loss at the spine, hip, or total body after 2 years. [18].

There have been other studies of concentrated forms of isoflavones extracted from soy protein.

In a 2-year study 403 postmenopausal women from North America, mean age 55 years, were randomized to isoflavone tablets 80 mg/day, 120 mg/day, or placebo. Only the data on total body density is presented in the paper. Total body density is total body calcium corrected for body size and represents about 80 % cortical and 20 % of the trabecular bone in the skeleton. There was a significant reduction ($P<0.05$) in the adjusted rate of bone loss using this measurement on the 120 mg dose compared to placebo; however bone loss was still negative; there was no significant difference between the 80 mg dose compared to placebo. Even though spine and hip BMD were primary outcomes the data was not presented although it states in the paper that there was no significant effect of isoflavones on spine or hip BMD [19].

In a 3-year double-blind placebo-controlled study [20], 224 postmenopausal women from North America, mean age 54 years, were randomized to isoflavone tablets, 80 or 120 mg. The ratio of genistein:daidzein:glycitein was similar to that in the natural soybeans (1.3:1.0:0.3). There was no significant effect of isoflavones on spine or hip (total and femoral neck) BMD (Fig. 9.1). In the complier analysis 120 mg marginally reduced the rate of bone loss at the hip ($p<0.024$). In comparison to the Italian studies that used 54 mg of genistein the highest isoflavone dose of 120 mg contained 46 mg of genistein. Recently a study in North America was performed that used an isoflavone dose of 200 mg containing 91 mg genistein. In this trial that was a 2-year double-blind placebo-controlled study of 248 postmenopausal women, mean age 53 years, soy isoflavones 200 mg/day given as two tablets twice daily were compared to placebo. There was no effect of isoflavones on bone mineral density at spine, total hip, and femoral neck [21].

In another large 2-year double-blind placebo-controlled study of 431 Chinese postmenopausal women, aged 55–56 years, from Taiwan [22], the highest dose yet evaluated of isoflavones, 300 mg/day containing 172.5 mg of genistein, was given in the form of three capsules, each with 50 mg taken two times a day; there was no significant effect on spine and hip BMD. In this study the baseline intake of isoflavones was high (up to 53 mg/day) and the authors suggested that the high-baseline soy intake could mask the effects of isoflavones on bone.

Table 9.4 1-Year randomized clinical trials of the effect of soy isoflavones on bone mineral density (BMD)

Study	Study design and population	Country	Dosage of soy isoflavones	BMD comparison		BMD results		
				Placebo	Treatment	Spine	Hip	Whole body
Morabito et al. (2002)	1-Year randomized and double-blinded study $N=90$ Age 47–57 years	Italy	*Three groups*: HRT, genistein 54 mg/day, or placebo	Spine: –1.6 % Femur neck: –0.65 %	*Genistein* Spine: +3.0 % Femur neck: +3.6 % *HRT* Spine: +3.8 % Femur neck: +2.4 %	Treatment Significant*	Treatment Significant*	NR[a]
Chen et al. (2003)	1-Year randomized and double-blinded study $N=203$ Early postmenopausal women Age 48–62 years	Hong Kong	*Three groups*: 40 mg/day soy isoflavones, 80 mg/day soy isoflavones, or placebo	Spine: –0.79 % Total hip: –0.63 % Femur neck: –0.12 % Trochanter: –0.34 % Total body: –0.55 %	*40 mg* Spine: –0.62 % Total hip: –0.44 % Femur neck: –0.50 % Trochanter: –0.51 % Total body: –0.70 % *80 mg* Spine: –0.99 % Total hip: –0.41 % Femur neck: –0.22 % Trochanter: –0.12 % Total body: –0.46 %	NS	BMD No significant difference No significance for femoral neck	NS
Kreijkamp-Kaspers et al. (2004)	1-Year randomized study $N=202$ Postmenopausal women Age 60–75 years	Holland	*Two groups*: 25.6 g of soy + 99 mg of isoflavones, or milk protein as a powder	*Milk protein* Spine: –0.002 g/cm² Total hip: –0.005 g/cm² Femur neck: –0.004 g/cm² Trochanter: –0.006 g/cm²	*Soy + isoflavones* Spine: +0.002 g/cm² Total hip: –0.001 g/cm² Femur neck: –0.004 g/cm² Trochanter: –0.001 g/cm²	NS	NS	NR
Arjmandi et al. (2005)	1-Year randomized and double-blinded study $N=87$ Postmenopausal women Age <65 years	USA	*Two groups*: 60 mg/day soy isoflavones or placebo	Spine: –0.008 g/cm² Total hip: –0.001 g/cm² Total body: –0.015 g/cm² Spine: –0.9 % Total body: –1.3 %	Spine: –0.010 g/cm² Total hip: –0.001 g/cm² Total body: –0.015/cm² Spine: –1.0 % Total body: –1.3 %	NS	NS	NS

(continued)

Table 9.4 (continued)

Study	Study design and population	Country	Dosage of soy isoflavones	BMD comparison		BMD results		
				Placebo	Treatment	Spine	Hip	Whole body
Newton et al. (2006)	1-Year randomized and double-blinded trial *N*=99 men and 16 women Age 50–80 years	USA	*Two groups*: Soy isoflavones 83 mg/day or control group (3 mg isoflavones)	Spine: +0.12 % Hip: –0.13 %	Spine: +1.20 % Hip: +0.54 %	NS	NS	NR
Brink et al. (2008)	1-Year randomized and double-blinded study *N*=237 Early postmenopausal women Age 50–56 years	The Netherlands, Italy, and France	*Two groups*: 110 mg/day soy isoflavones or placebo	Spine: NR Total body: NR	Spine: NR Total body: NR No difference in the rate of bone loss	NS	NS	NS
Kenny et al. (2009)	1-Year randomized and double-blinded trial *N*=131 postmenopausal women Age >60 years	USA	*Four groups*: Soy protein+105 mg of isoflavones, soy protein+placebo, control protein+105 mg isoflavones, control protein+placebo	Soy protein+placebo Spine: +0.001 g/cm^2 Total hip: –0.011 g/cm^2 Femur neck: +0.001 g/cm^2 Total body: –0.003/cm^2 Spine: + 0.010 g/cm^2 Fem neck: –0.003 g/cm^2 Total hip: –0.008 g/cm^2 Total Body –0.005/cm^2	Soy protein+isoflavones Spine: +0.004 g/cm^2 Total hip: +0.003 g/cm^2 Femur neck: +0.001 g/cm^2 Total body: –0.007/cm^2 Control protein+ isoflavones Spine: +0.018 g/cm^2 Total hip: –0.003 g/cm^2 Femur neck: –0.006 g/cm^2 Total body: –0.004/cm^2	NS	NS	NS

NS No significant difference
HRT hormone replacement therapy
[a]Not reported
* Should better than placebo *($P < 0.05$)*

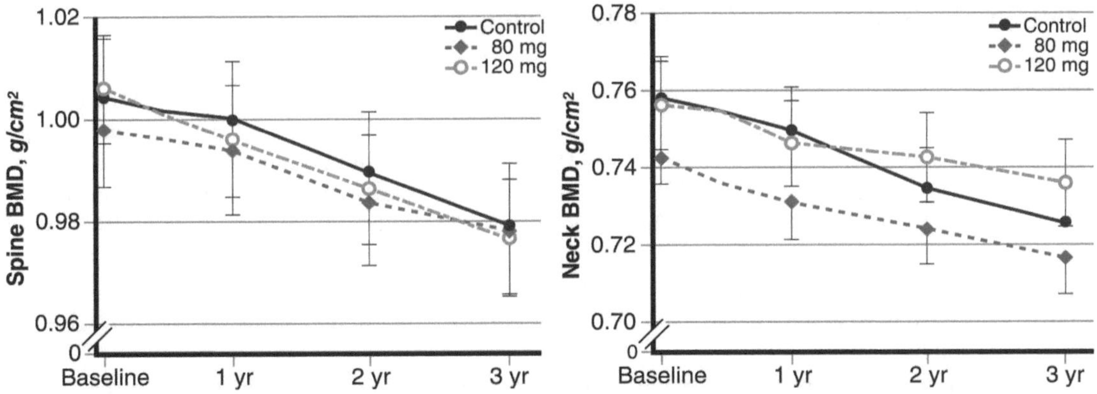

Fig. 9.1 Change in bone mineral density of spine and femoral neck between the soy treatment and control groups in a 3-year study by Alekel et al. (2010). Data adapted from the paper by Alekel et al. (2010) ([20])

There have been seven evaluable controlled studies lasting 1 year (Table 9.3) that evaluated the effect of soy isoflavones on bone density in postmenopausal women.

In a small trial from Italy [23] lasting 1 year genistein compound of 54 mg was used in 90 early menopausal women, aged 51years, randomized to genistein, estradiol 1 mg, or placebo. On genistein spine BMD increased 5.4 % and femoral neck BMD increased 4.2 % compared to placebo. The changes in BMD on estradiol were very similar to those of genistein and as expected bone markers decreased about 50 % on both genistein and estradiol. A study from Hong Kong studied 203 early postmenopausal women, mean age 54 years, using two doses of isoflavones 40 and 80 mg/day (18 and 36 mg genistein) derived from soy germ extracts and found no significant effects of isoflavones on spine, hip, or total body BMD compared with placebo [24].

In a 1-year randomized study in 87 postmenopausal women from North America of soy foods that contained either 60 mg/day isoflavones or none, there was no significant difference in spine, hip, and total body BMD between the treatment and control groups [25]. In another 1-year study of 123 men and 22 women from North America, subjects were given a soy drink containing 83 mg/day isoflavones or no isoflavones. There were no significant differences in the spine or hip BMD in men or women [26].

In a multicenter study conducted in four countries and lasting 1 year women with an average age of 53 years were randomized blindly to soy biscuits and bars containing 110 mg isoflavones (75 mg genistein) or no isoflavones. At the end of the year there were no significant differences in total body or spine BMD between the groups and hip BMD was not measured. A later analysis showed no difference between equol and non-equol producers [27].

In a 1-year study in North America, 131 women, mean age 73 years, were randomized to one of the four groups, soy protein isolate with or without 105 mg isoflavones (57 mg genistein) or control protein with or without the same isoflavones. At the end of 1 year there were no significant differences in the rates of bone loss at the spine, hip, or total body sites between the four groups. Nor were there any differences in the bone markers. A further analysis showed no differences in the BMD changes based on equol or non-equol producers [28].

A very small study in Taiwan of 43 women randomized to control, 100 or 200 mg isoflavones, failed to show consistent effects on spine or hip BMD probably because the groups were too small for a bone efficacy study [29]. In a large study from Holland, 202 women, average age 66 years, were randomized to a soy powder enriched with 99 mg isoflavone containing 52 mg genistein or matching milk protein as the control. At the end of 1 year there was no difference in the rates of bone loss at the spine or the hip between the groups [30].

Meta-analyses of Randomized Control Trials

Three meta-analyses examined the effect of soy isoflavones on bone mineral density. In a recent meta-analysis [31] of 12 RCTs with 1,433 women, it was reported that there was no effect of an average amount of 90 mg/day of soy isoflavones on BMD at lumbar spine in perimenopausal and postmenopausal Western women. The mean difference in spine BMD between treatment and placebo was 9.86 mg/cm^2 (95 % CI −2.64 to 22.36). This is consistent with another meta-analysis of ten RCTs with 896 women by Liu et al. [32] in which no difference is seen in lumbar spine, femoral neck, and total hip with an average dose of 87 mg/day. In their analysis the mean differences in BMD in mg/cm^2/year were 4.1 (CI −1.6, 9.8) at the lumbar spine, −1.5 (CI −7.2, 4.3) at the femoral neck, and 2.5 (CI −0.5, 5.4) at the total hip.

In contrast, a meta-analysis by Taku et al. [33] that included data on 1,240 menopausal women showed that a dose of 82 mg/day soy isoflavones significantly increased spine BMD by 22.25 mg/cm^2 (95 % CI: 7.62, 32.89; $p=0.002$) or by 2.38 % (95 % CI: 0.93, 3.83; $p=0.001$) compared with the control group. No significant effects on femoral neck, hip total, and trochanter BMD were found.

One of the reasons for the discrepancy between the meta-analyses by Taku and Ricci is that the studies included in the two analyses are quite different; only 3 of 12 studies were common to both analyses and 7 of the 12 studies by Taku et al. were from Asia compared to none of the 12 by Ricci et al. Also Taku et al. included studies only up to 2008. Since this last analyses there have been three more large well-controlled studies [19, 21, 22], all of which are essentially negative.

Soy Isoflavones in Premenopausal Women

There have been few studies that studied the relationship between soy and bone in premenopausal women. A study in young adult healthy females reported that isoflavone-rich soy supplementation (90 mg/day) had no effect on whole-body BMD. It was suggested that young women who still produce estrogen from their ovaries might not improve their BMD from the isoflavone "estrogenic" effect because endogenous estrogen may have stronger affinity to the receptors than isoflavones [34]. In a longitudinal study of young Korean women, soy isoflavone intake had a favorable effect on femoral neck [15]. But in Chinese study in women aged 19–86 years no effect of soy supplementation on BMD was seen on younger women [13].

Role of Equol

Equol is a product of the isoflavone daidzein and is formed in the colon from the action of microflora. Equol production occurs in about 25–30 % of the Western population [7], 38–58 % in the Asian population [35], and even higher in 60 % in vegetarians [36]. The difference between equol producers and non-producers after isoflavone supplementation in terms of bone has been reported in few studies.

In one study [16] a subgroup analysis of equol producers versus non-producers after isoflavone treatment showed slightly higher increase in spine BMD in producers but the numbers were small (10 vs. 12) and not significantly different amongst the two groups.

In a controlled study, 54 Japanese women were given 75 mg isoflavones/day or placebo for 1 year. When the data was analyzed by equol status the rate of change in spine BMD was the same in both groups but total hip and trochanter showed less bone loss in equol producers ($p<0.05$); however the group size was small (10 vs. 15), marginally significant, and inadequately powered for a bone study [37].

Other studies have not been able to show a difference in BMD between equol producers and non-producers [27, 28, 30].

To explore the importance of equol status further a randomized controlled study administered natural S-equol 2, 4, and 10 mg/day or placebo to 93 postmenopausal Japanese women who were non-equol producers. There was a 24 % decrease in urine deoxypyridinoline, which is a marker of bone resorption, but no effect on another bone resorption marker urine N-telopeptides. There was a significant decrease in total body BMD on the 10 mg dose versus placebo (−1.1 % vs. −1.88 %, $p < 0.05$) but no effect on spine or hip BMD [38]. The decrease in bone resorption markers is modest and about half that seen on low-dose estrogen suggesting that the dose of equol should be higher than 10 mg in order to prevent bone loss in women.

The difference between equol producers and non-producers remains largely unclear in terms of clinical benefits in Western women and further studies are needed. It is entirely possible that because of the lifelong high intake of soy in Asian people responses to equol may be different from those of Western people. An important issue for the future of equol research is to design bone studies that are statistically powered to detect differences in BMD between equol producers and non-producers.

Synthetic Isoflavones

Ipriflavone is a synthetic daidzein derivative of isoflavones that was shown in vitro to demonstrate an antiresorptive action in cell systems [39]. Despite earlier studies from Italy claiming efficacy of ipriflavone in preventing bone loss [40] a large multicenter controlled trial lasting 2 years that involved 474 women aged 61 years who were randomized to ipriflavone 600 mg/day or placebo did not show any significant difference in spine or hip BMD between the groups [41].

Conclusion

There is no compelling evidence for a beneficial effect of soy isoflavones on bone density in postmenopausal women. Altogether combining the 1- and 2-year studies there are 2,992 subjects in the negative studies and 568 in positive studies; 85 % of the positive results are from the same group in Italy. Although the two strongly positive studies from Italy were given the same dose of genistein 54 mg/day, 11 of the negative studies used either similar or doses greater than 54 mg of genistein (Table 9.2). It is difficult to explain these discrepant results from Italy. In the five largest randomized controlled trials totaling 1,510 postmenopausal women there was no consistent skeletal effect of isoflavones given in doses ranging from 80 to 300 mg/day on bone density of the spine, hip, or total body. Another study that was positive from Denmark [16] was very small with only 22–23 per group, did not show consistent results with the combination treatment, and was not adequately powered to detect significant bone loss in postmenopausal women; so the effect may have occurred by chance.

The issue that the proportion of equol producers versus non-producers in a study may affect the efficacy of isoflavones has not been demonstrated in a Western population. The difference in BMD between equol and non-equol producers in Asian women is restricted to two small studies and the results are marginal. Newer studies on the effects of S-equol and bone are very much in pilot stage and larger studies with other doses lasting at least 2 years with bone as an end point are necessary.

Acknowledgements The authors acknowledge Dr. D. Lee Alekel, Ph.D., and Dr. William W. Wong, Ph.D., C.N.S., F.A.C.N., for kindly providing data from their study.

References

1. Barkhem T, Carlsson B, Nilsson Y, Enmark E, Gustafsson J, Nilsson S. Differential response of estrogen receptor alpha and estrogen receptor beta to partial estrogen agonists/antagonists. Mol Pharmacol. 1998;54(1):105–12.
2. Adlercreutz H, Mazur W. Phyto-oestrogens and Western diseases. Ann Med. 1997;29(2):95–120.
3. Kuiper GG, Carlsson B, Grandien K, Enmark E, Häggblad J, Nilsson S. Comparison of the ligand binding specificity and transcript tissue distribution of estrogen receptors alpha and beta. Endocrinology. 1997;138(3):863–70.
4. Onoe Y, Miyaura C, Ohta H, Nozawa S, Suda T. Expression of estrogen receptor beta in rat bone. Endocrinology. 1997;138(10):4509–12.
5. Blair HC, Jordan SE, Peterson TG, Barnes S. Variable effects of tyrosine kinase inhibitors on avian osteoclastic activity and reduction of bone loss in ovariectomized rats. J Cell Biochem. 1996;61(4):629–37.
6. Fujioka M, Uehara M, Wu J, Adlercreutz H, Suzuki K, Kanazawa K. Equol, a metabolite of daidzein, inhibits bone loss in ovariectomized mice. J Nutr. 2004;134(10):2623–7.
7. Lampe JW, Karr SC, Hutchins AM, Slavin JL. Urinary equol excretion with a soy challenge: influence of habitual diet. Proc Soc Exp Biol Med. 1998;217:335–9.
8. Arjmandi BH, Smith BJ. Soy isoflavones' osteoprotective role in postmenopausal women: mechanism of action. J Nutr Biochem. 2002;13(3):130–7.
9. Register TC, Jayo MJ, Anthony MS. Soy phytoestrogens do not prevent bone loss in postmenopausal monkeys. J Clin Endocrinol Metab. 2003;88(9):4362–70.
10. Darling AL, Millward DJ, Torgerson DJ, Hewitt CE, Lanham-New SA. Dietary protein and bone health: a systematic review and meta-analysis. Am J Clin Nutr. 2009;90(6):1674–92.
11. Tsuchida K, Mizushima S, Toba M, Soda K. Dietary soybeans intake and bone mineral density among 995 middle-aged women in Yokohama. J Epidemiol. 1999;9(1):14–9.
12. Greendale GA, FitzGerald G, Huang MH, Sternfeld B, Gold E, Seeman T. Dietary soy isoflavones and bone mineral density: results from the study of women's health across the nation. Am J Epidemiol. 2002;155(8):746–54.
13. Mei J, Yeung SS, Kung AW. High dietary phytoestrogen intake is associated with higher bone mineral density in postmenopausal but not premenopausal women. J Clin Endocrinol Metab. 2001;86(11):5217–21.
14. Ho SC, Woo J, Lam S, Chen Y, Sham A, Lau J. Soy protein consumption and bone mass in early postmenopausal Chinese women. Osteoporos Int. 2003;14(10):835–42.
15. Song Y, Paik HY, Joung H. Soybean and soy isoflavone intake indicate a positive change in bone mineral density for 2 years in young Korean women. Nutr Res. 2008;28(1):25–30.
16. Lydeking-Olsen E, Beck-Jensen JE, Setchell KD, Holm-Jensen T. Soymilk or progesterone for prevention of bone loss–a 2 year randomized, placebo-controlled trial. Eur J Nutr. 2004;43(4):246–57.
17. Marini H, Minutoli L, Polito F, Bitto A, Altavilla D, Atteritano M. Effects of the phytoestrogen genistein on bone metabolism in osteopenic postmenopausal women: a randomized trial. Ann Intern Med. 2007;146(12):839–47.
18. Vupadhyayula PM, Gallagher JC, Templin T, Logsdon SM, Smith LM. Effects of soy protein isolate on bone mineral density and physical performance indices in postmenopausal women–a 2-year randomized, double-blind, placebo-controlled trial. Menopause. 2009;16(2):320–8.
19. Wong WW, Lewis RD, Steinberg FM, Murray MJ, Cramer MA, Amato P. Soy isoflavone supplementation and bone mineral density in menopausal women: a 2-y multicenter clinical trial. Am J Clin Nutr. 2009;90(5):1433–9.
20. Alekel DL, Van Loan MD, Koehler KJ, Hanson LN, Stewart JW, Hanson KB. The soy isoflavones for reducing bone loss (SIRBL) study: a 3-y randomized controlled trial in postmenopausal women. Am J Clin Nutr. 2010;91(1):218–30.
21. Levis S, Strickman-Stein N, Ganjei-Azar P, Xu P, Doerge DR, Krischer J. Soy isoflavones in the prevention of menopausal bone loss and menopausal symptoms: a randomized, double-blind trial. Arch Intern Med. 2011;171(15):1363–9.
22. Tai TY, Tsai KS, Tu ST, Wu JS, Chang CI, Chen CL. The effect of soy isoflavone on bone mineral density in postmenopausal Taiwanese women with bone loss: a 2-year randomized double-blind placebo-controlled study. Osteoporos Int. 2012;23(5):1571–80.
23. Morabito N, Crisafulli A, Vergara C, Gaudio A, Lasco A, Frisina N. Effects of genistein and hormone-replacement therapy on bone loss in early postmenopausal women: a randomized double-blind placebo-controlled study. J Bone Miner Res. 2002;17(10):1904–12.
24. Chen YM, Ho SC, Lam SS, Ho SS, Woo JL. Soy isoflavones have a favorable effect on bone loss in Chinese postmenopausal women with lower bone mass: a double-blind, randomized, controlled trial. J Clin Endocrinol Metab. 2003;88(10):4740–7.
25. Arjmandi BH, Lucas EA, Khalil DA, Devareddy L, Smith BJ, McDonald J. One year soy protein supplementation has positive effects on bone formation markers but not bone density in postmenopausal women. Nutr J. 2005;4:8.

26. Newton KM, LaCroix AZ, Levy L, Li SS, Qu P, Potter JD. Soy protein and bone mineral density in older men and women: a randomized trial. Maturitas. 2006;55(3):270–7.
27. Brink E, Coxam V, Robins S, Wahala K, Cassidy A, Branca F. Long-term consumption of isoflavone-enriched foods does not affect bone mineral density, bone metabolism, or hormonal status in early postmenopausal women: a randomized, double-blind, placebo controlled study. Am J Clin Nutr. 2008;87(3):761–70.
28. Kenny AM, Mangano KM, Abourizk RH, Bruno RS, Anamani DE, Kleppinger A. Soy proteins and isoflavones affect bone mineral density in older women: a randomized controlled trial. Am J Clin Nutr. 2009;90(1):234–42.
29. Huang HY, Yang HP, Yang HT, Yang TC, Shieh MJ, Huang SY. One-year soy isoflavone supplementation prevents early postmenopausal bone loss but without a dose-dependent effect. J Nutr Biochem. 2006;17(8):509–17.
30. Kreijkamp-Kaspers S, Kok L, Grobbee DE, de Haan EH, Aleman A, Lampe JW. Effect of soy protein containing isoflavones on cognitive function, bone mineral density, and plasma lipids in postmenopausal women: a randomized controlled trial. JAMA. 2004;292(1):65–74.
31. Ricci E, Cipriani S, Chiaffarino F, Malvezzi M, Parazzini F. Effects of soy isoflavones and genistein on glucose metabolism in perimenopausal and postmenopausal non-Asian women: a meta-analysis of randomized controlled trials. Menopause. 2010;17(5):1080–6.
32. Liu J, Ho SC, Su YX, Chen WQ, Zhang CX, Chen YM. Effect of long-term intervention of soy isoflavones on bone mineral density in women: a meta-analysis of randomized controlled trials. Bone. 2009;44(5):948–53.
33. Taku K, Melby MK, Takebayashi J, Mizuno S, Watanabe S, Ishimi Y. Effect of soy isoflavone extract supplements on bone mineral density in menopausal women: meta-analysis of randomized controlled trials. Asia Pac J Clin Nutr. 2010;19(1):33–42.
34. Anderson JJ, Chen X, Boass A, Symons M, Kohlmeier M, Renner JB. Soy isoflavones: no effects on bone mineral content and bone mineral density in healthy, menstruating young adult women after one year. J Am Coll Nutr. 2002;21(5):388–93.
35. Morton MS, Arisaka O, Miyake N, Morgan LD, Evans BA. Phytoestrogen concentrations in serum from Japanese men and women over forty years of age. J Nutr. 2002 Oct;132(10):3168–71.
36. Setchell KD, Cole SJ. Method of defining equol-producer status and its frequency among vegetarians. J Nutr. 2006 Aug;136(8):2188–93.
37. Wu J, Oka J, Ezaki J, Ohtomo T, Ueno T, Uchiyama S. Possible role of equol status in the effects of isoflavone on bone and fat mass in postmenopausal Japanese women: a double-blind, randomized, controlled trial. Menopause. 2007;14(5):866–74.
38. Tousen Y, Ezaki J, Fujii Y, Ueno T, Nishimuta M, Ishimi Y. Natural S-equol decreases bone resorption in postmenopausal, non-equol-producing Japanese women: a pilot randomized, placebo-controlled trial. Menopause. 2011;18(5):563–74.
39. Notoya K, Yoshida K, Taketomi S, Yamazaki I, Kumegawa M. Inhibitory effect of ipriflavone on pit formation in mouse unfractionated bone cells. Calcif Tissue Int. 1992;51:S1–6.
40. Gennari C, Adami S, Agnusdei D, Bufalíno L, Cervetti R, Crepaldi G. Effect of chronic treatment with ipriflavone in postmenopausal women with low bone mass. Calcif Tissue Int. 1997;61 Suppl 1Suppl 1:S19–22.
41. Alexandersen P, Toussaint A, Christiansen C, Devogelaer JP, Roux C, Fechtenbaum J. Ipriflavone multicenter european fracture study. Ipriflavone in the treatment of postmenopausal osteoporosis: a randomized controlled trial. JAMA. 2001;285(11):1482–8.
42. Somekawa Y, Chiguchi M, Ishibashi T, Aso T. Soy intake related to menopausal symptoms, serum lipids, and bone mineral density in postmenopausal Japanese women. Obstet Gynecol. 2001;97(1):109–15.

[illegible]

Chapter 10
S-equol, a Natural Metabolite of Soy Daidzein, for the Treatment of Menopausal Symptoms and Osteoporosis in Postmenopausal Women

Richard L. Jackson, Jeffrey S. Greiwe, and Richard J. Schwen

Key Points

- S-equol is a potent, nonhormonal, nonsteroidal estrogen receptor β agonist.
- S-equol is produced by the gut biotransformation of soy daidzein, an isoflavone present in soy.
- Individuals, particularly Asians, who are equol producers have fewer menopausal symptoms, osteoporosis, diseases of the prostate, and cardiovascular diseases.
- A soy-derived dietary supplement containing 10 mg S-equol has been shown to reduce menopausal symptoms and improve bone mineral density in postmenopausal women.
- A clinical study in men and women with doses of S-equol up to 320 mg/day demonstrated that the compound has an excellent safety and pharmacokinetic profile.

Keywords S-equol • Soy • Menopausal symptoms • Hot flashes • Women's health

Abbreviations

HT	Hormone therapy
WHI	Women's health initiative
VMS	Vasomotor symptoms
DRI	Daidzein-rich isoflavone
BMD	Bone mineral density
BMC	Bone mineral composition

Introduction

In 2002 the results of the Women's Health Initiative (WHI) were published [1]. Surprisingly, postmenopausal women on hormone therapy (HT), Premarin® (0.625 mg/day) plus medroxy-progesterone (2.5 mg/day), had significantly increased cardiovascular diseases, invasive breast cancer, stroke, and venous thromboembolism compared to the placebo group. The women on HT did have fewer hip

R.L. Jackson, Ph.D. (✉) • J.S. Greiwe, Ph.D. • R.J. Schwen, Ph.D.
Ausio Pharmaceuticals, LLC, 1776 Mentor Avenue, Suite 340, Cincinnati, OH 45212, USA
e-mail: richard@ausiopharma.com: jeff@ausiopharma.com: rick@ausiopharma.com

C.J.H. Martin et al. (eds.), *Nutrition and Diet in Menopause*, Nutrition and Health,
DOI 10.1007/978-1-62703-373-2_10, © Springer Science+Business Media New York 2013

fractures and there was a reduced incidence of colorectal cancer. Nonetheless, the findings of WHI have had a major impact on women's health. Women do not want HT as reflected in the reduced prescriptions for products containing estrogens, and as a result, the incidence of hip fractures has increased by 55 % since 2002 [2]. As an alternative to HT, many women have resorted to nonhormonal therapies for the treatment of menopausal symptoms, including antidepressants, herbal extracts, soy extracts, and soy isoflavones, also referred to as phytoestrogens [3–6]. It is well known that Japanese people consume large amounts of soy products and have fewer chronic diseases compared to Caucasians. Adlercreutz et al. [7] proposed that Japanese women have fewer menopausal symptoms based on their soy intake. The first report on the consumption of soy products and the incidence of hot flashes was by Nagata et al., 2001 [8]. In this study, a questionnaire was used to measure an individual's intake of soy foods. The tertiles for soy intake were low (44.5 g/day), middle (75.2 g/day), and high (115.9 g/day); the intake of total isoflavones was 20.5, 32.8, and 50.8 mg/day, respectively. A decrease in the hazard ratio for hot flashes was directly related to soy and total isoflavone intake ($p<0.005$).

Since these early findings, many controlled clinical studies have been carried out with soy and soy isoflavones to alleviate vasomotor symptoms (VMS) in menopausal women (for review, see [9–11]). The results of meta-analysis are for the most part inconclusive as to the clinical benefit of soy and soy extracts. For many studies, the sample size was too small and the duration of the study was too short (<4–6 weeks) to show a statistical difference between the treated and placebo groups. If the frequency of hot flashes was the primary end point, there was little or no response to soy isoflavone extracts in women who experienced four or fewer hot flashes per day. A complicating factor in many of the studies was the variability in the composition of the isoflavone supplement. The major isoflavones in soy beans are the glycoside conjugates of genistein, daidzein, and glycetin. The conjugated isoflavones are absorbed more slowly than the respective aglycone forms, with a different pharmacokinetic profile. The amount of each isoflavone also varies from each batch of soy bean. Finally, and as discussed below, most published studies have not considered the influence of intestinal bacteria to produce S-equol, a metabolite of daidzein. In this review, we have discussed those studies that have shown a positive effect of dietary isoflavone supplements on reducing menopausal symptoms and improving bone health.

Soy Isoflavones and Menopausal Symptoms

Table 10.1 summarizes the studies that show a decrease in hot flashes with dietary supplements. Han et al. [12] carried out a 4-month, double-blind study in Sao Paulo, Brazil, to determine the effects of isoflavones on menopausal symptoms, as well as cardiovascular risk factors. Postmenopausal women (aged 45–55 years) were divided into two groups, a placebo group ($n=40$) and an isoflavone group ($n=40$). The isoflavone group received 100 mg isoflavones/day, 18.6 mg as daidzein and 70.0 mg as genistein. A Kupperman Index questionnaire was used to assess the menopausal symptoms. Consumption of isoflavones was associated with a significant decrease in vasomotor symptoms from 11.3 to 8.2 hot flashes/day and an overall decrease in the Kupperman Index from 44.6 to 24.9.

Table 10.1 Effects of dietary soy supplementation on hot flashes

Treatment	Content (mg)		Population studied	Reduction in HF (treatment time)	References
	Daidzein	Genistein			
Isoflavone capsule (100 mg/day)	18.6	70	Brazil	27 % ↓ HF (4 months)	Han et al. [12]
Fruit drink containing isoflavones (60 mg/day)	ND	ND	Sweden	57 % ↓ HF (3 months)	Cheng et al. [13]
Isoflavone tablet (Previna®) (90 mg/day)	316	30	Brazil	50 % ↓ HF (4 months)	Carmignami et al. [14]

The equol producer status was not determined in this study. Total cholesterol and LDL-cholesterol were decreased significantly in the isoflavone group and HDL-cholesterol was increased, suggesting a clinical benefit for cardiovascular diseases.

Cheng et al. [13] carried out a double-blind prospective study in 51 postmenopausal women in Sweden. The women were between 49 and 69 years of age (mean 58.4±5.0) and received a fruit drink containing 60 mg isoflavones/day for 3 months. The equol producer status was not determined in this study. Women taking the isoflavones showed a significant 57 % lower score for hot flashes, 1.4±1.3 before treatment versus 0.6±0.7 after treatment ($p<0.05$). For night sweats, the change was from 1.4±1.3 to 0.8±0.8 ($p<0.05$). The isoflavone treatment did not affect plasma levels of lipids, follicle-stimulating hormone, or estradiol. Immunohistochemical staining of endometrial and breast biopsy tissues showed no differences in the expression levels of steroid, estrogen, or progesterone receptors or the proliferation marker K_i67, indicating that the isoflavones had no effect on the endometrium and breast.

Carmighani et al. [14] gave 20 postmenopausal women with moderate to severe hot flashes a dietary soy supplement (Previna®, Sanavita Functional Foods) for 16 weeks. The supplement consisted of 20 g of food powder containing 12 g of soy protein and a total of 45 mg of isoflavones (26.5 mg aglycones). The supplement was taken twice a day. Compared to the placebo group, the isoflavone supplement had a significant improvement in hot flashes and muscle pain. Based on these limited studies, it is difficult to conclude which of the isoflavones in soy accounts for the decrease in VMS. Williamson-Hughes et al. [15] reviewed earlier studies and concluded that the reduction in hot flashes was related to the genistein dose with >15 mg genistein (calculated as aglycone equivalents) giving positive results. However, in these earlier studies the equol-producing status was not determined.

S-equol-Producing Status and Menopausal Symptoms

S-equol is produced by gut bacteria from daidzein (Fig. 10.1). The equol hypothesis was first proposed by Setchell et al. [16]. Subsequently, Setchell et al. [17] determined the structure of equol and reported that it is only the S-enantiomer of equol that is produced by man and animals. S-equol is a potent, selective estrogen receptor β agonist with tenfold lesser activity for ERα, the estrogen receptor that is expressed in the breast and uterus. For this reason, it is anticipated that women taking S-equol will have fewer safety issues. Jackson et al. [18] have recently reviewed the literature on the health benefits of being an equol producer. In addition, an Equol, Soy, and Menoapausal Research Leadership Conference was held on June 16, 2009, and the proceedings were published [19]. Table 10.2 summarizes the menopausal studies in which the equol-producing status was determined in postmenopausal women receiving soy and soy isoflavones.

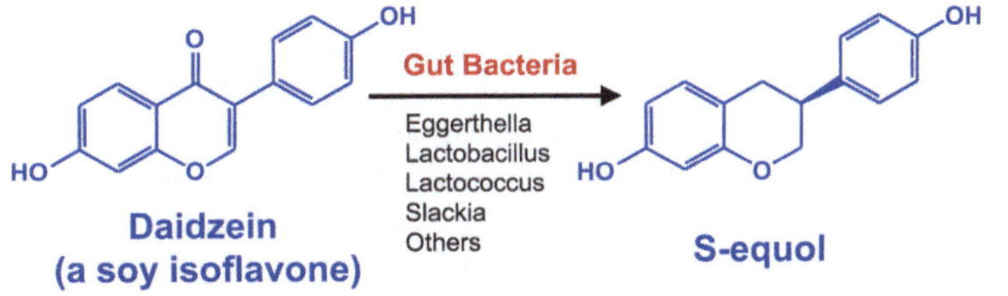

Fig. 10.1 Biotransformation of daidzein to S-equol. Various bacteria have been shown to carry out this process. Reprinted with permission from Jackson RL, Greiwe JS, Desai PB, Schwen RJ. Single-dose and steady-state pharmacokinetic studies of S-equol, a potent nonhormonal, estrogen receptor β-agonist being developed for the treatment of menopausal symptoms. Menopause. 2011;18:185–193

Table 10.2 Summary of the effects of isoflavones on hot flashes in equol producers

Treatment	Content of daidzein	Population studied	Reduction in HF (treatment time)	Equol determination	References
Effisoy™ (40 mg/day)	28 mg	Boston	52 % ↓ HF (12 weeks)	Plasma S-equol (8.89 ng/mL)	Khaodhiar et al. [22]
Effisoy™ (60 mg/day)	43 mg	Boston	51 % ↓ HF (12 weeks)	Plasma S-equol (13.19 ng/mL)	Khaodhiar et al. [22]
Isoflavone tablet (42 mg/day)	13.5 mg	Tokyo	65 % ↓ HF (8 weeks)	Equol producers	Uesugi et al. [23]
Soy germ extract powder (135 mg/day)	32.7 mg	Taipei	68 % ↓ HF (6 months)	Equol producers	Jou et al. [21]
Soyflour (45 g/day)	ND	Melbourne, Australia	40 % ↓ HF (12 weeks)	24-h urine (3.6 μmol equol)	Murkies et al. [20]

One of the first clinical trials to assess the effects of soy on menopausal symptoms in equol producers was reported by Murkies et al. [20]. Fifty-eight Australian postmenopausal women (mean age 53.8 years) were randomized to either a wheat flour (45 g/day) group or a soy flour (45 g/day) group. After 12 weeks, the soy group showed a significant reduction of 40 % in hot flashes; the number of hot flashes decreased from 6.0 to 3.5/day during the 12 weeks of treatment. The absolute amount of equol in a 24-h urine collection in the soy flour group was 3.6 ± 1.6 μmol (mean ± SEM) and could be accounted for by 5 of the 28 subjects indicating that 20 % of the population were equol producers.

A study [21] in menopausal women at Taiwan Adventist Hospital and National Taiwan University compared a placebo group ($n = 30$) to a treatment group ($n = 66$) consuming a daily dose of 6 g of soy germ extract powder containing 135 mg isoflavones of which 32.7 mg was daidzein. Those subjects who received the soy powder and were equol producers ($n = 34$) experienced a greater and more rapid improvement of their menopausal symptoms. After 6 months of treatment, the equol producer group had a lower total score for 17 different vasomotor symptoms than the equol nonproducers and placebo group (4.32 vs. 8.77 vs. 6.74), respectively. In this study, equol producer status was determined in urine by a positive chromatographic peak for equol in urine.

The effects of a daidzein-rich isoflavone (DRI) supplement (Effisoy,™ a dietary supplement containing 70 % daidzein) on hot flashes has been reported by Khaodhiar et al. [22]. Postmenopausal women (mean age 53 years) living in the Boston area were randomized into a placebo group ($n = 45$), a group receiving 40 mg DRI daily ($n = 48$) and a group receiving 60 mg DRI ($n = 49$). After 12 weeks of supplementation, the frequency of hot flashes in the 40 mg DRI group was reduced by 52 % and by 51 % in the 60 mg group; the reduction in the placebo group was 39 %. While the differences between the 40 and 60 DRI groups and placebo were not significant ($p = 0.07$ and 0.09, respectively), combining the two DRI treatment groups did show a significant reduction in hot flashes. The plasma levels of equol in the 40 and 60 mg DRI groups were 8.89 and 13.19 ng/mL, respectively. DRI supplementation did not produce any significant changes in serum levels of thyroid-stimulating hormone, thyroxine, luteinizing hormone, or estradiol.

A double-blind, placebo-controlled 28-day crossover study in 58 climacteric Japanese women (mean age 58 ± 7 years) was carried out with a daily isoflavone supplement containing 40.0 mg total isoflavones, as aglycones [23]. The subjects were also allowed to consume 20 mg isoflavones from their normal dietary intake of soy. The total isoflavone intake in the treated group was 51.1 mg/day versus 13.7 mg/day in the placebo arm. A significant reduction of 65 % in hot flashes from the placebo group was observed in the isoflavone-supplemented diet. There was no effect of the isoflavone supplement on plasma lipids or liver function. The equol producers showed a significant decrease in urinary deoxypyridinoline levels, a marker for a bone-sparing effect. In this study, equol producers were defined as those subjects who excreted equol in urine more than 0.01 nM/mM Cr throughout the study period.

S-equol-Producing Status and Osteoporosis

A number of reports in the literature describe the effects of isoflavone diets on bone health (for review, see [24]). In general, controlled clinical studies in humans have shown that soy isoflavone supplements have a positive effect on bone mineral density (BMD). The largest study comparing soy consumption and the risk of bone fracture is the Shanghai Women's Health Study where 75,000 Chinese women aged 40–70 years were followed for 4.5 years [25]. Soy intake was determined by a questionnaire and based on this information the subjects were divided into either low or high soy consumption groups. The mean daily intake of soy isoflavones was 8.5 and 38.0 mg, respectively. During the study, 1,770 incident fractures were reported. After adjustment for age and total caloric intake, higher isoflavone consumption was associated with lower risk of bone fractures. After the data were stratified by time since menopause, there was a pronounced positive benefit associated with women taking isoflavones in early menopause. In this study, plasma equol levels were not determined.

Six interventional studies have examined the effects of dietary isoflavones on bone, and equol levels were determined. Kreijkamp-Kaspers et al. [26] carried out a 12-month double-blind, randomized, placebo-controlled trial in 202 postmenopausal Dutch women (18 years past menopause) receiving 99 mg isoflavones/day (41 mg daidzein) versus placebo. Equol producer status was defined as a plasma equol concentration >83 nmol/L (approximately 20 ng/mL). The proportion of equol producers in the isoflavone group was 29.9 %. Both the treated and placebo groups showed a decrease in BMD after 1 year. There were no significant differences in hip and lumbar spine BMD between the two groups. However, the BMD in the intertrochanter region of the hip was significantly higher in the isoflavone-treated group. Subgroup analysis for the number of years since menopause showed that women in the lowest tertile with <14 years since menopause had the most improvement in BMD whereas those individuals with >22 years had a BMD no better than the placebo group. This study is important because it is one of the first intervention studies to consider time since start of menopause as a factor in the clinical outcome later in life.

A 2-year, double-blind study in postmenopausal Danish women (mean age 58.2 years) examined the effects of diet and isoflavones on markers of osteoporosis [27]. The diets consisted of (1) soymilk containing 76 mg isoflavones/day; (2) the same diet as (1) but with application of a topical progesterone cream; (3) the cream alone but without the isoflavones; and (4) soymilk alone. In the soymilk-alone group, there was a greater than 4 % decrease in BMD and bone mineral composition (BMC) in the lumbar spine over the 2-year period, which is typical for bone loss in women after menopause. The progesterone groups also showed a similar decrease in BMD. However, the isoflavone group showed an overall mean increase of 1.1 and 2.0 % for lumbar spine BMD and BMC, respectively. After the data were stratified in the isoflavone group into equol producers (serum equol >10 ng/mL) and non-producers, there was an increase of 2.4 % in BMD and 2.8 % in BMC in the equol producers. Serum equol levels in the equol producers were 44.0 ± 25.2 ng/mL. In contrast, only 0.6 and 0.3 % increases were observed in lumbar spine BMD and BMC of women in the nonproducers. Thus, the addition of isoflavones to the diet was associated with a bone-sparing effect in the equol nonproducer group. In this study, there were no differences in the isoflavone-treated group between baseline and after treatment in BMD and BMC in the hip. This was an important study since it is the first report to measure serum equol concentration status in a controlled clinical study, but more importantly, the data suggest that equol has bone building activity in younger postmenopausal women.

Wu et al. [28] carried out a 24-week placebo-controlled study in postmenopausal Japanese women who were within 5 years of their natural menopause. The isoflavone group (33 subjects) received a daily morning dose of 75 mg isoflavone conjugates (38.9 mg daidzein/daidzin) in two capsules; the placebo group (33 subjects) received capsules containing only dextrin. All subjects were allowed to consume their normal diet of soy, equivalent to 40–45 mg isoflavones per day. No significant differences in BMD were noted in any of the bone areas measured between the isoflavone and placebo groups after 24-week treatment. However, after the subjects were stratified into equol producers (defined as >10 % conversion of daidzein to equol after 96-h incubation in fecal culture) versus non-producers (0 % conversion of daidzein to equol in fecal culture) there was a significant positive effect on whole-body and hip BMD in the equol producer group. After 6 months of intervention, the mean plasma equol concentration in the isoflavone-supplemented group who were equol producers was approximately 350 nmol/L or 85 ng/mL, whereas in the isoflavone-supplemented group who were not equol producers the equol concentration was <2 ng/mL. In this study, the subjects were allowed to consume their daily diet of soy products. Thus, in the placebo group who were not given the supplement but were allowed to consume their normal diet and were equol producers the mean plasma concentration of equol was approximately 60 nmol/L or 14 ng/mL. Thus, one estimate for the plasma concentration of equol for Japanese people who are equol producers is 14 ng/mL.

In another study from the same group of investigators, Wu et al. [29] gave 75 mg of isoflavone conjugates to 25 postmenopausal Japanese women for 6 months and compared the results on BMD and whole-body fat mass to 29 placebo subjects; all subjects were allowed to consume their normal diet. At baseline, the serum concentration of equol in the placebo and isoflavone-supplemented group who were equol producers was 150 nmol/L or 34 ng/mL. After 1-year treatment, the equol concentration for the placebo group who were equol producers was 215 nmol/L (52 ng/mL) and for the isoflavone group 645 nmol/L (156 ng/mL). In the isoflavone group who were equol producers there was a significant increase in total hip and intertrochanter BMD.

A Dietary Supplement Containing S-equol (SE5-OH) and Menopausal Symptoms

The clinical effectiveness of a dietary supplement (SE5-OH) containing 10 mg equol per dose has been evaluated for menopausal symptoms and mood states in 127 peri- and postmenopausal Japanese women [30]. The equol supplement was produced from soy germ by fermentation with *Lactococcus garvieae*; the bacteria converts daidzein to S-equol. Although it was not determined in this study, it can be assumed that the product contains S-equol in addition to all the other components of soy. Prior to treatment, women (40–59 years of age) were stratified into equol producers and nonproducers. Equol producers were defined as those subjects that excreted more than 10 ng/mL equol in a 24-h urine sample after consuming a single dose of 50 mg isoflavones at dinner; plasma levels of equol were not determined. The subjects consumed the 10 mg equol supplement once a day ($n=28$) or three times a day ($n=29$). Study participants were allowed to consume 20 mg isoflavones daily from their meals. Menopausal symptoms and mood states were evaluated by a questionnaire at the beginning and at the end of the 12-week study. In those subjects who were equol producers, based on the isoflavone challenge, the once or three times a day supplement group did not show any significant differences from their baseline values for menopausal or mood symptoms after 12 weeks of treatment. In contrast, the subjects who were not equol producers after the isoflavone challenge showed a significant improvement but only in those subjects who were treated three times a day. The vasomotor score, which consisted of hot flashes, sweating, and chilliness, decreased from 2.4 ± 1.9 to 1.4 ± 1.3 ($p<0.05$) and the total menopausal score decreased from 20.2 ± 7.5 to 13.6 ± 6.2 ($p<0.01$). Why the equol producer group showed no significant difference in menopausal or mood symptoms from baseline is not evident. Those subjects would have had to have hot flashes in order to enter the study and yet there was no further benefit after consuming additional S-equol. One explanation is that the baseline scores for the equol producer group were lower than the nonproducers. Since the subjects were allowed to consume 20 mg isoflavones from meals, they probably had higher plasma levels of S-equol. Another explanation is that there was a significant placebo effect in the equol producer group; the vasomotor score decreased from 3.3 ± 2.2 to 1.8 ± 2.2 ($p<0.01$). Since the fermented supplement contained other components of soy, including soy protein, genistein, and unmetabolized daidzein, the decrease in VMS may have been due to these components of the fermented soy. However, a recent report using the ovariectomized rat suggests that it is S-equol in SE5-OH that accounts for its therapeutic effect [31]. In this study, ovariectomy was associated with approximately a 0.8 °C increase in tail temperature. SE5-OH containing 11.7 mg/kg as S-equol or pure S-equol (11.7 mg/kg) were administered orally once a day for 38 days beginning 3 days after overiectomy; conjugated estrogens (6 mg/kg) served as the positive control. Tail temperatures were taken on days 21, 28, and 35. At the first time point (day 21), estrogen, SE5-OH, and S-equol significantly decreased the tail temperature. Importantly, the decrease was the same for SE5-OH and S-equol suggesting that the effect seen with SE5-OH was due to S-equol. However, pure S-equol was more effective than SE5-OH in reducing plasma total cholesterol and deoxypyridinoline levels, a measure of bone sparing, suggesting that SE5-OH is less effective than pure S-equol.

In the Ishiwata et al. study [30], the number of hot flashes was not reported. In a follow-up study [32], SE5-OH (10 mg S-equol/day) was given to 160 equol nonproducing, postmenopausal Japanese women who experienced at least one hot flash/day. The 10 mg daily dose of the S-equol supplement was divided into portions with 5 mg consumed at breakfast and the other 5 mg at dinner. The participants were allowed to maintain their normal Japanese diet but since they were not equol producers it is unlikely that diet played any role in the outcome. Baseline hot flush frequency was 3.2 ± 2.4/day in the SE5-OH group and 2.9 ± 2.1/day in the placebo group. After 12 weeks of treatment, the decrease in hot flash frequency occurred only in women with ≥3 hot flashes/day (mean number of hot flashes was 4.9/day). In these 28 women, the decrease in hot flashes was 2.9 ± 2.0/day (−62.8 %) versus 1.2 ± 2.9/day (−23.6 %) in the placebo group ($p < 0.009$). A significant decrease between the treatment and placebo group in neck and shoulder muscle stiffness was also observed in this study. One limitation in this study was the high dropout rate in the placebo group (28 % vs. 14 % for the SE5-OH group). Nonetheless, the results demonstrated a positive effect of S-equol on mild hot flashes.

The only clinical study to date with oral S-equol and bone health is that by Tousen et al. [33]. These investigators performed a 1-year double-blind, randomized, placebo-controlled trial with the S-equol supplement described above in 93 non-equol-producing postmenopausal Japanese women. The four groups received 0, 2, 6, or 10 mg of S-equol per day; the supplement was formulated into 420-mg tablets containing 1.07 mg S-equol, 0.04 mg daidzein, 0.06 mg genistein, and 0.38 mg glycetin. The tablets were consumed at one time at breakfast and the subjects were allowed to consume their normal diet. The concentration of plasma S-equol after 12-month treatment was significantly higher in the 6 mg group (40 nM, 10 ng/mL) and the 10 mg group (70 nM, 18 ng/mL) compared to the placebo group. The percent decrease in urinary deoxypyridinoline, a measure of bone resorption, after 12 months was 23.9 % in the 10 mg group compared to 2.87 % in the placebo group ($p < 0.02$). There were no changes in osteocalcin or alkaline phosphatase. Whole-body BMD was significantly less in the 10 mg S-equol group but there were no differences in lumbar spine, hip, femoral neck, trochantes, Ward's triangle, or intertrochanter BMD. While these are small studies and there was no control over the diet (the subjects consumed 28.8–55.7 mg isoflavones per day), the results provide the first evidence that 10 mg of S-equol may improve bone health in postmenopausal women.

Pharmaceutical S-equol and Vasomotor Symptoms

S-equol has been synthesized in a pure form, and Phase 1 safety studies have been carried out in normal volunteers. Jackson et al. [34] reported that orally dosed pure S-equol was well tolerated up to a daily dose of 320 mg for 14 days (Table 10.3). Furthermore, plasma levels of S-equol were liner with dose (Fig. 10.2a, b) and repeat oral doses provided consistent steady-state levels of total S-equol in plasma (Fig. 10.3). A Phase 2a study in postmenopausal women with VMS is in progress. The results

Table 10.3 Adverse events related or possibly related to study drug

Placebo (N=26)	10 mg S-equol (N=21)	20 mg S-equol (N=12)	40 mg S-equol (N=12)	80 mg S-equol (N=12)	160 mg S-equol (N=12)	320 mg S-equol (N=6)
Nausea	Nausea	Diarrhea		Flatulence	Nausea	
Headache	Paraesthesia	Abdominal pain[a]		Anorexia	Flatulence	
Paraesthesia		Nausea[a]		Nightmare	Constipation	
Hot flush				Accommodation disorder		

The table includes AEs from both a single-rising dose study and a multi-rising dose study, at the doses indicated (see [34] for details, reprinted with permission). Each event listed represents only one occurrence except paraesthesia related to phlebotomy in the 10 mg group, in which case there were two adverse events

[a]Related to study drug (one subject)

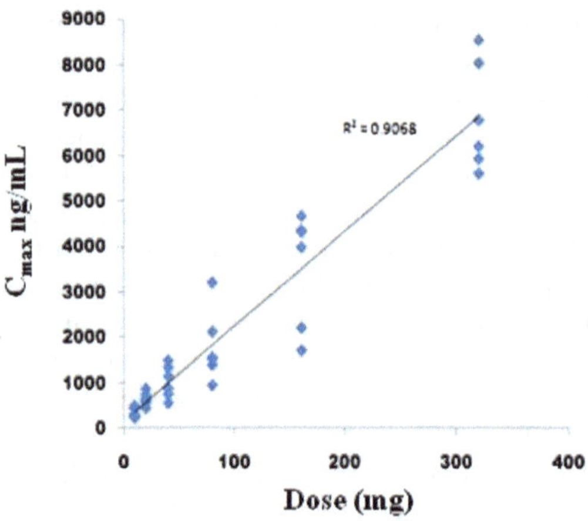

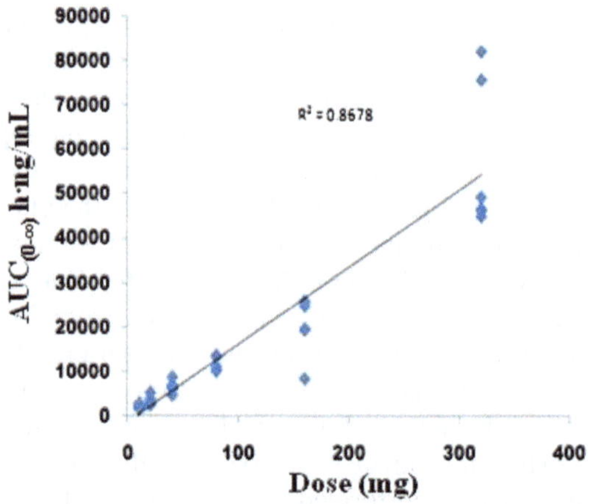

Fig. 10.2 (**a**) Dose proportionality of plasma total S-equol versus C_{max} following an oral single-rising dose (10, 20, 40, 80, 160, and 320 mg) of S-equol. Reprinted with permission from Jackson RL, Greiwe JS, Desai PB, Schwen RJ. Single-dose and steady-state pharmacokinetic studies of S-equol, a potent nonhormonal, estrogen receptor β-agonist being developed for the treatment of menopausal symptoms. Menopause. 2011;18:185–193. (**b**) Dose proportionality of plasma total S-equol $AUC_{(0-\infty)}$ following an oral single-rising dose (10, 20, 40, 80, 160, and 320 mg) of S-equol. Reprinted with permission from Jackson RL, Greiwe JS, Desai PB, Schwen RJ. Single-dose and steady-state pharmacokinetic studies of S-equol, a potent nonhormonal, estrogen receptor β-agonist being developed for the treatment of menopausal symptoms. Menopause. 2011;18:185–193

of this clinical trial, which includes measurement of plasma levels of S-equol, are expected to define the association between exposure to S-equol and a decrease in VMS. This study will also support the importance of ERβ as a viable target for treatment of VMS.

Conclusions

The importance of nutrition in women's health in the postmenopausal woman is complicated by the fact that estrogen production is greatly decreased after menopause. Estrogen is a key hormone for maintaining healthy skin and bone and cardiovascular health and preventing neurodegenerative diseases. Since the WHI study was reported, women are reluctant to take HT. As a result, there has been a decrease in breast cancer but in one study [2] a 55 % increase in hip fractures. The impact of WHI

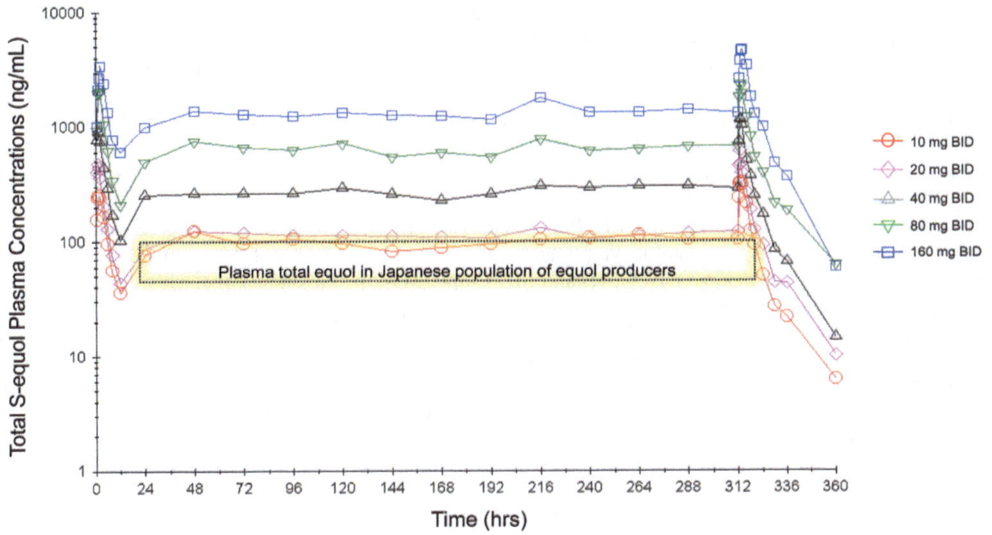

Fig. 10.3 Plasma total S-equol: Multi-dose phase 1 pharmacokinetics. Plasma total equol concentration appearance and disappearance curves were determined over 14 days of dosing; see [34] for details (reprinted with permission). At the initial dose and at day 14, multiple blood samples were taken to determine $T_{1/2}$. The other values represent trough levels of S-equol. The bar shows the concentration of total S-equol in a population of Japanese people who are equol producers. Reprinted with permission from Jackson RL, Greiwe JS, Desai PB, Schwen RJ. Single-dose and steady-state pharmacokinetic studies of S-equol, a potent nonhormonal, estrogen receptor β-agonist being developed for the treatment of menopausal symptoms. Menopause. 2011;18:185–193

on cardiovascular disease, cognitive function, and Alzheimer's disease remains to be determined. As discussed above, results of clinical trials of an S-equol soy supplement or a pure S-equol are expected to provide a new approach for treatment of menopausal symptoms and osteoporosis. These results are also expected to validate the use of ERβ-selective agonists for these symptoms.

References

1. Rossouw JE. For the writing group for the Women's Health Initiative Investigators. Risks and benefits of estrogen plus progestin in healthy postmenopausal women: principal results from the Women's Health Initiative randomized controlled trial. JAMA. 2002;288:321–33.
2. Karim R, Dell RM, Greene DF, Mack WJ, Gallagher JC, Hodis HN. Hip fracture in postmenopausal women after cessation of hormone therapy: results from a prospective study in a large health management organization. Menopause. 2011;18:1172–7.
3. Pinkerton JV, Stovall DW, Kightlinger RS. Advances in the treatment of menopausal symptoms. Womens Health. 2009;5:361–84.
4. Dog TL. Menopause: a review of botanical dietary supplements. Am J Med. 2005;118:98–108.
5. Clement YN, Onakpoys I, Hung SK, Ernst E. Effects of herbal and dietary supplements on cognition in menopause: a systematic review. Maturitas. 2011;68:256–63.
6. Newton KM, Reed SD, Lacroix AZ, Grothaus LC, Ehrlich K, Guiltinan J. Treatment of vasomotor symptoms of menopause with black cohosh, multibotanicals, soy, hormone therapy, or placebo. Ann Intern Med. 2006; 145:869–79.
7. Adlercreutz H, Hämäläinen E, Gorbach S, Goldin B. Dietary phyto-oestrogens and the menopause in Japan. Lancet. 1992;339:1233.
8. Nagata C, Takatsuka N, Kawakami N, Shimizu H. Soy product intake and hot flashes in Japanese women: results from a community-based prospective study. Am J Epidemiol. 2001;153:790–3.
9. Tempfer CB, Bentz EK, Leodolter S, Tscherne G, Reuss F, Cross HS, et al. Phyto-estrogens in clinical practice: a review of the literature. Fertil Steril. 2007;87:1243–9.

10. Jacobs A, Wegewitz U, Sommerfeld C. Efficacy of isoflavones in relieving vasomotor menopausal symptoms – a systematic review. Mol Nutr Food Res. 2009;53:1084–97.
11. Bolaños R, Del Castillo A, Francia J. Soy isoflavones versus placebo in the treatment of climacteric vasomotor symptoms: systematic review and meta-analysis. Menopause. 2010;17:660–6.
12. Han KK, Soares Jr JM, Haidar MA, deLima GR, Baracat EC. Benefits of soy isoflavone therapeutic regimen on menopausal symptoms. Obstet Gynecol. 2002;99:389–94.
13. Cheng G, Wilczek B, Warner M, Gustafsson JA, Landgren BM. Isoflavone treatment for acute menopausal symptoms. Menopause. 2007;14:468–73.
14. Carmignani LO, Pedro AO, Costa-Paiva LH, Pinto-Neto AM. The effect of dietary soy supplementation compared to estrogen and placebo on menopausal symptoms: a randomized controlled trial. Maturitas. 2010;67:262–9.
15. Williamson-Hughes PS, Flickinger BD, Messina MJ, Empie MW. Isoflavone supplements containing predominantly genistein reduce hot flash symptoms: a critical review of published studies. Menopause. 2006;13:831–9.
16. Setchell KDR, Brown NM, Lydeking-Olsen E. The clinical importance of the metabolite equol-a clue to the effectiveness of soy and its isoflavones. J Nutr. 2002;132:3577–84.
17. Setchell KDR, Clerici C, Lephart ED, Cole SJ, Heenan C, Castellani D, et al. S-equol, a potent ligand for estrogen receptor β, is the exclusive enantiomeric form of the soy isoflavone metabolite produced by human intestinal bacterial flora. Am J Clin Nutr. 2005;81:1072–9.
18. Jackson RL, Greiwe JS, Schwen RJ. Emerging evidence of the health benefits of S-equol, an estrogen receptor β agonist. J Nutr. 2011;69:432–48.
19. Shay N. (Editor) Equol, soy and menopause. J. Nutr. 2010;140:1350S–94S.
20. Murkies AL, Lombard C, Strauss BJG, Wilcox G, Burger HG, Morton MS. Dietary flour supplementation decreases post-menopausal hot flushes: effect of soy and wheat. Maturitas. 1995;21:189–1995.
21. Jou HJ, Wu SC, Chang FW, Ling PY, Chu KS, Wu WH. Effect of intestinal production of equol on menopausal symptoms in women treated with soy isoflavones. Int J Gynaecol Obstet. 2008;102:44–9.
22. Khaodhiar L, Ricciotti HA, Li L, Pan W, Schickel M, Zhou J, et al. Daidzein-rich isoflavone aglycones are potentially effective in reducing hot flashes in menopausal women. Menopause. 2008;15:125–32.
23. Uesugi S, Watanabe S, Ishiwata N, Uehara M, Ouchi K. Effects of isoflavone supplements on bone metabolic markers and climacteric symptoms in Japanese women. Biofactors. 2004;22:221–8.
24. Taku K, Melby MK, Kurzer MS, Mizuno S, Watanabe S, Ishimi Y. Effects of soy isoflavone supplements on bone turnover markers in menopausal women: systematic review and meta-analysis of randomized controlled trials. Bone. 2010;47:413–23.
25. Zhang X, Shu XO, Li H, Yang G, Li Q, Gao YT, et al. Prospective cohort study of soy food consumption and risk of bone fracture among postmenopausal women. Arch Intern Med. 2005;165:1860–95.
26. Kreijkamp-Kaspers S, Kok L, Grobbee DE, de Haan EH, Aleman A, Lampe JW, et al. Effect of soy protein containing isoflavones on cognitive function, bone mineral density, and plasma lipids in postmenopausal women. JAMA. 2004;292:65–74.
27. Lydeking-Olsen E, Beck-Jensen JE, Setchell KDR, Holm-Jensen T. Soymilk or progesterone for prevention of bone loss a 2 year randomized, placebo-controlled trial. Eur J Nutr. 2004;43:246–57.
28. Wu J, Oka J, Higuchi M, Tabata I, Toda T, Fujioka M, et al. Cooperative effects of isoflavones and exercise on bone and lipid metabolism in postmenopausal Japanese women: a randomized placebo-controlled trial. Metabolism. 2006;55:423–33.
29. Wu J, Oka J, Ezaki J, Ohtomo T, Ueno T, Uchiyama S, et al. Possible role of equol status in the effects of isoflavone on bone and fat mass in postmenopausal Japanese women: a double-blind, randomized, controlled trial. Menopause. 2007;14:1–9.
30. Ishiwata N, Melby M, Mizuno S, Watanabe S. New equol supplement for relieving menopausal symptoms: randomized, placebo-controlled trial of Japanese women. Menopause. 2009;16:141–8.
31. Yoneda T, Ueno T, Uchiyama S. S-equol and the fermented soy product SE5-OH containing S-equol similarly decrease ovariectomy-induced increase in rat tail skin temperature in an animal model of hot flushes. Menopause. 2011;18:814–20.
32. Aso T, Uchiyama S, Matsumura Y, Taguchi M, Nozaki M, Takamatsu K, et al. A natural S-(−) equol supplement alleviates hot flushes and other menopausal symptoms in equol nonproducing postmenopausal Japanese women. J Womens Health. 2011;20:1–9.
33. Tousen Y, Ezaki J, Fujii Y, Ueno T, Nishimuta M, Ishimi Y. Natural S-equol decreases bone resorption in postmenopausal, non-equol-producing Japanese women: a pilot randomized, placebo-controlled trial. Menopause. 2011;18:563–74.
34. Jackson RL, Greiwe JS, Desai PB, Schwen RJ. Single-dose and steady-state pharmacokinetic studies of S-equol, a potent nonhormonal, estrogen receptor β-agonist being developed for the treatment of menopausal symptoms. Menopause. 2011;18:185–93.

Chapter 11
Tofu in Menopause Therapy and Prevention

Wangjing Ke and Ronald Ross Watson

Key Points

- Tofu contains significant amount of bioactive isoflavones and calcium.
- The tofu matrix promotes the activity of isoflavones in vivo.
- Isoflavones and calcium have favorable effects on osteoporosis.
- Isoflavones are considered to be beneficial in releasing menopause-related hot flash, reducing cancer and cardiovascular disease risks.
- Consumption of tofu in a large amount shortly or in a reasonable dose regularly is recommended for keeping a relatively high level of isoflavones in serum.

Keywords Tofu • Menopause • Isoflavones • Osteoporosis • Hot flash • Cancer • Calcium • Hormone replacement

Introduction

Tofu was invented in China over 2,000 years ago and it has gradually become one of the most prevalent ingredients in Asian diets since then. Tofu is known in the Western world as an ideal vegetarian protein source as it is rich in high-quality protein, low in saturated fats and cholesterol, rich in minerals and vitamins, and low in cost [1]. In the last decades, studies have unveiled some previously overlooked characters of tofu, especially its richness in isoflavones [2]. Isoflavones are phytoestrogens produced by plants that are also bioactive in mammals because of the high similarity between them and their mammal counterparts [3]. Tofu, due to its high calcium and isoflavone concentration, is considered to be beneficial in preventing or releasing health threads resulted from menopause, such as osteoporosis,

W. Ke, M.P.H. • R.R. Watson, B.S., Ph.D. (✉)
Arizona Health Sciences Center, Mel and Enid Zuckerman College of Public Health and School of Medicine, University of Arizona, 1295 N. Martin Ave, P.O. Box 245155, Tucson, AZ 85724-5155, USA
e-mail: wke@email.arizona.edu; rwatson@u.arizona.edu

C.J.H. Martin et al. (eds.), *Nutrition and Diet in Menopause*, Nutrition and Health,
DOI 10.1007/978-1-62703-373-2_11, © Springer Science+Business Media New York 2013

hot flash, cancer, and cardiovascular diseases. It is recommended to consume tofu regularly to maintain the isoflavone concentration in serum at a sufficient level, so new phytoestrogen-rich recipes are necessary for a wider acceptance of tofu or other soy products in the Western diets.

History of Tofu

China is considered to be where tofu originated. The legendary inventor of tofu was Liu An (179–122 BC) in Han dynasty, but the first record about the procedure of making tofu was found as drawings in a Han tomb dated back to the first century [4]. There were not very much differences between the procedures depicted in the Han dynasty drawings and the ones we are following today, except for the missing of cooling soymilk. However, tofu was not commonly produced or consumed in China until the Tang dynasty (AD 618–907). It was then introduced to Japan, Korea, and Vietnam, soon becoming accepted as a localized dish [4]. Interestingly, the propagation of tofu corresponded quite well to the spread of Buddhism in eastern Asia, probably because tofu was the major protein source of monks, who may have missioned Buddhism as well as tofu production at the same time [1].

While tofu has a history in Asia for over 2,000 years, its history in the West has only just begun. About 100 years ago tofu made the leap westward to meet with the people in Europe and the United States [1], but it did not became prevalent in the Western diets because soybeans were not commonly produced or consumed in Europe at that time. Things have changed since the middle of the twentieth century when soybeans were produced in the United States on a larger and larger scale and people started to value the merits of soy protein [4].

Procedure of Tofu Production

Although the appearance of tofu products can vary dramatically from one to one, the basic manufacture process is universally consistent. It starts with the preparation of smashed soybean slurry, or soymilk, followed by boil and filtration at high temperature with coagulants. There are several options on the coagulants used in tofu production, such as salts (calcium sulfate), acids (glucono delta-lactone), or enzyme [5]. The curds resulted from protein precipitation are filtered and pressed in molds into shapes. This final product is known as tofu [6]. A firm tofu and a silken tofu are distinguished simply by the amount of water extracted from the tofu curds, and further processes such as fermentation, drying, frying, or freezing are sometimes conducted to endow tofu a variety in flavor and texture [1].

Nutritional or Dietary Value

1. Protein

   The studies on the nutritional value of tofu can be traced back decades ago, but most of them focused on the protein quality because tofu first came to people's sight as an ideal vegetarian protein source. A paper published in 1963 revealed data on the nutritional value of proteins of oriental soybean foods, which included tofu [7]. The results are shown in Table 11.1.

   The four brands of tofu used in this study were purchased from local grocery stores in Honolulu. Factory visits confirmed that all the tofu was produced in a similar way with calcium chloride as the coagulant. Equal portions of tofu of all brands were mixed before the mixture was tested for nutritional values. Test results suggest that tofu, compared to soybeans, contains fairly the same amount of water, protein, and fat, but significantly less carbohydrate. The same study also investigated the

Table 11.1 Composition of soybean products of oriental foods[a]

Foods	Moisture (%)	Protein[b] (%)	Fat (%)	Ash (%)	Carbohydrate[c] (%)
Edamame	64.6	14.0	7.9	2.3	11.2
Natto	55.3	25.7	11.4	2.4	5.2
Tofu	74.2	14.8	6.6	1.1	3.3
Soybean sprouts	84.9	7.6	2.4	0.9	4.2
Mung bean sprouts	93.3	2.2	2.2	0.3	2.1

[a]Modified from [7]
[b]By Kjeldahl method
[c]100 − (% protein + % fat + % ash)

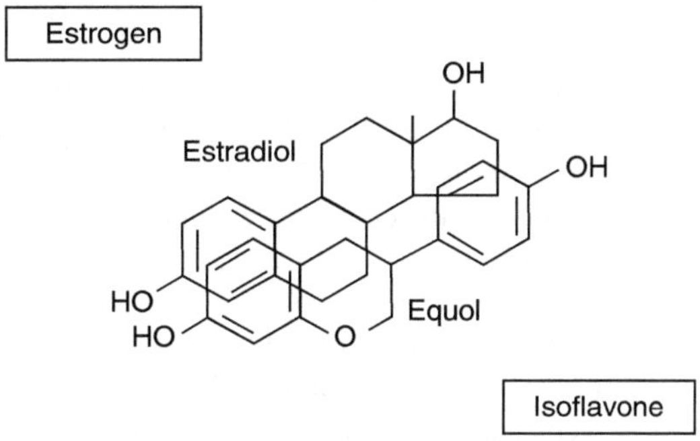

Fig. 11.1 Similarity of isoflavones to estrogens (modified from [3])

Net Protein Utilization (NPU) of tofu on an albino rat model and came up with the number of 65 %. The fact that tofu and chicken have same NPU values of 65 % suggests equivalence in digestibility and assimilability between them [6].

Approximately one-third of the original soybean mass, especially fibers, was lost during the first filtration step [6]. The major storage proteins in soybeans and tofu are glycinin (11S) and β-conglycinin (7S), accounting for about 70 and 30 % of the total tofu protein, respectively, and the exact number varies with the soybeans and processes used in the manufacture [8]. There are evidences suggesting that the 11S faction, the 7S faction, and their ratio may be related to tofu firmness, but conflicting results are commonly found among studies [9].

2. Calcium

The calcium levels in tofu were significantly increased by the addition of Ca^{2+}-rich coagulant mixture (calcium chloride or calcium sulfate). Depending on the concentration of calcium salts and type of soybeans used in the production, the calcium contents ranged from 200 to 1,940 mg per 100 g serving of tofu on a dry weight basis [10]. It has been long ago confirmed that artificially added calcium remains to have high bioavailability in tofu [11].

3. Isoflavones

The most interesting nutrients in tofu are isoflavones. Isoflavones are phytoestrogens produced naturally by plants, almost exclusively in legumes. Soybeans and its processed products, especially tofu, provide the most abundant source of isoflavones. Every 100 g tofu contains approximately 70 mg isoflavones, among which 26 % are daidzein and 35 % are genistin [2]. The average daily intake of isoflavones in typical Western diet is negligible (<1 mg/day), while it is about 20–59 mg/day in Japanese and Chinese diets [12].

Isoflavones share very high similarity with mammalian estrogens in terms of chemical structures (shown in Fig. 11.1), which explains the fact that isoflavones are capable of binding to estrogen receptors [3]. However, it has been discovered that isoflavones work as more than just estrogen agonists or antagonists, but a combination of both [3], a character that is well known in steroids.

A rat model showed the absorption and metabolism of isoflavones from tofu. Pressed tofu through a sieve as simulation of chewed material was then perfused into isolated but viable rat small intestine. There were in total 1,184.6 nmol genistein compounds and 572.8 nmol daidzein compounds in 1 g tofu suspension. However there were only about 8 % genistein compounds were absorbed by the small intestine, smaller than 17.2 %, the genistein compounds absorption ratio detected when genistin saline solution was perfused into isolated rat small intestine. This finding suggested that the content of tofu matrix, such as its fibers or proteins, may have interrupted the genistin absorption rate [13].

Although tofu matrix shows negative effect on the absorption of isoflavones [13], it may increase the activity of isoflavones in vivo. The antioxidant properties of soybean isoflavone extract and tofu were studied in vitro and in vivo [2]. The extract has shown strong in vitro antioxidant activity compared with vitamin E as a positive control. A dose-dependent response was observed at lower concentrations and the curve leveled off at higher concentrations. At 25 ppm isoflavone, the ratio between the induction time with and without isoflavone extract was about 1.4, and then the number rose gradually to 1.9 as the isoflavone concentration increased to 250 ppm. The ratio reached and stayed at its limit of 2.0 after the isoflavone concentration was over 300 ppm. Meanwhile, some intriguing results came out when the antioxidant properties of soybean isoflavone extract was compared with those of tofu extract in vivo. Rats were assigned randomly into six groups, and each group was fed on a designated diet (negative control, positive control (25 ppm vitamin E), tofu base, or three isoflavone diets: 50, 150, or 250 ppm). Then the enzyme levels of superoxide dismutase (SOD) and catalase in small intestine, kidney, liver, lung, and skin were recorded in 24 weeks and compared among groups because the activity level of antioxidant enzymes, typically SOD and catalase, is associated with cytotoxicity, genotoxicity, and carcinogenic processes. It turned out that the SOD activity in each group increased after the treatment and then reached a plateau. The amplitude of increase was positively correlated with the isoflavone concentration, and the most significant increase in SOD activity was observed in the group fed with tofu base. The results suggest that isoflavones may promote antioxidant enzyme levels at high concentrations or after a long time period. Meanwhile, despite the fact that there was only 50 ppm isoflavones in each tofu treatment, tofu, among the six groups of diets prepared, has shown the most significant effects in inducting the SOD activity in every organ tested, especially liver. A similar trend was also discovered in the tracing of catalase activity, but the distinction between tofu and the other groups was not as observable as that in the SOD activity measurements. This finding indicates that some unique molecule in tofu other than isoflavones may have a synergistic effect on the enhancement of in vivo antioxidant enzyme activity level [2]. In other words, tofu may be a better choice than isoflavone extracts in terms of the benefits of health and finance. It is not unreasonable to suspect that this synergistic effect by tofu may apply to other isoflavone biological effects, but no conclusions can be drawn without confirmation from further studies.

Tofu (Phytoestrogens) and Menopause

1. Osteoporosis

   There are results from both animal studies and human studies supporting the idea that isoflavone supplementation may prevent osteoporosis in postmenopausal women. However, the precise action mechanism remains veiled, waiting for further investigation [14].

   Several animal studies have presented data revealing the osteoprotective effect by isoflavones in rat models. In one study, 40 ovariectomized rats were randomly assigned into four groups and given diets that contained 0, 20, 40, or 80 μg/g body weight per day for 91 days [15]. Total femoral, diaphyseal, and metaphyseal bone mineral density were measured in initial controls and sham-operated

Table 11.2 A comparison of bone mineral density (mean ± SD) in postmenopausal Southern Chinese women analyzed according to the tertiles of isoflavone intake[a]

	Tertile of isoflavone intake			
	Low	Mid	High	*p*
L2-4 Bone mineral density (g/cm²)	0.77 ± 0.13	0.79 ± 0.15	0.82 ± 0.15	0.02
L2-4T score	−2.19 ± 1.14	−2.03 ± 1.37	−1.63 ± 1.18	<0.001
Ward's bone mineral density (g/cm²)	0.41 ± 0.14	0.42 ± 0.13	0.45 ± 0.15	0.05
Total hip T score	−2.05 ± 1.13	−1.96 ± 1.31	−1.68 ± 1.29	0.02

[a]Modified from [18]

and ovariectomized rats with or without isoflavone diet (IF 20, IF 40, and IF 80) at day 91. Ovariectomized rats with no isoflavone supplementation were found to have significant lower bone mineral density than rats in the other groups. Besides, 40 μg/g was considered to be an optimal dose due to the observable increase in total femoral bone mineral density and diaphyseal bone mineral density in IF 40 compared to IF 20 and IF 80, but the mechanism was unknown [15].

In humans, there is little information on the association of tofu intake and the prevention of osteoporosis, but the effect of isoflavones on osteoporosis has been widely investigated [16–18]. Results from a double-blind, randomized, controlled study conducted in Hong Kong show that isoflavones have a positive effect on bone loss [16, 17]. A total of 203 postmenopausal Chinese women, aged 48–62, were recruited. They were randomly assigned into three treatment groups: placebo (daily dose of 0 mg isoflavones), mid-dose (daily 40 mg isoflavones), and high dose (daily 80 mg isoflavones); all participants were given 500 mg calcium and 125 IU vitamin D_3 every day. Bone mineral density and bone mineral content at the whole body, spine, and hip were measured by dual-energy X-ray absorptiometry at baseline and 1 year post treatment. Some other parameters such as years since menopause, body weight, and individual dietary calcium intake were analyzed at the same time to evaluate whether they would affect the association between isoflavone supplementation and bone mineral density or bone mineral content changes. Results suggested that isoflavones have a strong positive effect on maintaining hip bone mineral content in women in later menopause, or those with lower body weight or calcium intake or low initial bone mass [16, 17].

Similar observations were reported by researchers in Hong Kong [18]. They enrolled 650 southern Chinese women, aged 19–86 years, in a study for the identification of genetic or environmental risk factors for osteoporosis. Participants completed a questionnaire regarding their diet, demographic characteristics, medical history, and the use of hormone replacement therapy. Their consumptions of 33 most common food items, including 9 soy items (soft tofu, firm tofu, fried tofu, dried soybean, canned soybean, soymilk skin, soybean sprout, soymilk, and soy drink) were recorded for the purpose of dietary phytoestrogen intake calculation. Bone mineral density was measured for each subject at lumbar spine, femoral neck, trochanter, Ward's triangle, and total hip using dual-energy X-ray absorptiometry. The results for all 357 postmenopausal women, adjusted for age, height, weight, years since menopause, smoking, alcohol consumption, hormone replacement therapy usage, and daily calcium intake, are summarized in Table 11.2, indicating that high dietary isoflavone intake is correlated to higher bone mineral density at the lumbar spine and hip region in postmenopausal women. On the other hand, results for 283 premenopausal subjects showed no association between bone mineral density and habitual isoflavone intake [18].

In another human study on soy isoflavones, two doses of soy isoflavones (55.6 mg/day or 90 mg/day) were given to postmenopausal women for 6 months, but only the group on higher dosage was reported to have gained bone mineral density after the treatment, suggesting that either isoflavones have a threshold effect or the effect of lower dosage isoflavones was not observable in such a short period of time [19]. Given the dosage used and effects observed in Chen's double-blind, randomized, controlled study [16, 17], the latter explanation was most likely.

Table 11.3 Measurements of weight, serum estradiol, and menopausal symptomatology scores of the phytoestrogen-rich diet group[a]

	Phytoestrogen group		Control group	
	Baseline	3 Months	Baseline	3 Months
Weight (kg)	70.7 ± 1.4	69.3 ± 2.1	69.7 ± 2.1	68.1 ± 2.0
Hot flash score	1.8 ± 0.1	0.8 ± 0.1[b]	1.7 ± 0.2	1.1 ± 0.1
Vaginal dryness score	1.5 ± 0.2	0.6 ± 0.1[c]	1.6 ± 0.3	1.2 ± 0.2
Estradiol (nmol/L)	179.7 ± 15.2	139.8 ± 1.1[b]	162.0 ± 4.1	140 ± 12.3[b]

[a]Modified from [22]
[b]$p \leq 0.05$
[c]$p \leq 0.005$

2. Hormone replacement
   Isoflavones, as nonsteroidal plant-derived compounds, exhibit estrogenic activity at several sites [20], which makes it possible to use them as an alternative to estrogen therapy. Compared to regular hormone replacement therapy, isoflavones or soy proteins so far have shown no adverse effects on humans [21], another advantage of using soy products as alternative hormone replacement. Japanese researchers have done a cross-sectional study with a study population of 3,704 female aged 45–55 in Japan (Nagata 02). They used a semiquantitative food frequency questionnaire to build up a diet history that can be used to analyze the average intake of specific nutrients. Data showed that postmenopausal women consume significantly more calcium and soy products than premenopausal women on average [12]. Importantly, the consumption of calcium and soy products was found to be positively related with the onset of menopause [12].
3. Hot flash, cognitive function, cardiovascular and cancer effects
   Phytoestrogen is also reported to have short-term effects in the reduction in hot flashes and vaginal dryness. Women, 145, with climacteric complaints were randomly assigned into a phytoestrogen-rich diet group or a control group [22]. Participants were required to evaluate the severity of their symptoms (hot flashes, night sweats, palpitations, headache, depression, vaginal dryness, urinary discomfort insomnia, and decreased libido) at baseline. Then the subjects in the intervention group were provided with phytoestrogen-rich diet, which included 80 g of tofu, soy drink (400 ml), one teaspoon of miso, and two teaspoons of ground flaxseed. Meanwhile, participants in the control group were on regular Israeli diet with no hormonal treatment. The dietary intervention lasted for 12 weeks, during which a few women dropped out of this study because they could not tolerate the soy foods. All baseline measurements were repeated for each participant when the study was finished. The results are listed in Table 11.3. Thus a short-term but large dose of dietary phytoestrogen supplementation can significantly relieve the severity of hot flashes and vaginal dryness in climacteric women [22].

   Dietary supplement of isoflavones benefited the cognitive function in postmenopausal women. To test this 56 women, aged between 55 and 74, were recruited for this double-blind, randomized, placebo-controlled clinical trial [23]. All participants were healthy postmenopausal women for at least 2 years, and were not on estrogen replacement therapy. They were randomly assigned into placebo group or intervention group. Subjects in the intervention group were provided with two soy-extracted isoflavone pills per day, which contained 100 mg isoflavones in total. Cognitive function tests were conducted at baseline and 6-month follow-up visits. The test included examining visuomotor tracking and attention, category fluency (testing verbal memory), and logical memory and recall (measuring immediate and delayed verbal memory). The changes of cognitive function from baseline to follow-up were compared between intervention and control groups. The data indicated that dietary isoflavone supplementation significantly promotes cognitive functions, particularly verbal memory, in postmenopausal women [23].

Phytoestrogens may have favorable effects on the prevention of cardiovascular disease. High dietary phytoestrogen intake and low cardiovascular disease rate in Asian populations relative to those in Western countries suggest benefits [24], which provides the first hint that soy product consumption may be beneficial in preventing cardiovascular diseases. To find out convincing evidence on this topic, researchers had 51 perimenopausal women aged 45–55 who were experiencing menopause participated in a randomized, double-blind crossover trial in investigating the effect of soy protein on cardiovascular diseases. Three diets were prepared for this study: 20 g of complex carbohydrate, 20 g of soy protein that contained 34 mg phytoestrogens. Participants were randomly assigned to be on one of the three diets for 6 weeks, and then subsequently randomly switched to the remaining two treatments. At the end of the study, the total cholesterol and low-density lipoprotein cholesterol levels of people on both soy diets reduced significantly in comparison with those of people on carbohydrate placebo diet [25]. These findings indicate an inverse relationship between soy product consumption and cardiovascular disease.

Another documented benefit of phytoestrogens, though not directly related to menopausal issue, is on prevention of cancer: breast cancer, endometrial cancer, and colon cancer [26]. In a case–control study, a reduction of breast cancer risk was found in women with high dietary phytoestrogen intake [27]. This conclusion was supported by a study in Asian-Americans that discovered an association between high tofu consumption and low breast cancer risk [28].

4. Contradictions

Information on the potential effects of tofu or isoflavones in menopause is growing. A potential confounding factor is the half-time of most phytoestrogens, which is about 3–4 h [29]. Thus phytoestrogen-rich foods have to be consumed on a daily basis to maintain an effective level of isoflavones in blood. However, soy products are not widely accepted in a Western diet at this point, making it a challenge to introduce tofu or other soy products as alternative sources for hormone replacement. In some studies, participants quit studies as they could not tolerate the phytoestrogen-rich diet [22]. There were also doubts on the association between isoflavones and hot flash prevention because sometimes participants in the control group experienced a decrease of hot flashes by 15–50 % due to a placebo effect [21]. Besides, the relationship between high dietary calcium intake and high bone mineral density was questioned [18].

Conclusions

Having been a traditional oriental food for thousands of years, tofu has gradually been accepted by Western diet as an ideal vegetarian protein source. Tofu is considered equivalent to chicken meat in terms of protein digestibility and assimilability but with less fat [6].

Tofu is also valued for phytoestrogen with more per unit than any other soy products or soy itself. Isoflavones, one of the most common phytoestrogens in soy products, are more bioavailable in tofu than those in soy because the tofu matrix may potentially promote the utilization of isoflavones in organisms. Besides, tofu receives a boost of calcium during its manufacture procedure by the use of calcium salt coagulants, making it one of the most efficient dietary calcium supplementation sources [2].

The intake of tofu benefits women in terms of menopause mainly because of the large amount of phytoestrogens (isoflavones) in it. Phytoestrogens are so similar to mammal estrogen in chemical structure and bioactivity that it is able to bind to mammal estrogen receptors, working in a way that compromises estrogen agonist and antagonist. Convincing evidence from epidemiological, clinical trials and basic science suggests that phytoestrogen has positive effect on the prevention or at least relief of menopausal symptoms, such as osteoporosis, hot flashes, and vaginal dryness. The calcium supplementation from tofu is also helpful in the prevention of osteoporosis in postmenopausal women with relatively low bone mineral density. In addition, phytoestrogen is reported to reduce cancer and cardiovascular disease risk, while it promotes cognitive function in postmenopausal women.

There is a possibility of using tofu or other soy products as an alternative to estrogen hormone replacement therapy, but a few issues should be taken into consideration: In order to benefit from dietary phytoestrogen, people have to consume a large dose of soy products in a short time or a reasonable dose almost every day because phytoestrogen has a relatively short half-time in human body. Besides, new phytoestrogen-rich recipes should be created adjusted to Western diet so that tofu and other soy products can be more widely accepted in the Western world.

Overall, it should be encouraged to introduce tofu to Western peri- or postmenopausal women as an economic and healthy protein source and alternative hormone replacement therapy to release them from menopausal symptoms.

References

1. Shurtleff W, Aoyagi A. Tofu as a food. In: The book of tofu. PA, USA: Ten Speed Press; 1983. Vol. 1, p. 21–9.
2. Liu J, Chang S, Wiesenborn D. Antioxidant properties of soybean isoflavone extract and tofu in vitro and in vivo. J Agric Food Chem. 2005;53:2333–40.
3. Setchell K, Cassidy A. Dietary isoflavones: biological effects and relevance to human health. J Nutr. 1999;129:758S–67.
4. Huang T. Early uses of soybean in Chinese history. In: Du Bois CM, Tan CB, Mintz S, editors. The world of soy. PA, USA: The University of Illinois Press; 2008. p. 45–55.
5. Berk Z. Tofu, tempeh, soy sauce and miso. In: Technology of production of edible flours and protein products from soybeans. Rome, PA: Food and Agriculture Organization of the United Nations; 1992. p. 121–34.
6. Van der Riet WB, Wight AW, Cilliers JJL, et al. Food chemical investigation of tofu and its byproduct okara. Food Chem. 1989;34:193–202.
7. Standal BR. Nutritional value of proteins of oriental soybean foods. J Nutr. 1963;81:279–85.
8. Cai T, Chang KC. Processing effect of soybean storage proteins and their relationship with tofu quality. J Agric Food Chem. 1999;47:720–7.
9. Mujoo R, Trinh D, Ng PK. Characterization of storage proteins in different soybean varieties and their relationship to tofu yield and texture. Food Chem. 2003;82:265–73.
10. Tsai SJ, Lan CY, Kao CS, Chen SC. Studies on the yield and quality characteristics of tofu. J Food Sci. 1981;46:1734–40.
11. Adolph WH, Chen SC. The utilization of calcium in soy bean diets. J Nutr. 1931;5:379–85.
12. Nagata C, Takatsuka N, Inaba S, Kawakami N, Shimizu H. Association of diet and other lifestyle with onset of menopause in Japanese women. Maturitas. 1998;29:105–13.
13. Andlauer W, Kolb J, Furst P. Isoflavones from tofu are absorbed and metabolized in the isolated rat small intestine. J Nutr. 2000;130:3021–7.
14. Arjmandi BH, Smith BJ. Soy isoflavones' osteoprotective role in postmenopausal women: mechanism of action. J Nutr Biochem. 2002;13:130–7.
15. Picherit C, Chanteranne B, Bennetau-Pelissero C, et al. Dose-dependent bone-sparing effects of dietary isoflavones in the ovariectomised rat. Br J Nutr. 2001;85:307–16.
16. Chen YM, Ho SC, Lam SS, et al. Beneficial effect of soy isoflavones on bone mineral content was modified by years since menopause, body weight, and calcium intake: a double-blind, randomized, controlled trial. Menopause. 2004;11(3):246–54.
17. Chen YM, Ho SC, Lam SS, et al. Soy isoflavones have a favorable effect on bone loss in Chinese postmenopausal women with lower bone mass: a double-blind, randomized, controlled trial. J Clin Endocrinol Metab. 2003;88(10):4740–7.
18. Mei J, Yeung SS, Kung AW. High dietary phytoestrogen intake is associated with higher bone mineral density in postmenopausal but not premenopausal women. J Clin Endocrinol Metab. 2001;86(11):5217–21.
19. Potter SM, Baum JA, Teng H, et al. Soy protein and isoflavones: their effects on blood lipids and bone density in postmenopausal women. Am J Clin Nutr. 1998;68:1375S–9.
20. Scheiber MD, Rebar RW. Isoflavones and postmenopausal bone health: a viable alternative to estrogen therapy. Menopause. 1999;6(3):233–41.
21. Vincent A, Fitzpatrick L. Soy isoflavones: are they useful in menopause. Mayo Clin Proc. 2000;75:1174–84.
22. Brzezinski A, Adlercreutz H, Shaoul R, et al. Short-term effects of phytoestrogen-rich diet on postmenopausal women. Menopause. 1997;4(2):89–94.

23. Kritz-Silverstein D, Von Muhlen D, Barrett-Connor E, et al. Isoflavones and cognitive function in older women: the soy and postmenopausal health in aging (SOPHIA) study. Menopause. 2003;10(3):196–202.
24. Keys A, Menotti A, Aravanis C, et al. The seven countries study: 2,289 deaths in 15 years. Prev Med. 1984;13:141–54.
25. Washburn S, Burke GL, Morgan T, et al. Effect of soy protein supplementation on serum lipoproteins, blood pressure, and menopausal symptoms in perimenopausal women. Menopause. 1999;6(1):7–13.
26. Warren M, Shortle B, Dominguez JE. Use of alternative therapies in menopause. Best Pract Res Clin Obstet Gynaecol. 2002;16(3):411–48.
27. Ingram D, Sanders K, Kolybaba M, et al. Case–control study of phyto-oestrogens and breast cancer. Lancet. 1997;350:990–4.
28. Wu AH, Horn-Ross PL, West DW, et al. Tofu and risk of breast cancer in Asian-Americans. Cancer Epidemiol Biomarkers Prev. 1996;5:901–6.
29. Busby MG, Jeffcoat AR, Bloedon LT, et al. Clinical characteristics and pharmacokinetics of purified soy isoflavones: single-dose administration to healthy men. Am J Clin Nutr. 2002;75:126–36.

Chapter 12
Dietary Phytoestrogens in Preventing Osteoporosis in Postmenopausal Women: Italian Aspects

Luigi Mario Chiechi

Key Points

- Following the increased life expectancy in industrialized countries, postmenopausal osteoporosis has become a serious social health problem.
- Drug prevention, mainly hormone replacement therapy, has been considered efficacious in preventing this disease but it is not harm-free, as the experience of the Women's Health Initiative study showed.
- Dietary phytoestrogens, food substances acting as natural selective estrogen receptor modulators, are able to prevent the main hormonal postmenopausal chronic diseases, including osteoporosis.
- Increasing evidence suggests that the Asiatic diet, rich in phytoestrogen isoflavones, and the Mediterranean diet, rich in phytoestrogen lignans, are the ideal healthy diets for menopausal women.
- Diet, sunlight, and weight-bearing activities are the pillars of a modern approach to preventing postmenopausal osteoporosis.

Keywords Phytoestrogens • Osteoporosis • Menopause • Diet • Prevention • Mediterranean diet

Abbreviations

ER	Estrogen receptor
SERMs	Selective estrogen receptor modulators
HRT	Hormonal replacement therapy
ET	Estrogen therapy
TSEC	Tissue-selective estrogen complex
DXA	Dual-energy X-ray absorptiometry
SD	Standard deviation
BMD	Bone mineral density
WHI	Women's Health Initiative
WB	Whole bone
ISTAT	Italian National Institute of Statistics
ESOPO	Epidemiological study on the prevalence of osteoporosis
QUS	Quantitative ultrasound

L.M. Chiechi, M.D. (✉)
Department of Bioethics, University of Bari, Corso A de Gasperi 495, 70125 Bari, Italy
e-mail: chiechi@ediself.it

C.J.H. Martin et al. (eds.), *Nutrition and Diet in Menopause*, Nutrition and Health,
DOI 10.1007/978-1-62703-373-2_12, © Springer Science+Business Media New York 2013

Introduction

One of the most neglected aspects of the diet is its potential to preserve or harm human health. Foods are not neutral substances; they can cause diseases, such as diabetes, or can cure, as in the case of pellagra. As well as being nourishing and enjoyable, foods are "functional," too, so their organoleptic aspect, although predominant today, is only a secondary feature of the diet, and can sometimes be dangerous. The diet is a complex process whereby culture influences biology; in humans foods are processed by each society, so the brain has become the organ of taste. Eating is a part of culture, a civilization trait built up by thousands of generations to optimize human life. Every single food has been selected first instinctively by our biology (by taste, eyesight, touch, digestion) and then wisely by our ancestors to ensure the best nutrition and health, finally being made pleasing by enhancing the best appreciated flavors. We, and obviously the next generation, are lucky because we have been given an advantage by our forebears, who selected the best diet for each people, while globalization is now imposing recognition in the world that two among these are the healthiest, namely, the Asiatic and the Mediterranean diet.

Why are they the best? Because they have excellent nutritive and health components, and because over the centuries these functional foods have been transformed into tasty foods while maintaining the unity of these two components after experiencing their safety. This is the modern diet.

Functional foods are natural foods (i.e., soy, fruits, vegetables) containing bioactive compounds that can positively influence human physiology or, as defined by Wildman, they are foods able to enhance physiological performance or to prevent or treat diseases and disorders [1].

A healthy diet is valid for all people, obviously; but there are some people who deserve special attention: children, the elderly, and, maybe in particular, women. In fact, the female body is special, because it has the supreme task of giving birth, and to do this it changes, increases, transforms, and even duplicates itself. So maternity, as well as the reproductive and the post-reproductive phase, has important different needs and, first of all, special dietary requirements.

Luckily, our assignment is simple today, because the bulk of work has already been done: we have only to recover what has already been created but, at times, unfortunately lost, as has occurred for some of the foods making up the Mediterranean diet.

Dietary Phytoestrogens

Although an estrogenic activity of plant extracts was first reported in 1927 [2], the concept that also plants can produce compounds with estrogenic effects is recent, having been established only in 1966 whereas before it was assumed that only synthetic or animal estrogens exclusively produced hormonal activity [3]. On the contrary, phytoestrogens are highly potent vegetal compounds that can induce infertility, abortions, and other hormone-related diseases in animals that feed on herbs with a rich content of these substances. In fact, their biological consequences were realized in the early 1940s as a result of the explosion of the so-called clover disease in Australian sheep grazing on pastures of *Trifolium subterraneum*, a species of clover native to Europe imported into Australia as more convenient forage. Therefore, the first scientific observation of the importance of phytoestrogens was a chance finding made in animals, reported more than 60 years ago, in February 1946 by H. W. Bennetts, on a veterinary journal.

For many years these compounds were considered as estrogens, in the belief that not only 17β-estradiol but also any compound able to bind ER, inducing receptor dimerization and subsequent binding to estrogen response elements, can act as an estrogen. Accordingly, they were defined as nonsteroidal plant compounds able to exert estrogenic effects. Now this concept has changed and, more appropriately, they are denominated natural selective estrogen receptor modulators (SERMs) [4].

There are many classes of phytoestrogens, and those of human interest among them are the isoflavones, lignans, coumestans, and the polyphenol resveratrol (Table 12.1). Their importance in the

Table 12.1 Phytoestrogens of human interest

Classes	Compound	Food source
Isoflavones	*Genistein*	Soy foods
	Daidzein	Beans
		Legumes
		Peanuts
		Walnut
Lignans	*Enterodiol*	Fruits
	Enterolactone	Vegetables
		Linseeds
		Seaweed
		Oilseeds
		Cereals
		Rye
		Whole grains
		Berries
Cumestran	*Coumestrol*	Mug beans
		Soy sprouts
		Alfa-alfa sprout
Polyphenols	*Resveratrol*	Red wines

The table shows the main compounds with a phytoestrogenic activity of human interest and their food source (unpublished)

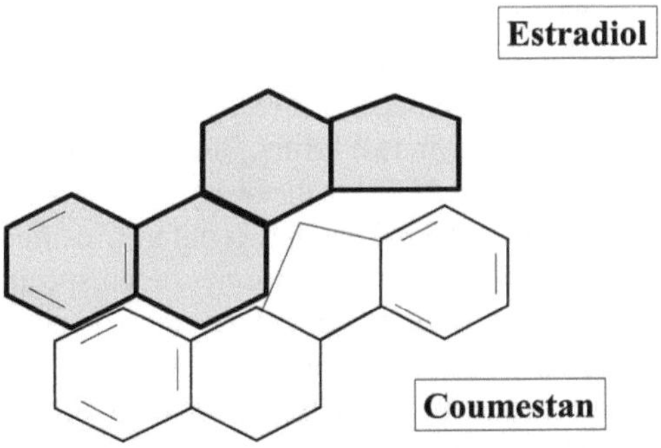

Fig. 12.1 Chemical structure of estradiol and coumestan. The figure shows the biochemical similarity of an endogenous estrogen and a phytoestrogen that allows them to occupy the same receptor site (unpublished)

medical field emerged from epidemiological studies that provided evidence of their importance in protecting against the development of numerous chronic diseases, such as hormonal related cancers, both male and female, cardiovascular disease, osteoporosis, and menopausal disturbances.

Although phytoestrogens are nonsteroidal compounds, they are structurally similar to estrogens (Fig. 12.1), both endogenous and synthetic, and to anti-estrogens such as tamoxifen; this biochemical similarity confers them a biological similarity, too. Phytoestrogens are very frequent in nature; those most widely distributed in plants are lignans, found in most fruits and vegetables, legumes, whole grains, and seeds, particularly flaxseed. Instead, isoflavones, biologically more potent than lignans, are present in few foods: beans and legumes, being present in the highest amounts only in soybeans and soy foods.

The metabolism of phytoestrogens is complex. Briefly, isoflavones are ingested in their glucosidic form (Fig. 12.2), and then they are metabolized by the glucosidases produced by intestinal bacteria to their corresponding aglycones, termed genistein, daidzein, and glycitein; these, in turn, are further metabolized to their isoflavone metabolites, specifically genistein to *p*-ethyl phenol, and daidzein to equol or *O*-desmethylangolensin (*O*-DMA), which are absorbed to be conjugated to glucuronic acid or sulfate in the liver. In the same way as estrogens, they undergo enterohepatic circulation, whereby they are deconjugated, reabsorbed, or excreted.

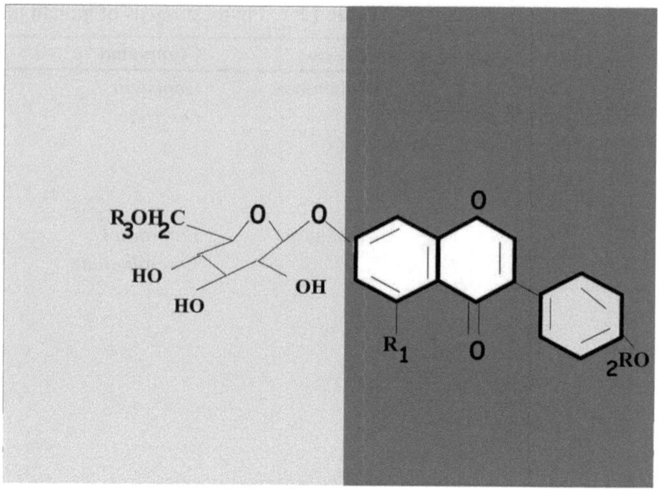

Fig. 12.2 Chemical structure of an isoflavone, as present in food in its glucosidic form [47]. In the *right* part of the figure aglycone isoflavone, the active form of the phytoestrogen after intestinal metabolism, is recognizable (unpublished)

Lignans have a similar metabolism; following oral ingestion the plant lignan, named secoisolariciresinol-diglucoside, is hydrolyzed by intestinal bacteria to secoisolariciresinol; then demethylated to enterodiol, which is absorbed or oxidized to enterolactone; and then reabsorbed. The lignan matairesinol is also converted via dehydroxylation and demethylation to enterolactone to be absorbed. Once absorbed, these mammalian lignans are conjugated to glucuronic acid or sulfate to enter the circulation and are finally excreted in the urine, or undergo enterohepatic circulation.

Because of their structural similarity to 17β-estradiol, phytoestrogens are able to bind estrogen receptors (ERs). ERs are intracellular receptors located primarily in the membrane of the nucleus; in the human body they are present in two forms, ERα and ERβ, with ERα playing a major role in the uterus, hypothalamus, and skeleton, and ERβ in the ovary, cardiovascular system, and brain. In most tissues ERα has proliferative effects, whereas ERβ has anti-proliferative effects; some studies have indicated an inhibitory effect of ERβ on ERα. In this view they are not organ specific as thought in the past, but balance each other in a Ying Yang fashion when present in the same organ. It seems logical, then, that a high ratio of ERα to ERβ may be correlated with high cellular proliferation and a low ratio with the opposite [5].

Interaction of phytoestrogens with ERs activates the classic genomic estrogen response: in this way phytoestrogens act as agonists of estrogens. Even if they have a much lower activity than 17β-estradiol, if they reach high levels (considered for genistein to be over 100 nmol/l) their effects may approach those of natural 17β-estradiol circulating at physiological level. Their affinity to the two ERs is not similar, however; for example, the affinity of genistein to ERβ is about 30–50 times higher than to ERα. As compared to 17β-estradiol the potency of phytoestrogens is much lower: for coumestrol it is 0.202, for genistein 0.086, for equol 0.061, for daidzein 0.013, for biochanin A 0.094, and for formononetin 0.084 [6]. Since phytoestrogens compete with estrogens for binding to the same receptor, their effect also depends on the levels of endogenous estradiol, acting as antagonists in premenopausal women (when estrogens reach high levels) and as agonists when endogenous estrogens are lacking, as happens in menopause (Fig. 12.3). This is the reason why phytoestrogens have been proposed as an alternative to hormonal replacement therapy (HRT).

The final activity of a phytoestrogen at a target site will consequently be related to:

1. The biological potency of the particular type of phytoestrogen involved.
2. Its level of affinity to ERα or ERβ.
3. The presence of ERα or ERβ in the target organ.
4. The ratio of ERα to ERβ.
5. The level of endogenous estrogens.

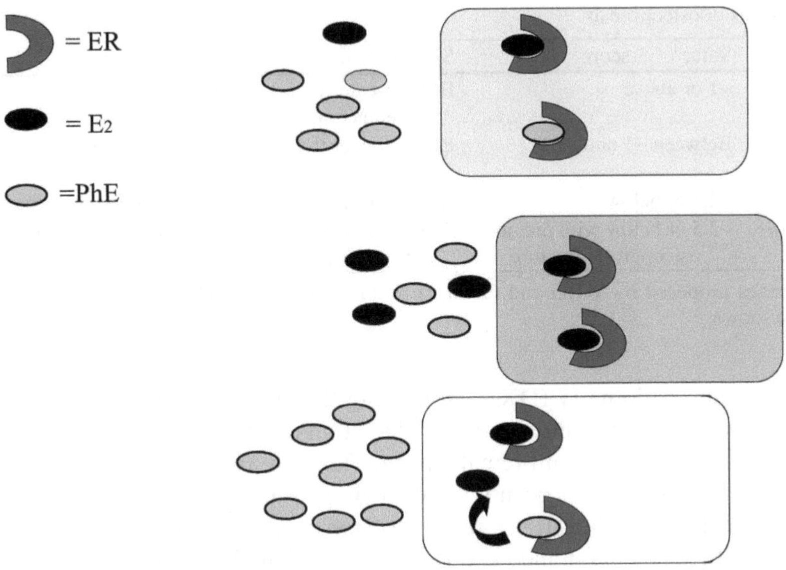

Fig. 12.3 Interaction between the endogenous estrogen estradiol (E_2) and phytoestrogens (PhE) with the same receptors (ER). At the *top*, a condition of normality is shown; in the *middle* part a hyper-estrogenic condition and at the *bottom* of the figure, a condition of hypoestrogenism, as it occurs in menopause

In this way the final biological effect of phytoestrogens can be estrogen-agonistic, estrogen-antagonistic, estrogen-agonistic in one tissue, and estrogen-antagonistic in another, and ultimately, a phytoestrogen will act as a SERM. SERMs are molecules able to bind to ERs determining mixed estrogen-agonist and -antagonist effects depending on the target tissue; their progenitor is the drug tamoxifen, used to treat breast cancer for over 35 years. Tamoxifen is a synthetic nonsteroidal agent that, after binding to ER, produces a specific activity of the receptor in relation to the characteristics of the tissue type. In this way tamoxifen reduces both the risk of invasive breast cancer (acting as an antagonist on breast tissue) and the incidence of osteoporotic fractures, acting as an agonist on bone tissue. But because of its estrogenic activity, the synthetic agent tamoxifen increases endometrial hyperplasia and cancer, making it by no means an ideal SERM for postmenopausal osteoporosis. Even if new SERMs have since been discovered, such as raloxifene, lasofoxifene, and bazedoxifene, no optimal SERM is yet available that could prevent both breast cancer and postmenopausal diseases [7] without inducing serious side effects.

Postmenopausal Osteoporosis

The term *osteoporosis* is now widely understood among the general public, since osteoporosis is considered a social health problem in industrialized countries, even if there is recent evidence of a declining incidence of hip fractures in the Western world [8]. In the USA, an estimated 55 % of people over the age of 50 years are believed to be at risk of developing this condition. Because 80 % of osteoporotic people are women, and because among them the risk of osteoporotic hip fractures is high, equaling the combined risk of breast, uterine, and ovarian cancer, this is above all a female problem. Osteoporosis has been defined as a "systemic skeletal disorder characterized by low bone mass and microarchitectural deterioration of bone tissue, with a consequent increase in bone fragility and susceptibility to fracture" [8]. It indicates a reduction in bone mass per unit volume and, basically, is caused when bone resorption exceeds bone formation. The diagnosis is easily made today by

Table 12.2 Diagnosis of osteoporosis

Definition	Value of T score	Significance
Normal	−1 or above	BMD greater than 1 SD below the young adult female reference mean
Low bone mass or osteopenia	Between −1 and −2.5	BMD greater than 1 SD below the young adult female mean but less than 2.5 SD below this value
Osteoporosis	−2.5 or below	BMD 2.5 SD or more below the young adult female mean
Severe osteoporosis	−2.5 or below with previous osteoporotic fracture	BMD 2.5 SD below the young adult female mean in the presence of one or more fragility fractures

Diagnostic categories proposed by WHO and modified by the International Osteoporosis Foundation. Assessments done by DXA are shown

dual-energy X-ray absorptiometry (DXA), following the criteria established by WHO, namely, a T-score ≤ −2.5 (Table 12.2), meaning a standard deviation (SD) of the bone mineral density (BMD) of 2.5 or more below the young adult female mean. There are two types of osteoporosis: Type I, or *postmenopausal osteoporosis*, that occurs in postmenopausal women aged 51–75 years, involving mainly trabecular bone, and Type II, or *senile osteoporosis*, that causes loss of both cortical and trabecular bone, and that occurs in men and women older than 70 years of age. For prevention purposes it is important to bear in mind that osteoporosis is not a disease in itself but poses a risk of disease. In fact, the true disease is the osteoporotic fracture, so the importance of osteoporosis is that it predisposes to fracture, as hypertension does to stroke.

From a clinical point of view postmenopausal osteoporosis is correctly defined as "a (silent) skeletal disorder characterized by compromised bone strength predisposing to an increased risk of fracture. Bone strength reflects the integration of two main features: bone density and bone quality" [9]. The pathogenetic process of bone thinning that conduces to postmenopausal osteoporosis is very long, starting long before the menopause after the peak bone density has been reached, which occurs in the woman at about 30 years, and then gradually declines. However, it is the menopausal lack of endogenous estrogen that increases bone loss up to one-third to one-half of the total bone loss, causing a steep step in the female lifeline. This menopausal related estrogen deficiency produces an accelerated *bone turnover*, the balanced remodeling process between bone resorption and formation during which osteoclasts resorb bone by acidification and proteolytic digestion, and osteoblasts fill the resorption cavity with new osteoid substance, to ensure a correct maintenance of the BMD. Because in postmenopause the rate of bone turnover is high and negative, the bone remodeling process being in balance only until the fifth decade of life, the final result is a progressive continuous bone loss. Estrogen therapy (ET) produces a net increase in bone density because estrogens inhibit osteoclast formation and prolong the life span of osteoblasts, thus reducing the rate of hip fracture as demonstrated by the WHI study [10]. For this reason HRT was very popular up to a decade ago, when the same WHI trial showed an increased incidence of some fearsome hormone-related diseases, mainly breast cancer. Moreover, once ET is discontinued the hormonal protection of bone is unfortunately lost within 5 years.

Therefore, preventive intervention strategies need to be reconsidered. One way is, of course, to identify high-risk women for hormonal treatment, such as those with thrombophilic Factor V Leiden, or women with additional hormonal risk factors for breast cancer. Another way is to use new drugs, such as TSEC. All these ways are being pursued by the pharmaceutical industry. But we also have an ethical option, a new concept of non-pharmacological prevention based on respect for the fundamental bioethical principles of the *person*, *beneficence*, and *non-maleficence* [11]. Respect not of an organ or a body but of a *person* implies respecting human biology as belonging to a human being, so not damaging it, and acting in harmony with our physiological features and functions. Ultimately, it means abandoning unhealthy lifestyle habits, such as drinking alcohol, smoking cigarettes, and adopting a sedentary lifestyle, in favor of a healthy diet and practical exercise. This should be considered not only as a way to prevent disease, but as a bioethical behavior in itself, according to which prevention is a logical, we could say mandatory, consequence. Dietary phytoestrogens therefore represent not an alternative to prevention by estrogen treatment, but simply the natural way to maintain bone health, in the same way as physical activity is the most efficacious way to prevent fractures, because the prevention of fractures relies on bone strength (both bone density and quality) certainly, but combined with alertness and a good reactivity to prevent falling. A drug may ensure only bone strength, at best, but cannot provide guarantees against pharmacological harm which, in bioethical terms, means violating the concept of *non-maleficence*. In fact, drug prevention is certainly not a harm-free intervention. In 1989, Lubsen and Tijssen proposed an illustrative model where they showed that any preventive drug treatment in healthy women does not follow a linear trend, but the benefit for the patient increases and decreases in parallel to the risk of disease. On the contrary, adverse events caused by drugs follow a fixed trend, equal for patients at risk or not, so that while patients at high risk will derive great benefit from the treatment, patients at low or no risk will suffer only pharmacological harm without gaining any benefit [12].

Dietary Phytoestrogens in Preventing Postmenopausal Osteoporosis

Interest in the beneficial effects of phytoestrogens in preventing postmenopausal osteoporosis was generated by observational studies showing a lower incidence of hip fractures in Asian women than Caucasian women, combined with a positive association between the soy intake of pre- and postmenopausal women and BMD [13].

Subsequently, many in vitro studies provided useful insights into the possible actions of isoflavones on individual bone cells; these results have been confirmed by in vivo studies where it is possible to evaluate more complex effects on bone, mainly variations of the BMD. The early studies examined the effects of soymilk and soy protein isolate compared with casein, and all found that the BMD was higher in soy-fed rats than in controls [14].

It has been shown that phytoestrogens enhance bone formation by stimulating osteoblastic activity via the activation of ERs and by promoting the production of insulin-like growth-factor-I (IGF-I) [3] and it now seems well established that a high content of phytoestrogens has the capacity to act positively on both osteoclasts and osteoblasts [15].

To confirm the results derived from epidemiological animal in vitro-based studies, many human trials have attempted to evaluate the effects of phytoestrogens in menopausal women. The data resulted conflicting, above all because of the great methodological variability, premenopausal or postmenopausal status, as well as early or late postmenopausal period, and the type of phytoestrogens used. There were also wide differences as regards dosage, duration of studies, sample size, intake analysis, different ethnicity, different outcome variables measured, and confounding factors, all of which make it difficult to understand the real efficacy of phytoestrogens [16].

Obviously, randomized controlled trials are the most indicative studies for assessing the effect of experimental interventions but they suffer from some drawbacks, above all because it takes a long time to observe the effect of the intervention on the clinical endpoint of interest, in our case the occurrence of osteoporotic fractures. Even surrogate endpoints, such as bone biomarkers, require long-term studies, because just one remodelling cycle lasts 30–80 weeks. Therefore, the efficacy of a phytoestrogen intervention on postmenopausal osteoporosis could be judged only on the basis of studies lasting many months, ideally 2–3 years. Because of all these reasons very few adequate studies have yet been reported.

In a double-blind randomized placebo-controlled trial, Kreijkamp-Kaspers et al. [17] found no significant effect on BMD of 99 mg of isoflavones taken daily by women aged 60 to 75 years, showing a scant efficacy of isoflavones in the late postmenopausal phase. Vupadhyayula et al. [18], in a 2-year randomized double-blind placebo-controlled trial, failed to show any efficacy on the BMD of the main bone sites. Potter et al. [19], in a randomized double-blind 3-intervention trial with isolated soy protein containing 56 or 90 mg of isoflavones, showed that BMD was increased with an intake of 90 mg of soy isoflavones but not with 56 mg, suggesting that there is a threshold of isoflavone intake required to achieve a positive effect on bone; this positive effect was not evident at the femoral level, in accordance with the known greater sensitivity of the spine to estrogens because of both the higher content of trabecular bone and the shorter time from exposure to reaction.

In a three-arm (HRT, phytoestrogen-rich diet, and control) 6-month randomized controlled trial, we evaluated the effects of dietary phytoestrogens on bone biomarkers and BMD in 187 asymptomatic postmenopausal healthy women aged 39–60 years [20]. Diet resulted effective (even if not as much as HRT) in reducing postmenopausal bone loss and bone turnover, but diet stimulated bone osteoblastic activity, too, as evidenced in the study by the significant increase of osteocalcin concentrations in the second group.

A recent meta-analysis [21] confirmed the ability of phytoestrogen intake in preventing bone resorption but no advantage resulted on bone formation; the authors hypothesized that higher doses are necessary to reverse bone loss. In a multicenter, randomized, double-blind, placebo-controlled 24-month trial conducted to assess the effects of daily supplementation with 80–120 mg of soy hypocotyl aglycone isoflavones plus 400 mg calcium and 400 IU vitamin D in 403 postmenopausal women, daily supplementation with 120 mg reduced whole-body (WB) bone loss, while supplementation with 80 mg of soy hypocotyl aglycone isoflavones reduced WB BMD but nonsignificantly [22]. Two meta-analyses of randomized controlled trials with a duration ranging from 3 to >24 months showed an increase in LS BMD with an isoflavone intake >90 mg/day in menopausal women [23, 24]. Moreover, the powerful prospective Shanghai Women's Health Study of a cohort of 24,403 menopausal women showed a bone fracture incidence inversely related to the quintiles of soy protein intake [25].

Contradictory results can also reflect a different individual biology. The end product of intestinal metabolism of the phytoestrogen isoflavone daidzein is equol that shows an 80 times higher estrogen receptor-β binding affinity as compared to its parent daidzein [26]. Because ER-β is dominant in bone, equol has been hypothesized as the main candidate in the prevention of postmenopausal osteoporosis [27]. Among humans however, only 30–50 % of the population possess the gut microflora needed for intestinal bacteria conversion of daidzein to equol; non-producers need more time and a gradual intake to be able to promote the growth of a proper bacterial flora that can metabolize equol, providing further evidence of the capacity of the environment to modify human biology.

As regards the class of phytoestrogens denominated coumestans, although they are plentifully present in nature, only coumestrol is important for humans. Clover and soybean sprouts, legumes, and to a lesser extent Brussel sprouts and spinach are the main dietary sources of coumestrol. Coumestrol has a higher binding affinity to ERs than genistein and it is able both to inhibit bone resorption and to stimulate bone formation. Even if some evidence showed an interesting capacity of coumestrol to inhibit bone resorption and, at the same time, to stimulate bone mineralization [28] there are not enough studies to assess its use in the human field.

Other human intervention studies assessed the positive effects of phytoestrogen consumption, not only isoflavones but also lignans, on BMD, specifically on the lumbar spine, and on biomarkers of both bone formation and resorption [29]. The effects on osteoporosis of the Mediterranean diet, which is very rich in phytoestrogen lignans, have recently been exhaustively reviewed [30]. Fruits and legumes have a bone-protective effect at every age, with an evident positive action on bone metabolism. This anti-osteoporotic activity of the Mediterranean diet is probably the result of many components, present and working together, the best known of which are:

1. Phytoestrogens, namely, lignans contained in fruits, vegetables, legumes, and seeds, with their known estrogenic properties described above.
2. Potassium, present in fruits and legumes, with its alkalinizing power that can prevent the urinary excretion of bone calcium.
3. Vitamin K, present particularly in green leafy vegetables, which improves the bone metabolism.

4. Vitamin C, present in fruits and fresh vegetables, which has been shown in vitro to improve osteoblastic differentiation.
5. β-carotene, present in raw carrots and cress, positively associated to lumbar BMD.
6. Vitamins B6 and B9, whose deficiencies produce bone alterations.
7. Vitamin E, oleic acid, and olive oil polyphenols, which have shown bone-protective effects in animals and anti-inflammatory properties in preventing rheumatoid arthritis in humans [30].

Another compound of the Mediterranean diet with prominent phytoestrogenic properties, apart from its long known antioxidant capacities, is resveratrol, renowned as responsible for the so-called French Paradox, the paradoxical phenomenon whereby Frenchmen, despite a diet rich in saturated fats, suffer a relatively low incidence of coronary heart disease by virtue of their high consumption of red wine that contains higher quantities of resveratrol (1.5 mg/l) than white wine (0.027 mg/l). Interestingly, resveratrol, a polyphenol compound found also in grapes, cranberries, mulberries, and peanuts, has the potential to antagonize osteoclasts and to promote osteoblasts; it inhibits the reabsorption activity of osteoclasts and promotes the formation of osteoblasts from mesenchymal precursors in vitro [31]. Moreover, in combination with vitamin D, it has been shown to be capable of preventing weight gain and bone loss in a postmenopausal rat model [32].

Lignans are structurally similar to tamoxifen, showing estrogenic, antioxidant, and anti-inflammatory properties that can reduce the rapid rate of bone loss in postmenopausal women. They are widely distributed in nature, being necessary components for the formation of the lignin constituent of the plant cell wall. Vegetables, legumes, and whole grain cereals, which are the main components of the Mediterranean diet, are good sources of lignans, but because lignans are localized in the outer fiber-containing layer, modern milling techniques that eliminate this layer in grain and cereals lower the overall lignan content, so the actual intake in Western populations is relatively low. Indeed, in the Framingham study a median daily intake of 578 μg of lignans was found in American postmenopausal women [33].

Italian Aspects

A clear north–south gradient has been observed in the epidemiology of osteoporosis (Fig. 12.4). Moreover, and much more worryingly, the incidence of hip fracture in women older than 50 years of age shows a great variability in the world, ranging from a minimum of 26/100,000/year in South Africa to 903/100,000/year in Norway [34]. The geographic influence on this disease could not be clearer, demonstrating the great importance of the sun.

Diet, sunlight, and weight-bearing activity are the three pillars that support the structure of the bone.

Italy is one of the countries with the highest life expectancy rates in the world. According to the Italian National Institute for Statistics (ISTAT) in this country life expectancy at birth has now reached the finish line of 87.4 years for women and at the last survey, 20 % of Italian people were more than 65 years old [35]. The main Epidemiological Study on the Prevalence of Osteoporosis (ESOPO) in Italy reported a prevalence of osteoporosis of 23 % among all women, ranging from 9 % (40–49-year-olds) up to 45 % (70–79 years or older) [36], but because the ESOPO study was conducted using quantitative ultrasound (QUS) densitometry measurements, an overestimation of this incidence has been suspected. Using DXA measurements, Andreoli et al. [37] found, instead, an incidence of osteopenia and osteoporosis of 43.9 and 8.5 %, respectively, in women aged 50–59 years, that increased to 45.4 and 36.6 %, respectively, at 70–79 years of age. The overall incidence of osteoporosis in women aged 30–79 years was 16.7 %. Interestingly, in another recent study [38] none of the main known risk factors for osteoporosis (a history of fragility fracture, a family history of hip fracture, current smoking) was present in two out of three postmenopausal women, demonstrating how difficult targeted prevention can be.

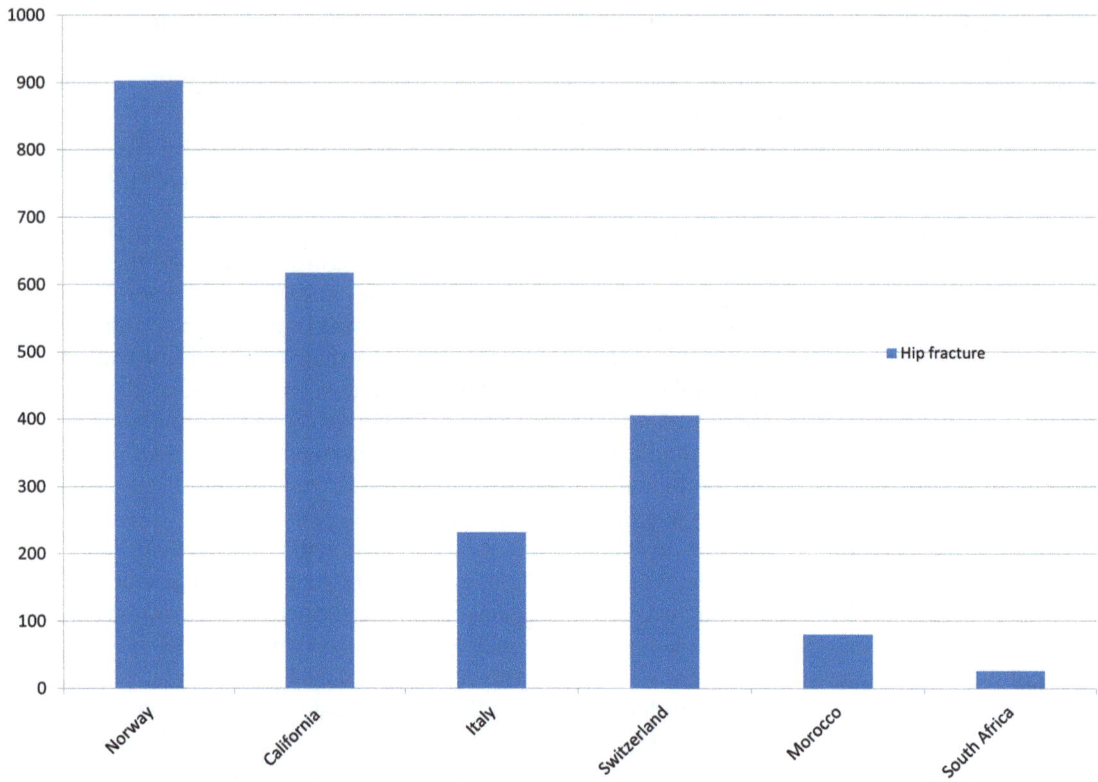

Fig. 12.4 Geographic variation in the incidence of hip fracture in the world. Variations in the incidence, as the number of people with hip fracture/100,000/year in the world, are shown. The chosen countries show the most significant differences among North, Center, and South of the world

Overall, a total of 3.5 million osteoporotic women and 1 million men have been estimated to be living in Italy today. The incidence of hip fractures, the most feared complication of osteoporosis, is more than 80,000 units/year in people >50 years of age [39] and it is 232/100,000/year in postmenopausal women [40]. Because we expect that the percentage of people aged over 65 years will increase by 25 % in the next years, we must expect a significant increase in the incidence of osteoporosis, too. Prevention seems every day to be more urgent, but at the same time more problematic and unsustainable if carried out by drug intervention.

The Mediterranean diet (Fig. 12.5), a diet rich in fruit, vegetables, and whole grain, and low in calories and saturated fat, has been judged, on the basis of current research, to be one of the key factors that can prevent postmenopausal chronic diseases, including osteoporosis [41]. This seems to us to be not a medical intervention, but simply the adoption of a course that respects the female biology and a modern concept of ethical medicine; it is, in fact, only bioethically sustainable behavior that automatically translates into a correct outcome for health. We need to change the medical organicist vision and to begin to see human health in a holistic way. It has been shown, and it is scientifically logical, that obesity significantly decreases the risk of osteoporosis, but no one could judge it to be a useful strategy to prevent a disease by inducing another disease. In any case, since the two diseases are caused basically by the same causes, i.e., improper diet and lack of exercise, there is only one way forward.

These problems also affect the Mediterranean countries. The increasing incidence of osteoporosis in Italy depends on many factors, of course, since it is a multifactorial disease, but the main reason is the increasing abandonment of the traditional Mediterranean diet [42], a healthy diet with a rich content of lignans, antioxidants, and anti-inflammatory and alkalinizing components.

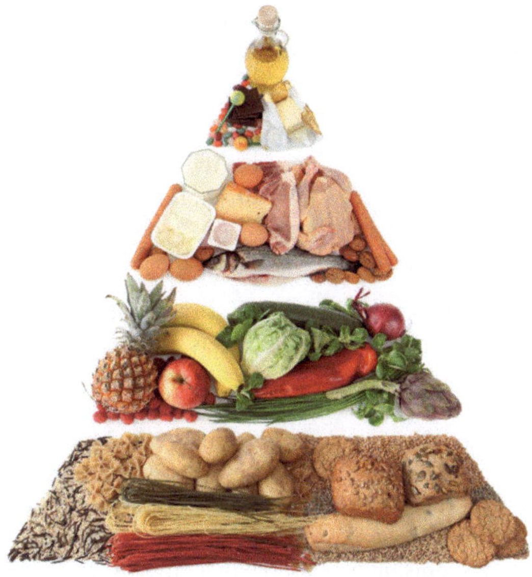

Fig. 12.5 The Mediterranean diet. The main foods of the Mediterranean diet are shown, placed according to the model of the Diet Pyramid (unpublished)

Conclusion

Diet can make us sick or maintain health, and foods have been used to prevent or even to treat diseases for centuries; thousands of sailors were saved from scurvy by citrus foods and the curse of beriberi was abolished by unpolished rice, so its importance for human health is unquestionable. But what is the role of the diet in the prevention of modern diseases?

The scientific interest in phytoestrogens has derived from their proposed capacity to influence human health, above all in relation to the so-called Western diseases. Despite the few trials of high quality and many contradictory results, it is possible to mark out some milestones today:

1. Phytoestrogens are efficacious natural compounds able to counteract postmenopausal bone loss.
2. Food phytoestrogens do not have relevant side effects if they are ingested in the traditional Mediterranean–Asiatic diet.
3. Dietary phytoestrogens have other important preventive effects apart from those on osteoporosis, mostly in preventing cardiovascular diseases, obesity, and breast, endometrial, and prostate cancers.

The history of β-carotene has made us suspicious of using supplements derived from foods on the presumption of established beneficial properties resulting from a plethora of in vivo, animal, and epidemiological data. In 1981 Sir Richard Peto, following numerous observational epidemiological studies showing a lower incidence of lung cancer in people eating carotenoid-rich foods, hypothesized a protective effect of β-carotene in preventing this cancer. Three large primary prevention trials tested this hypothesis in the early 1980s. The results were unexpected. The ATBC study showed an increase in the lung cancer incidence (16 %) and overall mortality (8 %) in the β-carotene intervention group, and the CARET study showed a 28 % increase in lung cancer and a 17 % increase in overall mortality after an average of 4 years of ingestion of 30 mg of β-carotene and 25,000 IU retinyl palmitate supplements versus placebo [43]. This puts a stop to medical arrogance. Foods contain thousands of substances endowed with biological properties, and these substances work together to produce the final effect. Often it is only an act of arrogance to believe that we have understood the complexity of these interactions. Dietary interventions are, instead, natural and basic in health promotion. Obviously, diet is only one component of lifestyle and, for Western medicine, learning to see our body in a holistic way is a more difficult challenge. The Shanghai Breast Cancer Survival Study, a large, population-based cohort study of 5,042 female breast cancer survivors, showed that soy food consumption was significantly associated with a decreased risk of death and recurrence [44].

The authors hypothesized a multifactorial mechanism of action:

1. Soy isoflavones compete with endogenous estrogens for binding to the same ERs.
2. Soy isoflavones increase the synthesis of sex hormone-binding globulin (SHBG), lowering the biological availability of sex hormones.
3. Soy isoflavones inhibit 17 β-hydroxysteroid dehydrogenases, thus reducing estrogen synthesis.
4. Soy isoflavones increase the clearance of steroids from the circulation.

It seems reasonable, then, to assume that some diets, like those rich in phytoestrogens, are able to produce pharmacological effects in the human body, counteracting simultaneously many of the modern diseases.

Phytoestrogens have a modest beneficial effect on bone, but they have been shown to be useful and sufficient in preventing postmenopausal bone loss [45]. Our opinion is that this is true, and that it is an ethical, not a medical, concept; a diet that can keep the human body healthy is only a natural attitude of respect toward human physiology. Phytoestrogens are natural components of some diets that thousands of generations have selected as the most healthy, such as the Mediterranean and Asiatic diets, and they are, it seems, indispensable in a physiological phase of deficiency of endogenous estrogens, such as the postmenopausal phase. It seems, also, reductive to limit the complex activity of these compounds to the prevention of postmenopausal osteoporosis. A phytoestrogen-rich diet, ideally a Mediterranean diet with components of the Asiatic diet, or vice versa, is tasty, healthy, safe, ethical, and protective against all the so-called Western diseases, i.e., cardiovascular and osteoporotic diseases; endometrial, breast, and prostate cancers; overweight and obesity; moreover promotes longevity. We hope to stimulate a reflection on the way to preserve human health. Prevention has been medicalized in the last years; but medicalization is not a harmless process. The experience of HRT in preventing menopause-related chronic diseases should serve as a lesson, as the net decrease of breast cancer paralleling that of the hormonal drug market has shown [46]. Medicalization is a cultural process involving biological, social, psychological, and conceptual aspects, with their obligations and timelines, and that can close us inside a cage. We have to liberate woman, and let her fly free under the power of her own body.

Acknowledgments I am grateful to Mary V.C. Pragnell, B.A., for careful proofreading.

References

1. Wildman REC, editor. Handbook of nutraceuticals and functional foods. Washington, DC: CRC Press; 2001. p. 2.
2. Loewe S, Lange F, Spohr E. Uber weiliche sexual hormone (Thelytropine). Biochem Zeitschr. 1927;180:1–26.
3. Bawa S. The significance of soy protein and soy bioactivity compounds in the prophylaxis and treatment of osteoporosis. J Osteoporos. 2010;2010:891058.
4. Marini H, Bitto A, Altavilla D, Burnett BP, Polito F, Di Stefano V, et al. Breast safety and efficacy of genistein aglycone for postmenopausal bone loss: a follow-up study. J Clin Endocrinol Metab. 2008;93:4787–96.
5. Jordan VC. Chemoprevention of breast cancer with selective oestrogen-receptor modulators. Nat Rev Cancer. 2007;7:46–53.
6. Campos MG, Matos MP. Bioactivity of isoflavones: assessment through a theoretical model as a way to obtain a "Theoretical Efficacy Related to Estradiol (THERE)". Int J Mol Sci. 2010;11:480–91.
7. Pickar JH, MacNeil T, Ohleth K. SERMs: progress and future perspectives. Maturitas. 2010;67:129.38.
8. Guidelines AACE. American Association of Clinical Endocrinologists Medical Guidelines for Clinical Practice for the diagnosis and treatment of postmenopausal osteoporosis. Endocr Pract. 2010;16 Suppl 3Suppl 3:1–37.
9. No authors listed. Consensus development conference: diagnosis, prophylaxis and treatment of osteoporosis. Am J Med. 1993;94:646–50.

10. The Women's Health Initiative Steering Committee. Effects of conjugated equine estrogen in postmenopausal women with hysterectomy: the Women's Health Initiative randomized controlled trial. JAMA. 2004;291:1701–12.
11. Beauchamp T, Childress J. Principles of biomedical ethics. New York: Oxford Unity Press; 1979.
12. Glasziou PP, Irwing LM. An evidence based approach to individualizing treatment. BMJ. 1995;311:1356–9.
13. Tsuchida K, Mizushima S, Toba M, Soda K. Dietary soybeans intake and bone mineral density among 995 middle-aged women in Yokohama. J Epidemiol. 1999;9:14–9.
14. Arjmandi BH, Alekel L, Hollis BW. Dietary soybean protein prevents bone loss in an ovariectomized rat model of osteoporosis. J Nutr. 1996;126:161–7.
15. Chen XW, Garner SC, Anderson JJ. Isoflavones regulate interleukin-6 and osteoprogesterin synthesis during osteoblast cell differentiation via an estrogen-receptor-dependent pathway. Biochem Biophys Res Commun. 2002;295:417–22.
16. Branca F. Dietary phytoestrogens and bone health. Proc Nutr Soc. 2003;62:877–87.
17. Kreijamp-Kaspers S, Kok L, Grobbee DE, de Haan EH, Aleman A, Lampe JW, et al. Effect of soy protein containing isoflavones on cognitive function, bone mineral density, and plasma lipids in postmenopausal women, a randomized controlled trial. J Am Med Assoc. 2004;292:65–74.
18. Vupadhyayula PM, Gallagher JC, Templin T, Logsdon SM, Smith LM. Effects Effects of soy protein isolate on bone mineral density and physical performance indices in postmenopausal women–a 2-year randomized, double-blind, placebo-controlled trial. Menopause. 2009;16(2):320–8.
19. Potter SM, Baum JA, Teng H, et al. Soy protein and isoflavones. Their effects on blood lipids and bone density in postmenopausal women. Am J Clin Nutr. 1998;68:1375S–9.
20. Chiechi LM, Secreto G, D'Amore M, Fanell M, Venturelli E, Cantatore F, et al. Efficacy of a soy rich diet in preventing postmenopausal osteoporosis: the Menfis randomized trial. Maturitas. 2002;42:295–300.
21. Salari Sharif P, Nikfar S, Abdollahi M. Prevention of bone resorption by intake of phytoestrogens in postmenopausal women: a meta-analysis. Age (Dordr). 2011;33(3):421–31.
22. Wong WW, Lewis RD, Steinberg FM, Murray MJ, Cramer MA, Amato P, et al. Soy isoflavone supplementation and bone mineral density in menopausal women: a 2-y multicenter clinical trial. Am J Clin Nutr. 2009;90:1433–9.
23. Ma DF, Qin LQ, Wang PY, Katoh R. Soy isoflavone intake increases bone mineral density in the spine of menopausal women: metanalysis of randomized controlled trials. Clin Nutr. 2008;27:57–64.
24. Liu J, Ho SC, Su YX, Chen WQ, Zhang CX, Chen YM. Effect of long-term intervention of soy isoflavones on bone mineral density in women: a meta-analysis of randomized controlled trials. Bone. 2009;44:948–53.
25. Zhang X, Shu XO, Li H, Yang G, Li Q, Gao YT, et al. Prospective cohort study of soy food consumption and risk of bone fracture among postmenopausal women. Arch Intern Med. 2005;165:1890–5.
26. Muthyala RS, Ju YH, Sheng S, Williams LD, Doerge DR, Katzenellendogen BS, et al. Equol, a natural estrogenic metabolite from soy isoflavones: convenient preparation and resolution of R- and S.equols and their differing binding and biological activity through estrogen receptors alpha and beta. Bioorg Med Chem. 2004;12:1559–67.
27. Weaver CM, Legette LCL. Equol, via dietary sources or intestinal production, may ameliorate estrogen deficiency-induced bone-loss. J Nutr. 2010;140:1377S–9.
28. Tsutsumi N. Effect of coumestrol on bone metabolism in organ culture. Biol Pharm Bull. 1995;18(7):1012–5.
29. Duncan AM, Phipps WR, Kurzer MS. Phyto-oestrogens. Best Pract Res Clin Endocrinol Metab. 2003;17(2): 253–71.
30. Puel C, Coxam V, Davicco MJ. Régime méditerranéen et ostéoporose. Medicine/Sciences. 2007;23:756–60.
31. Kupisiewicz K, Boissy P, Abdallah BM, et al. Potential of resveratrol analogues as antagonists of osteoclasts and promoter of osteoblasts. Calcif Tissue Int. 2010;87:437–49.
32. Rayalam S, Della-Fera MA, Baile CA. Synergism between resveratrol and other phytochemicals: implications for obesity and osteoporosis. Mol Nutr Food Res. 2011;55:1–9.
33. De Kleijn MG, Nan der Shouw YT, Wilson PW. Intake of dietary phytoestrogens in postmenopausal women is low in the United States. The Framingham study. J Nutr. 2001;131:1826–32.
34. El Maghraoui A, Koumba BA, Jroundi I, Achemlal L, Bezza A, Tazi MA. Epidemiology of hip fractures in 2002 in Rabat, Marocco. Osteoporos Int. 2005;16:597–602.
35. National Institute for Statistics. Italian Statistics 2005. Rome: National Institute for Statistics; 2005.
36. Tarantino U, Capone A, Planta M, D'Arienzo M, Letizia Mauro G, Impagliazzo A, et al. The incidence of hip, forearm, humeral, ankle, and vertebral fragility fractures in Italy: results from a 3-year multicenter study. Arthritis Res Ther. 2010;12:R226.
37. Andreoli A, Bazzocchi A, Celi M, Lauro D, Sorge R, Tarantino U, et al. Relationship between body composition, body mass index and bone mineral density in a large population of normal, osteopenic and osteoporotic women. Radiol Med. 2011;116(7):1115–23.
38. Pedrazzoni M, Girasole G, Giusti A, Barone A, Pioli G, Palummeri E, et al. Assessment of the 10-year risk of fracture in Italian postmenopausal women Using Frax : a North Italian Multicenter Study. J Endocrinol Invest. 2011;34(11):e386–91.

39. Linee guida per la diagnosi, prevenzione e terapia dell'osteoporosi. SIOMMMS. Reumatismo. 2005;61(4):1–25.
40. Mazzuoli GF, Gennari C, Passeri M, Celi FS, Acca M, Camporeale A, et al. Incidence of hip fracture: an Italian survey. Osteoporos Int. 1993;1:S8–9.
41. Schlienger JL, Pradignac A. Nutrition approaches to prevent chronic disease. Rev Prat. 2009;59(1):61–5.
42. Chiechi LM, Secreto G, Vimercati A, Greco P, Venturelli E, Pansini F, et al. The effects of a soy rich diet on serum lipids: the Menfis randomized trial. Maturitas. 2002;41:97–104.
43. Goodman GE. Prevention of lung cancer. Curr Opin Oncol. 1998;10(2):122–6.
44. Shu XO, Zheng Y, Cai H, Gu K, Chen Z, Zheng W, et al. Soy food intake and breast cancer survival. JAMA. 2009;302(22):2437–43.
45. Shedd-Wise KM, Alekel DL, Hofman H, Hanson KE, Schiferi DJ, Hanson LN, et al. The soy isoflavones for reducing bone loss study: 3-yr effects on pQCT bone mineral density and strength measures in postmenopausal women. J Clin Densitom. 2011;14(1):47–57.
46. Stang A. Decline in hormone replacement prescription and fall in breast cancer incidence. Dtsch Arztebl Int. 2008;105(16):303–9.
47. Reinli K, Block G. Phytoestrogen content of foods—a compendium of literature values. Nutr Cancer. 1996; 26:123–48.

Chapter 13
Curcumin and Its Potential Effects on the Development of Postmenopausal Osteoporosis

Joanna Folwarczna

Key Points

- Curcumin, a constituent of turmeric, is currently considered a potential treatment in numerous diseases, including osteoporosis.
- Curcumin has been reported to affect osteoclastogenesis and osteoblast proliferation and activity in vitro.
- Results of studies on curcumin effects on the skeletal system of estrogen deficient animals are inconsistent.
- There are no reports on the effects of curcumin on the skeletal system in humans.
- The available experimental data do not support the use of curcumin in the prophylaxis and treatment of postmenopausal osteoporosis.
- Future research is necessary in order to determine the benefit–risk ratio of curcumin.

Keywords Curcumin • Osteoporosis • Osteoblasts • Osteoclasts • Menopause

Abbreviations

AP-1	Activator protein-1
ERK	Extracellular signal-regulated kinase
Gpx-1	Glutathione peroxidase-1
GSK-3β	Glycogen synthase kinase-3β
HO-1	Heme oxygenase-1
IKK	IκB kinase
IL	Interleukin
JNK	c-Jun N-terminal kinase
MAPK	Mitogen-activated protein kinase
MMP	Matrix metalloproteinase
NFAT	Nuclear factor of activated T cells

J. Folwarczna, Pharm.D., Ph.D. (habil.) (✉)
Department of Pharmacology, School of Pharmacy with Division of Laboratory Medicine, Medical University of Silesia, Katowice, Jagiellońska 4, 41-200 Sosnowiec, Poland
e-mail: jfolwarczna@sum.edu.pl

C.J.H. Martin et al. (eds.), *Nutrition and Diet in Menopause*, Nutrition and Health,
DOI 10.1007/978-1-62703-373-2_13, © Springer Science+Business Media New York 2013

NF-κB	Nuclear factor-κB
RANK	Receptor activator of nuclear factor-κB
RANKL	RANK ligand
ROS	Reactive oxygen species
TNF-α	Tumor necrosis factor-α

Introduction

There is increasing interest in the discovery of natural compounds that could favorably affect the skeletal system and be used in the prophylaxis and treatment of postmenopausal osteoporosis. Active substances contained in plants may affect the skeletal system; however, the bone effects of the majority of them have never been investigated.

Curcumin, a plant polyphenol, is an active principle of turmeric—the dried ground rhizomes of the turmeric plant (*Curcuma longa* L.) [1]. Turmeric has been used for centuries as a dietary spice, as well as a traditional remedy to treat numerous common ailments in Indian Ayurvedic, Chinese, Arabic, and other traditional medicines [2]. In modern times, especially in the last decade, curcumin has focused interest on its multidirectional activities. The theoretical background and results of in vitro and in vivo experimental studies on the effects of curcumin on the skeletal system are reviewed in this chapter.

Curcumin

Curcuma longa L. (Fig. 13.1 [3]) belongs to the ginger family (Zingiberaceae). It is a short-stemmed perennial herb, growing to up to 100 cm in height, having white to colorful flower, curved, oblong, and ovate leaves, and cylindrical rhizomes [4]. *Curcuma longa* L. grows naturally throughout the

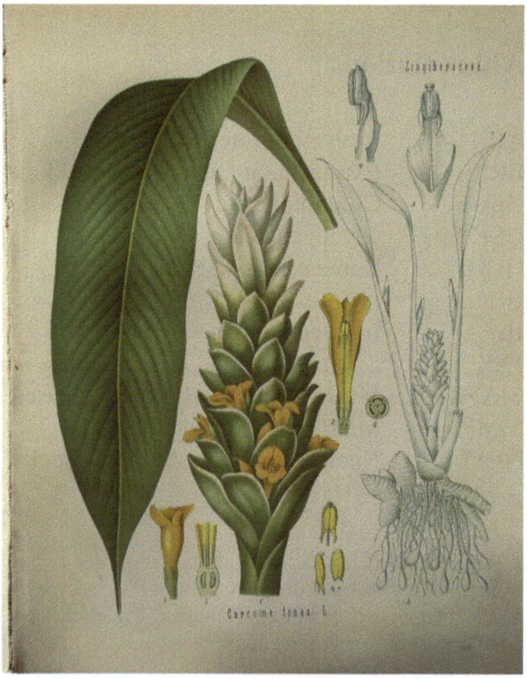

Fig. 13.1 *Curcuma longa* L. Reproduced from "Köhler's Medizinal-Pflanzen in naturgetreuen Abbildungen mit kurz erläuterndem Texte" [3]

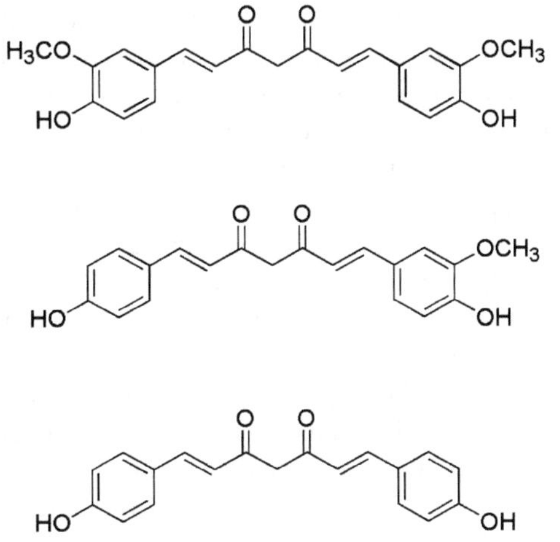

Fig. 13.2 Structure of main curcuminoids of turmeric. I—curcumin, II—demethoxycurcumin, III—bisdemethoxycurcumin

Indian subcontinent and in tropical climates, especially in Southeast Asia [1, 4]. Most of the World's supply of turmeric is produced and consumed in India [1].

In India and Southeast Asia fresh turmeric root is widely used in a similar way to ginger. In the West, turmeric is available as a dried powder [2]. Turmeric was first introduced to Europe by Arab traders in the thirteenth century. It was mentioned by Marco Polo in the writings concerning his 1280 journey to China and India. During the rule of British in India, turmeric was combined with various other spices and renamed "curry powder" [5].

The bright yellow color of turmeric originates mostly from fat-soluble, polyphenolic pigments: curcuminoids [6] (Fig. 13.2). Curcuminoids constitute 0.3–5.4 % of dried rhizomes of turmeric [1]. Curcumin (chemically diferuloylmethane) is the most abundant curcuminoid of turmeric, generally considered to be its most active constituent [6]. The other main curcuminoids of turmeric are demethoxycurcumin and bisdemethoxycurcumin. Moreover, turmeric contains volatile oils to which its aromatic properties are attributable (4–5 %), proteins (6 %), fat (1.7–3.3 %), resins (1 %), carbohydrates (65–70 %), and moisture (10 %) [1].

Commercially available preparations of "curcumin" usually are not pure and comprise curcumin itself and other curcuminoids [1, 2].

At present, curcumin is used worldwide as a cooking spice, flavoring agent and colorant. Dishes traditionally prepared with turmeric include most curries, pickles, relishes, and chutneys. Curcumin is used to color such products as mustards, margarines, mayonnaises, beverages [2, 4]. Curcumin, understood as a mixture of curcumin, demethoxycurcumin, and bisdemethoxycurcumin in varying proportions, is listed in the numbering system for food additives with the code E 100 [7].

In India, the average intake of turmeric in the diet has been reported to be even 2–2.5 g, which corresponds to a curcumin intake of approximately 60–100 mg daily [1, 8]. Some data on the daily intake of curcumin in Europe can be found in the expert opinion [7]. Evaluation of curcumin content in various sample blends of turmeric and curry powders purchased in grocery stores in the USA revealed the highest value of 3.14 % for one turmeric powder, with much lower values for curry powders [9]. In 2004 the Joint FAO/WHO Expert Committee on Food Additives allocated an acceptable daily intake (ADI) for curcumin (E 100) of 0–3 mg/kg body weight/day [7].

Most of the effects associated with curcumin therapeutic properties seem to be based on its ability to suppress inflammation [10]. Curcumin has been reported to exert anti-inflammatory, antioxidant but also pro-oxidant, pro-apoptotic and anti-apoptotic, anti-angiogenic, antiviral, antibacterial, antifungal, anticancer (both chemopreventive and chemotherapeutic), wound healing activities [1, 2, 4, 5]. In recent years, an enormous number of experimental studies on curcumin have been carried out, indicating very diverse mechanisms of its action.

Curcumin, at the cellular level, modulates important molecular targets: transcription factors, such as NF-κB, AP-1, β-catenin, peroxisome proliferator-activated receptor-γ; protein kinases (like MAPKs) and other enzymes, like cyclooxygenase-2, 5-lipoxygenase, inducible nitric oxide synthase, glutathione S-transferase, heme oxygenase-1, MMPs; cytokines (e.g., TNF-α, IL-1β, IL-6); growth factors (like fibroblast growth factor, transforming growth factor-β1, vascular endothelial growth factor); receptors (epidermal growth factor receptor, low density lipoprotein receptor, estrogen receptor-α, androgen receptor); cell cycle proteins, apoptosis-related proteins, adhesion molecules, and others (e.g., P-glycoprotein) [1, 2, 5, 6, 10–12]. Due to these effects, curcumin is now proposed to be a potential treatment for cancer, arthritis, cardiovascular diseases, inflammatory bowel disease, Alzheimer's disease, diabetes, psoriasis, and other illnesses, even to be an agent which could slow down ageing [2, 10, 11, 13, 14]. The targets and therapeutic potential of curcumin have been comprehensively reviewed in numerous publications [1, 2, 14, 15]. However, it must be pointed out that the potential of curcumin has not been confirmed through multicenter, randomized, double-blind, placebo-controlled clinical trials yet [5, 8]. The conducted and ongoing clinical trials of curcumin have been summarized in review articles [1, 6, 8, 15]. In fact, there is an increasing gap between numerous and often high level experimental studies and scarce clinical research [6, 8].

Although curcumin is regarded to be effective in some diseases and safe, it has not yet been approved as a therapeutic agent [8]. So far, low oral bioavailability of curcumin due to poor aqueous solubility and gastrointestinal absorption, efficient first pass metabolism, and rapid elimination [2] limit the possibility to establish its indications and safety.

An important issue is the possibility that curcumin, targeting so many cellular signaling pathways may act as a double-edged sword, and exert favorable or unfavorable effects. For example, due to its antioxidant properties, achievable in the body, curcumin can alleviate the symptoms of some diseases, but also induce the suppression of innate immune responses, making the host vulnerable to infections. Excess use of curcumin can damage the gut microbiota and thus alter host's physiology and immune response [16]. Under specific conditions, it may exert toxic and carcinogenic effects, it may also alter the effectiveness of radiotherapy and chemotherapy [17]. So far, adverse effects reported by patients taking part in clinical trials have been mainly nausea, diarrhea, allergic dermatitis [4].

Possible interactions of curcumin with drugs used concurrently should be taken into account. Curcumin administration with nonsteroidal anti-inflammatory or anticoagulant drugs may increase the risk of bleeding [1]. Curcumin and its derivatives have been shown to inhibit the activity of several drug-metabolizing enzymes such as cytochrome P450 (CYP3A4), glutathione-*S*-transferase, and UDP-glucuronosyltransferase, which may lead to an undesired increase in plasma concentrations of drugs metabolized by these enzymes [18]. Moreover, curcumin has been shown to inhibit function of gut P-glycoprotein, which may lead to increased bioavailability of other drugs [19].

Menopause and Curcumin

Due to numerous curcumin's targets and reports on possible health benefits, its use as a dietary supplement in menopause may be taken into consideration. So far there are no data on its effects concerning specific symptoms of estrogen deficiency. However, among pathologies potentially targeted by curcumin, osteoporosis has been enumerated [5, 10, 14, 20–22].

The issue whether and how curcumin may interfere with estrogenic pathways should be discussed in the context of menopause. It has been recently proposed that curcumin may act as a phytoestrogen, since it exerted estrogen-like transcriptional activity in the MCF7 breast cancer cell line [23]. Phytoestrogens are plant derived substances with estrogenic activity; they bind to estrogen receptors with an affinity much lower than estradiol. Phytoestrogens can both compete with estradiol, decreasing its effects, and activate the estrogen receptors; moreover, they may reduce local estradiol production by inhibiting activity of enzymes involved in its synthesis [23]. In our study, we observed that

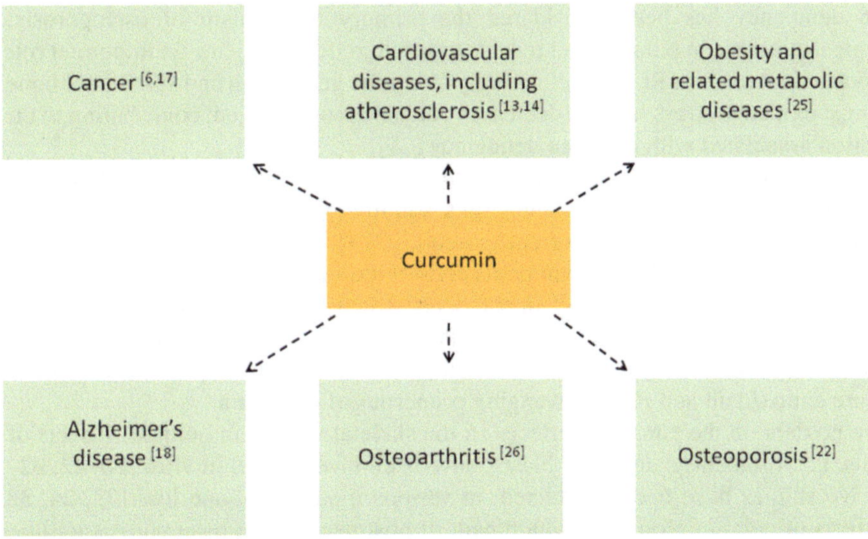

Fig. 13.3 Potential uses of curcumin in the prevention and treatment of diseases related to ageing (based on experimental research only, not confirmed in clinical trials)

administration of curcumin decreased serum estradiol levels in normal female rats [24]. To our knowledge, there are no data available on the effect of curcumin on the estrogen level in women.

Physiological menopause is inseparably related to ageing. It seems that the lifespan is regulated by genes controlling the activity of metabolism, antioxidant systems, DNA repair, cellular senescence and cell death [11]. Since it is thought that lesions accumulating with age are caused by increasing level of ROS and the low grade inflammatory process contribute to ageing, it is believed that ageing can be slowed down by some nutraceuticals. Curcumin, as an agent blocking the NF-κB-dependent inflammation, has been proposed to be potentially capable to slow ageing and consequently postpone the onset of age-related diseases [11]. However, it must be stated that the considerations on the curcumin role in ageing are purely theoretical. On the other hand, curcumin has been observed in experimental settings to have favorable effects in some age-related diseases [6, 13, 14, 17, 18, 22, 25, 26] (Fig. 13.3).

Many of the curcumin targets mentioned earlier take part in the regulation of bone remodeling, and curcumin may affect the skeletal system. The incidence of fractures related to osteoporosis is significantly lower in Southern and Eastern Asian women than in Western women. This fact may be attributed to Asian diets, which are typically rich in soy based foods, since soy isoflavones may have protective effects on the skeleton [27]. However, it is possible that other dietary constituents, like turmeric, may also be of value.

Osteoporosis and Potential Targets of Curcumin in the Skeletal System

Osteoporosis is the most common metabolic disorder of old age in humans [28]. Throughout the life, the skeletal system undergoes continuous regeneration—remodeling. During the process of remodeling, small quantities of old bone are removed by osteoclasts (bone resorbing cells) and replaced with new bone, due to activity of osteoblasts (cells responsible for bone formation). With ageing, the balance between the amounts of bone resorbed and bone formed during the process of remodeling becomes negative. The decreased bone mass is accompanied by disproportionally decreased bone strength; together they lead to development of osteoporosis [28].

Estrogen deficiency has been considered the primary mechanism of osteoporosis, however, epidemiological evidence in humans and recent studies in rodents indicate an important role of ageing and the associated increase in ROS. ROS strongly affect the generation and survival of bone cells. The defense against oxidative stress in bone decreases due to loss of estrogen, contributing to the increased bone resorption associated with estrogen deficiency [29].

In the treatment of osteoporosis, drugs slowing down bone resorption (bisphosphonates, raloxifene, denosumab, strontium ranelate) and drugs stimulating bone formation (parathormone, teriparatide, also strontium ranelate) are currently used [30, 31].

The most probable targets of curcumin in the cells of the skeletal system are downstream pathways of RANKL, including NF-κB signaling, in osteoclast precursors and osteoclasts, and Wnt signaling pathway in osteoblastic cells. Effects of curcumin on those pathways in other cell types have been relatively well recognized. Another, to some extent overlapping field of possible curcumin effects on bone cells, are antioxidant and ROS scavenging properties of curcumin.

There are no data on the curcumin effects on the skeletal system in humans. Effects of curcumin on bone cells, i.e., osteoclasts and osteoblasts, have been investigated in vitro [20–22, 32–37]. Also, several in vivo studies have been conducted, in various models of bone loss [22, 24, 38–41]. The potential effects of curcumin on the development of postmenopausal osteoporosis will be discussed based on the available preclinical research.

Effects of Curcumin on Osteoclasts and Bone Resorption In Vitro

The majority of in vitro studies on the skeletal curcumin effects concerns osteoclastogenesis. Osteoclasts are multinucleated cells that are formed by the fusion of monocyte-macrophage precursor cells. In regulation of osteoclast differentiation three principal cytokines expressed by osteoblasts and bone marrow stromal cells: macrophage colony-stimulating factor (M-CSF), RANKL, and osteoprotegerin (OPG) take part. M-CSF promotes the differentiation of hematopoietic stem cells into macrophages and osteoclasts, and RANKL is a key cytokine that stimulates osteoclastogenesis and bone resorption. OPG, as a decoy receptor for RANKL, inhibits the pathways activated by RANKL. Moreover, other cytokines, like TNF-α and IL-1, take part in osteoclast differentiation or activation of inflammatory osteolysis [35].

The interaction of RANKL and its receptor RANK activates several signaling pathways, including NF-κB, mitogen-activated protein kinases (MAPKs): ERK, p38 MAPK, and JNK, protein kinase C, phosphoinositide 3-kinase, and Ca^{2+}/calcineurin/NFAT [35, 42]. The activation of NF-κB by RANKL in osteoclast precursors occurs in two pathways: classical and alternative. In non-stimulated cells, NF-κB dimers are located in the cytoplasm due to their interaction with inhibitory proteins IκBs, and stimulation activates IκB kinases (IKKs). In the classical pathway, phosphorylation of IκBα by a complex of IKKα, β and γ leads to its proteasomal degradation, allowing NF-κB (primarily p50/p65 dimers) to translocate to the nucleus, where it affects transcription, leading to osteoclast survival. In the alternative pathway, activation of IKKα in consequence leads to nuclear translocation of NF-κB (primarily RelB/p52 dimers) and transcription of genes involved in osteoclast differentiation [43]. It has been also demonstrated that RANKL mediates generation of ROS which act as a second messenger that regulates several signaling cascades including JNK, p38 MAPK, and ERK pathways [35, 44].

Curcumin has been reported to dose-dependently inhibit parathormone-stimulated formation of osteoclast-like cells in mouse bone marrow cell cultures (even at 10^{-8} M) [33] and IL-1α-stimulated osteoclast formation in cocultures of mouse bone marrow stromal cells and whole bone marrow cells (at 2×10^{-6} and 4×10^{-6} M) [21]. Curcumin (5×10^{-6} and 10^{-5} M) suppressed RANKL-induced formation of osteoclasts in murine bone marrow-derived macrophages and monocytic cell line RAW 264.7.

In RAW 264.7 cells, curcumin prevented RANKL-stimulated osteoclastogenesis by inhibiting RANKL-induced IκB kinase activity, which led to the suppression of NF-κB activation [20]. An inhibitory effect of curcumin (10^{-6} and 10^{-5} M) on human osteoclast differentiation and function was also demonstrated. Inhibition of osteoclastogenesis in human preosteoclast cultures was accompanied with the inhibition of IκB phosphorylation and NF-κB activation [34]. Recent works indicate that suppressive effect of curcumin on osteoclastogenesis may have more complex mechanism. In RAW-D murine osteoclast precursor cells, curcumin (2.5×10^{-6}–10^{-5} M) inhibited RANKL-induced osteoclastogenesis, inducing heme oxygenase-1 and leading to suppression of release of high mobility group box 1, a chromatin protein, recently identified as one of osteoclast differentiation cytokines. Moreover, curcumin at 10^{-5} M enhanced RANKL-induced decrease in proliferation of RAW-D cells [35]. Curcumin also inhibited osteoclastogenesis by affecting other targets connected with oxidative stress defense [22]. Curcumin (4×10^{-6} M), in the culture of mouse bone marrow-derived macrophages, increased RANKL-induced Gpx-1 (an antioxidant enzyme responsible for intracellular degradation of ROS during osteoclastogenesis; its induction by RANKL could be a part of antioxidant defense mechanism induced in response to ROS) expression and activity, and decreased the stimulatory effect of homocysteine, which generates ROS, on osteoclastogenesis by increasing Gpx activity. Moreover, defective RANKL signaling generated by curcumin was also characterized by decreased expression of NFATc1 and reduced activation of MAPKs (ERK, JNK, and p38), contributing to decreased osteoclast formation [22]. In addition to the inhibitory effect on osteoclastogenesis in murine and human cell cultures, curcumin has been reported to stimulate apoptosis of rabbit osteoclasts (dose- and treatment time-dependently) [32].

The inhibitory effects of curcumin on osteoclastogenesis may be also indirect, since curcumin (4×10^{-6} M) has been reported to decrease expression of RANKL induced by IL-1α in mouse bone marrow stromal cells. It was proposed that reduction of RANKL expression could be explained by the activity of curcumin as a ROS scavenger [21]. Curcumin (5×10^{-6}–10^{-5} M) also decreased expression of RANKL mRNA in mouse osteoblasts infected with *Porphyromonas gingivalis* [45]. The effects of curcumin on RANKL-induced osteoclastogenesis are depicted in Fig. 13.4.

The data described above demonstrated that curcumin decreased number of osteoclasts, which should lead to inhibition of bone resorption. However, the reports on the effects of curcumin on bone resorption are equivocal. Although curcumin has been reported to inhibit *Porphyromonas gingivalis* fimbria-stimulated bone resorption by mouse embryonic calvarial cells [46] and resorption by mouse, rabbit, and human osteoclasts [20, 32, 34] in pit formation assays, it did not inhibit the stimulatory effect of parathormone on bone resorption in rat femoral tissue cultures in vitro. Addition of curcumin alone to culture media also did not affect the femoral calcium content in tissue cultures in vitro [33].

Effects of Curcumin on Osteoblasts and Bone Formation In Vitro

Osteoblasts are bone forming cells derived from mesenchymal stem cells [30]. Canonical Wnt/β-catenin signaling in osteoblastic cells is one of the most important mechanisms controlling bone formation and bone mass. In the absence of Wnt receptor activation, β-catenin is phosphorylated by a complex containing, among others, GSK-3β. The phosphorylation leads to ubiquitination and proteasomal degradation of β-catenin and keeping it at low cytoplasmic levels. In contrast, the degradation is inhibited in the presence of Wnt ligands, and β-catenin accumulates in the cytoplasm and nucleus where it induces transcription [47]. Activation of the canonical Wnt/β-catenin pathway promotes osteoblastic cell proliferation, differentiation and survival, and reduces adipogenic differentiation in mesenchymal stem cells [31].

Moreover, very recently, it has been recognized that NF-κB plays an important role in regulation of differentiation and activity not only of osteoclasts, but also of osteoblasts. It has been demonstrated

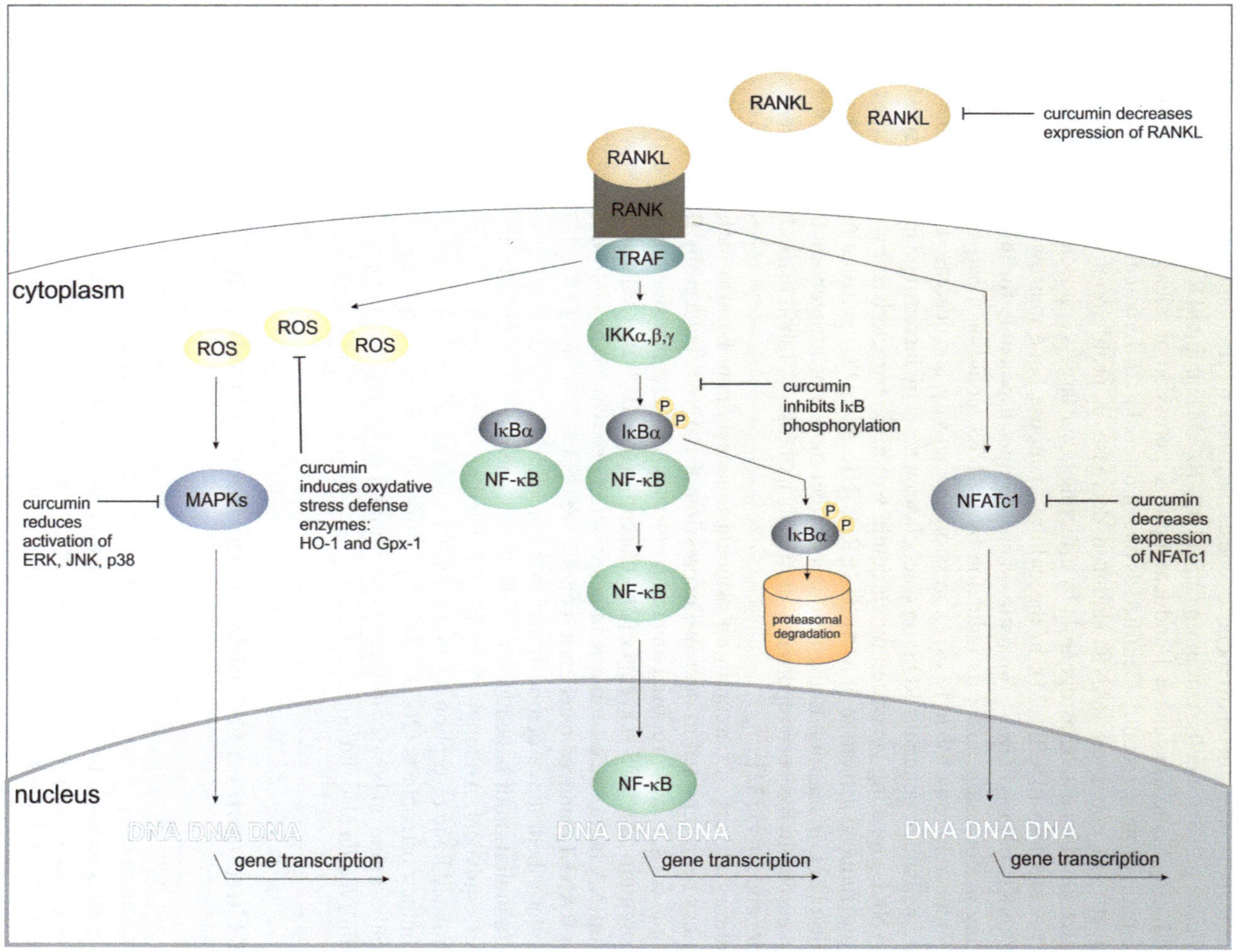

Fig. 13.4 Effects of curcumin on RANKL signaling in osteoclast precursors. RANKL (RANK ligand) is a key cytokine stimulating osteoclastogenesis and bone resorption [30, 42, 43]. Curcumin inhibits RANKL signaling in osteoclast precursor cells by several mechanisms, in consequence leading to decreased osteoclastogenesis [20–22, 34, 35, 45]. IκB —inhibitor of κB, IKK—IκB kinase, MAPKs—mitogen-activated protein kinases, NFAT—nuclear factor of activated T cells, NF-κB—nuclear factor-κB, ROS—reactive oxygen species

that a reduction in NF-κB activity in murine osteoblasts leads to an increase in bone formation via enhanced JNK activity, moreover, estrogen targeting (inhibiting) among others NF-κB signaling may increase osteoblast function [48]. Osteoblast maturation is affected by NF-κB acting in its classical pathway [43]. It has been proposed that targeting NF-κB could provide a novel treatment strategy for osteoporosis and other inflammatory bone diseases, which would not only inhibit bone resorption, but also increase bone formation [48]. Theoretically, curcumin as a potent inhibitor of NF-κB activation can be considered a candidate for such a treatment.

However, curcumin (5×10^{-6} and 10^{-5} M) significantly inhibited the proliferation of rat calvarial osteoblastic cells. Curcumin also affected osteoblast activity, reducing the rate of deposition of calcium and the formation of mineralized nodules. At 10^{-5} M, it did not induce osteoblastic cell apoptosis, but it arrested them in G_1 phase of cell cycle [36]. On the other hand, in human osteoblast cell line (HFOb 1.19), curcumin treatment induced two distinct types of cell death: apoptosis at concentrations of $1.25–2.5 \times 10^{-5}$ M and necrosis at concentrations greater than 5×10^{-5} M [37]. In human osteogenic sarcoma cell line (HOS), curcumin induced successive G_1/S and G_2/M phase arrest, and activated caspase-3 pathway leading to their apoptosis [49] (osteosarcoma is a sarcoma originating in bone-forming cells).

It seems possible that the curcumin effects on osteoblast proliferation and activity observed in vitro may be explained by inhibition of Wnt/β-catenin signaling in those cells. Excessive Wnt signaling has been implicated in cancer development [31], and curcumin anticancer properties have been attributed, among others, to blocking of Wnt/β-catenin signaling [50]. In human osteosarcoma U2OS cells, curcumin inhibited Wnt/β-catenin signaling and inhibited Wnt/β-catenin-induced cell invasiveness and MMP-9 expression. It was reported to disrupt the nuclear translocation of β-catenin in human osteosarcoma cells [51]. However, curcumin induced suppression of adipogenic differentiation of 3T3-L1 preadipocytes, which was accompanied by activation of Wnt/β-catenin signaling (among others by inhibited expression of GSK-3β and increased expression of Wnt10b mRNA) [52]; this process should lead to activation of osteoblastogenesis. Moreover, consistently, curcumin has been reported to inhibit expression of GSK-3β, thus activate Wnt/β-catenin signaling, in APPswe transfected SHSY5Y (human neuroblastoma) cells [53]. In fact, some results of in vivo studies indicate increased bone formation induced by curcumin [24, 38], although it is possible that those effects were due to inhibition of NF-κB signaling in osteoblasts. Potential effects of curcumin on canonical Wnt signaling in osteoblastic cells, based on the results of studies performed on other cell types, are demonstrated in Fig. 13.5.

It has been suggested that the treatment protocol (treatment period as well as the dosage) may determine the effects of curcumin on different cell types [37]. It must be strongly pointed out that majority of the in vitro curcumin effects was observed after using it at concentrations that are dietary not achievable in humans. Nevertheless, the results of the in vitro studies seem to indicate that curcumin may be a dietary factor which decreases bone turnover, decreasing number and activity of both osteoclasts and osteoblasts. However, the effects of curcumin administration to experimental animals do not fully confirm this conclusion.

Effects of Curcumin on the Skeletal System of Experimental Animals In Vivo

Effects of curcumin on the skeletal system of normal animals were investigated only in two studies [22, 24]. In our study [24], in non-ovariectomized female rats, curcumin (10 mg/kg *po* for 4 weeks) affected only the cancellous bone. The increased width of femoral trabeculae could result from inhibition of bone resorption, which agrees with the effects of curcumin on osteoclastogenesis in vitro [20, 33, 34]. Inconsistently with reports on the effect of curcumin on the proliferation and apoptosis of osteoblasts in vitro [36, 37], curcumin seemed to increase cancellous bone formation in vivo. However, although curcumin increased the mass of the vertebra, the mineralization of the vertebra was impaired,

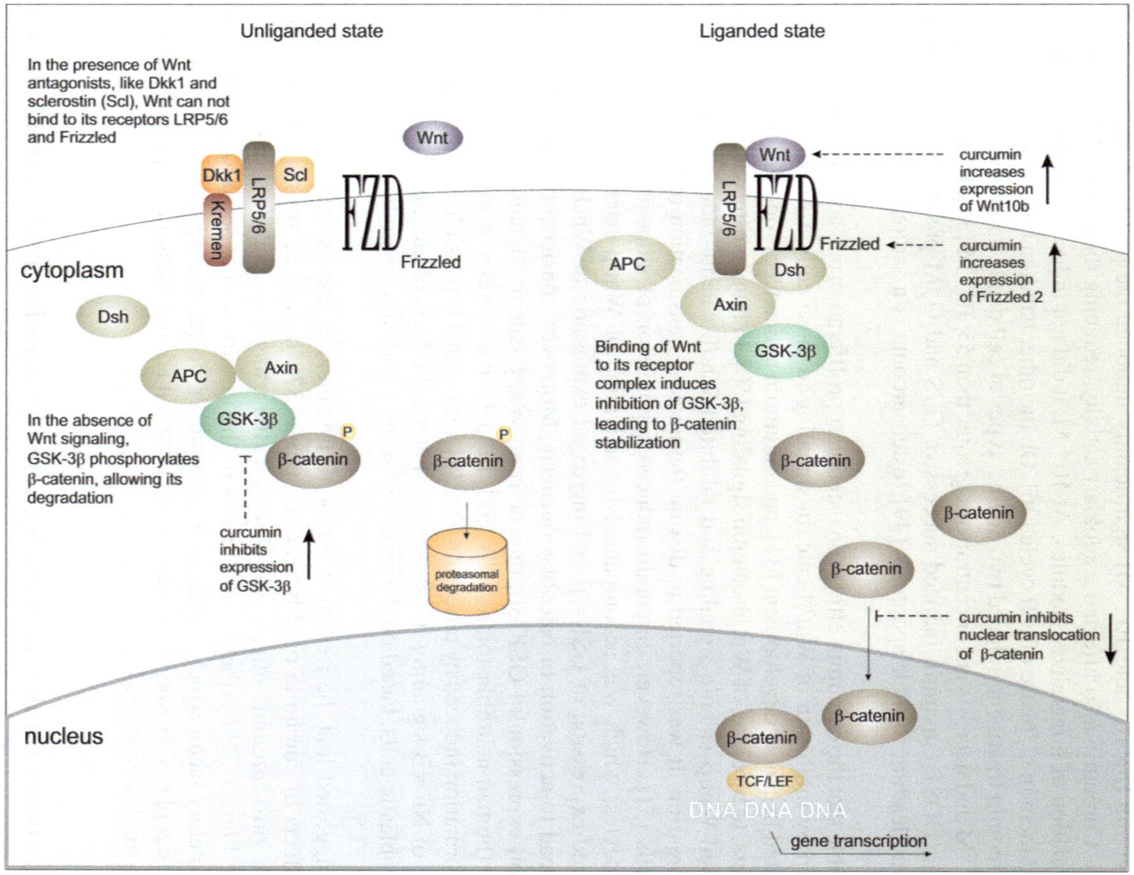

Fig. 13.5 Possible effects of curcumin on canonical Wnt signaling in osteoblastic cells based on the results from other cell types. Activation of Wnt/β-catenin pathway in osteoblastic cells leads to increased bone formation [30, 47]. There are no data on effects of curcumin on this pathway in osteoblasts. Potential curcumin effects on Wnt pathway were demonstrated in other cell types (osteosarcoma, preadipocytes) [51, 52]. *Arrows* ↑ and ↓, accompanying description of curcumin action, indicate potential increase or decrease in bone formation, respectively. GSK-3β—glycogen synthase kinase-3β

indicating decreased bone quality. Contrary to those results, curcumin did not unfavorably affect the skeletal system of non-ovariectomized (sham-operated) mice. In those mice, curcumin administered in a similar dose, but for a longer period (9.5 mg/kg *po* for 8 weeks), increased trabecular bone volume and did not significantly affect other investigated parameters [22].

Bilaterally ovariectomized animals are the commonly used experimental models of postmenopausal osteoporosis. Bilaterally ovariectomized rats present accelerated bone loss similar to that observed in postmenopausal women due to estrogen deficiency. Bone remodeling rate is increased, both bone resorption and formation, with an imbalance between them that favors the former [29]. So far, four reports on the curcumin effects on the development of estrogen deficiency-induced osteoporosis have been reported [22, 24, 38, 39].

French et al. [38], in a long-term experiment conducted on ageing ovariectomized rats (9–10-month-old at the beginning of experiment), found no significant differences in the markers of bone turnover, mineral density or mechanical properties between the rats receiving curcumin (1.5, 3, and 15 mg/day) for 6 months in the diet and the ovariectomized controls. The only significant change in the skeletal system was an increase in the size of the femur after a 6 month period of the highest curcumin dose administration. However, a significant positive correlation between curcumin dose and the energy to fracture of the femur was demonstrated, indicating some slight potential to favorably affect bone in estrogen-deficient animals [38].

In our study [24] on 3-month old ovariectomized rats, curcumin (10 mg/kg *po* for 4 weeks) did not counteract the effects of estrogen deficiency, manifested as decreased ratios of bone mass and bone mineral mass to the body mass and worsened bone mineralization (decreased ratio of bone mineral mass to bone mass). A slight, probably antiresorptive, effect was observed in the cancellous bone of the femur (increase in the width of trabeculae), but the effect was not confirmed by improvement in the mechanical properties of the femoral neck. In estrogen-deficient rats, curcumin also seemed to counteract the increased cortical bone formation indices, consistently with the reports from in vitro studies on osteoblasts suggesting the possibility of inhibition of bone formation [36]. Taken together, we have concluded that the favorable effects of curcumin on the bones of estrogen-deficient rats were negligible [24].

It should be noted, however, that intraperitoneal administration of curcuminoid mixture at high doses for 56 days (60 mg/kg three times a week) to 3-month-old ovariectomized rats counteracted trabecular bone loss [39].

Contrary to the results of studies on rats [24, 38], Kim et al. [22] have recently reported that curcumin (9.5 mg/kg *po* for 8 weeks) counteracted bone loss induced by estrogen deficiency in ovariectomized mice. Curcumin administration significantly increased femoral bone mineral density, trabecular number and bone volume, as well as reduced trabecular separation and the level of serum bone resorption marker: collagen-type I fragments. Based on those results and in vitro research, it was concluded that curcumin inhibited ovariectomy-induced bone loss through reducing osteoclastogenesis due to increased antioxidant activity and impaired RANKL signaling [22].

Two studies have been performed on other models of metabolic bone diseases [40, 41]. Hie et al. [40] studied the effects of curcumin (0.5 % in the standard laboratory diet, i.e., approximately 120 mg/day for 10 days) on bone biochemical markers in 10-week-old female rats with insulin-dependent diabetes mellitus induced by streptozotocin. Curcumin counteracted the streptozotocin effects manifested in increased osteoclastogenesis and bone resorption indices, and did not affect the decreased bone formation indices. Dietary supplementation of curcumin induced the inhibition of osteoclastogenesis in bone marrow cell culture from the diabetic rats. This effect was associated with inhibition of the expression of components of AP-1: c-Fos and c-Jun, which were increased in diabetic rats [40].

Yang et al. [41] investigated the effects of dietary supplementation with curcumin (0.06 %) in APP/PS1 transgenic mice, between 9 and 12 months of age. Those mice serve as an animal model of Alzheimer's disease. APP/PS1 transgenic mice had decreased bone mineral density and worsened microstructural parameters of cancellous bone in comparison with wild-type mice. Curcumin treatment led to improvement in the trabecular microstructural parameters and bone mineral density. It also decreased serum levels of TNF-α and IL-6, which were elevated in APP/PS1 transgenic mice [41].

Summing up, the results from the in vivo experiments on effects on the skeletal system not always were consistent with the results from in vitro assays. One possible explanation for those discrepancies is that by targeting numerous molecules, curcumin leads to specific effects in specific bone cells in vitro, but different effects may occur in vivo. It is possible that differential curcumin targets may be aimed depending on the animal model, age, hormone status, duration of treatment. For example, in our experiment [24] on non-ovariectomized rats, the increased cancellous bone formation and/or decreased bone resorption might have resulted from the inhibition of NF-κB, whereas the inhibition of the increased periosteal bone formation in ovariectomized rats might have been the effect of inhibition of Wnt signaling. Oppositely, after the long term treatment of much older ovariectomized rats with the highest curcumin dose, the increase in bone formation was observed [38]. Curcumin exerted much stronger positive effects in mice than in rats. In the studies on rats in which significant effects of curcumin were demonstrated [39, 40], curcumin was administered at very high doses. It is possible that there are species differences concerning the sensitivity to curcumin or its bioavailability.

Moreover, there is a problem of the identity of "curcumin" used in different studies. Commercial curcumin usually comprises also other curcuminoids [1]. It is unclear whether the analogs exhibit equal activity; in most studies curcumin was the most potent, but in some systems bisdemethoxycurcumin exhibited higher activity, and there were also suggestions that the mixture of curcumin, demethoxycurcumin, and bisdemethoxycurcumin is more potent than either one alone [5]. Most of authors have not mentioned the purity of the preparations they used.

Considerations for the Hypothetical Curcumin Use in the Prevention of Osteoporosis in Humans

The question arises whether in doses which are readily achievable by dietary intake curcumin can exert its effects observed in experimental settings. The local levels of curcumin possible to be achieved in bone would be much lower than the concentrations reported to be effective in the in vitro studies. In most of those studies on bone cell number and activity, the effects were observed with curcumin concentrations of at least micromolar range [20, 22, 32, 34–37, 45, 46]. In humans, very high curcumin doses, 4–8 g, are necessary to achieve average peak serum concentrations of $0.51 \pm 0.11 - 1.77 \pm 1.87 \times 10^{-6}$ M, respectively [54]. Nevertheless, some studies have suggested that even low concentrations of curcumin (physiologically achievable) may be sufficient to exert therapeutic activity [6].

As it was already mentioned, curcumin has been consumed as a dietary spice at doses of up to 100 mg/day [10], i.e., approximately 1.5 mg/kg/day, assuming that human body mass is 65–70 kg. Phase I clinical trials indicated that humans can tolerate curcumin even at a dose of 8 g/day [54]. Studies on better available pharmaceutical formulations of curcumin have been undertaken [4, 55]. However, the vital molecular targets of curcumin indicate that, achieving appropriate concentrations, it may seriously affect different body functions.

A summary of curcumin effects on the skeletal system is presented in Table 13.1. In in vitro studies curcumin inhibited osteoclastogenesis, but also decreased osteoblastic cell proliferation and activity. It should be emphasized that curcumin exerted those effects in the similar concentration range. In in vivo studies, curcumin counteracted the development of estrogen deficiency-induced osteoporosis in mice, whereas its effects in rats after oral administration were rather negligible. Stronger curcumin effects were observed in other models of metabolic bone disorders [40, 41], however the doses used there were much higher than those used in estrogen-deficient animals [22, 24, 38]. Their results may not be relevant to the situation of postmenopausal women.

Table 13.1 Summary of curcumin effects on the skeletal system

Type of research		Target (cells/animal model/species)		Effect	References
Experimental	In vitro	Osteoclasts/bone resorption	Mouse, human	Decreased osteoclastogenesis	[20–22, 33–35]
			Rabbit	Increased apoptosis	[32]
			Rabbit, mouse, human	Decreased bone resorption	[20, 32, 34, 46]
			Rat	No effect on bone resorption	[33]
		Osteoblasts/bone formation	Rat	Decreased proliferation and reduced calcium deposition. No pro-apoptotic effect	[36]
			Human	Induction of apoptosis/necrosis dependent on concentration	[37]
	In vivo	Healthy animals	Rats	Increased cancellous bone formation, but decreased mineralization	[24]
			Mice (sham-operated)	Increased trabecular bone volume	[22]
		Estrogen deficiency-induced osteoporosis	Rats (ageing)	Very slight/lack of effect	[38]
			Rats (young mature)	Very slight/lack of effect	[24]
			Rats (young mature)	Protection from bone loss	[39]
			Mice	Protection from bone loss	[22]
		Other models of osteoporosis	Rats with streptozotocin-induced diabetes	Decreased bone resorption indices	[40]
			APP/PS1 transgenic mice	Improvement of bone status	[41]
Human	Clinical			Not reported	–
	Population-based			Not reported	–

Possible curcumin use in the prevention of osteoporosis, as a long-term treatment, would only be of value if it was effective at doses that are safe and easily acceptable for patients. According to López-Lázaro, although curcumin use at the maximum tolerated dose is a valid approach in cancer chemotherapy, it may not be appropriate for cancer prevention because it may produce toxicity in the long term, and doses equivalent to those found in diets rich in turmeric should be used in future cancer chemoprevention clinical trials [17]. Similar careful approach is necessary for its potential use in other diseases.

Curcumin is readily available not only as a dietary spice, but also a dietary supplement [56]. It should be emphasized that uncontrolled use of such supplements, enabling intake of high doses, may potentially lead to unwanted effects. In fact, the benefit–risk ratio of curcumin needs to be established [57].

There is a possibility that turmeric, which is routinely used in diet, may exert other effects on the skeletal system than curcumin alone. Turmeric contains curcuminoids, and a number of other identified compounds, which effects have not been studied extensively. Balaji and Chempakam [58] performed a cheminformatics study of 200 compounds from turmeric to predict the toxicity (bacterial mutagenicity, rodent carcinogenicity, and human hepatotoxicity) from their chemical structure, and found that majority of them was potentially toxic. Moreover, other constituents of turmeric may affect curcumin absorption and metabolism. For example, differences in the curcumin distribution and activity concerning expression of pro-inflammatory genes after dietary supplementation with curcumin (0.07 % in the diet) and turmeric (1.4 % in the diet) were observed in rats [59]. Of two turmeric extracts examined, only the purified one (94 % curcuminoids) prevented bone loss after intraperitoneal administration at the same curcuminoid dose to ovariectomized rats [39]. This issue needs to be investigated further.

Taken together, further studies are necessary to establish the effects of curcumin on the skeletal system in humans; in fact currently available data indicate that they may be both favorable and deleterious. Despite the theoretical background, the preclinical studies performed so far are preliminary and do not sufficiently support the hypothesis that curcumin may counteract the development of postmenopausal osteoporosis.

Conclusions

Numerous original papers, mostly based on experimental data, and review articles on the beneficial effects of curcumin in many disorders have been published in the last years. Curcumin affects multiple targets, which may be of value in different diseases. Curcumin is poorly available after oral administration, but even low concentrations of curcumin may exert some activity. Not only efficacy of curcumin but also safety has been claimed. However, future research is necessary in order to establish the benefit–risk ratio of curcumin. Ambiguous results of the experimental studies and a complete lack of reports from human studies do not support the hypothesis that curcumin could be useful for the prophylaxis or treatment of postmenopausal osteoporosis.

References

1. Strimpakos AS, Sharma RA. Curcumin: preventive and therapeutic properties in laboratory studies and clinical trials. Antioxid Redox Signal. 2008;10:511–45.
2. Epstein J, Sanderson IR, MacDonald TT. Curcumin as a therapeutic agent: the evidence from in vitro, animal and human studies. Br J Nutr. 2010;103:1545–57.
3. Pabst G, ed. Köhler's Medizinal-Pflanzen in naturgetreuen Abbildungen mit kurz erläuterndem Texte. Vol. 1. Gera: Friedrich von Zezschwitz, ca 1885.
4. Basnet P, Skalko-Basnet N. Curcumin: an anti-inflammatory molecule from a curry spice on the path to cancer treatment. Molecules. 2011;16:4567–98.
5. Aggarwal BB, Sundaram C, Malani N, Ichikawa H. Curcumin: the Indian solid gold. Adv Exp Med Biol. 2007;595:1–75.
6. Bar-Sela G, Epelbaum R, Schaffer M. Curcumin as an anti-cancer agent: review of the gap between basic and clinical applications. Curr Med Chem. 2010;17:190–7.
7. EFSA Panel on Food Additives and Nutrient Sources added to Food (ANS). Scientific opinion on the re-evaluation of curcumin (E 100) as a food additive. EFSA J. 2010;8:1679 [46 pp.].
8. Schaffer M, Schaffer PM, Zidan J, Bar SG. Curcuma as a functional food in the control of cancer and inflammation. Curr Opin Clin Nutr Metab Care. 2011;14:588–97.
9. Tayyem RF, Heath DD, Al-Delaimy WK, Rock CL. Curcumin content of turmeric and curry powders. Nutr Cancer. 2006;55:126–31.
10. Shishodia S, Sethi G, Aggarwal BB. Curcumin: getting back to the roots. Ann N Y Acad Sci. 2005; 1056:206–17.

11. Sikora E, Bielak-Zmijewska A, Mosieniak G, Piwocka K. The promise of slow down ageing may come from curcumin. Curr Pharm Des. 2010;16:884–92.
12. Zhou H, Beevers CS, Huang S. The targets of curcumin. Curr Drug Targets. 2011;12:332–47.
13. Wongcharoen W, Phrommintikul A. The protective role of curcumin in cardiovascular diseases. Int J Cardiol. 2009;133:145–51.
14. Aggarwal BB, Harikumar KB. Potential therapeutic effects of curcumin, the anti-inflammatory agent, against neurodegenerative, cardiovascular, pulmonary, metabolic, autoimmune and neoplastic diseases. Int J Biochem Cell Biol. 2009;41:40–59.
15. Hatcher H, Planalp R, Cho J, Torti FM, Torti SV. Curcumin: from ancient medicine to current clinical trials. Cell Mol Life Sci. 2008;65:1631–52.
16. Marathe SA, Dasgupta I, Gnanadhas DP, Chakravortty D. Multifaceted roles of curcumin: two sides of a coin! Expert Opin Biol Ther. 2011;11:1485–99.
17. López-Lázaro M. Anticancer and carcinogenic properties of curcumin: considerations for its clinical development as a cancer chemopreventive and chemotherapeutic agent. Mol Nutr Food Res. 2008;52 Suppl 1:S103–27.
18. Mancuso C, Siciliano R, Barone E, Preziosi P. Natural substances and Alzheimer's disease: from preclinical studies to evidence based medicine. Biochim Biophys Acta. 2012;1822:616–24.
19. Zhang W, Han Y, Lim SL, Lim LY. Dietary regulation of P-gp function and expression. Expert Opin Drug Metab Toxicol. 2009;5:789–801.
20. Bharti AC, Takada Y, Aggarwal BB. Curcumin (diferuloylmethane) inhibits receptor activator of NF-κB ligand-induced NF-κB activation in osteoclast precursors and suppresses osteoclastogenesis. J Immunol. 2004;172: 5940–7.
21. Oh S, Kyung TW, Choi HS. Curcumin inhibits osteoclastogenesis by decreasing receptor activator of nuclear factor-κB ligand (RANKL) in bone marrow stromal cells. Mol Cells. 2008;26:486–9.
22. Kim WK, Ke K, Sul OJ, Kim HJ, Kim SH, Lee MH, et al. Curcumin protects against ovariectomy-induced bone loss and decreases osteoclastogenesis. J Cell Biochem. 2011;112:3159–66.
23. Bachmeier BE, Mirisola V, Romeo F, Generoso L, Esposito A, Dell'eva R, et al. Reference profile correlation reveals estrogen-like transcriptional activity of curcumin. Cell Physiol Biochem. 2010;26:471–82.
24. Folwarczna J, Zych M, Trzeciak HI. Effects of curcumin on the skeletal system in rats. Pharmacol Rep. 2010;62:900–9.
25. Aggarwal BB. Targeting inflammation-induced obesity and metabolic diseases by curcumin and other nutraceuticals. Annu Rev Nutr. 2010;30:173–99.
26. Henrotin Y, Clutterbuck AL, Allaway D, Lodwig EM, Harris P, Mathy-Hartert M, et al. Biological actions of curcumin on articular chondrocytes. Osteoarthritis Cartilage. 2010;18:141–9.
27. Ma DF, Qin LQ, Wang PY, Katoh R. Soy isoflavone intake inhibits bone resorption and stimulates bone formation in menopausal women: meta-analysis of randomized controlled trials. Eur J Clin Nutr. 2008;62:155–61.
28. Manolagas SC, Parfitt AM. What old means to bone. Trends Endocrinol Metab. 2010;21:369–74.
29. Manolagas SC. From estrogen-centric to aging and oxidative stress: a revised perspective of the pathogenesis of osteoporosis. Endocr Rev. 2010;31:266–300.
30. Rachner TD, Khosla S, Hofbauer LC. Osteoporosis: now and the future. Lancet. 2011;377:1276–87.
31. Marie PJ, Kassem M. Osteoblasts in osteoporosis: past, emerging, and future anabolic targets. Eur J Endocrinol. 2011;165:1–10.
32. Ozaki K, Kawata Y, Amano S, Hanazawa S. Stimulatory effect of curcumin on osteoclast apoptosis. Biochem Pharmacol. 2000;59:1577–81.
33. Yamaguchi M, Hamamoto R, Uchiyama S, Ishiyama K. Effects of flavonoid on calcium content in femoral tissue culture and parathyroid hormone-stimulated osteoclastogenesis in bone marrow culture in vitro. Mol Cell Biochem. 2007;303:83–8.
34. von Metzler I, Krebbel H, Kuckelkorn U, Heider U, Jakob C, Kaiser M, et al. Curcumin diminishes human osteoclastogenesis by inhibition of the signalosome-associated IκB kinase. J Cancer Res Clin Oncol. 2009;135:173–9.
35. Sakai E, Shimada-Sugawara M, Nishishita K, Fukuma Y, Naito M, Okamoto K, et al. Suppression of RANKL-dependent heme oxygenase-1 is required for high mobility group box 1 release and osteoclastogenesis. J Cell Biochem. 2012;113:486–98.
36. Notoya M, Nishimura H, Woo JT, Nagai K, Ishihara Y, Hagiwara H. Curcumin inhibits the proliferation and mineralization of cultured osteoblasts. Eur J Pharmacol. 2006;534:55–62.
37. Chan WH, Wu HY, Chang WH. Dosage effects of curcumin on cell death types in a human osteoblast cell line. Food Chem Toxicol. 2006;44:1362–71.
38. French DL, Muir JM, Webber CE. The ovariectomized, mature rat model of postmenopausal osteoporosis: an assessment of the bone sparing effects of curcumin. Phytomedicine. 2008;15:1069–78.
39. Wright LE, Frye JB, Timmermann BN, Funk JL. Protection of trabecular bone in ovariectomized rats by turmeric (*Curcuma longa* L.) is dependent on extract composition. J Agric Food Chem. 2010;58:9498–504.
40. Hie M, Yamazaki M, Tsukamoto I. Curcumin suppresses increased bone resorption by inhibiting osteoclastogenesis in rats with streptozotocin-induced diabetes. Eur J Pharmacol. 2009;621:1–9.

41. Yang MW, Wang TH, Yan PP, Chu LW, Yu J, Gao ZD, et al. Curcumin improves bone microarchitecture and enhances mineral density in APP/PS1 transgenic mice. Phytomedicine. 2011;18:205–13.
42. Raju R, Balakrishnan L, Nanjappa V, Bhattacharjee M, Getnet D, Muthusamy B, et al. A comprehensive manually curated reaction map of RANKL/RANK-signaling pathway. Database (Oxford). 2011:bar021 [9 pp.].
43. Novack DV. Role of NF-κB in the skeleton. Cell Res. 2011;21:169–82.
44. Lee NK, Choi YG, Baik JY, Han SY, Jeong DW, Bae YS, et al. A crucial role for reactive oxygen species in RANKL-induced osteoclast differentiation. Blood. 2005;106:852–9.
45. Okahashi N, Inaba H, Nakagawa I, Yamamura T, Kuboniwa M, Nakayama K, et al. *Porphyromonas gingivalis* induces receptor activator of NF-κB ligand expression in osteoblasts through the activator protein 1 pathway. Infect Immun. 2004;72:1706–14.
46. Naganuma K, Amano S, Takeda H, Kitano S, Hanazawa S. Role of transcriptional factor activation protein-1 in endogenous expression of the interleukin-1β gene involved in *Porphyromonas gingivalis* fimbria-stimulated bone resorption in the mouse calvarial system. Oral Microbiol Immunol. 2000;15:53–7.
47. Milat F, Ng KW. Is Wnt signalling the final common pathway leading to bone formation? Mol Cell Endocrinol. 2009;310:52–62.
48. Krum SA, Chang J, Miranda-Carboni G, Wang CY. Novel functions for NFκB: inhibition of bone formation. Nat Rev Rheumatol. 2010;6:607–11.
49. Lee DS, Lee MK, Kim JH. Curcumin induces cell cycle arrest and apoptosis in human osteosarcoma (HOS) cells. Anticancer Res. 2009;29:5039–44.
50. Sarkar FH, Li Y, Wang Z, Kong D. The role of nutraceuticals in the regulation of Wnt and Hedgehog signaling in cancer. Cancer Metastasis Rev. 2010;29:383–94.
51. Leow PC, Tian Q, Ong ZY, Yang Z, Ee PL. Antitumor activity of natural compounds, curcumin and PKF118-310, as Wnt/β-catenin antagonists against human osteosarcoma cells. Invest New Drugs. 2010;28:766–82.
52. Ahn J, Lee H, Kim S, Ha T. Curcumin-induced suppression of adipogenic differentiation is accompanied by activation of Wnt/β-catenin signaling. Am J Physiol Cell Physiol. 2010;298:C1510–6.
53. Zhang X, Yin WK, Shi XD, Li Y. Curcumin activates Wnt/β-catenin signaling pathway through inhibiting the activity of GSK-3β in APPswe transfected SY5Y cells. Eur J Pharm Sci. 2011;42:540–6.
54. Cheng AL, Hsu CH, Lin JK, Hsu MM, Ho YF, Shen TS, et al. Phase I clinical trial of curcumin, a chemopreventive agent, in patients with high-risk or pre-malignant lesions. Anticancer Res. 2001;21(4B):2895–900.
55. Anand P, Thomas SG, Kunnumakkara AB, Sundaram C, Harikumar KB, Sung B, et al. Biological activities of curcumin and its analogues (congeners) made by man and Mother Nature. Biochem Pharmacol. 2008;76:1590–611.
56. Goel A, Jhurani S, Aggarwal BB. Multi-targeted therapy by curcumin: how spicy is it? Mol Nutr Food Res. 2008;52:1010–30.
57. Burgos-Morón E, Calderón-Montaño JM, Salvador J, Robles A, López-Lázaro M. The dark side of curcumin. Int J Cancer. 2010;126:1771–5.
58. Balaji S, Chempakam B. Toxicity prediction of compounds from turmeric (*Curcuma longa* L). Food Chem Toxicol. 2010;48:2951–9.
59. Martin RC, Aiyer HS, Malik D, Li Y. Effect on pro-inflammatory and antioxidant genes and bioavailable distribution of whole turmeric vs curcumin: similar root but different effects. Food Chem Toxicol. 2012;50:227–31.

Chapter 14
Menopause and Sarcopenia: Dietary and Nutritional Aspects

Sébastien Barbat-Artigas and Mylène Aubertin-Leheudre

Key Points

- Nutrition plays a key role in maintaining skeletal muscle mass and preventing sarcopenia.
- Sufficient protein intake may be the cornerstone of a healthy nutrition, although standards need to be fixed in regard to the needs of an aging population.
- A dietary protein intake of 1.1–1.5 g/kg/day may be appropriate to prevent an excessive loss of skeletal muscle mass in postmenopausal women.
- Other nutrients, such as vitamin D and isoflavones appear promising, although more research is needed to demonstrate their effectiveness and determine the optimal dosage.
- 700–1,000 IU of vitamin D per day may be effective in improving muscle function and functional capacity in postmenopausal women.
- 50 mg/day of isoflavone, for a period of 6 months, may be sufficient to have significant endocrine effects.
- The primary objective of preventing sarcopenia being to limit the development of functional incapacities, an effective therapy should improve muscle function, not just mass.
- Data supporting improvements in muscle function following supplementation being limited, effective nutritional supplementation would require to be combined with other intervention aimed to improve muscle function such as physical activity.
- Resistance exercise combined with appropriately timed nutritional supplementation promotes gains in muscle mass and strength.

Keywords Menopause • Sarcopenia • Protein • Vitamin D • Phytoestrogen

Abbreviations

O-DMA	*O*-Desmethylangolensin
1,25(OH)2D	1,25-Dihydroxyvitamin D
AA	Amino acids
EAA	Essential amino acids

S. Barbat-Artigas, Ph.D. • M. Aubertin-Leheudre (✉)
Groupe de Recherche en Activité Physique Adaptée, Pavillon des Sciences Biologiques, Université du Québec à Montréal, 141 Avenue du Président Kennedy, Montréal, QC, Canada H2X 1Y4
e-mail: barbat.sebastien@gmail.com; aubertin-leheudre.mylene@uqam.ca

C.J.H. Martin et al. (eds.), *Nutrition and Diet in Menopause*, Nutrition and Health,
DOI 10.1007/978-1-62703-373-2_14, © Springer Science+Business Media New York 2013

ER	Estrogen receptor
IU	International unit
PPARs	Peroxisome proliferator-activated receptors
RDA	Recommended dietary allowance
VDR	Vitamin D receptor

Introduction

Menopause and Skeletal Muscle Mass

Menopause is widely associated with profound changes in body composition. Evidence suggests that women increase in body fatness with age, and that this change may be accelerated with the onset of menopause. Indeed, fat mass and lean mass appear to be stable in the premenopausal years, whereas a linear decline in lean mass is noted in postmenopausal women, along with an increase in fat mass. Moreover, the loss of lean mass (and by extrapolation skeletal muscle mass) is paralleled by changes in characteristics of muscle tissue. For instance, postmenopausal women have been reported to have twice the amount of non-contractile muscle tissue, such as intramuscular fat, compared to younger women [1]. Various mechanisms have been put forth to explain the change in total skeletal muscle mass. This is primarily due to an imbalance between muscle protein synthesis and muscle protein breakdown, and the increase of catabolic factors such as oxidative stress and inflammation, but other factors such as decline in hormonal levels, decreased resting metabolic rate, a loss of neuromuscular function, and apoptosis are thought to be implicated in this inevitable process. Controllable factors such as physical activity and diet are also involved. Although these factors are not specific to menopause, it appears that they are exacerbated by changes in this status. Nevertheless, the combination of these factors directly promotes the emergence of "sarcopenia" with advancing age in women.

The term sarcopenia is derived from the Greek words sarx (flesh) and penia (loss) and was created by Rosenberg in 1989 to refer to the age-related loss in skeletal muscle mass and size with normal aging [2]. Sarcopenia is determined by two factors: the initial amount of skeletal muscle mass and the rate at which it declines with age. Results from longitudinal studies indicate that muscle mass and size decrease by approximately 6 % per decade past the age of 50 years. Therefore, an 85-year-old woman will have a skeletal muscle mass that is three-quarters of what it was when she was 45 years old. Unfortunately, it appears that skeletal muscle mass loss is inevitable. However, it is important to note that there are considerable interindividual differences in both peak skeletal muscle mass and the rate at which it declines, depending on the lifestyle of the individual.

Rather than defining sarcopenia as a process that all aging individuals go through, it was proposed that an operational threshold be used to identify older persons who have low skeletal muscle mass values, qualifying them as sarcopenic [3]. Modeled on the definition of osteoporosis, type I sarcopenia was then defined as height-adjusted skeletal muscle mass of 1–2 standard deviations below the mean of a young adult reference population and type II sarcopenia as an index of 2 standard deviations or more below the same value. Since skeletal muscle mass is not routinely measured or measurable, other indices are then used. Total and appendicular lean mass are the main indices used. Although their definition is not strictly that of skeletal muscle, it is widely accepted that changes in lean mass are representative of changes in muscle mass (since bone mass only represents a small portion of lean body mass). Depending on the studies cited in this chapter, the two terms can be used. Type II sarcopenia is very common in older women with a prevalence from 5 to 13 % in the sixth decade and of 11–50 % in the eighth decade. Furthermore, it was reported that the prevalence of type I and type II sarcopenia was 50 % and 7 % respectively in women aged between 50 and 59 years old. This is a 15 % increment in the prevalence of type I sarcopenia compared to women aged 40–49 years [4], suggesting again a concordance between the increase in the prevalence of sarcopenia increases and significant changes in the hormonal status that occur in women at menopause.

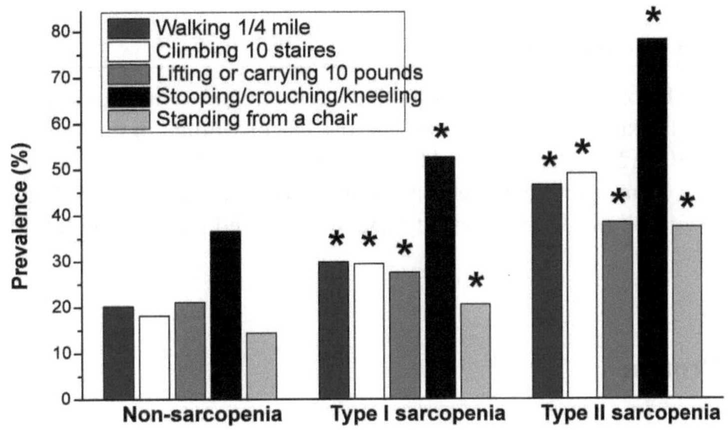

Fig. 14.1 Prevalence of functional impairment and physical disability in sarcopenic women aged 60 years and over. *Significantly greater than non-sarcopenia ($p<0.05$). Figure adapted from Janssen et al. [4]

Sarcopenia and Its Consequences

A primary rationale for studying the age-related loss in skeletal muscle mass is the belief that the loss of skeletal muscle mass is indicative of a loss of skeletal muscle strength and function. Thus, in the causal chain, sarcopenia was thought to cause a loss in muscle strength, which in turn would cause functional impairment and physical disability. Most research on the health implication of sarcopenia focused on physical function outcomes, such as the difficulty to perform activities of daily living (self-care tasks) and instrumental activities of daily living (tasks necessary for an individual to live independently in a community). The first evidence, based on cross-sectional studies, suggested that the association between sarcopenia and physical function were moderate to strong in magnitude (Fig. 14.1). However, findings from recent longitudinal studies showed that the effects of sarcopenia on functional impairment and physical disability were overestimated. While it has been postulated that sarcopenia contributes to metabolic and cardiovascular diseases, such as insulin resistance, type II diabetes, dyslipidemia, and hypertension, the literature is also mixed and, in general, does not support this assumption. For instance, it has been reported that sarcopenic postmenopausal women may have more favorable lipoprotein profiles than those without sarcopenia [5] and results of the Cardiovascular Health Study showed that sarcopenia was not a risk factor for the development of cardiovascular disease over an 8-year follow-up period [6]. However, there is evidence that accelerated loss of skeletal muscle mass might be a risk factor for early mortality in older persons. Indeed, it appears that individuals with sarcopenia are twice likely to contract infection during a hospital stay than older patients with a normal skeletal muscle mass [7], suggesting a decreased immunity in these individuals.

Two main strategies are used to prevent or counteract sarcopenia; exercise and nutritional interventions. To this point, numerous resistance training studies have successfully shown gains in skeletal muscle mass in postmenopausal women. Physical activity, particularly resistance training, currently represents the cornerstone of prevention and treatment of sarcopenia. A recent meta-analysis revealed that after an average of 20.5 weeks of resistance training, aging men and women experienced an average increase in lean mass of 1.1 kg. These findings bear clinical significance, given the exaggerated rate of skeletal muscle atrophy that occurs among sedentary individuals after the age of 50 years [8]. Alone or in combination with physical activity, the nutritional factor also appears to be crucial to efficiently treat sarcopenia. In this chapter, we try to summarize the state of knowledge concerning the association between diet and sarcopenia, as well as the debates in this field. We then address the issue of protein intake (total, creatinine, and essential amino acids (EAAs)), vitamin D, and isoflavone, three nutrients that appear to play key roles. We also present exercise and dietary recommendations for the elderly and touch upon different types of diets (vegetarian vs. omnivore).

Take-Home Message

Menopause is associated with changes in body composition, including decreased muscle mass, also known as sarcopenia. Up to 13 % of women in the sixth decade and 50 % of women aged 80 and over are affected by sarcopenia

Sarcopenia has been associated with various adverse health outcomes such as functional disabilities, early mortality and an increased risk to contract infections.

Protein

Dietary Protein Needs of Elderly People

Over the last 20 years, scientific evidence has provided new information on the role and impact of nutritional status on functional capacity and health of the aging population. Studies have pointed to protein as a key nutrient for the elderly. Proteins are essential parts of the organism and participate in virtually every intracellular process. The current adult Recommended Dietary Allowance (RDA) for protein is 0.8 g/kg//day [9]. Most individuals do not consider the RDA for protein when preparing meals or selecting foods to eat. In fact, most adults do not know what the RDA is, or how to calculate their daily protein intake even if they were trying to meet the RDA. For instance, 32–41 % of women older than 50 years ingested less than the RDA [10]. The RDA is nonetheless of great importance, because national and international policies regarding food programs are based on this value as the target level of protein that should be eaten. It was also recommended that protein constitute between 10 and 35 % of the daily energy intake, but virtually no older persons ingest the highest acceptable macronutrient distribution of 35 %. Accordingly, in the Health, Aging and Body Composition Study, even persons in the highest quintile of protein intake lost appendicular lean mass than, indicating that their intake of protein failed to counteract the loss of lean mass [11]. It is however interesting to note that for an increase of 0.1 g/kg of daily protein intake, the drop in skeletal muscle mass would be reduced by 0.62 kg [12]. Nevertheless, there is evidence that this recommendation may not be suitable for elderly people. In a study that examined the long-term consequences of consumption of the protein RDA, Campbell et al. [13] showed that over a 14-week period, the subjects (men and women aged 55–77 years) demonstrated a significant reduction in the cross-sectional area of the thigh skeletal muscle. These data suggest that the protein RDA for elderly people is not adequate, even while consuming a weight maintenance diet.

The etiology of this increased need for dietary protein is not well understood. Because of metabolic changes, older persons may produce less muscle protein than younger persons from the same amount of dietary protein. However, larger amounts of protein may produce responses similar to those of younger persons [14]. A protein intake of 1 g/kg//day seems to be the minimal amount required to maintain skeletal muscle mass in elderly women. For these reasons, expert recommendations for optimal protein intake in the elderly range from 1.0 to 2.0 g/kg//day or higher. These conclusions are reinforced by results demonstrating that older individuals whose consumption levels approach the RDA are at greater risk for disease than those consuming more than the RDA [15]. In addition, it is recommended that the amount of protein ingested should be spread equally throughout the day (e.g., equivalent amounts at breakfast, lunch, and dinner).

High protein diets are accused of constituting a favorable environment for kidney stones and renal diseases (through the increase of acid and calcium excretion [16]). In healthy subjects, no damaging effect of high protein diets on kidneys has been found in either observational or interventional studies, and it seems that high protein diets might be deleterious only in patients with preexisting metabolic renal dysfunction [16]. However, since aging is accompanied by a decrease in renal activity and in water consumption, potential damage is never totally excluded.

Essential Amino Acids

Proteins contained in food are broken down by the digestive juices in stomach and intestine into basic units called amino acids (AA). The quality of a protein is relative to its capacity to deliver AAs to the individual. AAs are the building blocks of protein in the body, and thus are critical elements of the diet. They can be reused to make the proteins body needs to maintain skeletal muscles, bones, blood, and body organs. A shortfall of any one of these AAs would be a limiting factor in protein synthesis. Of the 22 standard AAs, nine are called EAAs because they cannot be synthesized by the organism, and therefore must be supplied in the diet.

Muscle protein metabolism alternates between periods of net catabolism in the postabsorptive state and net anabolism in the postprandial states. Although muscle protein anabolism decreases with aging, it can nonetheless be directly stimulated by increased AAs availability. In fact, over 80 % of the stimulatory effect on protein synthesis observed after a meal may be attributed to AAs [17]. Specifically, hyperaminoacidemia acutely stimulates muscle protein synthesis by increasing the AA transport into muscle. Muscle protein synthesis is an energy-consuming process and if additional energy (from extra food intake or supplements) had any influence on muscle protein synthesis, such an effect should have been positive rather than negative. Insulin is also a potent anabolic stimulus for muscle protein, and a number of studies [14] have reported that hyperinsulinemia can increase muscle protein synthesis, particularly when AAs availability is increased. However, such an anabolic effect of insulin is absent in older subjects [14], suggesting that muscle protein synthesis is resistant to the anabolic action of insulin or that a higher insulin level is required to obtain similar results in older. This also suggests that age-associated insulin resistance of muscle proteins pays a role in the reduced muscle anabolic response to feeding, and in the development of sarcopenia. Evidence indicate that the anabolic response of skeletal muscle proteins to mixed feeding decreases with age despite the fact that AAs alone can normally stimulate protein synthesis in older muscle.

Among the EAAs, leucine has been recognized to have a crucial role in enhancing the insulin sensitivity of protein synthesis, bringing about a stimulation of muscle protein synthesis [18]. Furthermore, besides the insulin dependent stimulation, leucine may have a direct effect on protein metabolism [19] by partly inhibiting muscle protein breakdown. Aged skeletal muscle may be less sensitive to the stimulatory effect of AAs at low physiologic concentrations, but this impairment may be overcome by the provision of a larger amount of leucine [18]. For instance, no differences exist in protein balance in the elderly relative to the young postabsorptive or following administration of either 30 g of beef protein or 15 g of EAAs. However, when given half this amount of EAAs (6.7 g), the overall protein synthetic response is blunted in the elderly relative to the young [20]. Furthermore, the anabolic stimulus afforded by a nutritional supplement is influenced by the type and composition of the AA–protein mixture ingested. It appears that the anabolic response to an AA supplementation given to elderly subjects is blunted by the ingestion of carbohydrate, whereas in a young population, this combination elicits an anabolic response greater than achieved by AA supplementation alone [21]. This compromised interaction between carbohydrates and AAs may also partly explain why some dietary supplements fail to produce beneficial anabolic effects in the elderly.

In conclusion, to achieve the highest anabolic efficiency, it is not only important to deliver the nutrients that are absolutely necessary for the stimulation of muscle protein metabolism, but it is also crucial to provide them in sufficient quantity (a dose of 15 g/day of EAA appears effective in stimulating protein synthesis). Particularly, leucine may play a key role in the formulation of any AA/protein supplement for reversing attenuated response of muscle protein synthesis in the elderly. Furthermore, a supplementation of leucine may have a sparing effect on muscle glycogen degradation during endurance exercise and result in an increased deposition of lean mass and an increase in strength during intensive resistance exercise training [22].

It is however important to note that a role for leucine as an enhancer of insulin sensitivity also implies the possibility that prolonged very high intakes of leucine may lead to insulin resistance. In addition, some AAs (methionine, cystein, and histidine) are thought to result in toxic effects at high doses. Evidence exists that they can cause tissue damage and increase homocysteine and/or cholesterol levels and so may be associated with chronic diseases if taken over long periods of time. Nonetheless, the data relevant to humans are very limited, so unanticipated adverse consequences of consuming large amounts cannot be completely ruled out [23]. Dietary supplements should then be consumed with caution.

Animal and Vegetal Protein Intake

Proteins can be separated in two broad categories; animal and vegetal proteins. These two types of proteins do not necessarily have the same properties. For instance, proteins from vegetal sources tend to have a relatively low "biological value", in comparison to protein from eggs, meat, or milk [24]. Biological value is a measure of the proportion of absorbed protein from a food which becomes incorporated into the proteins of the organism's body. It summarizes how readily the broken down protein can be used in protein synthesis in the cells of the organism. However, the biological value does not take into account how readily the protein can be digested and absorbed. Nevertheless, vegetal proteins are "complete" in that they contain at least trace amounts of all of the AAs that are essential in human nutrition. Content of all EAAs in selected items of vegetal commodities (legumes, nuts, oil seeds, grains) is 62–81 % in comparison to reference animal proteins [24]. On the other hand, vegetal proteins are richer in nonessential AAs (111–129 %) compared with animal proteins.

The main limiting AAs in vegetal proteins are methionine, lysine, and tryptophan [25]. These AAs are not specifically critical to the process of protein synthesis, but since all acidic AAs are required to complete the process, a shortfall of any one of the AAs would be a limiting factor [24]. This may explain why 20 % of adults vegans are thought to have a hypoproteinemia. Evidence also shows differences in the bioavailability of these proteins. For an equivalent protein intake, vegetal proteins from cereals and legumes may be less digested and absorbed than animal proteins. A decrease in the amount or bioavailability of EAAs could alter their ability to be used for growth. Finally, it appears that elderly women experience a greater inhibition of protein degradation and a higher net protein balance when consuming a diet high in animal protein as compared to those consuming a diet high in vegetal protein. It is then not surprising that a strong positive association has been repeatedly observed between animal protein intake and skeletal muscle mass or skeletal muscle mass index in postmenopausal women [26] (Fig. 14.2), while the relationship between vegetal protein intakes or total protein intake and skeletal muscle mass or skeletal muscle mass index may be weaker or nonexistent.

This could suggest that diet (omnivore, ovo-lacto vegetarian, or vegan) directly impacts muscle mass. An omnivorous diet includes both plant and animal foods. It is the most common diet among humans in Western countries. Vegetarianism is the voluntary abstinence from eating meat, including seafood. Ovo-lacto-vegetarians supplement their diet with dairy (lactose) products and eggs (ovo). Veganism is a type of vegetarian diet that excludes meat, eggs, dairy products, and all other animal-derived ingredients. Recent estimates suggest that approximately 2.5 % of American adults and 4 % of Canadian adults report following a vegetarian diet [27].

The literature is consistent in reporting that vegetarians' protein intakes are lower than those of omnivores [28]. One would then expect that vegans or vegetarians have a lower skeletal muscle mass

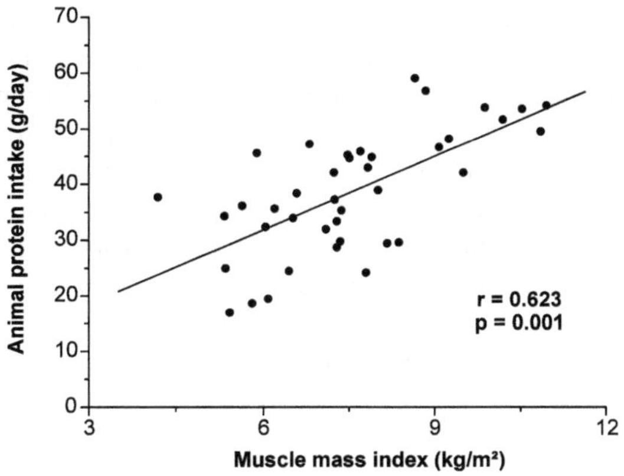

Fig. 14.2 Partial correlation between animal protein intake and skeletal muscle mass index. Correlation was controlled for sex hormone-binding globulin and plant protein intake. Figure adapted from Aubertin-leheudre et al. [26]

compared with omnivores. However, to date, the literature is too poor in this regard to state on the effect of diet on the development of sarcopenia. Some observed that vegetarians have a lower skeletal muscle mass than omnivores while others did not. In fact, eating various vegetal foods in combination can provide a protein of higher biological value, without the need to intentionally combine different foods for this purpose necessarily. However, as a preventive measure, because animal proteins are higher in EAAs, the elderly are suggested to consume a diet rich in lean source of meat-based and milk products in order to achieve sufficiently high doses. In premenopausal women, diet- and exercise-induced weight loss with higher protein and increased dairy product intakes promotes lean mass maintenance and fat loss [29]. Between minimum benefits and potential adverse effects, a dietary protein intake of 1.1–1.5 g/kg/day may be appropriate to prevent an excessive loss of skeletal muscle mass in postmenopausal women.

Creatine

Creatine is naturally produced or synthesized half in the human body from certain AAs (glycine, arginine, and methionine), the other half comes from food (mainly from meat and fish). Approximately 95 % of creatine contained in the human body is stored in skeletal muscle [30]. In skeletal muscle, a fraction of the total creatine binds to phosphate. The reaction is catalyzed by creatine kinase, and results in phosphocreatine (PCr). PCr then binds to adenosine biphosphate (ADP), to convert it back to adenosine triphosphate (ATP), an important source of energy. An increase in PCr from creatine supplementation should theoretically increase PCr resynthesis during muscle contraction leading to greater exercise training intensity and subsequently skeletal muscle mass. Indeed, creatine supplementation during exercise training has been shown to be effective in increasing skeletal muscle mass, but also appears to slow the loss of skeletal muscle mass and strength during immobilization in young adults [31]. Increasingly, there is research showing a positive effect from creatine supplementation (5–20 g/day for 5 days–6 months) on muscle accretion in postmenopausal women [32]. Based on these results, a low supplementation (5 g/day) over a long period (6 months) appears to more effective that an important supplementation (20 g/day) for a very short duration (5 days). Interestingly, this increase in skeletal muscle mass was paralleled by an increase in muscle strength, which is significant in terms of maintenance of functional capacity. While the mechanistic actions remain to be determined, it has been theorized that creatine has the ability to regulate osmosis within the working cell and could potentially elevate intracellular osmolarity. The anabolic signal induced by cellular hydration may increase the expression of myogenic transcription factors which augment the up-regulation of muscle specific-genes (such as myosin heavy chain), thereby facilitating an increase in skeletal muscle hypertrophy and strength [32]. Furthermore, the timing of creatine supplementation appears to be crucial for creating an anabolic environment for muscle growth. Creatine ingestion in close proximity to resistance training sessions (before and after exercise) may be more beneficial than ingesting creatine at other times of the day [32]. Postmenopausal women, but also the elderly in general, may thus be recommended to consume creatine (5 g/day for at least 6 months) or food products containing creatine (red meat or sea food), particularly in close proximity to resistance training sessions, which may enhance functional capacity through increased muscle mass and strength. However, in spite of these studies, there is a need for long-term studies on the effects of creatine on sarcopenia and aging muscle biology.

Take-Home Message

A protein intake of 1 g/kg/day seems to be the minimal amount required to maintain skeletal muscle mass in elderly women. An optimal protein intake in postmenopausal would range from 1.1 to 1.5 g/kg//day or higher.
Particularly, leucine may play a key role in the formulation of any AA/protein supplement for reversing attenuated response of muscle protein synthesis in the elderly.

Vitamin D

Definition and Mechanism of Action of vitamin D

Vitamin D is both a fat-soluble vitamin and a prohormone which has the distinction of being synthesized by the epidermis when exposed to sunlight. In fact, up to 80 % of vitamin D is produced following ultraviolet B light exposure, the other 20 %being provided by food [33]. 10–15 min of sunshine three times weekly may be enough to produce the body's requirement of vitamin D. Vitamin D can be found in dairy products (Cheese, butter, cream, fortified milk), fatty fish (such as tuna, salmon, and mackerel), oysters, fortified breakfast cereals, margarine, and soy milk. Vitamin D consists of a set of substances sometimes called provitamin D. These include the provitamin ergocalciferol (D2; plant form) and cholecalciferol (D3; animal form). The body partly transforms these compounds in calcitriol, which generates the majority of the health benefits. Vitamin D can accumulate in fat and liver where it is placed in reserve. Depending on the needs of the body, it can be put back in circulation and metabolized.

It has been well-established that vitamin D plays an essential role in the regulation of calcium and phosphate homeostasis and in bone development and maintenance. Over the last two decades, however, there has been increasing evidence that vitamin D plays an important role in many other tissues including skeletal muscle. The identification of vitamin D receptors (VDR) on muscle cells provided further support for a direct effect of vitamin D on skeletal muscle tissue [34]. It has been suggested that the VDR in skeletal muscle tissue is a nuclear receptor that binds 1,25-dihydroxyvitamin D (1,25(OH)2D) with high affinity and elicits its actions to regulate protein synthesis. This may be confirm by results showing an association between 1,25(OH)2D and skeletal muscle mass [35] (Fig. 14.3).

The mechanisms by which vitamin D and its metabolic pathways may affect muscle function are quite complex [36]. A physiologic explanation for the beneficial effect of vitamin D on muscle strength is that 1,25(OH)2D, the active vitamin D metabolite, binds to a vitamin D-specific nuclear receptor in muscle tissue, which leads to enhanced transcription of a range of proteins, including those involved

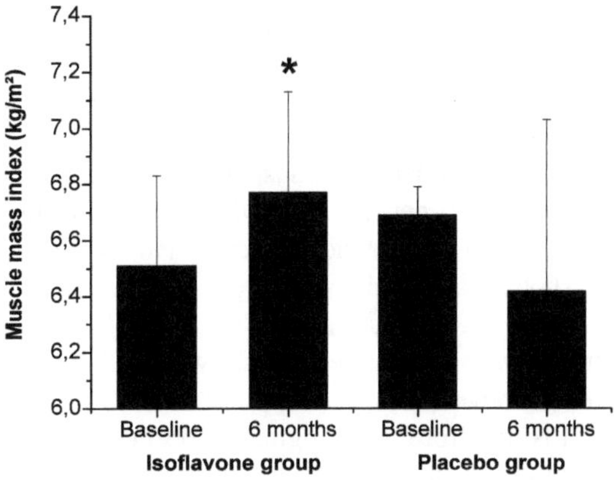

Fig. 14.3 Effect of a 6 months supplementation of isoflavone or placebo on muscle mass index. *Significantly different from baseline values ($p<0.05$). Figure adapted from Aubertin-leheudre et al. [62]

in calcium metabolism, a critical modulator of skeletal muscle function. 1,25(OH)2D may affect skeletal muscle function through both calcium-related protein transcription and total body calcium levels. However, it has been suggested that 1,25(OH)2D also has a transcription-enhancing role on proteins other than those involved directly in calcium metabolism. Briefly, 1,25(OH)2D may promote IGFP-3 expression, a component which bind IGF-1 with high affinity and specificity, limiting its clearance. This mechanism is of importance since IGF-1 has been recognized as a potential means for addressing sarcopenia. Accordingly, IGF-1 is known to induce proliferation, differentiation, and hypertrophy of skeletal muscle.

While the vast majority of food components (proteins, carbohydrates, vitamin A, etc.) standards are defined in terms of quantity to absorb daily, the fact that vitamin D is mainly synthesized by the body invalidates this approach. Then, to determine whether an individual is in the standard or not, we refer to a concentration (measured in the blood, in nmol/L) rather than a quantity provided by food.

The consensus threshold for defining vitamin D deficiency is currently set at 25 nmol/L, and the threshold selected by the World Health Organization to define vitamin D insufficiency is 50 nmol/L. However, more recently, it has been suggested that the most advantageous target concentration of 25(OH)D begins at 75 nmol/L and that the optimum concentrations are between 90 and 100 nmol/L [37]. If 75–100 nmol/L were the target range of a revised RDA, the new RDA should meet the requirements of 97 % of the population.

It is currently estimated that at least 1 billion people through the world have a vitamin D deficiency [33]. More precisely, Vitamin D insufficiency and deficiency may be particularly prevalent in people who live at higher latitudes where the winters are prolonged. Thus, at latitudes above 40° (e.g., Europe or the USA), 40–90 % of community dwelling elderly have a hypovitaminosis D. Even if all adults can be affected by hypovitaminosis D, those most at risk are the elderly, especially if they live in institutions or are hospitalized. Also, over 50 % of women taking treatment for osteoporosis have been reported to be deficient [38].

Aging and Vitamin D

This high prevalence of hypovitaminosis D in the elderly is due to different mechanisms directly associated with aging, foremost among them the decreased skin synthesis. Hypovitaminosis D may also be the consequence of the altered metabolism of vitamin D (renal and hepatic insufficiency), inadequate food intake, reduction in bioavailability (malabsorption, obesity with sequestration of vitamin D in the fat), increased catabolism (anticonvulsants, glucocorticoids, immunosuppressants) and urinary losses of vitamin D. Furthermore, this decreased vitamin D synthesis/intake with aging is paralleled by a diminished Vitamin D receptor expression in muscle tissue [39]. Over time, this may impair protein synthesis in muscle cells, resulting in a decrease in muscle fibers (mostly type II fibers), and eventually sarcopenia. Also, vitamin D and its metabolites are transported in blood by an α-globulin called Vitamin D-Binding Protein whose synthesis is increased in the presence of estrogen. The decrease in estrogen production at menopause therefore directly impairs the transport of vitamin D. It is however interesting to note that, in men, this relationship may also depend on VDR polymorphisms [40]. These results suggest that the VDR locus may contribute to interindividual variation in skeletal muscle mass and susceptibility to sarcopenia. A few studies showed associations of allelic variants at the VDR locus with muscle strength in postmenopausal women [41]. To date, no study has established a relationship between VDR polymorphism and skeletal muscle mass in postmenopausal women. However, it appears that such a relationship does not exist in young women [42].

It is therefore quite logical to observe that Vitamin D deficiency has been widely associated with functional disabilities. In an analysis of men and women age 60 and over who participated in the cross-sectional NHANES III survey, individuals with higher serum 25(OH)D levels up to 94 nmol/L were able to walk faster (8-ft walk test) and to get out of a chair faster (sit-to-stand test) than subjects with lower levels, particularly in the subset with 25(OH)D levels under 60 nmol/L [43]. Time of the 8-ft-walk test in subjects in the highest quintile of 25(OH)D was 5.6 % lower than the results in subjects in the lowest quintile of 25(OH)D. Time of the sit-to-stand test in subjects in the highest quintile of 25(OH)D was 3.9 % lower than the results in subjects in the lowest quintile of 25(OH)D. This finding is supported by data from the Longitudinal Aging Study Amsterdam that included 1,351 Dutch men and women aged 65 years and more. In that study [44], a physical performance score (chair stands, a walking test, and a tandem stand) showed the greatest improvement from very low concentrations of serum 25(OH)D up to 50 nmol/L and had less pronounced but continuous improvement at concentrations >50 nmol/L. low 25(OH)D levels (less than 25 nmol/L) were also associated with an increased risk of repeated falling over the subsequent year. Finally, lower serum 25(OH)D levels predicted decreased grip strength and appendicular skeletal muscle mass in elderly men and women over the subsequent 3 years [44]. All these phenomenon being closely linked, a poor vitamin D status may play a role in the risk of developing incapacities through an effect on muscle function (skeletal muscle mass and strength).

Vitamin D Supplements

If standards are based on 25(OH)D blood levels, supplements, however, are expressed in terms of quantity (International Unit, IU) to absorb daily. Oral supplementation is the most effective way to treat vitamin D deficiency. Vitamin D found in supplements and fortified foods comes in two different forms (D3 and D2), the D_3 form appearing to have a superior efficacy compared with the D_2 form. Studies suggest that 700–1,000 IU vitamin D per day may bring 50 % of younger and older adults up to a concentration of 90–100 nmol/L [37]. The current intake recommendation for older persons (600 IU/day) may bring concentrations in most subjects to 50–60 nmol/L, but not to 90–100 nmol/L. Because of seasonal fluctuations in 25(OH)D concentrations, some persons may be in the target range during the summer months, but not during the winter months, even in sunny latitudes. Several studies even suggest that many older persons will not achieve optimal serum 25(OH)D concentrations during the summer months. However, it is important to note that although vitamin D is relatively rare in food, some foods are particularly rich and can largely achieve doses provided by supplementation. Among the richest foods in vitamin D are pure cod liver oil (1,360 IU for one tablespoon), salmon (360 IU for 100 g), mackerel (345 IU for 100 g), tuna fish (200 IU for 100 g), milk (whole, skimmed or low-fat; 100 IU for 1 cup), or eggs (20 IU for a whole egg).

Intakes of 700–800 IU vitamin D/day (with or without calcium) could prevent approximately one-fourth of all hip and nonvertebral fractures in both ambulatory and institutionalized older persons [45]. Furthermore, because the positive association between 25(OH)D concentrations and bone mineral density in younger adults is consistent with the concept that higher concentrations of serum 25(OH)D may contribute to peak bone mass, maintenance of high 25(OH)D concentrations in younger adulthood could further protect against fractures at older ages [46].

Also, a few studies have examined the effect of vitamin D supplementation on balance and gait performance [37, 47]. Specifically, vitamin D with calcium, compared to calcium alone, improved body sway in ambulatory elderly women with serum 25(OH)D levels less than 50 nmol/L within 8 weeks and improved musculoskeletal function in institutionalized elders with serum 25(OH)D levels less than 50 nmol/L within 12 weeks. A recent meta-analysis showed that the efficacy of supplemental vitamin D for fall prevention depended on dose and achieved 25(OH)D concentrations among individuals aged 60 years and older. No fall reduction was observed for a daily dose of less than 700 IU vitamin D or achieved serum 25(OH)D concentrations below 60 nmol/L. Daily vitamin D doses in the range of 700–1,000 IU or achieved serum concentrations between 60 and 95 nmol/L reduced the risk of falling by 19 %. The benefit was sustained for 12–36 months [48], partly through improved muscle function.

700–1,000 IU per day may thus be recommended to improve muscle function and functional capacity in postmenopausal women. Furthermore, contrary to high doses of vitamin E and C, vitamin D supplements do not seem to increase risks of cancers. However, it is important to note that excessive intake of vitamin D may lead to hypercalcemia, which may cause nausea, vomiting, loss of appetite, and weakness. In case of chronic hypercalcemia, kidney stones as well as deposits of calcium and phosphorus in the organs and soft tissues can be observed.

Take-Home Message

Vitamin D deficiency has been widely associated with functional disabilities.
Intakes of 700–1,000 IU vitamin D/day may be recommended to prevent falls and to improve muscle function and functional capacity in postmenopausal women

Phytoestrogen

Estrogen and Muscle Mass

Estrogens are the primary female sex hormones. Natural estrogens are steroid hormones which readily diffuse across the cell membrane. Once inside the cell, they bind to and activate estrogen receptors (ERs) which in turn modulate the expression of many genes. Although it can cause women to retain fluid, and early exposure through early menses can increase a woman's risk of developing breast cancer, estrogen has its benefits. It can contribute to increase high density lipoprotein and lower the low density lipoprotein. At menopause, women experience a reduction in estrogen. This can lead to vaginal dryness, memory problems, hot flashes, fatigue, irritability, and possibly one of the most devastating problems, a decrease in bone mineral density. Furthermore, there is evidence that a decreased estrogen production in women at menopause may be associated with a loss of skeletal muscle mass [49]. The mechanisms by which a decrease in estrogen levels may have a negative effect on skeletal muscle mass are not well understood but it has been suggested that decreases in estrogen concentrations may be associated with increased pro-inflammatory cytokines, such as tumor necrosis factor alpha (TNF-α)

or interleukine-6 (IL-6), which might be implicated in the apparition of sarcopenia [50]. Furthermore, estrogen could have a direct effect on skeletal muscle mass since it has been shown that skeletal muscle has ERs on the cell membrane, in the cytoplasm and on the nuclear membrane, implying that estrogen could have a direct influence on protein synthesis, similar to its effects on transcription in bone cells [49].

Estrogens are used as part of some oral contraceptives and in estrogen replacement therapy for postmenopausal women. It is thus not surprising that hormone therapy has been reported to be associated with skeletal muscle mass and has been hypothesized to prevent sarcopenia [51]. The Women's Health Initiative study randomized a large number ($n = 835$) of postmenopausal women to hormone therapy or placebo for 3 years and evaluated changes in lean mass [52]. Women randomized to receive hormone therapy lost 0.04 kg of lean mass, which was significantly less than the 0.44 kg lost by women on placebo, indicating that hormone therapy can have a small beneficial effect on muscle mass. Hormone therapy given over 10 months to postmenopausal women also increased blood concentrations of growth hormone and insulin-like growth factor-1, both of which have an anabolic effect on skeletal muscle. Unfortunately, the Women's Health Initiative also showed that the risks of hormone therapy (estrogen and progesterone) outweigh its benefits. The study found statistically significant increases in rates of breast cancer, coronary heart disease, strokes, and pulmonary emboli. Because of the increased knowledge of these risks, many women are thus seeking alternatives to estrogen or hormone therapy [53].

Phytoestrogens as Alternatives to Hormone and Estrogen Therapies

One such alternative is the class of plant-based compounds termed phytoestrogens. The presumption that phytoestrogens may have beneficial effects on menopausal symptoms arose from the observation that Asian women are thought to suffer from fewer hot flashes than women in Western countries. Phytoestrogens are plant-derived xenoestrogens (environmental hormones that imitate estrogen) functioning as estrogens. Also called "dietary estrogens," they are a diverse group of naturally occurring nonsteroidal plant compound that, because of their structural similarity with estrogens, have the ability to mildly mimic and sometimes act as antagonists of estrogen. Phytoestrogens may have protective action against diverse health disorders, such as prostate, breast, bowel, and other cancers, cardiovascular disease, brain function disorders, and osteoporosis. Evidence also suggests that a sufficiently large quantity of phytoestrogens (70 mg/day for 4 months) may reduce symptoms of menopause [54] while effects are mixed for smaller quantities.

Phystoestrogens cannot be considered as nutrients, given that the lack of these in diet does not produce any characteristic deficiency syndrome, nor do they participate in any essential biological function. The coumestans (an organic compound that is a derivative of coumarin), prenylated flavonoids (a subclass of plant secondary metabolites), and isoflavones are three of the most active in estrogenic effects in this class. In a cohort of 946 healthy US postmenopausal women [55], the intake of phytoestrogens was estimated to be less than 1 mg/day. Median total intake of isoflavones, which main sources were beans and peas, was 154 μg. The estimated daily intake of coumestans was 0.6 μg, with broccoli as the main source and the median total intake of lignans was 578 μg, primarily from fruits.

Rates of absorption and bioavailability of phytoestrogens depend on many factors including the absolute quantity in a foodstuff, processing in food preparation and chemical structure. Concerning the bioavailability of commercial soy isoflavone supplements, overall high levels of absorption but marked qualitative and quantitative differences between types of supplements have been reported. Furthermore, metabolism of dietary components can result in the production of metabolites that are more biologically active than their precursors, which could ultimately influence their effect on host health. For instance, the predominant daidzein (isoflavone compound) metabolites produced by human are dihydrodadzein, equol, and

O-desmethylangolensin (*O*-DMA) and their production appears to be associated with reduced risk of certain cancers and other diseases [56]. Interestingly, the prevalence of equol-producer phenotype may be higher (51 % vs. 36 %), and the *O*-DMA-producer phenotype lower (84 % vs. 92 %), in Korean than in Caucasian women. The prevalence of the combinations of equol- and *O*-DMA-producer phenotypes also differed between Korean and Caucasian women (41 % and 35 %, respectively) [57]. Nevertheless, little evidence is currently available and larger studies are needed to confirm or refute relationships between daidzein-metabolizing phenotypes and disease risk.

Phytoestrogens and Muscle Mass

Phytoestrogens may exert a beneficial effect on skeletal muscle mass because of their affinity for ERs, which are found on muscle [51]. There are two variants of the estrogen receptor, alpha (ER-α) and beta (ER-β) and many phytoestrogens display somewhat higher affinity for ER-β compared to ER-α. Phytoestrogens may also influence skeletal muscle mass through their effects on reducing inflammation [51]. Indeed, chronic low-grade inflammation is related to decreased skeletal muscle mass and strength with age [58]. Interleukin-6, one of the main inflammatory cytokines, has been associated with a decrease in skeletal muscle mass, strength, and fiber number in older adults. Studies relating phytoestrogens to prevention of inflammation and muscle protein degradation are limited, but one study in rats subjected to intense exercise resulting in muscle damage revealed that a chronic high soy protein diet was effective for reducing activation of pathways involved in muscle protein degradation [59].

In addition to interaction with ERs, phytoestrogens may also modulate the concentration of endogenous estrogens by binding or inactivating some enzymes, and may affect the bioavailability of sex hormones by binding or stimulating the synthesis of sex hormone binding globuline (SHBG) [60]. Plasma SHBG is the major plasma transport protein for biologically active androgens and estrogens, and changes in the blood levels of SHBG widely influence their distribution and access to target tissues and cells.

Finally, emerging evidence shows that some phytoestrogens bind to and transactivate peroxisome proliferator-activated receptors (PPARs) [61], a group of nuclear receptor proteins that function as transcription factors regulating the expression of genes. PPARs play essential roles in the regulation of cellular differentiation, development and metabolism (carbohydrate, lipid, protein).

Isoflavones

Isoflavones belong to a class of phytoestrogens and is the most studied of these. A few studies have investigated changes in skeletal muscle mass or lean mass in older individuals with either isolated isoflavones or soy protein, which contains isoflavones. Isoflavones on their own result in a small increase in lean mass; however, it is unclear whether they would result in a significant increase when added to an exercise program. Aubertin-Leheudre et al. investigated the effect of a 70 mg/day of soy isoflavone supplementation for 24 weeks on muscle mass in obese-sarcopenic postmenopausal women and observed that isoflavone supplementation was associated with a significant increase in appendicular lean mass (+0.5 kg), but this increase was not enough to reverse sarcopenia [62] (Fig. 14.4). Another study randomized postmenopausal women to receive either isoflavone-rich soy protein (40 g), isoflavone-poor soy protein or whey protein (control) for 24 weeks [63]. It was reported that changes in total lean mass were not different between groups; however, lean mass at the hip increased to a greater extent in the isoflavone-rich group (+3.4 %) than in the isoflavone-poor (+1 %) or control

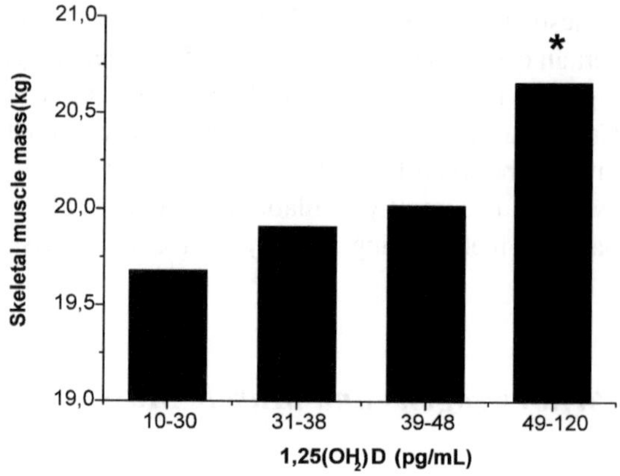

Fig. 14.4 Relationship between 1,25(OH)$_2$D and skeletal muscle mass. *Higher 1,25(OH)$_2$D value was associated with a higher skeletal muscle mass ($p=0.012$). Analyses were adjusted for age, height, physical activity, season, and fat mass. Figure adapted from Marantes et al. [35]

(0 %) groups. Studies of soy protein combined with 12–16 weeks of resistance training in postmenopausal women or older men (age 65 years) did not result in greater increases in strength or muscle mass compared with either placebo or beef protein.

Thus, although currently limited, the results obtained with isoflavones are encouraging and deserve some attention to better characterize their effects and determine the optimal dosages. To date, studies indicate that 50 mg/day, for a period of 6 months, is sufficient to have significant endocrine effects, whereas half this dose appears biologically inactive [64].

Take-Home Message

Phytoestrogens are currently considered as potential alternatives to hormone and estrogen therapies.

Phytoestrogens are still under investigation, and evidence of their effectiveness are limited. However, 50 mg/day of isoflavone, for a period of 6 months, may be sufficient to have significant endocrine effects.

Conclusion

In conclusion, nutrition clearly appears to play a key role in maintaining skeletal muscle mass, and thus in the prevention and treatment of sarcopenia. In particular, a sufficient protein intake may be the key of a healthy nutrition, even if standards need to be fixed in regard to the needs of an aging population. We have to admit that our understanding of the relationship between nutrition and sarcopenia is still limited, but interesting alternatives to proteins, as well as supplements, emerge in the literature. Among them, vitamin D and isoflavones appear promising, although much research is needed to demonstrate their effectiveness and determine the optimal dosage. Nevertheless, the primary objective of preventing sarcopenia being to limit the functional incapacities associated with this condition, we should keep in mind that an effective therapy to counteract the negative consequences of muscle wasting should improve function, not just mass. Data supporting an improvement in muscular function following supplementation are limited, which bring into question the functionality of any lean mass gain. In this regard, effective nutritional intervention would then require to be combined with other interventions aimed to improve muscle function such as physical activity. Indeed, Little and Phillips [65] have highlighted the potential of resistance exercise combined with appropriately timed nutritional supplementation to promote gains in muscle mass and strength. Particularly, a combination of leucine, insulin, or carbohydrate, and contractile activity may have the greatest potential for increasing muscle protein synthesis. Thus, for optimal results, in addition to providing energy to the muscle, it is important to stimulate it.

References

1. Jubrias SA, Odderson IR, Esselman PC, Conley KE. Decline in isokinetic force with age: muscle cross-sectional area and specific force. Pflugers Arch. 1997;434(3):246–53.
2. Rosenberg IH. Summary comments. Am J Clin Nutr. 1989;50(5):1231–3.
3. Baumgartner RN, Koehler KM, Gallagher D, Romero L, Heymsfield SB, Ross RR, et al. Epidemiology of sarcopenia among the elderly in New Mexico. Am J Epidemiol. 1998;147(8):755–63.
4. Janssen I, Heymsfield SB, Ross R. Low relative skeletal muscle mass (sarcopenia) in older persons is associated with functional impairment and physical disability. J Am Geriatr Soc. 2002;50(5):889–96.
5. Aubertin-Leheudre M, Lord C, Goulet EDB, Khalil A, Dionne IJ. Effect of sarcopenia on cardiovascular disease risk factors in obese postmenopausal women. Obesity. 2006;14(12):2277–83.
6. Stephen WC, Janssen I. Sarcopenic-obesity and cardiovascular disease risk in the elderly. J Nutr Health Aging. 2009;13(5):460–6.
7. Cosqueric G, Sebag A, Ducolombier C, Thomas C, Piette F, Weill-Engerer S. Sarcopenia is predictive of nosocomial infection in care of the elderly. Br J Nutr. 2006;96(5):895–901.
8. Peterson MD, Sen A, Gordon PM. Influence of resistance exercise on lean body mass in aging adults: a meta-analysis. Med Sci Sports Exerc. 2011;43(2):249–58.
9. Trumbo P, Schlicker S, Yates AA, Poos M. Dietary reference intakes for energy, carbohydrate, fiber, fat, fatty acids, cholesterol, protein and amino acids. J Am Diet Assoc. 2002;102(11):1621–30.
10. Kerstetter JE, O'Brien KO, Insogna KL. Low protein intake: the impact on calcium and bone homeostasis in humans. J Nutr. 2003;133(3):855S–61.
11. Houston DK, Nicklas BJ, Ding J, Harris TB, Tylavsky FA, Newman AB, et al. Dietary protein intake is associated with lean mass change in older, community-dwelling adults: the Health, Aging, and Body Composition (Health ABC) Study. Am J Clin Nutr. 2008;87(1):150–5.
12. Bopp MJ, Houston DK, Lenchik L, Easter L, Kritchevsky SB, Nicklas BJ. Lean mass loss is associated with low protein intake during dietary-induced weight loss in postmenopausal women. J Am Diet Assoc. 2008;108(7):1216–20.
13. Campbell WW, Trappe TA, Wolfe RR, Evans WJ. The recommended dietary allowance for protein may not be adequate or older people to maintain skeletal muscle. J Gerontol A Biol Sci Med Sci. 2001;56(6):M373–80.
14. Fujita S, Volpi E. Amino acids and muscle loss with aging. J Nutr. 2006;136(1):277S–80.
15. Rousset S, Mirand PP, Brandolini M, Martin J-F, Boirie Y. Daily protein intakes and eating patterns in young and elderly French. Br J Nutr. 2003;90(6):1107–15.
16. Calvez J, Poupin N, Chesneau C, Lassale C, Tome D. Protein intake, calcium balance and health consequences. Eur J Clin Nutr. 2012;66(3):281–95.
17. Volpi E, Kobayashi H, Sheffield-Moore M, Mittendorfer B, Wolfe RR. Essential amino acids are primarily responsible for the amino acid stimulation of muscle protein anabolism in healthy elderly adults. Am J Clin Nutr. 2003;78(2):250–8.
18. Garlick PJ. The role of leucine in the regulation of protein metabolism. J Nutr. 2005;135(6):1553S–6.
19. Anthony JC, Reiter AK, Anthony TG, Crozier SJ, Lang CH, MacLean DA, et al. Orally administered leucine enhances protein synthesis in skeletal muscle of diabetic rats in the absence of increases in 4E-BP1 or S6K1 phosphorylation. Diabetes. 2002;51(4):928–36.
20. Katsanos CS, Kobayashi H, Sheffield-Moore M, Aarsland A, Wolfe RR. Aging is associated with diminished accretion of muscle proteins after the ingestion of a small bolus of essential amino acids. Am J Clin Nutr. 2005;82(5):1065–73.
21. Volpi E, Mittendorfer B, Rasmussen BB, Wolfe RR. The response of muscle protein anabolism to combined hyperaminoacidemia and glucose-induced hyperinsulinemia is impaired in the elderly. J Clin Endocrinol Metab. 2000;85(12):4481–90.
22. Mero A. Leucine supplementation and intensive training. Sports Med. 1999;27(6):347–58.
23. Garlick PJ. The nature of human hazards associated with excessive intake of amino acids. J Nutr. 2004;134(6 Suppl):1633S–9.
24. Krajcovicova-Kudlackova M, Babinska K, Valachovicova M. Health benefits and risks of plant proteins. Bratisl Lek Listy. 2005;106(6–7):231–4.

25. Metges CC, Petzke KJ, Young VR. Dietary requirements for indispensable amino acids in adult humans: new concepts, methods of estimation, uncertainties and challenges. Ann Nutr Metab. 1999;43(5):267–76.
26. Aubertin-Leheudre M, Adlercreutz H. Relationship between animal protein intake and muscle mass index in healthy women. Br J Nutr. 2009;102(12):1803–10.
27. Barr SI, Rideout CA. Nutritional considerations for vegetarian athletes. Nutrition. 2004;20(7–8):696–703.
28. Messina M, Messina V. Vegetarian diets for athletes. In: Messina V, Messina M, editors. The dietitian's guide to vegetarian diets: issues and applications. Gaithersburg (MD): Aspen; 1996. p. 124–35. 354–367.
29. Josse AR, Atkinson SA, Tarnopolsky MA, Phillips SM. Increased consumption of dairy foods and protein during diet- and exercise-induced weight loss promotes fat mass loss and lean mass gain in overweight and obese premenopausal women. J Nutr. 2011;141(9):1626–34.
30. Green AL, Hultman E, Macdonald IA, Sewell DA, Greenhaff PL. Carbohydrate ingestion augments skeletal muscle creatine accumulation during creatine supplementation in humans. Am J Physiol. 1996;271(5 Pt 1):821–6.
31. Johnston AP, Burke DG, MacNeil LG, Candow DG. Effect of creatine supplementation during cast-induced immobilization on the preservation of muscle mass, strength, and endurance. J Strength Cond Res. 2009;23(1):116–20.
32. Candow DG. Sarcopenia: current theories and the potential beneficial effect of creatine application strategies. Biogerontology. 2011;12(4):273–81.
33. Holick MF. Vitamin D, deficiency. N Engl J Med. 2007;357(3):266–81.
34. Ceglia L. Vitamin D, and skeletal muscle tissue and function. Mol Aspects Med. 2008;29(6):407–14.
35. Marantes I, Achenbach SJ, Atkinson EJ, Khosla 3rd S, Melton LJ, Amin S. Is vitamin D a determinant of muscle mass and strength? J Bone Miner Res. 2011;26(12):2860–71.
36. Hamilton B. Vitamin D, and human skeletal muscle. Scand J Med Sci Sports. 2010;20(2):182–90.
37. Bischoff-Ferrari HA, Giovannucci E, Willett WC, Dietrich T, Dawson-Hughes B. Estimation of optimal serum concentrations of 25-hydroxyvitamin D for multiple health outcomes. Am J Clin Nutr. 2006;84(1):18–28.
38. Lips P, Hosking D, Lippuner K, Norquist JM, Wehren L, Maalouf G, et al. The prevalence of vitamin D inadequacy amongst women with osteoporosis: an international epidemiological investigation. J Intern Med. 2006;260(3):245–54.
39. Bischoff-Ferrari HA, Borchers M, Gudat F, Durmuller U, Stahelin HB, Dick W. Vitamin D receptor expression in human muscle tissue decreases with age. J Bone Miner Res. 2004;19(2):265–9.
40. Roth SM, Zmuda JM, Cauley JA, Shea PR, Ferrell RE. Vitamin D receptor genotype is associated with fat-free mass and sarcopenia in elderly men. J Gerontol A Biol Sci Med Sci. 2004;59(1):10–5.
41. Geusens P, Vandevyver C, Vanhoof J, Cassiman JJ, Boonen S, Raus J. Quadriceps and grip strength are related to vitamin D receptor genotype in elderly nonobese women. J Bone Miner Res. 1997;12(12):2082–8.
42. Grundberg E, Brandstrom H, Ribom EL, Ljunggren O, Mallmin H, Kindmark A. Genetic variation in the human vitamin D receptor is associated with muscle strength, fat mass and body weight in Swedish women. Eur J Endocrinol. 2004;150(3):323–8.
43. Bischoff-Ferrari HA, Dietrich T, Orav EJ, Hu FB, Zhang Y, Karlson EW, et al. Higher 25-hydroxyvitamin D concentrations are associated with better lower-extremity function in both active and inactive persons aged>or =60 y. Am J Clin Nutr. 2004;80(3):752–8.
44. Visser M, Deeg DJH, Lips P. Low vitamin d and high parathyroid hormone levels as determinants of loss of muscle strength and muscle mass (sarcopenia): the longitudinal aging study Amsterdam. J Clin Endocrinol Metab. 2003;88(12):5766–72.
45. Bischoff-Ferrari HA, Willett WC, Wong JB, Giovannucci E, Dietrich T, Dawson-Hughes B. Fracture prevention with vitamin D supplementation: a meta-analysis of randomized controlled trials. JAMA. 2005;293(18):2257–64.
46. Tabensky A, Duan Y, Edmonds J, Seeman E. The contribution of reduced peak accrual of bone and age-related bone loss to osteoporosis at the spine and hip: insights from the daughters of women with vertebral or hip fractures. J Bone Miner Res. 2001;16(6):1101–7.
47. Annweiler C, Schott AM, Berrut G, Fantino B, Beauchet O. Vitamin D-related changes in physical performance: a systematic review. J Nutr Health Aging. 2009;13(10):893–8.
48. Bischoff-Ferrari HA, Dawson-Hughes B, Staehelin HB, Orav JE, Stuck AE, Theiler R, et al. Fall prevention with supplemental and active forms of vitamin D: a meta-analysis of randomised controlled trials. BMJ. 2009;339:b3692.
49. Messier V, Rabasa-Lhoret R, Barbat-Artigas S, Elisha B, Karelis AD, Aubertin-Leheudre M. Menopause and sarcopenia: a potential role for sex hormones. Maturitas. 2011;68(4):331–6.
50. Roubenoff R. Origins and clinical relevance of sarcopenia. Can J Appl Physiol. 2001;26(1):78–9.
51. Chilibeck PD, Cornish SM. Effect of estrogenic compounds (estrogen or phytoestrogens) combined with exercise on bone and muscle mass in older individuals. Appl Physiol Nutr Metab. 2008;33(1):200–12.
52. Chen Z, Bassford T, Green SB, Cauley JA, Jackson RD, LaCroix AZ, et al. Postmenopausal hormone therapy and body composition–a substudy of the estrogen plus progestin trial of the Women's Health Initiative. Am J Clin Nutr. 2005;82(3):651–6.
53. Rossouw JE, Anderson GL, Prentice RL, LaCroix AZ, Kooperberg C, Stefanick ML, et al. Risks and benefits of estrogen plus progestin in healthy postmenopausal women: principal results from the Women's Health Initiative randomized controlled trial. JAMA. 2002;288(3):321–33.

54. Faure ED, Chantre P, Mares P. Effects of a standardized soy extract on hot flushes: a multicenter, double-blind, randomized, placebo-controlled study. Menopause. 2002;9(5):329–34.
55. de Kleijn MJ, van der Schouw YT, Wilson PW, Adlercreutz H, Mazur W, Grobbee DE, et al. Intake of dietary phytoestrogens is low in postmenopausal women in the United States: the Framingham study(1–4). J Nutr. 2001;131(6):1826–32.
56. Atkinson C, Frankenfeld CL, Lampe JW. Gut bacterial metabolism of the soy isoflavone daidzein: exploring the relevance to human health. Exp Biol Med (Maywood). 2005;230(3):155–70.
57. Song KB, Atkinson C, Frankenfeld CL, Jokela T, Wahala K, Thomas WK, et al. Prevalence of daidzein-metabolizing phenotypes differs between Caucasian and Korean American women and girls. J Nutr. 2006;136(5):1347–51.
58. Schaap LA, Pluijm SMF, Deeg DJH, Visser M. Inflammatory markers and loss of muscle mass (sarcopenia) and strength. Am J Med. 2006;119(6):526.e9–17.
59. Nikawa T, Ikemoto M, Sakai T, Kano M, Kitano T, Kawahara T, et al. Effects of a soy protein diet on exercise-induced muscle protein catabolism in rats. Nutrition. 2002;18(6):490–5.
60. Ibarreta D, Daxenberger A, Meyer HH. Possible health impact of phytoestrogens and xenoestrogens in food. APMIS. 2001;109(3):161–84.
61. Ricketts ML, Moore DD, Banz WJ, Mezei O, Shay NF. Molecular mechanisms of action of the soy isoflavones includes activation of promiscuous nuclear receptors. A review. J Nutr Biochem. 2005;16(6):321–30.
62. Aubertin-Leheudre M, Lord C, Khalil A, Dionne IJ. Effect of 6 months of exercise and isoflavone supplementation on clinical cardiovascular risk factors in obese postmenopausal women: a randomized, double-blind study. Menopause. 2007;14(4):624–9.
63. Moeller LE, Peterson CT, Hanson KB, Dent SB, Lewis DS, King DS, et al. Isoflavone-rich soy protein prevents loss of hip lean mass but does not prevent the shift in regional fat distribution in perimenopausal women. Menopause. 2003;10(4):322–31.
64. Setchell KD, Cassidy A. Dietary isoflavones: biological effects and relevance to human health. J Nutr. 1999; 129(3):758S–67.
65. Little JP, Phillips SM. Resistance exercise and nutrition to counteract muscle wasting. Appl Physiol Nutr Metab 2009;34:817–28.

Part III
Cardiovascular System, Metabolism and Cancer

Chapter 15
Effects of Flaxseed on Cardiovascular Disease Risk Factors in Menopause

Maureen Meister, Brenda J. Smith, Bahram H. Arjmandi, and Edralin A. Lucas

Key Points

- Both animal and human studies indicate that flaxseed may reduce CVD risk factors in ovarian hormone deficiency.
- Most of the observed positive effect of flaxseed in postmenopausal women is on their ability to improve lipid profile.
- Whole flaxseed seems to be more beneficial than its isolated components such as the lignan, secoisolariceresinol diglucoside (SDG), its oil, or fiber.
- Results of clinical studies demonstrate that flaxseed can be a part of a heart healthy diet of postmenopausal women.
- Further research is needed to understand the mechanism(s) by which flaxseed lowers CVD risk factors in ovarian hormone deficiency.

Keywords Flaxseed • Cardiovascular disease • Menopause • Lignans • α-Linolenic acid • Secoisolariciresinol diglucoside

Abbreviations

CVD	Cardiovascular disease
LDL	Low-density lipoprotein
HDL	High-density lipoprotein
HRT	Hormone replacement therapy

M. Meister, B.S.
Nutritional Sciences Department, Oklahoma State University, 301 Human Sciences, Stillwater, OK 74078, USA
e-mail: mmeist@okstate.edu

B.J. Smith, Ph.D.
Nutritional Sciences Department, Oklahoma State University, 420 Human Sciences, Stillwater, OK 74078, USA
e-mail: bjsmith@okstate.edu

B.H. Arjmandi, Ph.D.
Department of Nutrition, Food and Exercise, Florida State University, 436A Sandels Building, Tallahassee, FL 32306, USA
e-mail: barjmandi@fsu.edu

E.A. Lucas, Ph.D. (✉)
Nutritional Sciences Department, Oklahoma State University, 422 Human Sciences, Stillwater, OK 74078, USA
e-mail: edralin.a.lucas@okstate.edu

C.J.H. Martin et al. (eds.), *Nutrition and Diet in Menopause*, Nutrition and Health,
DOI 10.1007/978-1-62703-373-2_15, © Springer Science+Business Media New York 2013

SDG	Secoisolariciresinol diglucoside
ALA	α-Linolenic acid
sVCAM	Soluble cell adhesion molecules
vWF	von Willebrand factor
Ovx	Ovariectomized
TG	Triglycerides
WF	Whole flaxseed
FO	Flaxseed oil
Lp(a)	Lipoprotein (a)
CRP	C-Reactive protein
EPA	Eicosapentanoic acid

Introduction

Cardiovascular disease (CVD) is considered a major public health issue worldwide [1]. It continues to be the leading cause of death in the USA each year and the health care costs associated with CVD were $411 billion in 2011 [2]. The number of deaths per year resulting from cardiovascular related disease was 823,804 individuals in 2007. Of these deaths 51.8 % were females and CVD is the major cause of mortality of almost half a million women, which is more than any other disease [2].

Menopausal status in women plays a significant role to their increased risk for CVD. While the incidence of CVD in premenopausal women is relatively low compared to men of the same age, as serum estrogen decreases, this advantage in women dissipates, placing them at equal risk for CVD as their male counterparts [1, 3, 4]. The decrease in estrogen that occurs during perimenopause and menopause brings about metabolic changes that are somewhat independent of aging. In the perimenopausal and menopausal state, many traditional CVD risk factors are exacerbated, including changes in body composition, reduced glucose tolerance, abnormal plasma lipids, increased blood pressure, endothelial dysfunction, and vascular inflammation [4]. In terms of lipid profile, the onset of menopause is associated with the elevation in total cholesterol and low-density lipoprotein (LDL)-cholesterol concentrations and a decrease in high-density lipoprotein (HDL)-cholesterol, which put postmenopausal women at an increased risk for developing CVD [4]. An increase in age and a decrease in estrogen levels have been blamed for this increased CVD risk during menopause; however, the exact mechanism remains unknown.

Hormone replacement therapy (HRT) has been traditionally used to relieve menopausal symptoms and reduce the risk of CVD [3]. However, findings from the Women's Health Initiative Studies have shown that the risks involved in HRT outweighs the benefits and consequently, the use of HRT for the prevention of CVD is no longer recommended [3]. In addition to maintaining or improving healthy lifestyle practices, pharmacological options such as aspirin, beta blockers, and agents focused in the treatment of hyperlipidemia, hypertension, and diabetes are also being used to reduce CVD risk factors in postmenopausal women. While some of these pharmacological options are effective, they are often cost-prohibitive for long-term treatment and may be associated with side effects and contraindications. Therefore, alternative strategies for reducing CVD risk factors in postmenopausal women are continuously being explored.

Lifestyle and nutritional factors play an important role in the maintenance of cardiovascular health. In the past two decades, there has been considerable interest in exploring the health benefits of plant-based bioactive compounds. One of these products that have gained popularity in recent years is flaxseed. Flaxseed is one of the oldest known crops, dating back to as early as 5,000 B.C. Flaxseed was traditionally used for the production of industrial linseed oil and was not widely recognized as an edible grain [5]. Flaxseed and its components have become increasingly popular around the 1980s

Table 15.1 Typical composition of flaxseed and other products used in animal and human studies to investigate postmenopausal cardiovascular disease (CVD) [10]

Product	Energy (kcal)	Carbohydrate (g)	Fat (g)	Protein (g)	Total dietary fiber (g)	18:3 fatty acids (g)	SDG (mg)[a]
Amount/100 g product							
Flaxseed	492	34.2	34	19.5	27.9	18.1	324
Wheat germ	360	51.8	9.7	23.2	13.2	0.723	NA
Wheat bran	216	64.5	4.2	15.6	42.8	0.167	0.1
Oat, whole grain	389	66.2	6.9	16.9	10.6	0.121	0.02
Sesame seed	573	23.4	49.7	17.8	11.8	0.415	0.24
Sunflower seed	570	18.8	49.6	22.8	10.5	0.069	0.6

Flaxseed oil provides about 886 kcal and 60 g of 18:3 fatty acids for every 100 g product
SDG secoisolariciresinol diglucoside, *NA* not available
[a]Adapted from Bloeden et al. [9]

as dietary supplements because of its role in promoting cardiovascular health and other potential health benefits [6].

Flaxseed is a very rich source of the lignan secoisolariciresinol diglucoside (SDG), α-linolenic acid (ALA), and fiber (Table 15.1), all of which play an important role in improving cardiovascular health. Lignans belong to one of the three major groups of phytoestrogens and have been shown to have similar effects on lipid metabolism as endogenous estrogen [7, 8]. SDG is converted by colonic bacteria to the bioactive mammalian lignans, enterodiol and enterolactone [6, 8]. SDG is suspected of being one of the components in flaxseed responsible for reducing total- and LDL-cholesterol as well as increasing HDL-cholesterol by modulating enzymes involved in cholesterol metabolism [6, 7]. Flaxseed contains approximately 30–40 % lipids and is one of the richest sources of ALA [9]. ALA reduces the risk of CVD through its anti-inflammatory and antioxidant properties [9]. Flaxseed is also a good source of dietary fiber (Table 15.1) which is known to decrease fecal transit time, hence, a reduction in fat absorption.

Over the past two decades, results from several preclinical and clinical trials have demonstrated the effects of flaxseed and its bioactive components on CVD risk factors associated with the postmenopausal state. In the following sections the findings from these studies will be discussed along with their potential implications for the reduction of cardiovascular risk in postmenopausal women.

Effects of Flaxseed on CVD Risk Factors in Animal Models of Menopause

Animal models including monkeys, swine, sheep, rabbits, mice, rats, and genetically modified mice have been used to investigate changes in the vascular system during menopause and the effects of pharmacological options and dietary interventions [11–14]. Animal studies that investigated the cardio-protective properties of flaxseed have utilized the LDL-receptor deficient mice and hypercholesterolemic rats and rabbits [13, 14]. Limited animal studies have been conducted that investigated the effects of flaxseed using animal models of postmenopausal CVD. The ovariectomized animal model has been considered a suitable model for mimicking the effects of hormone deficiency associated with menopause [11, 15].

The ovariectomized hamster and rat are the two animal models that have been used to study the effects of flaxseed on postmenopausal CVD risk factors. Elevated LDL and total cholesterol along with changes in body composition are observed in these animal models, consistent with changes associated with menopause [11, 15]. Additionally, cost, ethical considerations, and ease of handling of these small laboratory animals make them a popular choice. Using these animal models, researchers have been able to determine the effects of flaxseed supplementation on lipid parameters and other CVD risk factors that develop with menopause (Table 15.2).

Table 15.2 Effects of flaxseed on animal models of postmenopausal CVD

Animal model	Treatment groups/dosage	Study duration (n)	Outcomes/major findings	References
Aged (16–19 m) albino rats	Control diet Ovestin (12 μg/kg b.wt.) Flaxseed (10 g/kg b.wt) Flaxseed (15 g/kg b.wt) Flaxseed (20 g/kg b.wt)	3 months (n = 10/group)	10 and 15 g flaxseed/ kg b.wt ↓ total- and LDL-cholesterol , and triglycerides ↑HDL-cholesterol	Osman et al. [12]
Ovariectomized (Ovx) hamsters	Sham (control diet) Ovx (control diet) Ovx (control diet) + 17β-estradiol injection Ovx + 7.5 % (w/w) flaxseed diet Ovx + 15 % (w/w) flaxseed diet Ovx + 22.5 % (w/w) flaxseed diet	4 months (n = 10/group)	All doses of flaxseed prevented the ↑ in total cholesterol due to Ovx, similar to 17β-estradiol All doses of flaxseed ↓aortic fatty streaks and incidence of lesion, similar to the sham group	Lucas et al. [16]
Ovx Wistar rats	Sham and ovx divided into 3 subgroups: Standard diet Fat rich Fat rich + flaxseed	9 months	Flaxseed modestly ↓ circulating soluble adhesion molecules of endothelial origin (sVCAM) and von Willebrand factor (vWF)	Ciurea et al. [17]
Ovx hamsters	Sham (control diet) Ovx (control diet) Ovx + 15 % (w/w) flaxseed (WF) diet Ovx + flaxseed oil (FO; equivalent oil to the flaxseed diet)	3 months (n = 12/group)	↑ cholesterol in Ovx vs. sham hamsters WF was more effective than FO in ↓ total cholesterol WF and FO ↑ 7α-hydroxylase protein levels	Lucas et al. [23]

One of the first studies to report the effects of flaxseed supplementation on CVD using an animal model of ovarian hormone deficiency was by Lucas and colleagues [16]. In this study with ovariectomized hamsters, the effects of flaxseed supplementation (i.e., three different doses) on lipid metabolism and atherosclerotic lesion formation were compared to animals receiving estrogen replacement [16]. All three doses of flaxseed prevented the rise in total cholesterol associated with ovarian hormone deficiency [16]. However, the decrease in total cholesterol was not proportional to the amount of flaxseed in the diet, implying that a low dose of flaxseed may provide as much of a cardioprotective effects as higher dose in this animal model. In addition to the reduction in serum total cholesterol, this study also demonstrated that flaxseed had a considerable impact on the prevention of atherosclerotic lesion formation due to ovarian hormone deficiency. This study provided important evidence that supplementing the diet with flaxseed may not only be beneficial in terms of the lipid profile, but also prevents the actual development of atherosclerotic plaque.

Similar research has also been performed using ovariectomized and aged rats as a model of postmenopausal CVD [16, 17]. However, these rat models may not be ideal for lipid studies as they are associated with a number of shortcomings including high HDL to LDL ratio, requirement of high cholesterol diets with supplemental bile acids and thiouracil to develop hypercholesterolemia, and bile acid secretion and the organ contribution of cholesterol synthesis varies significantly from humans [18]. Nonetheless, rat models have been used for investigating the effects of flaxseed on postmenopausal CVD.

Osman and colleagues used aged albino rats as a model of postmenopausal ovarian hormone deficiency [12]. In their study, they compared the effects of four different doses of flaxseed (0, 10, 15, 20 g/kg b. wt) to that of estradiol (Ovestin) on lipid parameters. The results of this study were in agreement with the findings of Lucas and colleagues [16], in that a significant decrease in total cholesterol, triglycerides and LDL cholesterol also occurred in the groups supplemented with the lower doses of flaxseed [12]. These findings indicate that even lower doses of flaxseed may confer cardiovascular benefits.

Ciurea and colleagues [17] has investigated the effects of flaxseed together with high fat diet on endothelial dysfunction and atherosclerosis using ovariectomized Wistar rats (Table 15.2). Endothelial dysfunction as indicated by an increase concentration of circulating adhesion molecules was observed in this animal model when given a diet rich in saturated lipid. Dietary supplementation with flaxseed was able to modestly reduce plasma concentrations of circulating soluble adhesion molecules of endothelial origin (sVCAM) and von Willebrand factor (vWF). The authors concluded that flaxseed can delay or prevent endothelial dysfunction associated with high fat diet in estrogen deficient animals through its anti-inflammatory actions.

The promising findings related to flaxseed have lead to investigation into the component of flaxseed responsible for its cardiovascular protective effects. Jenkins and colleagues [19] attributed the cholesterol lowering effect of flaxseed primarily to the flaxseed gum. However, other constituents present in flaxseed may also play an essential role in lipid metabolism. For example, flaxseed is a rich source of ALA which has been reported to improve lipid profile in both animal models and human studies [6, 18]. ALA in flaxseed is thought to contribute to the prevention of atherosclerosis due to its anti-proliferative and anti-inflammatory properties [18]. The lignan precursor present in flaxseed, SDG, may also play an important role in lipid metabolism by modulating enzymes involved in cholesterol metabolism (i.e., 7α-hydroxylase and acyl CoA cholesterol transferase) [20]. The fiber in flaxseed has also been considered an important contributor to the health benefits by decreasing postprandial glucose absorption and increasing fecal excretion [21, 22]. Any one or all of these components may be responsible for the cardiovascular health benefits of flaxseed, but at the present time the bioactive component(s) remain uncertain.

In an attempt to determine whether flaxseed oil is the contributing factor to the hypocholesterolemic properties of flaxseed in ovarian hormone deficiency, Lucas and colleagues compared ground flaxseed to flaxseed oil [23]. The results of this study showed that ground flaxseed prevented the increase in circulating levels of cholesterol due to ovariectomy to a greater extent than flaxseed oil, indicating that other components are also involved [23]. Additionally, increased hepatic protein levels 7α-hydroxylase suggests that increased bile acid synthesis is one of the major cholesterol-lowering mechanisms of flaxseed.

While the research using animal model is limited, the results clearly suggest that flaxseed has a cardioprotective role in animal models of menopause by modulating lipid profile and/or improving endothelial function. Additionally, flaxseed may also delay or prevent atherosclerotic plaque formation associated with estrogen deficiency. Bassett and colleagues [24] attributed the anti-atherogenic action of flaxseed to three possible cellular mechanisms: (1) the powerful antioxidative effects of lignan, (2) the anti-inflammatory properties of ALA, and/or (3) the inhibition of cell proliferation. One may also extrapolate from the findings of the other animal models to further understand the role of flaxseed in reducing CVD risk factors associated with ovarian hormone deficiency. For example, flaxseed may modulate blood glucose in ovarian hormone deficiency as SDG from flaxseed was shown to prevent the development of diabetes in animal models of diabetes [25, 26]. SDG was also shown to significantly reduced high-fat diet-induced visceral and liver fat accumulation, hyperlipidemia, hypercholesterolemia, hyperinsulinemia, and hyperleptinemia in mice [25]. Additionally, ALA has been shown to have blood pressure lowering properties in spontaneously hypertensive rats [27]. Clearly, these animal studies demonstrate that flaxseed is beneficial to the heart and can reduce CVD risk factors in ovarian hormone deficiency. The clinical trials discussed in the next section will review the existing evidence related to the effects of dietary flaxseed supplementation in postmenopausal women.

Clinical Trials in Postmenopausal Women on the Effects of Flaxseed on CVD Risk Factors

Interestingly, there has been greater emphasis on the study of flaxseed on postmenopausal CVD in clinical trials compared to those using animal models (Table 15.3). Most of these clinical studies have incorporated flaxseed into breads, muffins, or food bars and the amounts of flaxseed have ranged from 25 to 50 g daily. Another distinguishing feature of these studies is that the duration of supplementation has ranged from 6 weeks, which was the shortest study duration, to 1 year as the longest.

The study by Arjmandi and colleagues [28] was one of the first clinical trials that investigated the effects of daily flaxseed supplementation on lipid profile of hypercholesterolemic postmenopausal women (Table 15.3). In a double-blind cross-over study, participants consumed bread and muffins containing either flaxseed or sunflower seed (38 g/day) for 6 weeks with a 2-week washout period between treatments. They reported that both flaxseed and sunflower seed treatments lowered serum total cholesterol, but only flaxseed was effective in lowering lipoprotein (a) [Lp(a)] concentration, which is considered a strong predictor of CVD because it interferes with fibrinolysis and promotes foam cell formation and atherosclerotic lesion [29, 30]. They attributed this positive effect of flaxseed on Lp(a) to be due to its lignan content which have been shown to exhibit some estrogenic activity [31]. Based on the evidence that estrogen is effective in lowering serum Lp(a) in postmenopausal women, flaxseed's lignan may act through a similar mechanism [32].

In a follow-up study, this same group investigated the effect of 3 months supplementation of ground flaxseed (40 g/day) compared to wheat-based control in Caucasian postmenopausal women [33]. Flaxseed lowered both serum total- and non-HDL cholesterol concentrations as well as apolipoprotein A-1 and B [33]. Jenkins and colleagues [19] also found that supplementation with 50 g of defatted flaxseed for 3 weeks reduced total- and LDL-cholesterol, apolipoprotein B and A-1 in hyperlipidemic men and postmenopausal women. Bloeden and colleagues [34] also observed a reduction in Lp(a) and improvement in insulin sensitivity in hyperlipidemic men and postmenopausal women that was given 40 g of ground flaxseed per day for 10 weeks coupled with a low fat and low cholesterol diet. In addition to reductions in total cholesterol, Dodin and colleagues [35] show that daily consumption flaxseed (40 g/day) for 1 year slightly reduces body weight and blood pressure in healthy French Canadian postmenopausal women.

The effect of flaxseed supplementation was investigated by Patade and colleagues [36] on Native American postmenopausal women. Approximately 60 % of this population has one or more CVD risk factors including high blood cholesterol, diabetes, hypertension and obesity, which make them a high risk group for CVD [37]. Flaxseed also lowered total- and LDL-cholesterol in Native American postmenopausal women. Their findings indicate that Native American postmenopausal women will also benefit from flaxseed consumption similar to what has been seen in Caucasian postmenopausal women.

Although most of the clinical studies on flaxseed show positive effects on lipid profile, a few studies have shown that flaxseed supplementation has no effect on serum lipids of postmenopausal women [38–40]. The longest duration of flaxseed supplementation (i.e., 1 year) in French-Canadian women who were approximately 5 years postmenopause demonstrate that flaxseed affected apo A-1 and apo B (4.4 % and 3 % increase in the flaxseed group vs. 11.6 % and 7 % increase in the wheat germ group in apo A-1 and apo B concentration, respectively) but has no effects on LDL particle size, markers of hemostatic balance, inflammatory mediators or glucose metabolism in comparison to wheat germ [38]. Similarly, recent studies by Simbalista et al. [39] in Brazilian postmenopausal women and Coulman et al. [40] on Canadian postmenopausal women show that flaxseed is not more effective than placebo in improving lipid profile and biomarkers of oxidative stress. Both these studies supplemented postmenopausal women with 25 g of flaxseed daily for 4–12 weeks. The lower amount of flaxseed in these two studies may be one reason that they did not observe an effect with flaxseed supplementation.

Table 15.3 Clinical trials in postmenopausal women investigating the effects of whole or ground flaxseed on risk factors of cardiovascular disease

Subject characteristics/study design and duration	Treatment groups (*n*)	Outcomes	References
Positive effects			
Hyperlipidemic (men = 22; postmenopausal women = 7) Double-blind, cross-over design 3 weeks treatment and >2 weeks washout	4 muffins daily containing: ~50 g partially defatted flaxseed meal + white flour Wheat bran flour + whole-meal flour	Flaxseed ↓ total- and LDL-cholesterol, apolipoprotein B and A-1	Jenkins et al. [19]
Hypercholesterolemic American women Double-blind, cross-over design 6 weeks treatment and 2 weeks washout	4 slices of bread and 3 muffins daily containing (38 g/day) of (*n* = 23): Flaxseed or Sunflower seed	↓ total cholesterol in both treatments ↓ LDL-cholesterol and lipoprotein (a) only with flaxseed	Arjmandi et al. [28]
American women single-blind, placebo control 3 m treatment	40 g daily of: Ground flaxseed (*n* = 20), or Wheat based control (*n* = 16)	Flaxseed ↓ total cholesterol and non-HDL cholesterol	Lucas et al. [33]
Hypercholesterolemic American adults (postmenopausal women and men) Single-blind, placebo control 10 weeks treatment	Following a low fat and low cholesterol diet and daily consumption of breads and muffins containing: 40 g/day ground flaxseed (men = 16; women = 14) or Matched wheat bran (men = 15; women = 17)	Flaxseed ↓LDL at 5 weeks but not sustained at 10 weeks Flaxseed ↓HDL but not in women Flaxseed improves insulin sensitivity No effect on markers of inflammation (i.e., C-reactive protein and interleukin-6) or oxidative stress (i.e., oxidized LDL and urinary isoprostanes)	Bloeden et al. [34]
French-Canadian women ~5 year postmenopause Double-blind, placebo control 12 m treatment	2 slices of bread + powder daily containing (total of 40 g/day): Ground flaxseed (21,071 μg total lignans daily; *n* = 85), or Wheat germ (196 μg total lignan daily; *n* = 94)	Flaxseed ↓ total- and HDL-cholesterol Mild decrease in body weight and blood pressure	Dodin et al. [35]
Mildly to moderately hypercholesterolemic Native American women Single-blind, placebo control 3 m treatment	Daily consumption of: Control (2 slices white bread + 2 muffins; *n* = 9) 35 g flaxseed (2 slices bread + 2 muffins + 2 tbsp flax powder; *n* = 17) 35 g flaxseed + 8 g oat bran soluble fiber (2 slices bread + 2 muffins + 2 tbsp flax powder; *n* = 16)	↓ in total- and LDL-cholesterol in both flaxseed groups No changes in C-reactive protein, hematological parameters	Patade et al. [36]
Modest to no effects			
French-Canadian women ~5 year postmenopause Double-blind, placebo control 12 m treatment	2 slices of bread + powder containing (total of 40 g/day) daily: Ground flaxseed (21,071 μg total lignans daily; *n* = 85), or Wheat germ (196 μg total lignan daily; *n* = 94)	Modest effect on apolipoprotein B and A-1 No effect on LDL electrophoretic characteristics, glucose, insulin, fibrinogen, and C-reactive protein	Dodin et al. [38]
Brazilian women 1–10 year postmenopause Double-blind, placebo control 12 weeks treatment	2 slices of bread daily containing: Flaxseed (25 g/day; 46 mg/day lignan; *n* = 20), or Wheat bran (<1 mg lignan; *n* = 18)	No significant difference in lipid profile or climacteric symptoms compared to the control	Simbalista et al.[39]
Canadian women (*n* = 16) >10 year postmenopause Cross-over design 4 weeks treatment and 4 weeks washout	Food bars containing: Flaxseed (25 g) Sesame seeds (25 g) Flaxseed + sesame seeds (12.5 g each)	No effect on plasma Lipids Antioxidant markers (total antioxidant power, LDL and protein oxidation)	Coulman et al. [40]

Table 15.4 Clinical trials in postmenopausal women investigating the effects of the flaxseed lignan complex (secoisolari-ciresinol diglucoside, SDG) on cardiovascular disease risk factors

Subject characteristics/ study design and duration	Treatment groups (*n*)	Outcomes	References
Healthy European women Double-blind, cross-over design 6 weeks treatment and 6 weeks washout	1 low-fat muffin daily containing (*n* = 22): Lignan complex (500 mg SDG/day), or No lignan complex	↓ in CRP concentrations with lignan complex No effect on other inflammatory markers (i.e., interleukin-6, tumor necrosis factor-α) and adhesion molecules (i.e., soluble intercellular adhesion molecules-1, sICAM-1; soluble vascular cell adhesion molecule-1, sVCAM-1; monocyte chemotactic protein-1, MCP-1)	Hallund et al. [7]
Healthy European women Double-blind, cross-over design 6 weeks treatment and 6 weeks washout	1 low-fat muffin daily containing (*n* = 22): 500 mg/day lignan complex SDG No lignan	Lignan has no effect on plasma lipid concentrations, serum lipoprotein oxidation resistance, or plasma antioxidant capacity	Hallund et al. [41]
Healthy European women Double-blind, cross-over design 6 weeks treatment and 6 weeks washout	1 low-fat muffin daily containing (*n* = 22): Lignan complex (500 mg SDG/day), or No lignan complex	Lignan has no effect on endothelial function (i.e., plasma nitrite and nitrate, endothelin-1, and asymmetric diarginine)	Hallund et al. [42]

Despite some example of studies which have not supported cardiovascular protective effects of flaxseed, the preponderance of the evidence supports benefits in some populations. In light of these potential beneficial effects, the question remains as to what bioactive compound(s) in flaxseed is responsible. In an attempt to determine whether it is the lignan in flaxseed responsible for its cardiovascular effects, Hallund and colleagues [41, 42] supplemented postmenopausal women with muffins containing 500 mg SDG for 6 weeks (Table 15.4). In their first paper [41], they reported that SDG has no effect on plasma lipid, lipoprotein oxidation resistance, and antioxidant capacity. A second report [42] from this group from the same study show that plant lignans isolated from flaxseed has no effect on endothelial function in healthy postmenopausal women. The final report from the same group examined the effects of lignan on inflammatory markers [7]. Their results show that C-reactive protein increased in both the lignan and the placebo groups but the increase was higher in the placebo group. The results of these three studies show that the lignan in flaxseed had a modest effect on inflammation marker, but no effects on plasma lipid concentrations, antioxidant capacity, and endothelial function in healthy postmenopausal women (Table 15.4). Some possible explanation for the modest effect of lignan on CVD risk factors from these three studies include the following: (1) the short duration of the study (i.e., 6 weeks) might not be sufficient to observe significant changes particularly in endothelial function; (2) participants were generally healthy and it is hard to observe distinct effects of flaxseed; and (3) lignans may work synergistically with the other components to improve CVD risk factors.

Another component of flaxseed that is thought to be responsible for its health benefit is its oil content that is rich in ALA. To our knowledge, there are no studies that investigate the effects of flaxseed oil specifically in postmenopausal women. However, a study by Allman et al. [43] showed that the platelet eicosapentanoic acid (EPA) is more than doubled in healthy young males consuming flaxseed oil in comparison to those supplemented with sunflower oil. The increase in EPA can lead to a decrease in platelet aggregation which may offer protection against thrombus formation and the associated acute cardiovascular event. Other investigators have also shown reduction in inflammatory markers and adhesion molecules with flaxseed oil supplementation [44, 45]. Whether these cardiovascular effects of flaxseed oil will be similar in postmenopausal women is not clear at this time.

Conclusion

In general, both animal and human studies demonstrate that in ovarian hormone deficiency, regular consumption of flaxseed may reduce CVD risk factors. Most of the observed positive effect of flaxseed in postmenopausal women is on their ability to improve lipid profile. These changes include lowering total cholesterol, LDL-cholesterol and triglyceride concentrations. However, some positive effects were also noted on endothelial function, antioxidant status, body weight, inflammatory markers, blood pressure and glucose. To date, the findings discussed from studies attempting to identify the bioactive components in flaxseed show that isolated components have modest effects in modifying CVD risk factors in postmenopausal women. Postmenopausal women may benefit more from incorporating whole flaxseed into their diet as opposed to adding individual components of flaxseed such as the fiber, ALA, and lignan. However, further studies are warranted to understand the mechanism by which flaxseed alters CVD risk and these studies may provide new insight into the bioactive components. Taken together, the results of clinical studies demonstrate that flaxseed can be a part of a heart healthy diet of postmenopausal women.

References

1. Zhang Y. Cardiovascular diseases in American women. Nutr Metab Cardiovasc Dis. 2010;20:386–93.
2. Roger VL, Go AS, Lloyd-Jones DM, Benjamin EJ, Berry JD, Borden WB, et al. Heart disease and stroke statistics—2012 update: a report from the American Heart Association. Circulation. 2012;125:e2–220.
3. Yang X, Reckelhoff JF. Estrogen, hormonal replacement therapy and cardiovascular disease. Curr Opin Nephrol Hypertens. 2011;20(2):133–8.
4. Rosano GM, Vitale C, Marazzi G, Volterrani M. Menopause and cardiovascular disease: the evidence. Climacteric. 2007;10:19–24.
5. Singh KK, Mridula D, Rehal J, Barnwal P. Flaxseed: a potential source of food, feed and fiber. Crit Rev Fod Sci Nutr. 2011;51(3):210–22.
6. Cunnane SC, Hamadeh MJ, Liede AC, Thompson LU, Wolever TM, Jenkins DJ. Nutritional attributes of traditional flaxseed in healthy young adults. Am J Clin Nutr. 1995;61:62–8.
7. Hallund J, Tetens I, Bügel S, Tholstrup T, Brunn JM. The effect of a lignan complex isolated from flaxseed on inflammation markers in healthy postmenopausal women. Nutr Metab Cardiovasc Dis. 2008;18:497–502.
8. Peterson J, Dwyer J, Adlercreutz H, Scalbert A, Jacques P, McCullough MJ. Dietary lignans: physiology and potential for cardiovascular disease risk reduction. Nutr Rev. 2010;68(10):571–603.
9. Bloedon LT, Szapary PO. Flaxseed and cardiovascular disease. Nutr Rev. 2004;62(1):18–27.
10. U.S. Department of Agriculture, Agricultural Research Service. USDA National Nutrient Database for Standard Reference, Release 24. Nutrient Data Laboratory Home Page; 2011. http://www.ars.usda.gov/ba/bhnrc/ndl.
11. Russell RG. Ibandronate: pharmacology and preclinical studies. Bone. 2006;38(4):S7–12.
12. Osman HF, Yousef Ayad SK, Abdel-Aziz EL-Mahdy A. The potential effect of flaxseed on female postmenopausal rats. Nature Sci. 2011;9(4):1–8.
13. Dupasquier CM, Dibrov E, Kneesh AL, Cheung PK, Lee KG, Alexander HK, et al. Dietary flaxseed inhibits atherosclerosis in the LDL receptor-deficient mouse in part through antiproliferative and anti-inflammatory actions. Am J Physiol Heart Circ Physiol. 2007;293(4):H2394–402.
14. Prasad K. Reduction of serum cholesterol and hypercholesterolemic atherosclerosis in rabbits by seciosolariciresinol diglucoside isolated from flaxseed. Circulation. 1999;99:1355–62.
15. Sohn E, Daggy BP, Arjmandi BH. Ovariectomized hamster: a potential model of postmenopausal hypercholestolemia. J Nutr Biochem. 1999;10:660–3.
16. Lucas EA, Lightfoot SA, Hammond LJ, Devareddy L, Khalil DA, Daggy BP, et al. Flaxseed reduces plasma cholesterol and atherosclerotic lesion formation in ovariectomized golden Syrian hamsters. Atherosclerosis. 2004;73:223–9.
17. Ciurea E, Mocanu V, Haliga R, Obroceanu D, Iamandei GL, Luca V, et al. Nutritional antioxidant effects on endothelial dysfunctions in experimental atherosclerosis by ovariectomy. Rev Med Chir Soc Med Nat Iasi. 2009;113(3):726–31.
18. Harris WS. n3 fatty acids and serum lipoproteins: animal studies. Am J Clin Nutr. 1997;65:1611S–6.

19. Jenkins DJA, Kendall CW, Vidgen E, Agarwal S, Rao AV, Rosenberg RS, et al. Health aspects of partially defatted flaxseed, including effects on serum lipids, oxidative measures and ex vivo androgen and progestin activity: a controlled crossover trial. Am J Clin Nutr. 1999;69:395–402.
20. Sanghvi A, Divven W, Seltman H. Inhibition of rat liver cholesterol 7-alpha hydroxylase and acetyl CoA:cholesterol aceyl transferase activities by entrodiol and enterolactone. In: Kritchevsky D, editor. Proceedings of the symposium on drugs affecting lipid metabolism. New York: Plenum Press; 1984. p. 311–22.
21. Kritchevsky D. Fiber effects of hyperlipidemia. In: Cunnane SC, Thompson LUE, editors. Flaxseed in human nutrition. Champaign, IL: AOCS Press; 1995. p. 174–86.
22. Wolever T. Flaxseed and glucose metabolism. In: Cunnane S, Thompson LU, editors. Flaxseed in human nutrition. Champaign, IL: AOCS Press; 1995. p. 157–64.
23. Lucas EA, Mahajan SS, Soung do Y, Lightfoot SA, Smith BJ, Arjmandi BH. Flaxseed but not flaxseed oil prevented the rise in serum cholesterol due to ovariectomy in the Golden Syrian hamsters. J Med Food. 2011;14(3): 261–7.
24. Bassett CMC, Rodriguez-Leyya D, Pierce GN. Experimental and clinical research findings on the cardiovascular benefits of consuming flaxseed. Appl Physiol Nutr Metab. 2009;34:965–74.
25. Fukumitsu S, Aida K, Ueno N, Ozawa S, Takahashi Y, Kobori M. Flaxseed lignan attenuates high-fat diet-induced fat accumulation and induces adiponectin expression in mice. Br J Nutr. 2008;6:1–8.
26. Prasad K. Secoisolariciresinol diglucoside from flaxseed delays the development of type 2 diabetes in Zucker rat. J Lab Clin Med. 2001;138:32–9.
27. Ogawa A, Suzuki Y, Aoyama T, Takeuchi H. Dietary alpha-linolenic acid inhibits angiotensin-converting enzyme activity and mRNA expression levels in the aorta of spontaneously hypertensive rats. J Oleo Sci. 2009; 58(7):355–60.
28. Arjmandi BH, Khan DA, Juma S, Drum M, Venkatesh S, Sohn E, et al. Whole flaxseed consumption lowers serum LDL-cholesterol and lipoprotein (a) concentrations in postmenopausal women. Nutr Res. 1998;18(7):1203–14.
29. Loscalzo J, Weinfeld M, Fless GM, Scanu AM. Lipoprotein(a), fibrin binding, and plasminogen activation. Arteriosclerosis. 1990;10:240.
30. Zioncheck TF, Powell LM, Rice GC, Eaton DL, Lawn RM. Interaction of recombinant apolipoprotein(a) and lipoprotein(a) with macrophages. J Clin Invest. 1991;87:767–71.
31. Setchell KDR, Adlercrutz H. Mammalian lignans and phytoestogens. Recent studies on their formation, metabolism and biological role in health and disease. In: Rowland IA, editor. The role of gut microflora in toxicity and cancer. New York: Academic Press; 1988. p. 315–45.
32. Shewmon DA, Stock JL, Rosen CJ, Heiniluoma KM, Hogue MM, Morrison A, et al. Tamoxifen and estrogen lower circulating lipoprotein (a) concentrations in healthy postmenopausal women. Aterioscler Thromb. 1994;14(10):1586–93.
33. Lucas EA, Wild RD, Hammond LJ, Devareddy L, Khalil DA, Daggy BP, et al. Flaxseed improves lipid profile without altering biomarkers of bone metabolism in postmenopausal women. J Clin Endocrinol Metab. 2002;87(4):1527–32.
34. Bloedon LT, Balikai S, Chittams J, Cunnane SC, Berlin JA, Rader DJ, et al. Flaxseed and cardiovascular disease risk factors: results from a double blind, randomized, controlled clinical trial. J Am Coll Nutr. 2008;27(1):65–74.
35. Dodin S, Leman A, Jacques H, Legare F, Forest JC, Masse B. The effects of flaxseed dietary supplement on lipid profile, bone mineral density and symptoms in menopausal women: a randomized, double-blind, wheat germ placebo-controlled clinical trial. J Clin Endocrinol Metab. 2005;90(3):1390–7.
36. Patade A, Devareddy L, Lucas EA, Korlagunta K, Daggy BP, Arjmandi BH. Flaxseed reduces total and LDL cholesterol concentrations in Native American postmenopausal women. J Womens Health (Larchmt). 2008;17(3): 355–66.
37. Sjoberg L, Kaaja R, Tuomilehto J. Epidemiology of postmenopausal hypertension. Int J Clin Pract Suppl. 2004; 139:4.
38. Dodin S, Cunnae SC, Masse B, Lemay A, Jacques H, Asselin G, et al. Flaxseed on cardiovascular disease markers in healthy menopausal women: a randomized, double-blind, placebo-controlled trial. Nutrition. 2008;24:23–30.
39. Simbalista RL, Sauerbronn AV, Aldrighi JM, Areas JAG. Consumption of a flaxseed-rich food is not more effective than a placebo in alleviating the climacteric symptoms of postmenopausal women. J Nutr. 2010;140:293–7.
40. Coulman KD, Liu Z, Michaelides J, Quan Hum W, Thompson LU. Fatty acids and lignans in unground whole flaxseed and sesame seed are bioavailable but have minimal antioxidant and lipid-lowering effects in postmenopausal women. Mol Nutr Food Res. 2009;53:1366–75.
41. Hallund J, Tetens I, Bügel S, Tholstrup T, Tetens I. A lignan complex isolated from flaxseed does not affect plasma lipid concentrations or antioxidant capacity in healthy postmenopausal women. J Nutr. 2006;136:112–6.

42. Hallund J, Tetens I, Bügel S, Tholstrup T, Ferrari M, Terrlink T, et al. Daily consumption for six weeks of a lignan complex isolated from flaxseed does not affect endothelial function in healthy postmenopausal women. J Nutr. 2006;136:2314–8.
43. Allman MA, Pena MM, Pang D. Supplementation with flaxseed oil versus sunflower seed oil in healthy young men consuming a low fat diet: effects on platelet composition and function. Eur J Clin Nutr. 1995;49(4):169–78.
44. Gillingham LG, Gustafson JA, Han SY, Jassal DS, Jones PJ. High-oleic rapeseed (canola) and flaxseed oils modulate serum lipids and inflammatory biomarkers in hypercholesterolaemic subjects. Br J Nutr. 2011;105(3):417–27.
45. Rallidis LS, Paschos G, Papaioannou ML, Liakos GK, Panagiotakos DB, Anastisiadis G, et al. The effect of diet enriched with alpha-linolenic acid on soluble cellular adhesion molecules in dyslipidaemic patients. Atherosclerosis. 2004;174(1):127–32.

Chapter 16
Magnesium Metabolism in Menopause

S.S. Avinash, Sreekantha, and B.K. Manjunatha Goud

Key Points

- Magnesium is a major mineral which is regulated at the level of kidney, bone and intestine.
- Parathormone (PTH), calcitonin, vitamin D, estrogen and cytokines are involved in regulation of magnesium.
- Menopause is associated with various endocrine changes and also alterations in magnesium metabolism.
- Oestrogen deficiency associated with menopause causes alteration in the metabolism of magnesium at the level of kidney, bone and intestine.
- Oestrogen deficiency induces various molecular and genetic changes which affect the uptake, intracellular transport and basolateral extrusion of magnesium in kidney and intestine.
- Oestrogen deficiency in menopause, also induces alteration in maturation, differentiation, activity, lifespan and cytokine secretion of osteoblasts and osteoclasts, leading to increased bone resorption and hence alteration in the metabolism of the bone mineral—magnesium.

Keywords Menopause • Oestrogen • Magnesium • Osteoporosis • Metabolism

Abbreviation

PTH	Parathormone
TRPM	Transient receptor potential melastatin
TRPV	Transient receptor potential vanilloid

S.S. Avinash, M.B.B.S., M.D. (✉)
Department of Biochemistry, Father Muller Medical College, Father Muller Road Kankanady, Mangalore, Karnataka 575002, India
e-mail: dravinash.ss@gmail.com; dravinashshimoga@yahoo.co.in

Sreekantha, M.B.B.S., M.D.
Department of Biochemistry, Navodaya Medical College, Raichur, Karnataka 584103, India
e-mail: grsreekantha@yahoo.com

B.K.M. Goud, M.B.B.S., M.D.
Department of Biochemistry, RAK College of Medical Sciences, RAK Medical and Health Sciences University, 11172, Ras Al Khaimah, United Arab Emirates
e-mail: drmanjunathag@gmail.com

C.J.H. Martin et al. (eds.), *Nutrition and Diet in Menopause*, Nutrition and Health,
DOI 10.1007/978-1-62703-373-2_16, © Springer Science+Business Media New York 2013

PCT	Proximal convoluted tubule
DCT	Distal convoluted tubule
CD	Collecting duct
ECF	Extracellular fluid
ICF	Intracellular fluid
CB	Calbindin
VDR	Vitamin D receptor
RXR	Retinoid receptor
VDRE	Vitamin D responsive element
RNA	Ribonucleic acid
DNA	Deoxyribonucleic acid
IGF	Insulin like growth factor
ER	Oestrogen receptor
KO	Knockout
GH	Growth hormone
IL	Interleukin
MCSF	Macrophage colony stimulating factor
TNF	Tumour necrosis factor
IFN	Interferon
ROS	Reactive oxygen species
REA	Repressor protein of oestrogen receptor activity
PDGF	Platelet-derived growth factor
OPG	Osteoprotegerin
RANK	Receptor activator of nuclear factor kappa beta
RANKL	Receptor activator of nuclear factor kappa beta ligand
RDA	Recommended daily allowance

Introduction

Menopause is associated with various hormonal changes and alterations in homeostasis of bone and mineral metabolism. Magnesium homeostasis is regulated directly or/and indirectly by hormones like parathormone (PTH), calcitriol, calcitonin and oestrogen at the levels of intestinal absorption, bone formation, bone resorption and renal reabsorption. Various cytokines also play an important role in the regulation. Nutrition, physiology and metabolism of these hormones in postmenopausal women are vastly different from healthy premenopausal women, predominantly due to deficiency of oestrogen observed in menopause. This article is intended to review various changes in the metabolism of magnesium at the molecular level, secondary to hormonal and other changes observed in menopause compared to the nutrition, physiology, diet and metabolism of normal healthy premenopausal women.

Magnesium Metabolism

Magnesium is the fourth most abundant cation in the body and second most abundant cation in the intracellular fluid. It plays an essential role in the intracellular regulation of metabolism since it is required as a cofactor to about more than 300 enzymes [1]. It also regulates several membrane channels, neuromuscular excitability, and cardiac rhythm, and is required for secretion of hormones like insulin, maintenance of immune function, and also in bone mineral density [1]. By forming stable ternary

Table 16.1 Magnesium distribution in the body

Total body magnesium	20–28 g
Bones	60 % of total body magnesium (14,600 mg) (30 % of bone magnesium in stable compartment) (70 % of bone magnesium in mobile compartment)
Muscle	4,250 mg
Other	2,070 mg
RBC	145 mg
ECF	270 mg

Source: Adapted from [1]
60 % of the total body magnesium is present in bones which serve as a major reservoir. Magnesium present in bones is distributed in a stable slowly exchangeable compartment as a complex of salts and a mobile, easily exchangeable compartment as a surface mineral. About 25 % is distributed in skeletal muscle. The remaining is distributed in organs with high metabolic rates such as myocardium, nervous tissue, digestive tract and kidney (*RBC* red blood cell, *ECF* extra cellular fluid)

Table 16.2 Requirement of magnesium

Age group	RDA of magnesium (mg)
1–3 years	80
4–8 years	130
9–13 years	240
14–18 years (boys)	410
14–18 years (girls)	360
Females adult	310–320
Pregnancy	350–400
Lactation	310–360
Males adult	400–420

Source: Adapted from [2]
Recommended daily allowance (RDA) of magnesium differs according to age and physiological conditions. RDA gradually increases with age in both males and females peaking at 14–18 years. Males have more RDA compared with females. RDA also increases during special physiological conditions like pregnancy and lactation

Table 16.3 Magnesium levels in serum

Serum level of magnesium	1.7–2.2 mg/dl
Ionic magnesium	65 % of serum magnesium
Complex to albumin	21 % of serum magnesium
Complex to globulin	9 % of serum magnesium
Complex to citrate, oxalate and phosphate	5 % of serum magnesium

Source: Adapted from [1]
Magnesium present in serum is in various forms. Ionic form: This is an active form. Non-ionic form: Magnesium complex with serum protein albumin, citrate, oxalate and phosphate. Non-ionic form is inactive

complex with nucleotides magnesium regulates transcription, translation and replication of DNA. Magnesium is distributed in various compartment of the body [1] (Table 16.1). Sources of magnesium are green leafy vegetables like spinach, legumes like beans and peas, nuts and seeds and whole unrefined grains. Magnesium requirement varies with age gender and physiological requirements [2] (Table 16.2). Magnesium is present in various forms in the serum [1] (Table 16.3).

Table 16.4 Normal metabolism magnesium in intestine

Average daily intake of magnesium	300 mg/day
Daily intestinal absorption of magnesium	125 mg/day
Daily intestinal secretion of magnesium	2.5 mg/day
Daily secretion of magnesium in faeces	170 mg/day

Source: Adapted from [5]
Part of the magnesium present in the diet is absorbed through intestine. Small amount of magnesium is also secreted into the intestine. The unabsorbed magnesium is excreted if faeces

Regulation of Magnesium at the Level of Intestine

Intestinal regulation of magnesium is absent or minor [3]. Regulation of intestinal absorption of magnesium is not related to magnesium status, physiological status or magnesium requirement of the body [4]. Metabolism of magnesium at the level of intestine is similar to calcium but not well regulated as calcium [5] (Table 16.4). Available data on the site and type of intestinal magnesium absorption are conflicting. Magnesium is absorbed throughout the intestine but predominantly in small intestine. It is absorbed by paracellular transport, transcellular transport and solvent drag [3] (Fig. 16.1). The passive paracellular transport of magnesium across the tight junctions is important only in a leaky epithelium and the passive diffusion is driven by chemical gradient of magnesium across intestinal lumen. At low dietary intake levels transcellular pathway is predominant whereas at usual dietary intake levels paracellular and solvent drag mode of absorption is operational [6]. Fractional intestinal absorption of magnesium is directly proportional to dietary intake of magnesium indicating the existence of paracellular pathway [7].

The active transcellular pathway in intestine includes luminal uptake of magnesium, the intracellular transport and basolateral extrusion of magnesium from the epithelium into the blood vessel (Fig. 16.1). Growing body of evidence suggests that the luminal uptake of magnesium in intestinal epithelium is presumably due to a magnesium carrier channel TRPM6 or a magnesium/2 cation exchange or magnesium/anion cotransport [7] (Fig. 16.1). The intracellular transport is regulated putatively by a yet to be characterised magnesium binding protein (Fig. 16.1). Basolateral extrusion of magnesium is supposedly by a magnesium/sodium exchange a secondary active transport driven by gradient created through Na–K ATPase (Fig. 16.1). Further research is needed to characterise the involved proteins. Recent studies have shown that TRPM6 is expressed predominantly in distal intestine and is involved in the regulation of magnesium absorption [7].

Studies in humans on the effect of calcitriol and magnesium absorption have yielded conflicting results, ranging from increase in magnesium absorption to no effect on magnesium absorption by the calcitriol administration. Significant vitamin D independent magnesium absorption seems to exist in humans. However, collective data in animals and humans suggest that in conditions of vitamin D deficiency, the magnesium absorption can be increased though in small amounts by pharmacologic doses of calcitriol and the physiological variations in the levels of calcitriol had no effect on magnesium absorption [8, 9].

Menopause and Intestinal Regulation of Magnesium

Not much is known in detail regarding the specificities of absorption of magnesium by the intestinal epithelium and the effect of various hormonal changes associated with menopause on the absorption mechanism of magnesium in intestine.

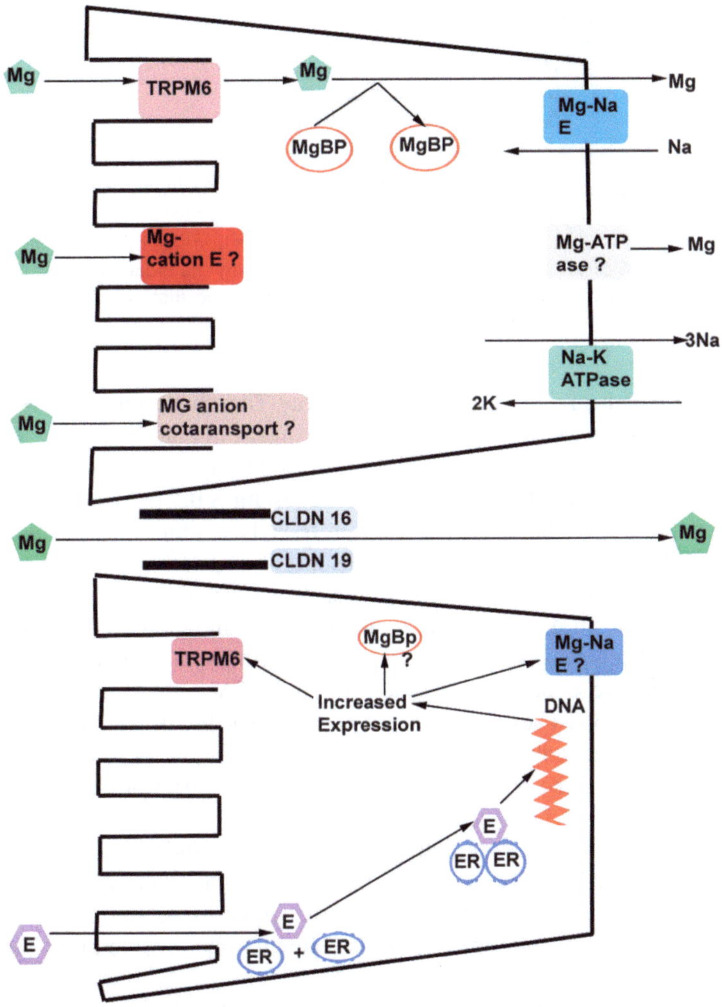

Fig. 16.1 Magnesium transport and effect of oestrogen on magnesium transport. Magnesium is transported by an active transcellular pathway; passive paracellular pathway and solvent drag [3]. Transcellular pathway involves uptake of magnesium by TRPM6 in intestine and kidney. TRPM7 is involved in the metabolism of magnesium in other cells. Role of magnesium/2 cation exchange protein and magnesium/anion cotransporter in the uptake of magnesium are yet to be elucidated completely [7]. The magnesium inside the cell is transported from apical to basolateral membrane by a yet to be elucidated magnesium binding protein similar to calcium binding protein [10]. At the basolateral membrane the magnesium is extruded by magnesium/sodium exchange protein, which is driven by the sodium gradient caused by sodium–potassium ATPase [10]. A magnesium ATPase is also proposed to be involved in basolateral extrusion [10]. Claudin 16 and claudin 19 are the tight junction proteins which are proposed to be involved in paracellular transport of magnesium. Oestrogen binds to intracellular oestrogen receptor which dimerises and binds to hormone responsive elements of genes involved in magnesium transport and increases the transcriptional expression of TRPM6 [12]. Role of oestrogen in regulation of expression of magnesium binding protein and magnesium/sodium exchange protein are yet to be elucidated [10] (*Mg* magnesium, *TRPM6* transcellular receptor potential melastatin 6, *Mg-Cation E* Magnesium/2 cation exchange protein, *MgBP* magnesium binding protein, *Na* sodium, *Mg–Na E* magnesium sodium exchange protein, *K* potassium, *CLDN* claudin, *E* oestrogen, *ER* oestrogen receptor)

Regulation of Magnesium at the Level of Kidney

Kidney plays a major role in the regulation of magnesium homeostasis [1] (Table 16.5). There is no evidence of secretion of magnesium in human kidneys. The reabsorption of magnesium in the cortical TAL is paracellular and driven by changes in transcellular voltage, whereas superficial portions of DCT

Table 16.5 Normal metabolism of magnesium in kidney

Filtered magnesium	3,400 mg/day
PCT	20–30 % of filtered magnesium
Loop of Henle	60–65 % of filtered magnesium
DCT	4 % of filtered magnesium
Magnesium excreted in urine	1–20 % of filtered magnesium depending upon dietary intake (about 120 mg/day)

Source: Adapted from [1]
80 % of the serum magnesium is ultra-filterable. With a glomerular filtration rate of 125 ml/min, almost 3,400 mg of magnesium is filtered. 90–99 % of the filtered magnesium is reabsorbed by the kidney tubules. Majority of the filtered magnesium is absorbed by the loop of henle. Unabsorbed fraction of magnesium is excreted in urine (*PCT* proximal convoluted tubule, *DCT* distal convoluted tubule)

reabsorbs magnesium through an active transcellular pathway. This transcellular pathway is well regulated. The transcellular active pathway in kidney involves apical uptake of magnesium by the proteins TRPM6, TRPM7, the gatekeepers of magnesium absorption followed by intracellular transport and basolateral extrusion [10] (Fig. 16.1). Paracellular absorption of magnesium is likely to be similar to that of calcium and sodium. The details are yet to be identified. Claudin 16 and Claudin 19 are the tight junction proteins which are proposed to be involved in paracellular transport of magnesium (Fig. 16.1).

Dietary magnesium restriction in humans increases the renal reabsorption of magnesium and decreases the urinary magnesium, whereas high dietary intake and increased plasma levels of magnesium decreases the renal reabsorption and increases the urinary magnesium level [11] (Fig. 16.2). Adaptation to dietary intake occurs mainly in PCT and cTAL. Paracellular transport in PCT is enhanced by dietary restriction by several unknown and yet to be identified mechanisms. Transcellular transport in TAL and DCT are enhanced by up regulation of several genes involved in transcellular pathway (Fig. 16.2). Studies done on mice shows that dietary restriction of magnesium increase the expression of TRPM6 mRNA in DCT cells [11].

Several hormones like PTH, calcitonin, arginine vasopressin and glucagon increases the magnesium reabsorption in both cTAL and DCT by affecting paracellular and transcellular pathways respectively. Many of these steroid, peptide hormones, prostaglandins act by formation of CAMP and involve protein kinase A [5]. Phospholipase C is also shown to be involved indicating intricate interrelated intracellular pathways.

ECF volume contraction increases the magnesium reabsorption and ECF volume expansion decreases the magnesium reabsorption in the loop of Henle [12]. Metabolic alkalosis increases the magnesium reabsorption in loop of Henle and DCT, whereas metabolic acidosis, hypokalaemia decreases the reabsorption in them [13]. Decreased phosphate levels can decreases the magnesium reabsorption by increased mobilisation from bone, suppression of PTH and altered tubular transport [14].

TRPM6 activity and expression are increased by a hormone EGF. EGF combines with EGFR expressed in basolateral membrane of DCT and activates the post receptor signalling which includes SrC family of tyrosine kinases, ERK/MEK pathway and PI3K, leading to activation Akt and later RACK1. This leads to mobilisation of TRPM6 towards the plasma membrane [15].

TRPM6 and TRPM7 are associated with an alpha kinase domain. Intracellular ATP binds to ATP binding motif in the alpha kinase domain of TRPM6 and modulates its activity [16]. Receptor associated c kinase 1 (RACK1) inhibits TRPM6 activity by phosphorylation of the fused alpha kinase domain [17].

Menopause and Renal Regulation of Magnesium

Serum levels of Mg^{2+} and total magnesium are inversely correlated with the oestrogen concentration in menopausal women. Oestrogen increases both activity and expression of TRPM6 in renal DCT cells [12] (Figs. 16.1 and 16.2). REA (repressor associated with oestrogen receptor activity) protein

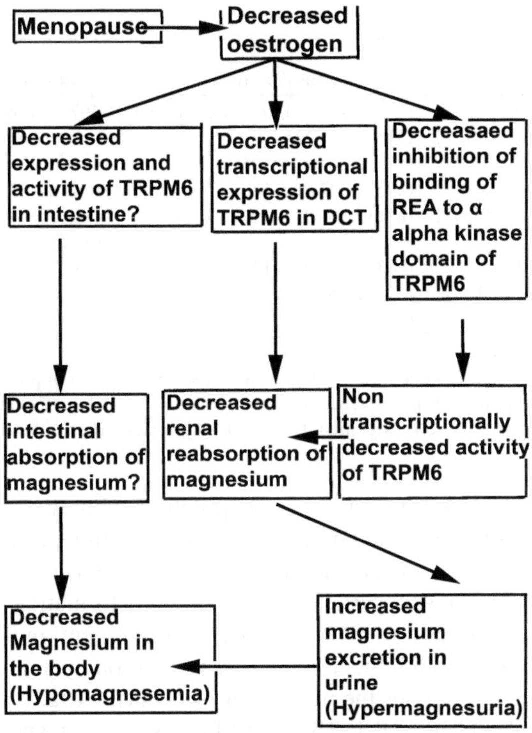

Fig. 16.2 Effect of menopause and oestrogen on the metabolism of magnesium in intestine and kidney. Oestrogen increases the activity and expression of TRPM6 in DCT of kidney [12]. Effect of oestrogen on regulation of expression and activity of TRPM6 present in intestine is yet to be completely elucidated. Oestrogen increases the expression of TRPM6 by increasing the rate of transcription of the gene coding TRPM6. Oestrogen inhibits the binding of REA to alpha kinase domain of TRPM6 and increases the activity of TRPM6 nontranscriptionally [18]. Menopause is associated with decreased oestrogen. Decrease in oestrogen causes decreased activity and expression of TRPM6 in intestine and DCT of kidney leading to decrease in renal reabsorption of magnesium and hypermagnesuria. Oestrogen supplementation increases the renal reabsorption of and decreases the magnesuria [11, 19]. All the above factors are responsible for hypomagnesaemia seen in menopause (*TRPM6* transcellular receptor potential melastatin 6, *DCT* distal convoluted tubule, *REA* repressor protein of oestrogen receptor activity)

co expressed with TRPM6 in DCT cells inhibits the TRPM6 activity by binding to the alpha kinase domain associated with TRPM6 in a phosphorylation dependant manner. Apart from a slow transcriptional increase in TRPM6 expression, oestrogen also exhibits a rapid non transcriptional stimulation of TRPM6 activity by inhibiting the binding of REA with alpha kinase domain of TRPM6 [18] (Fig. 16.2). TRPM6 expression decreases in ovariectomised rats and oestrogen supplementation increases the expression of TRPM6 in DCT cells [11].

Hypermagnesuria due to decreased renal reabsorption secondary to reduced oestrogen is observed in postmenopausal women (Table 16.6) (Fig. 16.2). Oestrogen replacement therapy in postmenopausal women decreases urinary magnesium indicating the positive effect of oestrogen on magnesium reabsorption in kidneys [19].

Regulation of Magnesium at the Level of Bone

Epidemiologic studies conducted on humans have revealed a positive correlation between low dietary intake of magnesium and rate of bone loss. Magnesium deficiency is one of the strong independent risk factor along with age in the development of osteoporosis especially in postmenopausal women.

Table 16.6 Magnesium levels in serum and urine in menopause

	Reference, year and type of study	Premenopausal women	Postmenopausal women	*p* value
Urinary magnesium	McNair P, 1984 (cross-sectional) [19]	355 ± 13 mmol/mol of creatinine (Mean ± SEM) (n = 48)	467 ± 20 mmol/mol of creatinine (Mean ± SEM) (n = 54)	$p < 0.01$
Serum magnesium	Naveenta G, 2011 (cross-sectional) [31]	0.95 ± 0.07 mmol/L (Mean ± SD) (n = 50)	0.81 ± 0.03 mmol/L (Mean ± SD) (n = 50)	$p < 0.05$
	Sreekantha, 2011 (cross-sectional) [32]	0.83 ± 0.14 mmol/L (Mean ± SD) (n = 28)	0.540 ± 0.063 mmol/L (Mean ± SD) (n = 32)	$p < 0.001$

Source: Adapted from [19], [31] and [32]

Increased magnesium excretion in urine and decreased magnesium in serum are seen in postmenopausal women compared to premenopausal women (*SEM* standard error of mean, *SD* standard deviation, *n* number of samples, *p* probability of significance of difference between the two means, $p < 0.05$—significant, $p < 0.01$—highly significant, $p < 0.001$—very highly significant)

Osteoporosis occurs with greater frequency in a population who are associated with magnesium deficiency such as in diabetes mellitus, alcoholism and malabsorption syndromes [20]. Dietary restriction of magnesium in humans is associated with decrease in PTH and or increased end organ resistance to PTH and decrease in calcitriol responsible for decreased bone formation (Fig. 16.3). Mild to moderate dietary restriction of magnesium (10–50 % of nutrient requirement) in mice which is in accordance with the level of dietary intake found in general human population, increases the bone loss, decreases the number of osteoblasts and increases the number of osteoclasts (Fig. 16.3). It is associated with an increase in levels of skeletal substance P, IL1β and TNFα. Skeletal substance P stimulates increase in cytokine production in the bone milieu. These cytokines are responsible for osteoclastogenesis and bone resorption (Fig. 16.3). RANKL which is a surface associated protein expressed on osteoblast binds to RANK a receptor for RANKL expressed on osteoclast. This RANKL–RANK interaction between osteoblast and osteoclast promotes osteoclast differentiation and activity. Several other assessments have also shown that magnesium restriction increases the RANKL and decreases its decoy receptor OPG, promoting the osteoclast activity and hence bone resorption [21] (Fig. 16.3). Magnesium restriction in mice is associated with decreased extracellular magnesium which stimulates the NMDA receptor causing an increase in release of substance P, followed by TNFα and ILβ [22, 23] (Fig. 16.3).

Magnesium is also mitogenic to osteoblasts [24]. Extracellular magnesium and TRPM7 are essential for PDGF induced osteoblast proliferation, migration and maturation. In magnesium deficiency osteoblast are resistant to PDGF induced stimulation [25] (Fig. 16.3). Magnesium restriction in mice is associated with decreased osteocalcin, osteocalcin mRNA serum and bone alkaline phosphatase, collagen and sulfation of glycosaminoglycan, indicating that decreased osteoblast function during magnesium deficiency is an important factor causing osteoporosis [26] (Fig. 16.3).

Studies done in humans showed a low dietary intake is associated with high urinary pyridinoline suggesting increase bone resorption. The above mechanisms of increased bone resorption and decreased bone formation associated with chronic magnesium deficiency could also be operating in humans, causing osteoporosis [27] (Fig. 16.3).

Menopause and Skeletal Regulation of Magnesium

Substance P, ILβ and TNFα are demonstrated to have an osteoclastogenic and bone resorptive function in postmenopausal women. The levels of these cytokines are increased in magnesium deficiency, secondary to oestrogen deficiency and decreased dietary intake in postmenopausal women (Fig. 16.3).

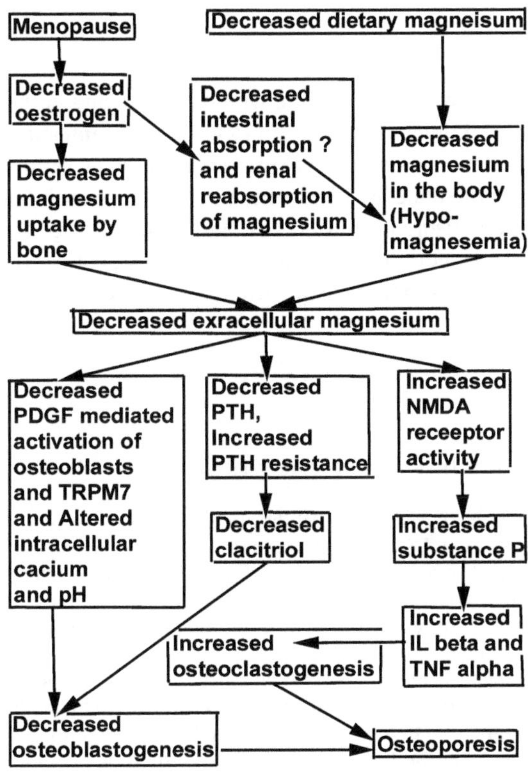

Fig. 16.3 Effect of menopause, oestrogen and magnesium on bone metabolism. Oestrogen deficiency in menopause causes decreased intestinal absorption, decreased renal reabsorption and increased excretion of magnesium in urine causing hypomagnesaemia [11, 19]. Dietary restriction of magnesium also causes hypomagnesaemia. Magnesium uptake to bone is decreased in menopause [30]. All the above factors causes decreased extracellular magnesium. Extracellular magnesium is required to maintain the PDGF mediated activation of osteoblasts, activity of TRPM7 that regulates the magnesium metabolism in bone cells, regulation of intracellular calcium and pH, secretion of PTH, action PTH and indirectly the synthesis of calcitriol [24, 25]. Magnesium deficiency causes alteration in all the above factors and hence decreased osteoblastogenesis. Magnesium deficiency increases the NMDA receptor activity and hence increases the substance P, which stimulates the secretion of osteoclastogenic IL beta and TNF alpha [22, 23]. Decreased OPG/RANKL ratio seen in magnesium deficiency also promotes osteoclast synthesis and activity [21]. Increased osteoclast synthesis and activity as well as decreased osteoblast synthesis and activity are responsible for the osteoporosis and decrease in BMD associated with menopause, decreased oestrogen and hypomagnesaemia [20, 26–30] (*PDGF* platelet-derived growth factor, *TRPM* transcellular receptor potential melastatin, *PTH* parathormone, *NMDA* *N*-methyl D-aspartate, *OPG* osteoprotegerin, *RANKL* receptor activated nuclear factor kappa beta ligand, *TNF* tumour necrosis factor, *IL* interleukin, *BMD* bone mineral density)

Magnesium supplementation in postmenopausal women increased the bone density and arrested bone resorption. Dietary supplementation of magnesium in ovariectomised rats improved the bone formation, bone mineral density and bone strength, as shown by an increase in osteocalcin synthesis and decrease in urinary pyridinoline and reversed the changes seen with oestrogen loss secondary to ovariectomy [28]. Studies conducted in postmenopausal women also have revealed a similar result [29]. Magnesium and calcium supplementation in ovariectomised rats improved the OPG/RANKL ratio. Oestrogen supplementation in postmenopausal women increased the magnesium uptake by bone [30].

Conclusions

Menopause is associated with decreased oestrogen, which directly and indirectly affects the magnesium metabolism in postmenopausal women. Magnesium absorption by intestine is decreased during menopause due to yet to be identified mechanisms. Hypomagnesemia in the serum (Table 16.6) and decreased magnesium mineral content of the bone are observed in postmenopausal women. Postmenopausal have increased osteoclastogenesis and decreased osteoblastogensis favouring the occurrence of osteoporosis [27] (Fig. 16.3). Decreased oestrogen in menopause also causes decreased renal reabsorption of magnesium and hypermagnesuria in postmenopausal women (Table 16.6) (Fig. 16.2).

References

1. Maria JL, Cristina PM, Manuel B. Role of cellular magnesium in health and human disease. Front Biosci. 2004;9:262–76.
2. Food and Nutrition Board, Institute of Medicine. DRI dietary reference intakes for calcium, phosphorus, magnesium, vitamin D, and fluoride. Washington, DC: National Academy Press; 1997.
3. Hardwick LL, Jones MR, Brautbar N, Lee DB. Site and mechanism of intestinal magnesium absorption. Miner Electrolyte Metab. 1990;16:174–80.
4. Fine KD, Santa ACA, Porter JL, Fordtran JS. Intestinal absorption of magnesium from food and supplements. J Clin Invest. 1991;88:396–402.
5. Quamme GA, Christian DR. Epithelial magnesium transport and regulation by kidney. Front Biosci. 2000;5:d694–711.
6. Brink EJ, Beynen AC. Nutrition and magnesium absorption: a review. Prog Food Nutr Sci. 1992;16:125–62.
7. Schweigel M, Martens H. Magnesium transport in the gastrointestinal tract. Front Biosci. 2000;1:D666–77.
8. Anast C, Kennedy R, Volk G, Adamson L. Studies of active transport of calcium, magnesium, and sulfate by the small intestine. J Pediatr. 1964;65:1105.
9. Wilz DR, Gray RW, Dominguez JH, Lemann Jr J. Plasma 1,25-(OH)2-vitamin D concentrations and net intestinal calcium, phosphate, and magnesium absorption in humans. Am J Clin Nutr. 1979;32:2052–60.
10. Qi X, Hoenderop JG, Bindels RJ. Regulation of magnesium reabsorption in DCT. Pflugers Arch. 2009;458:89–98.
11. Groenestege WTM, Hoenderop JG, Lambertus VDH, Nine K, Bindels RJ. The epithelial Mg^{2+} channel transient receptor potential melastatin 6 is regulated by dietary Mg^{2+} content and oestrogens. J Am Soc Nephrol. 2006;17:1035–43.
12. Quamme GA, de Rouffignac C. Epithelial magnesium transport and regulation by the kidney. Front Biosci. 2000;5:D694–711.
13. Wong NLM, Quamme GA, Dirks JH. Effects of acid–base disturbances on renal handling of magnesium in the kidney. Clin Sci. 1986;70:277–84.
14. Domingues JH, Gray RW, Leman JJR. Dietary phosphate deprivation in women and men: effect on mineral and acid balance, parathyroid hormone and metabolism of 25-OH-vitamin D. J Clin Endocrinol Metab. 1976;43:1056–68.
15. Theobalt S, Alexander RT, Groenestege WMT, Hoenderop JG, Bindels RJ. EGF increases TRPM6 activity and surface expression. J Am Soc Nephrol. 2009;20:78–85.
16. Theobault S, Gang C, Veneseelar H, Qi X, Bindels RJ, Hoenderop JG. Role of the alpha kinase domain in transient receptor potential melastatin 6 channel and regulation by intracellular ATP. J Biol Chem. 2008;283(29):19999–20007.
17. Gang C, Theobault S, van der Wijst J, van der Kemp A, Lasonder E, Bindels RJ, et al. RACK1 inhibits TRPM6 activity via phosphorylation of the fused alpha-kinase domain. Curr Biol. 2008;18(3):168–76.
18. Gang C, Van der Wijst J, Vann der Kemp A, Van Zeeland F, Bindels RJ, Hoenderop JG, et al. Regulation of the epithelial Mg^{2+} channel TRPM6 by oestrogen and the associated repressor protein of oestrogen receptor activity (REA). J Biol Chem. 2009;284(22):14788–95.
19. McNair P, Christiansen C, Transbol I. Effect of menopause and estrogen substitutional therapy on magnesium metabolism. Miner Electrolyte Metab. 1984;10(2):84–7.
20. Tucker K, Kiel DP, Hannan MT, Felson DT. Magnesium intake is associated with bone mineral density in elderly women. J Bone Miner Res. 1995;10:S466.
21. Rude RK, Singer FR, Gruber HE. Skeletal and hormonal effects of magnesium deficiency. J Am Coll Nutr. 2009;28(2):131–41.

22. McIntosh TK. Novel pharmacologic therapies in the treatment of experimental traumatic brain injury: a review. J Am Chem Soc. 1993;89:2719–25.
23. Weglicki WB, Dickens BF, Wagner TL, Chemielinska JJ, Phillips TM. Immunoregulation by neuropeptides in magnesium deficiency: ex vivo effect of enhanced substance P production on circulation T lymphocytes from magnesium-deficient mice. Magnes Res. 1996;9:3–11.
24. Liu CC, Yeh JK, Aloia JF. Magnesium directly stimulates osteoblast proliferation. J Bone Miner Res. 1988;3:S104.
25. Elie A, Robert M. Importance of melastatin-like transient receptor potential 7 and magnesium in the stimulation of osteoblast proliferation and migration by platelet-derived growth factor. Am J Physiol Cell Physiol. 2009;297:C360–8.
26. Creedon A, Flynn A, Cashman K. The effect of moderately and severely restricted dietary magnesium intakes on bone composition and bone metabolism in the rat. Br J Nutr. 1999;82:63–71.
27. New SA, Robins SP, Campbell MK, Martin JC, Garton MJ, Bolton SC, et al. Dietary influences on bone mass and bone metabolism: further evidence of a positive link between fruit and vegetable consumption and bone health. Am J Clin Nutr. 2000;71:142–51.
28. Yasuhiro T, Yasutaka K, Ritsuko M, Yukihiro T, Kazuharu S, Seiichiro A. Dietary magnesium supplementation affects bone metabolism and dynamic strength of bone in ovariectomized rats. J Nutr. 2000;130:216–20.
29. Hasan A, Oguzhan D, Dilek Y, Hulya G, Nilgun M, Isik K, et al. Short-term oral magnesium supplementation suppresses bone turnover in postmenopausal osteoporotic women. Biol Trace Elem Res. 2010;133(2):136–43.
30. Robert KR, Helen EG, Livia YW, Angelica F. Immunolocalization of RANKL is increased and OPG decreased during dietary magnesium deficiency in the rat. Nutr Metab. 2005;2:24.
31. Naveenta G, Kushdeep Singh A. The status of trace elements after menopause: a comparative study. J Clin Diagn Res. 2011;5(4):795–7.
32. Sreekantha, Satisha TG, Avinash SS, Manjunatha Goud BK, Remya, Sudhakar GK, Rangaswamy R, Raghavendra VT. Magnesium and calcium levels in early surgical menopause. J Clin Diagn Res. 2011; 5(1):55–7.

Chapter 17
Effect of Folic Acid Supplementation in Postmenopausal Women

Giancarlo Paradisi, Francesca Ianniello, Francesca Basile, Cristina Di Cesare, Lorena Quagliozzi, Laura Donati, and Alessandro Caruso

Key Points

- Folic acid is very important for postmenopausal women's health.
- Folic acid may offer a more acceptable alternative to the conventional HRT for postmenopausal women with hot flushes.
- Supplementation of folic acid to prevent depression symptoms in postmenopausal women is recommended.
- The effectiveness and safety of folic acid supplementation as chemopreventive agent against cancer in postmenopausal women is not established.
- Clinical trials should provide a more definitive answer whether folic acid is beneficial for the prevention or treatment of cardiovascular disease in postmenopausal women.

Keywords Folic acid • Menopause • Cardiovascular risk • Depression • Hot flushes • Cancer • Women • Diet

Abbreviations

HRT	Hormone replacement therapy
SAM	S-Adenosylmethionine
RDA	Recommended dietary allowance
DFE	Dietary folate equivalent
Hcy	Homocysteine
MTHFR	Methylenetetrahydrofolate reductase
CVD	Cardiovascular disease
CAD	Coronary artery disease
HTN	Hypertension
NO	Vascular nitric oxide
LDL	Low-density lipoprotein

G. Paradisi, M.D. (✉) • F. Ianniello, M.D. • F. Basile, M.D. • C. Di Cesare, M.D. • L. Quagliozzi, M.D. • L. Donati, M.D. • A. Caruso, M.D.
Department of Obstetrics and Gynecology, Catholic University of Sacred Hearth, Largo Agostino Gemelli, Rome, Italy
e-mail: giancarlo.paradisi@tin.it; giancarlo.paradisi@alice.it; francesca.ianniello@yahoo.it; francescab24@libero.it; cristinadicesare9@gmail.com; lorenaquagliozzi@gmail.com; laura.donati81@gmail.com; acaruso@rm.unicatt.it

C.J.H. Martin et al. (eds.), *Nutrition and Diet in Menopause*, Nutrition and Health,
DOI 10.1007/978-1-62703-373-2_17,

CRC	Colorectal cancer
ER	Estrogen receptor
PR	Progesterone receptor
HPV	Human papillomavirus
FR	Folate receptor
AD	Alzheimer disease

Introduction

Description and Functions

Folic acid is one of the eight vitamins that belong to the group that we know as vitamin B.

As enzyme cofactor is involved in numerous reactions in several metabolic processes.

It aids the production of the body's genetic material, and is especially important when cells and tissues are growing rapidly, such as in infancy, adolescence, and pregnancy. Folate coenzymes play a vital role in DNA metabolism through the synthesis of DNA from its precursors (thymidine and purines). An appropriate concentration of folate is essential for the synthesis of nucleic acids for cell division. Low levels of folate will result in a wrong uracil incorporation into DNA in the place of thymine, increasing the risk of DNA damage.

A folate coenzyme is required for the synthesis of methionine, and methionine is required for the synthesis of S-adenosylmethionine (SAM) (Figs. 17.1, 17.2, and 17.3).

The Recommended Dietary Allowance

Traditionally, the dietary folate requirement was defined as the amount needed to prevent a deficiency severe enough to cause symptoms like anemia. The most recent recommended dietary allowance (RDA) (1998) was based primarily on the adequacy of red blood cell folate concentrations at different levels of folate intake, as judged by the absence of abnormal hematological indicators. Red cell folates have been shown to correlate with liver folate stores (Table 17.1).

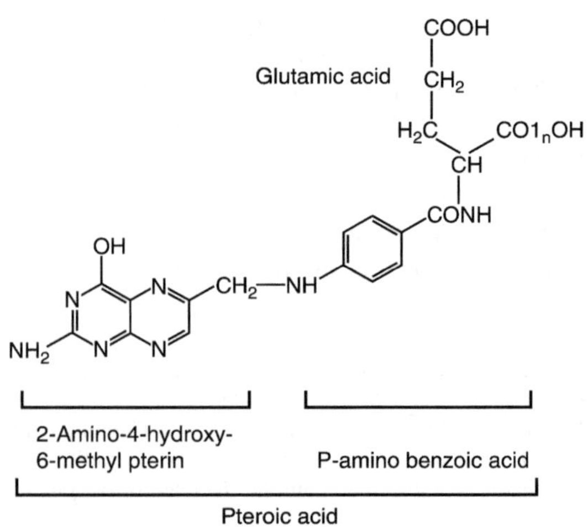

Fig. 17.1 Folic acid structure

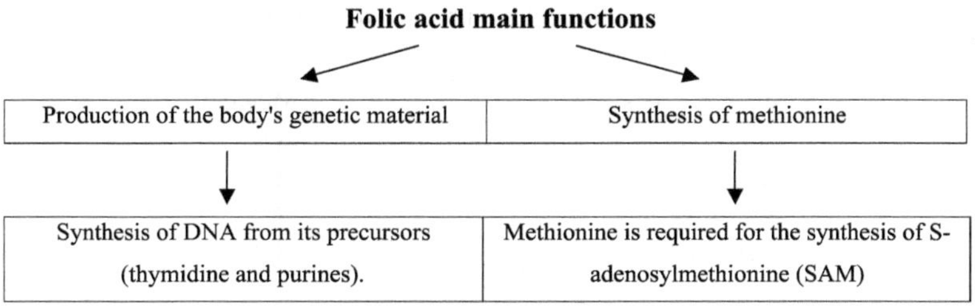

Fig. 17.2 Folic acid main functions

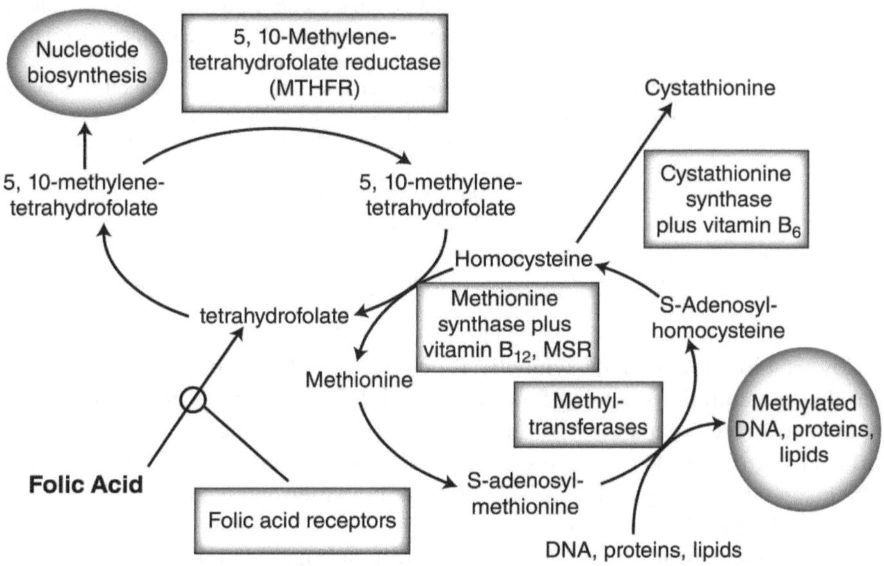

Fig. 17.3 Folic acid as coenzyme

Table 17.1 Folic acid amount present in common foods

Food	Serving	Folate (mcg)
Fortified breakfast cereal	1 cup	200–400
Orange juice	6 ounces	83
Spinach	½ cup	132
Asparagus	½ cup	134
Lentils	½ cup	179
Pasta	1 cup	60
Bread	1 slice	20
Rice	1 cup	60

The serum folatemia is between 6 and 19 ng/ml in adults and is about 2–3 times higher in infants. The amount of folic acid in the body can satisfy the need of the vitamin only for 2–4 months without a steady flow outside. Blood levels below 4 ng/ml indicate a deficiency state. To replenish stocks of folate, a daily oral intake of 1 mg is sufficient for about three weeks if there are problems of malabsorption (Table 17.2).

When the Food and Nutrition Board of the Institute of Medicine set the new dietary recommendation for folate, they introduced a new unit, the Dietary Folate Equivalent (DFE). Use of the DFE

Table 17.2 Folic acid requirement during different women life stage

Women' life stage	Mcg/day
Childbearing age	400
Pregnancy	600
Breast-feeding	500
Menopause	400

Table 17.3 Different folate requirement in women's life stage

Requirement of folic acid differs in women's life stage	
Childbearing age	It's important to compensate the loss that occurs during menstruation taking this vitamin
Pregnancy	Folate requirements increase during pregnancy. There is a dramatic acceleration in cell division and red blood cell development as the uterus enlarges, the placenta develops, maternal blood volume expands, and the fetus grows. The mother also transfers folate to the fetus. Evidence supports a RDA of 600 mcg DFEs per day to maintain normal folate status during pregnancy. Moreover folate can prevent neural tube defects, including spina bifida, if taken before conception and early in pregnancy
Lactation	There is an increased need for nutrients, including folic acid, for the production of breast milk, so the diet must be as varied and balanced
Postmenopausal women	In the intake of folic acid has the purpose to reduce homocysteine levels. High levels of homocysteine can lead to heart problems, depression, mood swings, and osteoporosis

reflects the higher bioavailability of synthetic folic acid found in supplements and fortified foods compared to that of naturally occurring food folates [1]. DFEs adjust for the nearly 50 % lower bioavailability of food folate compared with that of folic acid: 1 μg of dietary folate equivalent = 0.6 μg of folic acid from fortified food or as a supplement taken with meals = 1 μg of food folate = 0.5 μg of a supplement taken on an empty stomach. The RDA for both men and women is 400 μg/day of dietary folate equivalents (DFEs) (Table 17.3).

In general, postmenopausal women do not differ from premenopausal women in folate intake.

Genetic Variation in Folate Requirements

Methylenetetrahydrofolate reductase (MTHFR) is an enzyme that in humans is encoded by the MTHFR gene. MTHFR catalyzes the conversion of 5,10-methylenetetrahydrofolate to 5-methyltetrahydrofolate, a co-substrate for homocysteine remethylation to methionine. If there is a mutation in the MTHFR gene, homocysteine levels may not be regulated properly. Genetic mutations in MTHFR are the most commonly known inherited risk factor for elevated homocysteine levels. About 3 % of the population present MTHFR mutation: more of 50 % of individuals have inherited one copy of the mutate gene (heterozygous MTHFR) and from 5 to 25 % of individuals have inherited two copies of the abnormal gene (homozygous MTHFR) Although these mutations do impair the regulation of homocysteine, adequate folate levels essentially "cancel out" this defect. The amount of each of these supplements should be adjusted on the basis of the degree of homocysteine elevation, not on the basis of genetic status. The research of mutation MTHFR gene is widespread both in premenopausal women both in postmenopausal women because it is thought that this abnormal gene and its consequent hyperhomocysteinemia should interfere with the woman's health. Testing for genetic variants of MTHFR should be performed in all women with adverse pregnancy outcomes and personal or familiar history of venous thromboembolism prior to prescribing estrogen preparations (oral contraceptives or hormone replacement therapy).

Table 17.4 Effect of MTHFR mutation in premenopausal and postmenopausal women

Premenopausal women	Menopausal women
Neural tube defect	Thromboembolism
Preeclampsia	Ischemic stroke
Placental abruption	
Recurrent pregnancy loss	
Intrauterine growth restriction	
Thromboembolism	
Ischemic stroke	

In many studies on premenopausal women, MTHFR mutation has been linked to an increased chance of having a baby with a neural tube defect (spina bifida) [2]. Recent research has implied that risks vary, based on the nutritional status of the mother (folate levels, vitamin intake) rather than based on mutations of this gene [3]. Although further studies are needed, in women with two MTHFR mutations extra folate supplementation (usually 4 mg) during pregnancy is recommended. There is also conflicting evidence on the relation between homozygous MTHFR mutations and pregnancy complications (including preeclampsia, placental abruption, recurrent pregnancy loss, and intrauterine growth restriction, as described earlier). A recent meta-analysis, which combined all of the data from these studies, found that there was no association between MTHFR and recurrent pregnancy loss [4]. It seems that homozygous MTHFR may moderately increase the risk of preeclampsia and placental abruption, but more research in this area is necessary.

Homozygous MTHFR gene is considered a heritable risk factor for venous thromboembolism. It is known that exposure to hormonal therapy may increase the risk of ischemic stroke both in premenopausal both in postmenopausal women. It is still controversial whether in homozygous MTHFR women, the use of oral contraceptives and hormonal replacement therapy could be considered an additional risk factor (Table 17.4).

Folic Acid Benefits

Folic acid is very important for women's health. It is beneficial in a series of disease such as: anemia, headaches, rheumatoid arthritis, infertility, acne, and AIDS. Folic acid can also protect from the following:

- Heart attacks and stroke
- Cancers
- Osteoporosis
- Depression and other mental problems

Main Text

Cardiovascular Disease and Folic Acid

Cardiovascular disease (CVD), such as coronary artery disease (CAD) and hypertension (HTN), is more common in men than in premenopausal women of the same age, suggesting cardiovascular benefits of estrogens. Heart disease is rare in young women, but in industrialized countries it becomes

Table 17.5 Cardiovascular risk factors in menopause

Decrease estrogen levels
High homocysteine levels
Smoking
Cholesterol
Body mass index
High blood pressure
Diabetes

Table 17.6 Effects of hyperhomocysteinemia in postmenopausal women

Hyperhomocysteinemia	
Endothelial injury	Atherogenesis
Reduction of vascular nitric oxide	
Oxidative modification of LDL	
Increase of platelets adhesiveness	
Affection of several factors involved in the clotting cascade	
Increase H_2O_2 production	Cytotoxic effect
Affection of antioxidant defense systems	
Promotion of lipid peroxidation	
Trigger of apoptosis via mitochondrial oxidant production	

the leading cause of morbidity and mortality among postmenopausal women. Together, CVD and cerebrovascular disease account for the majority of deaths in postmenopausal women (75–76 %), a significantly higher proportion than breast cancer (6–8 %) [5]. The increased risk of CVD in postmenopausal women has been linked to the decrease in plasma estrogen levels, thus prompting further investigation of the effects of estrogen on the cardiovascular system. Strategies to prevent CVD in this population should therefore be a primary objective for health-care providers. Regarding lifestyle, change can be significant in the light of recent research suggesting that lifestyle changes can be considered as a primary prevention and treatment of CVD in postmenopausal women. A healthy lifestyle is an important strategy for the whole community, and it includes a balanced diet (Table 17.5).

Epidemiologic studies have shown a link between high plasma homocysteine concentration and increased risk of cardiovascular disease (CVD), but causality of the association is not yet proven. There is evidence that hyperhomocysteinemia is a risk factor for CVD independent of other known risk factors such as smoking, cholesterol, body mass index, age, high blood pressure, and diabetes [6]. Despite the direct association between homocysteine levels and increased risk of cardiovascular diseases, it is not yet clear whether lowering homocysteine levels will reduce this risk. On the other hand, the mechanism by which elevated homocysteine might increase the risk of developing vascular disease is unclear (Table 17.6).

Experimental studies suggest that homocysteine promotes atherogenesis by producing endothelial injury, reduction of vascular nitric oxide (NO) production, and bioavailability as well as oxidative modification of low-density lipoprotein (LDL) [7]. Vitro studies have shown that homocysteine can directly exert a cytotoxic effect to endothelial cells at higher than normal levels by increasing H_2O_2 production [8] affecting antioxidant defense systems [9], and promoting lipid peroxidation [10], as well as by triggering apoptosis via mitochondrial oxidant production [11]. Homocysteine causes a direct damage on endothelial cells and promotes the growth of smooth muscle cells, leading to atherosclerotic lesions. It can also increase adhesiveness of platelets and affect several factors involved in the clotting cascade [12]. In brief, it seems likely that homocysteine can cause cellular injury via oxidative damage [13] and that this mechanism is a major cause for vascular dysfunction in animals and in humans. After menopause, basal Hcy levels increase progressively [14]. Supplementation with folic acid has shown to reduce plasma Hcy levels, thus diminishing the hyperhomocysteine-induced generation of oxygen radicals, and the extent of LDL oxidation in postmenopausal women [15] at high risk for cardiovascular disease. Interestingly, this favorable effect is present not only in subjects at high risk for macro vascular disease, but also in healthy normo-homocysteinemic postmenopausal women [16]. Furthermore, folic acid supplementation improves insulin sensitivity and lipid metabolism, helping to reduce the risk of cardiovascular diseases in these women. On the basis of the above described experimental evidences, folate supplementation should be performed in all postmenopausal women. However, recent large, randomized, controlled trials reported conflicting data on the benefit of FA supplementation. The Heart Outcomes Prevention Evaluation (HOPE)-2 trial reported a 24 % decrease in stroke risk after 5 years of FA supplementation [17] in contrast, the Women's Antioxidant and Folic Acid Cardiovascular Study (WAFACS), reported a relative risk for stroke incidence comparing FA supplementation to placebo of 1.14 (0.83–1.57). More recently, two meta-analyses which include recent trials do not support the hypothesis that FA supplementation decreases risk of stroke (relative risk 0.95, 95 % CI 0.84–1.08, P = 0.43) and coronary heart disease despite 13–52 % reductions in plasma homocysteine concentrations [18].

There are many factors that may contribute to the discrepancy in results of observational studies and clinical trials of folic acid supplementation for the secondary prevention of vascular disease. First among them is the possibility of confounding in observational studies. Despite the most comprehensive measurement and adjustment strategies, the uncontrolled dietary intake or supplementation is always a concern. Therefore, whether increasing intake of folate could reduce the risk of vascular disease remains to be demonstrated. Consequently, the American Heart Association removed the recommendation of using folic acid to prevent cardiovascular diseases in high-risk women. The guidelines now encourage lifestyle changes to help manage blood pressure which include weight control, increased physical activity, alcohol moderation, sodium restriction, and an emphasis on eating fresh fruits, vegetables, and low-fat dairy products.

Completion of the ongoing clinical trials should provide a more definitive answer whether folic acid is beneficial for the prevention or treatment of heart disease or stroke.

Cancer and Folic Acid

Folates are essential substances for the synthesis of nucleic acids and for cell division.

Consequently, folate deficiency in tissues with rapidly replicating cells results in ineffective DNA synthesis.

In neoplastic cells, in which DNA replication and cell division occur at an accelerated rate, interruption of folate metabolism causes ineffective DNA synthesis, resulting in inhibition of tumor growth. Indeed, this has been the basis for cancer chemotherapy with several antifolate agents (i.e., methotrexate).

Epidemiological, clinical, and experimental evidence suggests that folate deficiency in normal tissues appears to predispose them to neoplastic transformation and folate supplementation suppresses the development of tumors in normal tissues [19].

Several observers have suggested that a positive relationship exists between the occurrence of menopause and the risk of cancer. Advanced age and hormonal changes are believed to be the main risk factors which are added those related to lifestyle.

In fact several studies have suggested an inverse association of folate with the risk of cancer of the colorectal, lungs, pancreas, esophagus, stomach, cervix, ovary, breast, neuroblastoma, and leukemia.

Colon-Rectal Cancer

Colorectal cancer (CRC) is the third most common malignancy among women in the USA, with 69.360 new cases projected in 2011 [20]. Lifestyle, diet, hormonal, and genetic status are considered the main CRC risk factors. Postmenopausal women result more susceptible to the development of colon-rectal cancer than premenopausal woman, as consistently demonstrated by some epidemiologic studies, thus supporting the hypothesis that female hormones are protective for developing colorectal cancer [21].

Further confirmations were found by the Women's Health Initiative trials that showed a decrease of the 40 % of colorectal cancer risk an in postmenopausal women undergoing to continuous combined hormone therapy, but not unopposed estrogen therapy [22].

Also the evidence linking low folate status with an increased risk of colorectal cancer (CRC) is strong. Data from the majority of human studies (retrospective, case–control, and prospective) suggested that people who regularly consume the highest level of folate or with the highest blood folate concentrations, had a significantly reduced risk of developing colon polyps or cancer [23]. In a large cohort study, Giovannucci et al. found that increased folate intake appeared to be protective against colon cancer. They observed a 30 % decrease in the risk of colon cancer for women with total folate intake exceeding 400 mcg/day when compared to women with an intake of 200 mcg/day. This research suggests that supplemental folate intake may have a causal relationship with decreased risk for colon cancer in the women.

The specific mechanism whereby folate influences colorectal carcinogenesis is unclear, but various experiments indicate that deficiency of folate in either form leads to abnormalities in DNA synthesis and methylation.

Breast Cancer

Breast cancer is the commonest cause of cancer death in women worldwide.

There are one million new cases in the world each year, breast cancer accounts for 18 % of all female cancers. The incidence of breast cancer increases with age, doubling about every 10 years until menopause, when the rate of increase slows dramatically.

Women who start menstruating early in life or who have a late menopause have an increased risk of developing breast cancer. Women who have a natural menopause after the age of 55 are twice as likely to develop breast cancer as women who experience the menopause before the age of 45.

Null parity and late age at first birth both increase the lifetime incidence of breast cancer, instead women who breastfeed have a risk reduced by 4 % for every 12 months of breastfeeding [24].

Higher levels of endogenous hormones have long been hypothesized to increase breast cancer risk. Some studies showed that postmenopausal women with the highest levels of estrogen and testosterone have 2–3 times the risk of women with the lowest levels [25].

The link between these hormones and premenopausal breast cancer risk is less clear.

The use of oral contraceptives (Oc) increases the risk of breast cancer in current and recent users, but there is no significant excess risk ten or more years after stopping use. Women currently taking HRT have a 66 % increased risk of breast cancer compared to nonusers [26]. The risk increase is temporary, with risk returning to that of a never-user within 5 years.

There has been a lot of research into the effects of dietary factors on breast cancer risk, but the findings are generally inconsistent and inconclusive. The strongest evidence seems to be the correlation between fat intake and breast cancer. Also phyto-estrogens, plant compounds that are structurally similar to estrogen, have been extensively studied in relation to breast cancer risk. A meta-analysis showed a 15 % reduction in breast cancer risk for postmenopausal women with the highest intakes [27].

Retrospective and prospective studies on folic acid supplementation suggest that high folate intake may be associated with a lower risk for postmenopausal breast cancer, particularly in women with moderate or high alcohol consumption. Although increases in sex hormones have been proposed to explain the association of alcohol and breast cancer, chronically high alcohol consumption, such as that of alcoholics, is also associated with inadequate folate status [28]. Therefore, the deficiency of this vitamin may explain the role of folate in the breast cancer prevention in women who are alcoholics.

In a recent study Martha J et al. evaluated baseline dietary intake of folate, vitamin B_6–B_{12} and breast cancer risk and whether the associations varied by menopausal status and estrogen receptor (ER) and progesterone receptor (PR) status. They showed that high folate intake was related to a lower risk of premenopausal and possibly ER_/PR_ breast cancer [29].

However, a recent report from the Lung, Colorectal, Prostate, and Ovarian Cancer Screening Trial (PLCO) study population suggests that a very high folate status, attributable to excessive supplement use, may generally be harmful rather than beneficial in breast cancer development.

So an increase in folate intakes may be beneficial in a deficient population, higher intakes may result in no further benefit or could be harmful in women whose folate status is already sufficient. Thus, the optimal folate intake for breast cancer prevention has not yet been defined and will differ depending on alcohol consumption and genetic susceptibility.

Cervical Cancer

Cervical cancer is the second most frequent cancer in women worldwide between the age of 15 and 44 years and the most common in developing countries [30]. Thus, premenopausal women are more frequently affect than postmenopausal women. The key factor in cervical cancer causation is infection with human papillomavirus (HPV).

Out of over 100 HPV types, Types 16, 18, 31, 33, and 45 account for up to 83 % of all cervical cancers cases [31]. HPV is established as a necessary but not as a sufficient cause for cervical cancer. Endogenous and exogenous cofactors might influence the risk of developing cervical cancer in combination with HPV.

Cofactors include long-term use of oral contraceptives, sexually transmitted infections such as human immunodeficiency virus, Chlamydia, and herpes simplex virus Type 2, high parity, smoking, and diet. Until now, only a small number of case–control and cohort studies looked at the role of diet intake as a cofactor for cervical cancer or as a risk factor for HPV persistence [32].

Folates have been considered as plausible protective factors in some case–control studies, prospective cohort studies, and small intervention trials, and although several of these studies suggest that increased consumption of folate reduces the relative risk of cervical neoplasia [33], statistical significance was not attained in these studies after adjustments were made for confounding variables. These studies had several limitations: folate intake was assessed with a food frequency instrument that had not been validated for folate intake; subjects were not stratified for HPV infections (1992); subjects were not stratified for stage of disease—advanced stages of neoplasia that may be unresponsive to folate [34]. Therefore, actually the effect of folate status on carcinogenesis in the cervix remains uncertain.

Ovarian Cancer

Ovarian cancer is the fourth most frequent cause of cancer death and the most lethal of all gynecologic tumors in women from North America and Northern and Western Europe [35]. The majority of cases are sporadic, and only 5–10 % of ovarian cancers are familial. The etiology of ovarian cancer is poorly understood. Models of ovarian carcinogenesis include the theory of incessant ovulation, in which a person's age at ovulation, lifetime number of ovulatory cycles, are an index of ovarian cancer risk. The main risk factors for ovarian cancer are: family history of ovarian cancer, previous cancer diagnosis especially breast, colon, rectum or uterus, increasing age, no pregnancy and hormone replacement therapy for menopause even if findings about the possible link between postmenopausal

Table 17.7 Folic acid effects in different cancer

Colon rectal cancer	Some human studies (prospective, retrospective, and case–control): high level of folate in the serum had a significantly reduced risk of developing colon polyps or cancer
	Giovannucci et al. (large cohort study): increased folate intake appeared to be protective against colon cancer
Breast cancer	Retrospective and Prospective studies: high folate intake may be associated with a lower risk for postmenopausal breast cancer, particularly in women with moderate or high alcohol consumption
	In a recent study (Martha J et al.): high folate intake was related to a lower risk of premenopausal and possibly ER_/PR_ breast cancer
	Recent report from the Lung, Colorectal, Prostate and Ovarian Cancer Screening Trial (PLCO) study population: high folate status, attributable to excessive supplement use, may generally be harmful rather than beneficial in breast cancer development
Cervical cancer	Some case–control studies, prospective cohort studies and small intervention trials: that increased consumption of folate reduces the relative risk of cervical neoplasia, but statistical significance was not attained in these studies [48]
Ovarian cancer	Four case–control studies: no association between folate intake and the risk of ovarian cancer
	Recent study (Kotsiopoulos et al.): modest levels of dietary folate may reduce the risk of ovarian cancer, while higher levels of folate (supplemental and dietary) may increase risk but given the small sample size, these data require replication in future studies

use of hormone replacement therapy and risk of ovarian cancer are still unclear. Also lifestyle like alcohol use, smoke and diet are considered important risk factors. Some studies have shown a reduced rate of ovarian cancer in women who ate a diet high in vegetables, but other studies disagree. Four case–control studies have generally reported no association between folate intake and the risk of ovarian cancer [36]; whereas the results from three of four prospective cohort studies, including one from the Nurses' Health Study (NHS), have suggested an inverse relationship with dietary folate intake, although none of the associations reached statistical significance [37]. The inconsistencies in the results for ovarian cancer have been attributed to the modification by other factors including alcohol consumption, intake of other folate cofactors involved in one-carbon metabolism (i.e., methionine, vitamins B_6 and B_{12}) and genetic variation in cellular folate metabolism.

Many epithelial ovarian tumors over express folate receptor (FR). FR expression has been associated with higher stage, grade, and worse survival [38].

However, it is not clear whether FR expression is an early or late event in tumorigenesis and whether the timing of intake of folate or other methyl donors influences the risk of developing FR positive ovarian tumors.

Kotsiopoulos et al. in a recent study suggest that modest levels of dietary folate may reduce the risk of ovarian cancer, while higher levels of folate (supplemental and dietary) may increase risk but given the small sample size, these data require replication in future studies. It is imperative to clarify these relationships because folate intake in the United States has increased dramatically with mandated food fortification. More importantly the authors observed increased risk at levels similar to the current recommended daily intake of 400 mcg/day.

Few modifiable risk factors for ovarian cancer exist, so the potential role of dose and formulation of this nutrient in the etiology of ovarian cancer risk should be considered seriously.

In conclusion, folic acid supplementation should not be adopted as a chemopreventive agent against the cancers previously described both in premenopausal and postmenopausal women, until definitive evidence indicates that such supplementation is indeed safe and effective. Although folic acid fortification may prevent the development of new cancers in persons without preexisting premalignant lesions or neoplastic foci, it may promote the progression of these lesions in persons harboring them. Further research is needed to elucidate the mechanisms by which folate interact with neoplastic process (Table 17.7).

Depression and Folic Acid

Depression is considered the most common cause of disability in the USA [39]. According to the National Institutes of Health, clinical depression will affect up to 25 % of women in their lifetimes. People with depression suffer in many areas of their lives, including sleep, eating, relationships, school, work, and self-image.

Depression is a clearly defined disorder that affects both mind and body.

The influence of female hormones on mood has been the subject of much investigation: probably a decrease of estrogen and progesterone could be related to the onset of symptoms in susceptible women.

In fact both the early postpartum and the menopause are phases of the women's life markedly associated to mood disorder. Epidemiologic studies established that about 10 % of women develop severe depressive symptoms as complications of the delivery, while between 8 and 15 % of menopausal women suffer from some form of depression, especially during the perimenopause [40].

Interestingly, studies have shown that elevated homocysteine is associated with depressive disorders and anger attacks caused by depression [41]. Thus, in addiction to sex hormones also the increase of Hcy in the serum may be linked to the development of mood disorders in the women.

Clinical trials have demonstrated that folic acid relieves depression on its own and enhances the antidepressant effect of conventional antidepressants. In one study, patients given 500 mcg folic acid daily in conjunction with fluoxetine experienced a significant improvement in depressive symptoms compared with patients receiving the antidepressant alone [42]. Because relapse is associated with low serum folate, it is important to maintain folate supplementation for a year following a depressive episode.

As well as for reducing the Hcy levels, folate are important also for the cells of nervous system at all ages and there is growing evidence of their involvement in the ageing brain, especially in mood and cognitive function.

An important study on the folate supplementation in depression showed the benefits of this vitamin even when folate status was not low [43]. This may be because serum folate concentrations do not reflect concentrations in the CNS or, as Shea and Rogers have suggested, folate requirements are increased in neuropsychiatric diseases [44].

The association of folate deficiency with depression and dementia has also been confirmed in epileptic, neurological, psychiatric, geriatric and psycho geriatric patients and is supported by neuropsychological, neuropathological, and neurochemical studies. Controlled treatment studies confirm an etiological link with specific effects of the vitamin on mood, drive, initiative, alertness, concentration, psychomotor speed, and social activity.

Several of the earliest reports of neurological disease associated with severe folate deficiency emphasize the importance of vitamin therapy for the treatment of dementia and depression.

For example, Botez et al. [45] described 16 patients whose impaired intellectual function, confirmed on neuropsychological testing, was strikingly improved after 6–12 months of folic acid therapy. Clearly, further clinical trials in precisely defined clinical categories are needed, but they should be long term (at least 6 months to 1 year) as the impact of folate is slow and cumulative over many months, perhaps because blood–brain barrier mechanisms limit entry to the brain. Small doses over the long term may be preferable to larger doses in the short or long term, not least because of risks to the nervous system.

In conclusion, supplementation of folic acid to prevent depression symptoms in postmenopausal women especially in the women with low folate levels in the serum is recommended, even if further studies are needed to establish the dosage and the risk groups.

Alzheimer Disease and Folic Acid

Alzheimer Disease is defined as a progressive, degenerative disease of the brain that leads to dementia. At present it is the most common cause of dementia.

Age represents the main risk factor for Alzheimer Disease, no association between AD and sex was found. A relative increase of AD is highest in the 75–84-years age group.

Some epidemiological studies found associations between hyperhomocysteinemia and histologically confirmed Alzheimer Disease and disease progression. They also revealed that dementia in AD was associated with evidence of brain infarcts on autopsy.

Thus, hyperhomocysteinemia and AD could be linked by stroke or micro vascular disease.

Another study found that dementia was worse in the presence of brain infarcts; therefore, hyperhomocysteinemia may contribute to AD dementia by induction of vascular changes [46].

However, a recent prospective study [47] showed that hyperhomocysteinemia was also a strong, independent risk factor for dementia and AD.

In a study Ho Pi et al. established that homocysteine was directly cytotoxic to cortical neurons in cell culture, which suggests a likely causal role for the amino acid in the cholinergic deficit characteristic of AD [48]. Alternatively neuronal death through apoptosis could result from folate deficiency via S-adenosyl-methionine (SAM) depletion and resultant hypomethylation, and hyperhomocysteinemia may be an epiphenomenon. Actually the links between homocysteine, folate, and AD result to be complex.

Whether AD is more likely to result from homocysteine toxicity or a deficiency of folate or micro vascular disease Hcy-related is still unclear but certainly acid folic supplementation seems to be a valid preventive opportunity for postmenopausal women.

Hot Flushes and Folic Acid

The most common symptom of menopause is hot flashes: the sensation of sudden flushing and sweating followed by chills. Almost two-thirds of postmenopausal women have hot flashes and nearly 20 % find them to be nearly intolerable. The experience of hot flashes can be very uncomfortable and can have a very negative impact upon the individual's quality of life energy and sleep. It was also reported that one-third of women with hot flashes described embarrassment and 20 % described a general sense of a loss of control In addition, hot flashes are associated with decreased libido. Several hormonal and nonhormonal therapies are claimed to alleviate hot flashes. Hormone therapy (HT) (estrogen with or without progestin) remains the gold standard treatment for hot flashes, but replacement therapy is a concern for some patients due to an associated increase in the risk of breast cancer.

As previously described, folate inadequacy was found to be associated with psychiatric symptoms such as mild depression, irritability, altered sleep pattern, and abnormal intellectual functioning. These symptoms, which can occur in the absence of any severe changes at routine hematological testing, are responsive to folate therapy [45]. It was reported that folic acid supplementation produced an antidepressant-like effect mediated by an interaction with the noradrenergic receptors (a1 and a2) and serotonergic receptors (5-HT1A and 5-HT2A/2C) [49]. It significantly reduced norepinephrine secretion and increased serotonin (5-hydroxytryptamine, 5-HT) activity [50].

It's hypothesized that folic acid supplementation may ameliorate hot flushes by the same mechanism as estrogen replacement, by lowering the increased central noradrenergic activity, interacting with monoamine neurotransmitters in the brain, namely, norepinephrine and serotonin.

Folic acid may offer a cheaper, safer, and more acceptable alternative to the conventional HRT for postmenopausal women with hot flushes.

Conclusions

Since its discovery as a protective factor, folic acid captured the interest of numerous clinicians.

The available scientific evidence shows that adequate folate intake prevents neural tube defects and other poor outcomes of pregnancy; it is helpful in lowering the risk of some forms of cancer, cardiovascular diseases, depression, dementia and osteoporosis.

The recommendation for 400 mcg/day of folic acid is especially important for postmenopausal women because blood homocysteine levels tend to increase with age.

Supplementation of folic acid to prevent cardiovascular disease and cancer in postmenopausal women actually is not recommended, although further studies are needed to provide a more definitive answer about the beneficial of folic acid for the prevention or treatment of heart disease or cancer.

In contrast, supplementation of folic acid to prevent climacteric symptoms like depression and hot flushes is recommended, even if further studies are needed to establish the dosage and the risk groups. Thus, folic acid may offer a valid alternative to the conventional HRT for postmenopausal women who have a reduced quality of life caused by the decrease in estrogen.

In conclusion, folic acid supplementation should be considered by clinicians as a possible treatment for postmenopausal symptoms in women, considering each individual case.

References

1. Bailey LB. Dietary reference intakes for folate: the debut of dietary folate equivalents. Nutr Rev. 1998;56(10):294–9.
2. Botto LD, Yang Q. 5,10-Methylenetetrahydrofolate reductase gene variants and congenital anomalies: a HuGE review. Am J Epidemiol. 2000;151:862–77.
3. Steegers-Theunissen RP, Van Iersel CA, Peer PG, Nelen WL, Steegers EA. Hyperhomocysteinemia, pregnancy complications, and the timing of investigation. Obstet Gynecol. 2004;104:336–43.
4. Rey E, Kahn SR, David M, Shrier I. Thrombophilic disorders and fetal loss: a meta-analysis. Lancet. 2003;361:901–8.
5. Eberhardt VMS. Health, United States, 2001. Hyattsville, MD: National Center for Health Statistics; 2001. p. 189–92.
6. Clarke R, Daly L, Robinson K, Naughten E, Cahalane S, Fowler B, et al. Hyperhomocysteinemia: an independent risk factor for vascular disease. N Engl J Med. 1991;324(17):1149–55.
7. Van Der Gried R, Biesma DH, Haas FJLM, Faber JAJ, Duran M, Meuwissen OJATH, et al. The effect of different treatment regimens in reducing fasting and postmethionine-load homocysteine concentrations. J Intern Med. 2000;248:223–9.
8. Righetti M, Serbelloni P, Milani S, Ferrario G. Homocysteine-lowering vitamin B treatment decreases cardiovascular events in hemodialysis patients. Blood Purif. 2006;24:379–86.
9. Bonaa KH, Njolstad I, Ueland PM, Schirmer H, Tverdal A, Steigen T, et al. Homocysteine lowering and cardiovascular events after acute myocardial infarction. N Engl J Med. 2006;354:1578–88.
10. Lonn E, Yusuf S, Arnold MJ, Sheridan P, Pogue J, Micks M, et al. Homocysteine lowering with folic acid and B vitamins in vascular disease. N Engl J Med. 2006;354:1567–77.
11. Liem A, Reynierse-Buitenwerf GH, Zwinderman AH, Jukema JW, van Veldhuisen DJ. Secondary prevention with folic acid: results of the Goes extension study. Heart. 2005;91:1213–4.
12. Harpel PC, Zhang X, Borth W. Homocysteine and hemostasis: pathogenic mechanisms predisposing to thrombosis. J Nutr. 1996;126(4 Suppl):1285S–9.
13. Lange H, Suryapranata H, De Luca G, Börner C, Dille J, Kallmayer K, et al. Folate therapy and in-stent restenosis after coronary stenting. N Engl J Med. 2004;350:2673–81.
14. Hak AE, Polderman KH, Westerdorp ICD, Jacobs C, Hofman A, Witteman JCM, et al. Increased plasma hormones homocysteine after menopause. Atherosclerosis. 2000;149:163–8.
15. De Leo V, La Marca A, Morgante G, Ciani F, Zammarchi E, Setacci C. Low dose folic acid supplementation reduces plasma levels of the cardiovascular risk factor homocysteine in postmenopausal women. Am J Obstet Gynecol. 2000;183:945–7.
16. Paradisi G, Cucinelli F, Mele MC, Barini A, Lanzone A, Caruso A. Endothelial function in post-menopausal women: effect of folic acid supplementation. Hum Reprod. 2004;19(4):1031–5.

17. Saposnik G, Ray JG, Sheridan P, McQueen M, Lonn E, Heart Outcomes Prevention valuation 2 Investigators. Homocysteine-lowering therapy and stroke risk, severity, and disability: additional findings from the HOPE 2 trial. Stroke. 2009;40:1365–72.
18. Bazzano LA, Reynolds K, Holder KN, He J. Effect of folic acid supplementation on risk of cardiovascular diseases: a meta-analysis of randomized controlled trials. JAMA. 2006;296(22):2720–6.
19. Kim YI. Role of folate in colon cancer development and progression. J Nutr. 2003;133:3731S–9.
20. Siegel R, Ward E, Brawley O, Jemal A. Cancer statistics, 2011: the impact of eliminating socioeconomic and racial disparities on premature cancer deaths. CA Cancer J Clin. 2011;61:212–3.
21. La Vecchia C, Franceschi S. Reproductive factors and colorectal cancer. Cancer Causes Control. 1991;2(3):193–200.
22. Rossouw JE, Anderson GL, Prentice RL, LaCroix AZ, Kooperberg C, Stefanick ML, et al. Risks and benefits of estrogen plus progestin in healthy postmenopausal women: principal results from the Women's Health Initiative randomized controlled trial. JAMA. 2002;288(3):321–33.
23. Kim YS, Milner JA. Dietary modulation of colon cancer risk. J Nutr. 2007;137(11 Suppl):2576S–9.
24. Collaborative Group on Hormonal Factors in Breast Cancer. Breast cancer and breastfeeding: collaborative reanalysis of individual data from 47 epidemiological studies in 30 countries, including 50302 women with breast cancer and 96973 women without the disease. Lancet. 2002;360(9328):187–95.
25. Key T, Appleby P, Reeves G. Endogenous sex hormones and breast cancer in postmenopausal women: reanalysis of nine prospective studies. J Natl Cancer Inst. 2002;94:606–16.
26. Beral V. Breast cancer and hormone-replacement therapy in the Million Women Study. Lancet. 2003;362(9382): 419–27.
27. Velentzis LS, Cantwell MM, Cardwell C, Keshtgar MR, Leathem AJ, Woodside JV, et al. Lignans and breast cancer risk in pre- and post-menopausal women: meta-analyses of observational studies. Br J Cancer. 2009;100(9): 1492–8.
28. Zhu K, Davidson NE, Hunter S, Yang X, Payne-Wilks K, Roland CL, et al. Methyl-group dietary intake and risk of breast cancer among African-American women: a case–control study by methylation status of the estrogen receptor alpha genes. Cancer Causes Control. 2003;14:827–36.
29. Shrubsole MJ, Xiao Ou Shu, Hong-Lan Li, Hui Cai, Gong Yang, Yu-Tang Gao, Jin Gao, Wei Zheng. Dietary B vitamin and methionine intakes and breast cancer risk among Chinese women American. J Epidemiol. 2011; 173:10.
30. Parkin M. Global cancer statistics in the year 2000. Lancet Oncol. 2001;2:533–43.
31. Munoz N, Bosch FX, Castellsague X, Diaz M, de Sanjose S, Hammouda D, et al. Against which human papillomavirus types shall we vaccinate and screen? The international perspective. Int J Cancer. 2004;111:278–85.
32. World Cancer Research Fund and American Investigation of Cancer Research. Food, nutrition, physical activity and the prevention of cancer: a global perspective. Washington, DC: American Investigation of Cancer Research; 2007.
33. Potischman N, Brinton LA, Laiming VA, Reeves WC, Brenes MM, Herrero R, et al. A case–control study of serum folate levels and invasive cervical cancer. Cancer Res. 1991;51(18):4785–9.
34. Mason JB, Levesque T. Folate: effects on carcinogenesis and the potential for cancer chemoprevention. Oncology (Williston Park). 1996;10(11):1727–36. 1742–3; discussion 1743–4.
35. Ferlay J, Bray F, Pisani P, Parkin DM. GLOBOCAN 2000: cancer incidence, mortality and prevalence worldwide. Version 1.0. Lyon: IARC Press; 2001.
36. Bidoli E, La Vecchia C, Talamini R, Negri E, Parpinel M, Conti E, et al. Micronutrients and ovarian cancer: a case–control study in Italy. Ann Oncol. 2001;12:1589–93.
37. Kelemen LE, Sellers TA, Vierkant RA, Harnack L, Cerhan JR. Association of folate and alcohol with risk of ovarian cancer in a prospective study of postmenopausal women. Cancer Causes Control. 2004;15:1085–93.
38. Toffoli G, Cernigoi C, Russo A, Gallo A, Bagnoli M, Boiocchi M. Overexpression of folate binding protein in ovarian cancers. Int J Cancer. 1997;74:193–8.
39. Norman TR. Prospects for the treatment of depression. Aust N Z J Psychiatry. 2006;40(5):394–401.
40. Avis NE, Crawford S, Stellato R, Longcope C. Longitudinal study of hormone levels and depression among women transitioning through menopause. Climacteric. 2001;4:243–9.
41. Chen CS, Tsai JC, Tsang HY, Kuo YT, Lin HF, Chiang IC, et al. Homocysteine levels, MTHFR C677T genotype, and MRI hyperintensities in late-onset major depressive disorder. Am J Geriatr Psychiatry. 2005;13(10):869–75.
42. Morris MS, Fava M, Jacques PF, Selhub J, Rosenberg IH. Depression and folate status in the US Population. Psychother Psychosom. 2003;72(2):80–7.
43. Passeri M, Cucinotta D, Abate G, Senin U, Ventura A, Stramba Badiale M, et al. Oral 5'-methyltetrahydrofolic acid in senile organic mental disorders with depression: results of a double-blind multicenter study. Aging (Milano). 1993;5:63–71.
44. Shea TB, Rogers E. Homocysteine and dementia. N Engl J Med. 2002;346:2007.
45. Botez MI, Young SN, Bachevalier J, Gauthier S. Folate deficiency and decreased brain 5-hydroxytryptamine synthesis in man and rat. Nature. 1979;278:182–3.

46. Snowdon DA. Brain infarction and the clinical expression of Alzheimer disease: the Nun Study. JAMA. 1997;277:813–7.
47. Seshadri S, Beiser A, Selhub J, Jacques PF, Rosenberg IH, D'Agostino RB, et al. Plasma homocysteine as a risk factor for dementia and Alzheimer's disease. N Engl J Med. 2002;346(7):476–83.
48. Ho PI, Ortiz D, Rogers E, Shea TB. Multiple aspects of homocysteine neurotoxicity: glutamate excitotoxicity, kinase hyperactivation and DNA damage. J Neurosci Res. 2002;70:694–702.
49. Brocardo PS, Budni J, Kaster MP, Santos AR, Rodrigues AL. Folic acid administration produces an antidepressant-like effect in mice: evidence for the involvement of the serotonergic and noradrenergic systems. Neuropharmacology. 2008;54:464–73.
50. Lucock MD, Green M, Levene MI. Methylfolate modulates potassium evoked neuro- secretion: evidence for a role at the pteridine cofactor level of tyrosine 3-hydroxylase. Neurochem Res. 1995;20:727–36.

Chapter 18
Use of Diet and Myoinositol in Postmenopausal Women: A New Approach to the Metabolic Syndrome

Rosario D'Anna and Maria Lieta Interdonato

Key Points

- The menopause transition or perimenopause begins several years before the menopause, when the ovaries gradually begin to produce less estrogen, and it ends on the first year after menopause, when a woman has gone 12 months without having her period.
- Decreasing endogenous estrogens after menopause may be the critical factor in removing the relative protection against cardiovascular diseases (CVDs) that women have in their premenopausal years.
- CVD risk in women until menopause is considerably less than in men, after menopause the risk is overlapped. So that CVD represents the leading causes of morbidity and mortality for both men and women in developed countries.
- Deep metabolic changes involving women in the menopause transition are responsible for the onset of metabolic syndrome. It is characterized by hyperinsulinemia with underlying insulin resistance, and a cluster of other CVD risk factors including impaired glucose regulation, elevated levels of triglycerides, decreased levels of HDL-cholesterol, raised blood pressure, and centrally distributed obesity.
- First-line intervention in the management of metabolic syndrome is to reduce the modifiable, underlying risk factors (obesity, physical inactivity, and atherogenic diet) through lifestyle changes, including low-caloric diet and physical activity.
- A new chance in pharmacological treatment may be myoinositol, which is a natural supplement, capable of reducing insulin resistance and all other features of metabolic syndrome.

Keywords Menopause • Metabolic syndrome • Diet • Myoinositol • Perimenopause

R. D'Anna, M.D. (✉)
Department of Obstetrics and Gynecology, University Hospital,
Via Consolare Valeria, n.1, Messina, Italy
e-mail: rosariodanna@tin.it; rdanna@unime.it

M.L. Interdonato, Dr.
Department of Obstetrics and Gynecology, Policlinico Universitario "G. Martino", Via consolare Valeria,
Via C/da Saitta compl. "La Zagara", Messina 98100, Italy
e-mail: lietainterdonato@hotmail.it

C.J.H. Martin et al. (eds.), *Nutrition and Diet in Menopause*, Nutrition and Health,
DOI 10.1007/978-1-62703-373-2_18, © Springer Science+Business Media New York 2013

Abbreviations

CVD	Cardiovascular disease
CHD	Coronary heart disease
LDL	Low-density lipoprotein
HDL	High-density lipoprotein
NCEP	National cholesterol education program expert panel
ATP III	Adult treatment panel III
WHO	World Health Organization
FFA	Free fatty acids
VLDL	Very low-density lipoprotein
IL-6	Interleukine-6
AHA	American Heart Association
NHLBI	National Heart, Lung, and Blood Institute
CRP	C-reactive protein
IGT	Impaired glucose tolerance
IPG	Inositol phosphoglycan
DCI	d-chiro-inositol
PCOS	Polycystic ovary syndrome
OGTT	Oral glucose tolerance test
HOMA	Homeostasis model assessment
BMI	Body mass index

Introduction

The menopause transition or perimenopause is the stage of women's reproductive life that begins several years before the menopause, when the ovaries gradually begin to produce less estrogen. Perimenopause ends the first year after menopause, when a woman has gone 12 months without having her period. In the last 1–2 years of menopause transition, estrogen decline accelerates and many women experience menopausal symptoms: hot flushes, irregular periods, fatigue, vaginal dryness, mood swings, difficulty in sleeping, etc. These are symptoms that characterize the first period of postmenopause too; but at the same time important modifications affect many metabolic processes with consequences that are usually revealed in the late postmenopausal period in terms of CVDs and osteoporosis.

Menopause Transition and Cardiovascular Risk

Traditionally, CVD, and above all coronary heart disease (CHD), have been considered predominantly to affect men and for a long time women were not included in cardiovascular research programs. Women are still not fully aware of their CHD risk and realize the chance of dying of breast cancer as far more likely than that of CHD.

In the early postmenopausal period and until 60 years old, malignant tumors principally influence female mortality rate; instead, after sixty, myocardial infarction and stroke determine a number of deaths five and two times more than breast cancer, respectively. Furthermore, if CHD risk in women until menopause is considerably less than in men, after menopause the risk is overlapped. So that CVD represents the leading causes of morbidity and mortality for both men and women in developed countries.

In both men and women, CHD risk depends on risk factors, which are divided into modifying and non-modifying ones. The main modifying factors are hypertension, obesity, diabetes, dyslipidemia, cigarette smoking, and physical inactivity; non-modifying risk factors are: genetics, sex and age. A significantly lower CHD incidence in premenopausal women suggests that estrogens have a protective effect on the development of the disease. Decreasing endogenous estrogens after menopause may be the critical factor in removing the relative protection against CHD that women have in their premenopausal years. During menopause transition estrogen decrease affects metabolism and body fat distribution. Women tend to put on weight either for less energy waste or for an imbalance between estrogens and androgens, which determines an androgenic fat distribution with truncal obesity. It's well known that independent of overall obesity, the distribution of body fat is a determining factor of CVD risk. It has been shown that truncal obesity, the so called android habitus, confers a far higher risk than the peripheral or "gynecoid" body fat distribution. Waist—hip ratio and waist circumference are highly correlated to the risk of CHD [1]; and weight reduction was associated with an improvement in risk factors and positive changes in triglycerides, high (HDL) and low-density lipoprotein (LDL) levels, and in blood pressure too [2]. These observations suggest a beneficial effect of weight reduction, and because of the difficulty in achieving and maintaining weight loss, the prevention of obesity is of great importance.

Endogenous estrogens exert important effects on metabolism and affect the atherosclerotic process through a variety of mechanisms. It has been reported that estrogens have a lowering effect on total cholesterol and LDL-cholesterol as they are effective LDL receptor up-regulating agents [3]. In the presence of low endogenous estrogen levels, LDL receptor activity is reduced: this leads to the elevated LDL concentrations observed in postmenopausal women. Elevated levels of LDL-cholesterol are correlated with an increased risk of atherosclerosis, and consequently an increased risk of CHD. HDL-cholesterol levels have also been reported to correlate closely and inversely with the risk of CHD [4]; furthermore, a decrease in HDL-Cholesterol levels following the menopause has also been reported [5]; indeed, they play an important role in capturing free cholesterol from circulating cells and lipoproteins, carrying it to the places of its use and excretion. With regards to triglycerides, their concentration depends on enzyme activity, in particular a liver lipase, which in the fertile period is inhibited by estrogens. After menopause this protection ends and then elevated triglycerides levels may increase CVD risk more in women than in men, implying a gender difference in the role of triglycerides in atherosclerosis [5]. Moreover, this risk is further increased when high triglycerides concentrations are associated with lower HDL-Cholesterol levels [6]. Another important parameter is lipoprotein (a): it consists of an LDL particle bound by a disulfide bridge to apolipoprotein (a). Even if its levels are independent of other lipid parameters, it has been reported that in women, circulating lipoprotein (a) levels increase after the menopause just like the other lipid parameters (triglycerides, LDL levels and total cholesterol) [7]. So it can be considered as a cardiovascular risk factor, but the evidence in women is not so strong as in men [5]. Estrogens also have an acute direct vasodilator effect on the vessel wall and a protective effect on atherosclerosis by inhibiting smooth-muscle cell proliferation [8]. The vasodilator effect is endothelium dependent through nitric oxide release stimulation [9], and not endothelium dependent through a calcium antagonist-like effect on smooth muscle vascular cells directly [10]. Consequently, a postmenopausal drop of estrogen concentrations reduce nitric oxide production and then vasodilation, triggering some atherogenic events, such as platelet aggregation, which leads to atheromatous plaque formation. Another substance involved in cardiovascular risk is homocysteine; many studies have stated that an elevated level of homocysteine is an independent risk factor for atherosclerosis; in fact, free oxygen species derive from homocysteine oxidation, which may damage the endothelium. Furthermore, homocysteine acts on coagulation factors inducing thrombogenesis [11]; it stimulates smooth muscle vascular cell proliferation and inhibits nitric oxide production [12]. A homocysteine lowering effect of estrogens has been reported in some studies [13], and it has been suggested that the lower levels of homocysteine in premenopausal women contribute to the lower incidence of vascular disease in this period.

In menopause transition changes in insulin and glucose concentrations do not occur, but only a progressive decrease in pancreatic reactivity, which leads to an insulin resistance condition, together with increased triglycerides levels and decreased HDL-cholesterol production. For this reason, there is a greater incidence of diabetes mellitus type 2 in postmenopause, with CVD increased risk.

During fertile age, female blood pressure levels are lower than in males; while after menopause, systolic and diastolic blood pressure are higher in women than in men. Isolated systolic hypertension is a common finding in elderly women, with a prevalence of 30 % in women over 65 years of age. These observations suggest that the menopausal failure of ovaries could also influence blood pressure increase.

Menopause Transition and Metabolic Syndrome

Deep metabolic changes involving women in the menopause transition are responsible for the onset of metabolic syndrome, even if this syndrome is not currently clearly defined. It consists of a constellation of metabolic abnormalities strictly associated with an increase risk of CVD and diabetes mellitus. In fact, it has been reported that cardiovascular mortality risk in people with metabolic syndrome was almost three times more compared to people without it [14].

The concept of metabolic syndrome was introduced by Reaven in 1988 [15], and it is characterized by hyperinsulinemia with underlying insulin resistance, and a cluster of other CVD risk factors including impaired glucose regulation, elevated levels of triglycerides, decreased levels of HDL-cholesterol, raised blood pressure, and centrally distributed obesity. The pathogenesis of the syndrome is complex and so far not completely understood; but the interaction of obesity, sedentary lifestyle, dietary habits, and genetic factors are known to contribute to its development.

Clinical and epidemiological research on the metabolic syndrome has been hampered by a lack of agreement on the definition of the syndrome and on the cut off points defining its components.

To resolve these problems the WHO consultation for diabetes and its complications and the National Cholesterol Education Program Expert Panel (NCEP) have formulated definitions for it.

Today the NCEP-ATPIII (Adult Treatment Panel III) [16] definition is developed for clinical use. It does not include any estimation of insulin resistance and is based on the presence of three or more of the following components:

1. Fasting plasma glucose concentration greater than 110 mg/Dl
2. A triglyceride concentration of 150 mg/Dl or greater
3. HDL-cholesterol concentration less than 40 mg/Dl in men and less than 50 mg/Dl in women
4. Blood pressure of 130/85 mmHg or greater
5. Waist-circumference greater than 102 cm in men and 88 cm in women.

The prevalence of metabolic syndrome varies across the globe, in part reflecting the age and ethnicity of the populations studied and the diagnostic criteria applied. Metabolic syndrome is more prevalent with increasing age, affecting half of adults aged 60 years and over; ethnicity also influences metabolic syndrome prevalence. With regard to the pathophysiology of metabolic syndrome, the most accepted and unifying hypothesis to describe it, is insulin resistance, caused by an incompletely understood defect in insulin action [17]. The onset of insulin resistance is heralded by postprandial hyperinsulinemia, followed by fasting hyperinsulinemia and, ultimately, hyperglycemia. Free fatty acids (FFA) are released in abundance from an expanded adipose tissue mass. In the liver, FFA result in an increased production of glucose, triglycerides and secretion of very low density lipoproteins (VLDL). Associated lipid/lipoprotein abnormalities include reductions in HDL-cholesterol occur, also for an increased clearance from the circulation. LDL are also modified in composition; with fasting serum triglycerides >180 mg/Dl, there is almost always a predominance of small dense LDL, and small dense LDL are thought to be more atherogenic. FFA also reduce insulin sensitivity in muscle by inhibiting insulin-mediated glucose uptake. Increases in circulating glucose, and to some extent FFA, increase pancreatic insulin secretion, resulting in hyperinsulinemia; and this may also result in enhanced sodium reabsorption and increased sympathetic nervous system activity contributing to hypertension. Finally, insulin resistance is characterized by pathway-specific impairment in phosphatidylinositol 3-kinase signalling. In the endothelium, this may cause an imbalance between the production of nitric oxide and secretion of endothelin-1, leading to decreased blood flow. The pro-inflammatory state is superimposed and contributory to the insulin resistance excessive FFA. The enhanced secretion of interleukin 6 (IL-6) and tumor necrosis factor produced by adipocytes and monocyte-derived macrophages results in more insulin resistance and lipolysis of adipose tissue triglyceride stores to circulating FFA. IL-6 and other cytokines also enhance hepatic glucose production, VLDL production by the liver, and insulin resistance in muscle. Cytokines and FFA also increase the hepatic production of fibrinogen and adipocyte production of plasminogen activator inhibitor 1, resulting in a prothrombotic state. Higher levels of circulating cytokines also stimulate the hepatic production of C-reactive protein (CRP). Reduced production of the anti-inflammatory and insulin sensitizing cytokine adiponectin are also associated with the metabolic syndrome.

Diet and Physical Activity for the Management of Metabolic Syndrome

Management of metabolic syndrome has been stated by the American Heart Association (AHA) and the National Heart, Lung, and Blood Institute (NHLBI) [18]. The predominant underlying risk factors for the syndrome appear to be abdominal obesity, insulin resistance and other associated conditions can be physical inactivity, aging and cigarette smoking. Not all insulin-resistant women are clinically obese, but they commonly have an abnormal fat distribution that is characterized by predominant upper body fat. Upper-body obesity correlates strongly with insulin resistance, and excess upper body fat can accumulate either intraperitoneally (visceral fat) or subcutaneously.

The AHA/NHLBI statement [18] maintained the ATP III criteria since ATP III criteria were simple to use in a clinical setting. The primary goal of clinical management in individuals with metabolic syndrome is to reduce risk for clinical atherosclerotic disease. First-line intervention in the management of metabolic syndrome is to reduce the modifiable, underlying risk factors (obesity, physical inactivity, and atherogenic diet) through lifestyle changes. An effective change in lifestyle will reduce all of the metabolic risk factors. Then, if absolute risk is high enough, consideration can be given to incorporating drug therapy to the regimen. The priority of drug therapy is elevations of LDL-Cholesterol, blood pressure, and glucose. Moreover, efforts should be made to encourage nonsmoking in cigarette smokers. Although many people may be genetically susceptible to the metabolic syndrome, rarely does it become clinically manifested in the absence of some degree of obesity and physical inactivity. The reason to modify underlying risk factors is to prevent or delay onset of CVD; and if type 2 diabetes mellitus is not already present, a concomitant goal is to prevent it as well. Weight reduction deserves first priority in individuals with abdominal obesity and metabolic syndrome. Both weight reduction and maintenance of a lower weight are best achieved by a combination of reduced calorie intake and increased physical activity. The first aim of weight loss is to achieve a decline of about 7–10 % from baseline total body weight during a period of 6–12 months. This requires decreasing calorie intake by 500–1,000 calories per day. Achieving the recommended amount of weight loss will reduce the severity of most or all of the metabolic risk factors. Maintenance of a lower weight is just as important; this requires long-term follow-up and monitoring. Currently available weight-loss drugs possess limited use in the management of obesity. Nevertheless, in some patients they may be helpful. Increasing physical activity assists in weight reduction; it also has beneficial effects on metabolic risk factors; and importantly, it reduces overall CVD risk. Current recommendations provide at least >30 min of moderate-intensity exercise, such as brisk walking, preferably every day of the week; even more exercise adds more benefit [19]. The author's suggestions went beyond current recommendations, and might be particularly beneficial for people with metabolic syndrome: 60 min or more of continuous or intermittent aerobic activity, preferably done every day, promotes weight loss or weight-loss maintenance. Preference is given to 60 min of moderate intensity brisk walking to be supplemented by other activities. The latter include multiple short (10–15 min) bouts of activity (walking breaks at work, gardening, or household work), using simple exercise equipment (e.g., treadmills), jogging, swimming, biking, golfing, team sports, and engaging in resistance training. The authors suggest, at the same time, avoiding common sedentary activities in leisure time (watching television and computer games). Self-monitoring of physical activity can help to achieve adherence to an activity program. For high-risk patients (e.g., those with recent acute coronary syndromes or recent revascularization), physical activity should be carried out under medical supervision.

Beyond weight control and reduction of total calories, the diet should be low in saturated fats, cholesterol, sodium, and simple sugars. In addition, there should be a large intake of fruit, vegetables, and whole grains; fish intake should be encouraged with recognition of concerns about the mercury content of some fish. A very high carbohydrate intake can exacerbate the dyslipidemia of the metabolic syndrome. ATP III [16] recommended that for individuals entering cholesterol management the diet should contain 25–35 % of calories as total fat. If the fat content exceeds 35 %, it is difficult to sustain the low intakes of saturated fat required to maintain a low LDL-cholesterol. On the other hand, if the fat content falls below 25 %, triglycerides can rise and HDL-cholesterol levels can decline; thus, very-low-fat diets may exacerbate atherogenic dyslipidemia. Effective weight loss requires a combination of calorie restriction, physical activity, and motivation; effective lifelong maintenance of weight loss essentially requires a balance between calorie intake and physical activity. The statement of AHA/NHLBI also included recommendations about hypertension: when overt hypertension is present without diabetes or chronic kidney disease, the goal for antihypertensive therapy is a blood pressure of <140/90 mmHg. In the presence of diabetes or chronic kidney disease, the blood pressure goal is <130/80 mmHg. The aim was to reduce blood pressure as much as possible even in the absence of overt hypertension and to obtain other metabolic benefits of lifestyle change. Mild elevations of blood pressure often can be effectively controlled with lifestyle therapies: weight control, increased physical activity, alcohol moderation, sodium reduction, and increased consumption of fresh fruit and vegetables and low-fat dairy products, in accord with the dietary approaches to stop hypertension diet [20]. If hypertension cannot be adequately controlled by lifestyle therapies, antihypertensive drugs are usually necessary to prevent long-term adverse effects, like myocardial infarction, stroke, and chronic kidney disease. People with metabolic syndrome typically manifest elevations of fibrinogen, plasminogen activator inhibitor-1, and other coagulation factors. These abnormalities, however, are not routinely detected in clinical practice. In metabolic syndrome patients who are at moderately high risk for CVD events, aspirin prophylaxis is a therapeutic option to lower vascular events. Measurement of C-reactive protein is the simplest way to identify a pro-inflammatory state in clinical practice. CRP levels >3 mg/L can be taken to define such a state in a person without other detectable causes. If CRP is measured, the finding of an elevated level supports the need for lifestyle changes. The latter, particularly weight reduction, will reduce CRP levels and will presumably mitigate the underlying inflammatory stimulus. The importance of diet plus exercise intervention for preventing diabetes was highlighted in a recent statement from the Cochrane Library [21].

Italian recommendations for diet treatment are included in the "Italian Standards for Diabetes Mellitus" [22]. In these guidelines, it has been confirmed that avoiding overweight and performing regular physical exercise is the most appropriate way of reducing the risk of type 2 diabetes mellitus in subjects with impaired glucose tolerance (IGT). Consequently, subjects with IGT must be given counselling concerning weight loss and indications to increase physical exercise. A moderate reduction in calorie intake (300–500 kcal/day) and a moderate increase in energy consumption (200–300 kcal/day) ensure slow but progressive weight loss (0.45–0.90 kg/week). Moderate physical exercise must be recommended to suit the patient's inclination and capacity when the program starts. This exercise must then gradually increase in duration and frequency to 30–45 min a day of moderate aerobic exercise for 3–5 days a week (goal: 150 min/week). Higher levels of physical exercise: at least 1 h a day of moderate activity (walking) or 30 min a day of more vigorous exercise (jogging), can be required to obtain effective long-term weight loss. The daily intake of carbohydrates in the diet must provide 45–60 % of total daily calories. Vegetables, pulses and fruit typical of the Mediterranean diet must be added to the diet of people with IGT and diabetes mellitus. People with IGT and diabetes mellitus must be encouraged to introduce food with a high-fiber content. The ideal fiber intake with the diet should be more than 40 g/day (or 20 g/1,000 kcal/day). In patients with no history of nephropathy, the protein intake should provide 10–20 % of the total energy daily supplied by food. Subjects with IGT must be encouraged to change their diet habits: reduce the total intake of fat and especially of saturated fatty acids. Fat intake must not contribute over 30 % of the total energy daily supplied by food. The daily intake of saturated fat must be less than 10 % of the total calories. A lesser amount (<7 %) can be useful if LDL cholesterol is <100 mg/dl. Oils rich in monounsaturated fatty acids are an important source of fat. Depending on the patient's preferences, they can provide 10–20 % of the total energy introduced with food daily. The intake of trans fatty acids must be minimized (<1 %). Polyunsaturated fatty acids must not contribute over 10 % of the total energy daily supplied by food. Cholesterol introduced with the diet must not exceed 300 mg/day. It can be further reduced if LDL cholesterol is >100 mg/dl. In overweight patients, a fat intake below 30 % of the total energy daily introduced can facilitate weight loss. A moderate intake of alcohol (up to 10 g/day in women and 20 g/day in men) is acceptable, if the patient wishes to take alcoholic drinks. Finally, like the population at large, IGT and diabetics must be recommended to take less than 6 g/day of salt.

Inositol as Insulin Second Messanger

Some of the actions of insulin may involve low molecular-weight inositol phosphoglycan (IPG) mediators. When insulin binds to its receptor, mediators of this class are generated by the hydrolysis of glycosylphosphatidylinositol lipids located at the cell membrane. An IPG molecule containing D-chiro-inositol (DCI) and galactosamine is known to have a role in activating key enzymes that control the oxidative and non-oxidative metabolism of glucose [23]. A deficiency of the DCI phosphoglycan mediator of the action of insulin may result in resistance to insulin. In fact, insulin resistance has been linked to decreased urinary excretion of chiro-inositol in primates, in humans with impaired glucose tolerance or type 2 diabetes mellitus, and in nondiabetic first-degree relatives of people with diabetes [24]. The amount of chiro-inositol in muscle is lower in subjects with type 2 diabetes mellitus than in normal subjects [25]. Administration of DCI decreased hyperglycemia in rats with diabetes and improved glucose tolerance in normal rats [26]. In a study of monkeys with varying degrees of insulin resistance, DCI accelerated the disposal of glucose and decreased insulin secretion [24]. These observations suggest that the administration of DCI, which is then presumably used in the formation of the active DCI phosphoglycan mediator, may increase insulin sensitivity and improve the action of insulin in insulin-resistant subjects. A syndrome characterized by insulin resistance is the polycystic ovary syndrome (PCOS); insulin resistance and/or compensatory hyperinsulinemia appear to play a key role in the pathophysiology of this disorder [27]. Insulin-resistant and hyperinsulinemic women with or without PCOS display increased urinary clearance of DCI and decreased insulin-stimulated release of DCI-IPG during an oral glucose tolerance test (OGTT), as compared to control cases [28, 29], and the higher DCI urinary clearance correlates with insulin resistance and hyperinsulinemia [28]. In 22 PCOS women, Nestler et al. [30] administered 1,200 mg/die of DCI improving insulin action and ovulatory function, while decreasing at the same time blood pressure, serum androgen, and plasma triglyceride concentrations [30]. A deficiency in this mediator could result from a defect in an epimerase-type enzyme responsible for the intracellular conversion of myoinositol to chiro-inositol

[31] or, alternatively, from accelerated catabolism of DCI before renal filtration. Unfortunately, Nestler's group in 2008, and in a small number of PCOS women, failed to repeat previous results [32]. Indeed, despite the rise in plasma DCI concentration, DCI administration compared to placebo did not change BMI, fasting insulin and glucose levels, total and free testosterone concentrations. It is unclear whether obese women with PCOS are simply deficient in DCI and DCI-IPG or whether some women may also display defective coupling of DCI-IPG to insulin, resulting in relative inactivity of this pathway in response to insulin. This latter possibility is supported by evidence that the administration of metformin to obese PCOS women enhances insulin-stimulated release of DCI-IPG during an OGTT [33]. Thus, it has been hypothesized that obese women with PCOS are insulin resistant in part due to defective coupling between insulin action and release of the DCI-IPG mediator. To test this hypothesis, insulin secretion was suppressed by administration of diazoxide and then insulin was exogenously administered in a dose-dependent manner via a two-step euglycemic–hyperinsulinemic clamp, during which the insulin-mediated release of bioactive DCI-IPG was determined both in obese PCOS women and non-obese normal women [34]. The study showed that, when plasma glucose is maintained at stable levels and plasma insulin is acutely raised and maintained at constant levels, the circulating DCI-IPG insulin mediator is released rapidly and briefly in normal women. In marked contrast, this early coupling between insulin action and DCI-IPG release was entirely absent in obese women with PCOS, despite the fact that higher insulin levels were attained in the obese PCOS women than in the control cases [34]. In contrast again to the normal women, DCI-IPG bioactivity tended to decrease progressively throughout the high-insulin clamp studies, falling below the baseline, suggesting an exhaustion of the ability to release DCI-IPG in obese PCOS women after approximately 4 h of continuous insulin stimulation [34]. Collectively, these findings strongly suggest that the ability of insulin to induce the release of the DCI-IPG mediator of insulin action is defective in women with obese PCOS, which may contribute to their insulin resistance [34]. Possible explanations for these findings are a deficit in intracellular DCI, the substrate for DCI-IPG, and/or a defect in incorporation of the substrate DCI with membrane phosphoglycans to generate the DCI-IPG mediator. Indeed, increased urinary clearance of DCI, with resultant decreased plasma DCI levels has been reported, in two populations of hyperinsulinemic women with or without PCOS [29]. The possibility that a deficit in circulating DCI, or its precursor myoinositol, is responsible for a defective insulin-stimulated release of DCI-IPG mediator in PCOS is further supported by the findings that oral supplementation with DCI [30, 35] or myoinositol [36, 37] in both lean and obese PCOS women improved their insulin resistance and clinical features. This finding suggests that defective insulin-mediated release of the DCI-IPG mediator may contribute to the insulin resistance that characterizes obese PCOS women.

Myoinositol Supplementation and Diet in Postmenopausal Women with Metabolic Syndrome

Recently, the interest in inositol was moved to the other isomer: myoinositol. Administration of myoinositol in PCOS women has restored spontaneous menstrual cycles during treatment in over 80 % of cases, with about 40 % of pregnancies [37, 38]. It's worth noting that PCOS features such as insulin resistance and obesity are very similar to the metabolic syndrome, so an Italian group wondered whether the improvement in insulin resistance could have been the same in a group of postmenopausal women affected by the metabolic syndrome, receiving myoinositol [39]. After menopause, women are at increased risk for obesity, insulin resistance and compensatory hyperinsulinemia with consequent dyslipidemia and hypertension. All these conditions are features of metabolic syndrome, which has been shown to increase the risk of CVD [40]. In fact, cardiovascular events are a rare occurrence in premenopausal women, but their incidence increases most markedly at the time of menopause [41]. Eighty outpatient postmenopausal women affected by metabolic syndrome were enrolled in a 6-month study. To define metabolic syndrome, NCEP/ATP III criteria was used [16], and all 80 women satisfied at

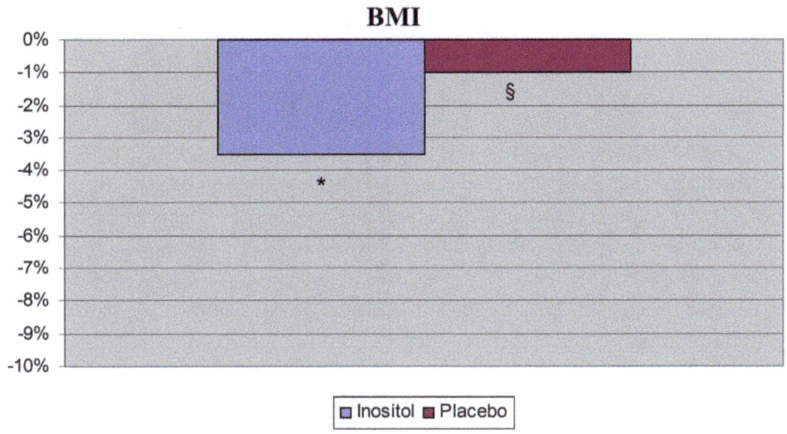

Fig. 18.1 Percentage reduction of BMI (body mass index) in myoinositol and placebo group after 6 months of treatment. The histograms show the significant statistical difference of: §Placebo group mean basal value versus 6 months $P=0.004$, *Inositol group mean basal value versus 6 months $P<0.0001$. Figure was created using the results from *Giordano D et al., Menopause, 2011*

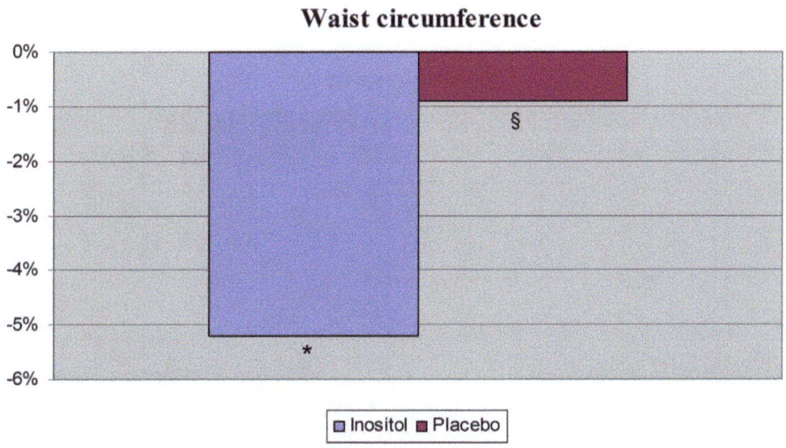

Fig. 18.2 Percentage reduction of waist circumference in myoinositol and placebo group after 6 months of treatment. The histograms show the significant statistical difference of: §Placebo group mean basal value versus 6 months $P=0.0001$, *Inositol group mean basal value versus 6 months $P<0.0001$. Figure was created using the results from *Giordano D et al., Menopause, 2011*

least three of the five criteria reported. At the time of the recruitment, all women were treated with a low-energy diet following the Italian guidelines [22], and were then assigned randomly to myoinositol 2 g twice daily (n.40) or to placebo (n.40) for 6 months. A computer randomization and an allocation of 1:1 in each group was used. All the women were hypertensive and were treated with various antihypertensive agents. They were evaluated for serum glucose, insulin, HOMA (Homeostasis Model Assessment), a marker of insulin resistance [42], triglycerides, total and HDL cholesterol, body mass index (BMI), and blood pressure at baseline and after 6 months of treatment.

At baseline, there was no difference between the two groups in maternal age, BMI, waist circumference, glucose, insulin, HOMA, blood pressure levels, serum triglycerides, total and HDL-cholesterol concentrations. After 6 months, no significant difference in BMI (Fig. 18.1) and waist circumference (Fig. 18.2) between groups occurred, but only inside each group; instead, a very significant difference of all other parameters between groups was highlighted. Furthermore, an important decrease in glucose

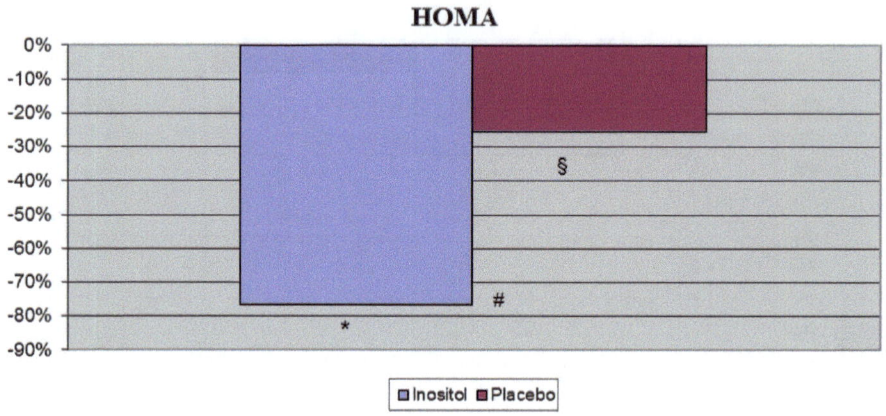

Fig. 18.3 Percentage reduction of HOMA (homeostasis model assessment) in myoinositol and placebo group after 6 months of treatment. The histograms show the significant statistical difference of: #Inositol versus placebo group mean values after 6 months $P<0.0001$, §Placebo group mean basal value versus 6 months $P=0.0001$, *Inositol group mean basal value versus 6 months $P<0.0001$. Figure was created using the results from *Giordano D et al., Menopause, 2011*

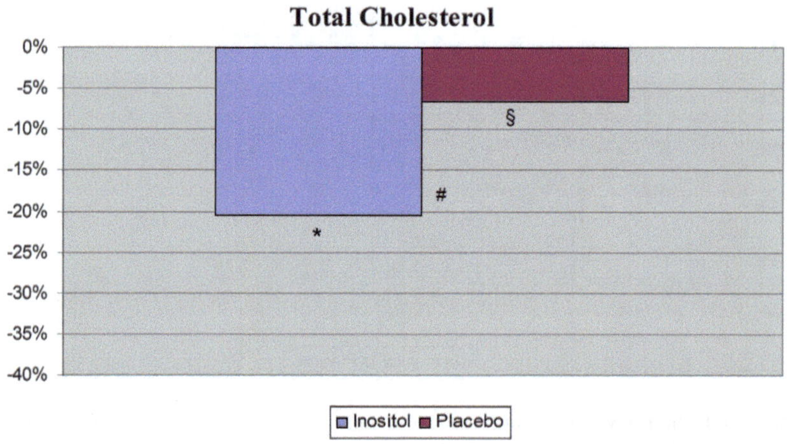

Fig. 18.4 Percentage reduction of total cholesterol in myoinositol and placebo group after 6 months of treatment. The histograms show the significant statistical difference of: #Inositol versus placebo group mean values after 6 months $P<0.0001$, §Placebo group mean basal value versus 6 months $P=0.02$, *Inositol group mean basal value versus 6 months $P<0.0001$. Figure was created using the results from *Giordano D et al., Menopause, 2011*

(–8 %), insulin (–69 %), and consequently HOMA (Fig. 18.3) mean value occurred in the treated group. The lipid profile was also improved in the myoinositol group: total cholesterol (–20.4 %) (Fig. 18.4), HDL-cholesterol (+27.9 %) (Fig. 18.5) and triglycerides (–21.3 %) (Fig. 18.6). Finally, the blood pressure mean value was also reduced in the treated group, either in systolic (Fig. 18.7) or diastolic values (Fig. 18.8). Furthermore, six women (15 %) no longer had metabolic syndrome. Instead, in the placebo group (Figs. 18.1–18.8), from baseline there was no significant difference in insulin, HDL-cholesterol and triglycerides concentrations, but also in blood pressure mean values [39]. Recently, the same Italian group has published a follow-up study [43], that lasted for another 6 months, confirming the results

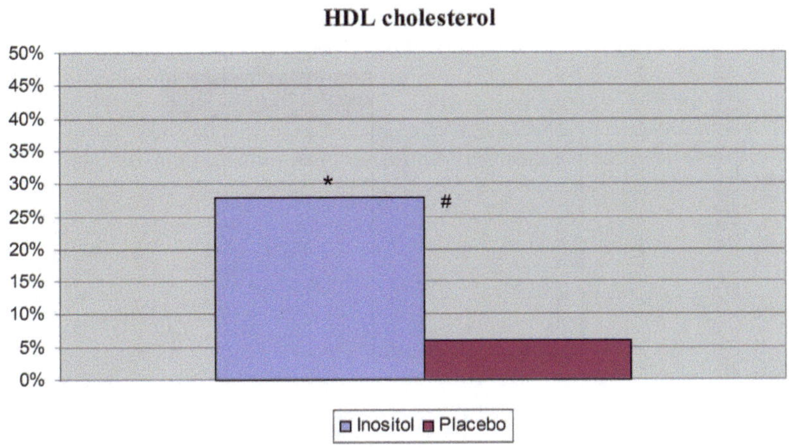

Fig. 18.5 Percentage reduction of HDL (high-density lipoprotein) cholesterol in myoinositol and placebo group after 6 months of treatment. The histograms show the significant statistical difference of: #Inositol versus placebo group mean values after 6 months $P<0.0001$, *Inositol group mean basal value versus 6 months $P<0.0001$. Figure was created using the results from *Giordano D et al., Menopause, 2011*

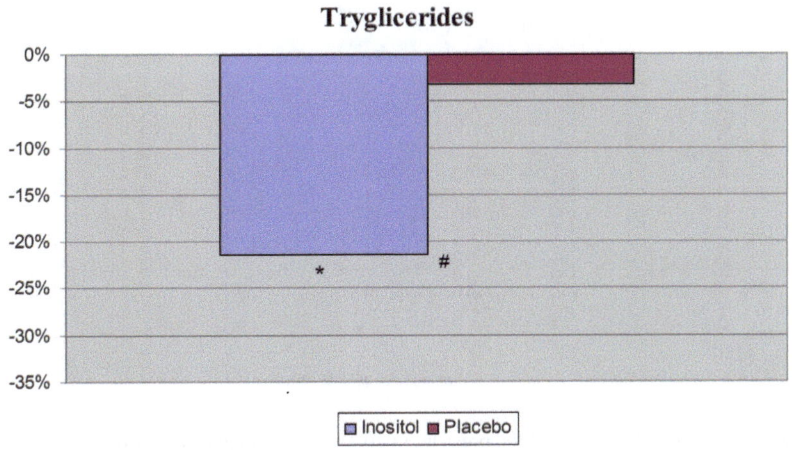

Fig. 18.6 Percentage reduction of triglycerides in myoinositol and placebo group after 6 months of treatment. The histograms show the significant statistical difference of: #Inositol versus placebo group mean values after 6 months $P<0.0001$, *Inositol group mean basal value versus 6 months $P<0.0001$. Figure was created using the results from *Giordano D et al., Menopause, 2011*

obtained in the 6-month study, with an increased amount of women without metabolic syndrome after 12 months of myoinositol treatment.

Comparing myoinositol with other insulin-sensitizing substances, pioglitazone seemed to be the most effective in reducing serum triglycerides by about 50 % [44], better than in the myoinositol study (−34 %) and by 20 % with rosiglitazone [45]. In a study performed with metformin for 12 months, no change in triglycerides was noted [46], but only a slight improvement of HDL-cholesterol (+2.4 %). In the study with myoinositol, the improvement in HDL-cholesterol concentrations (+21 %) was also better compared to others obtained with pioglitazone [44] and rosiglitazone [45]. With regard to blood

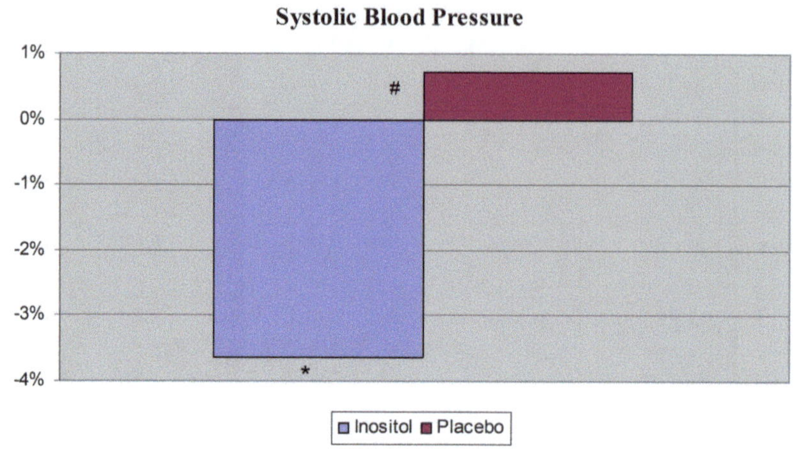

Fig. 18.7 Percentage reduction of systolic blood pressure in myoinositol and placebo group after 6 months of treatment. The histograms show the significant statistical difference of: #Inositol versus placebo group mean values after 6 months $P<0.0001$, *Inositol group mean basal value versus 6 months $P=0.002$. Figure was created using the results from *Giordano D et al., Menopause, 2011*

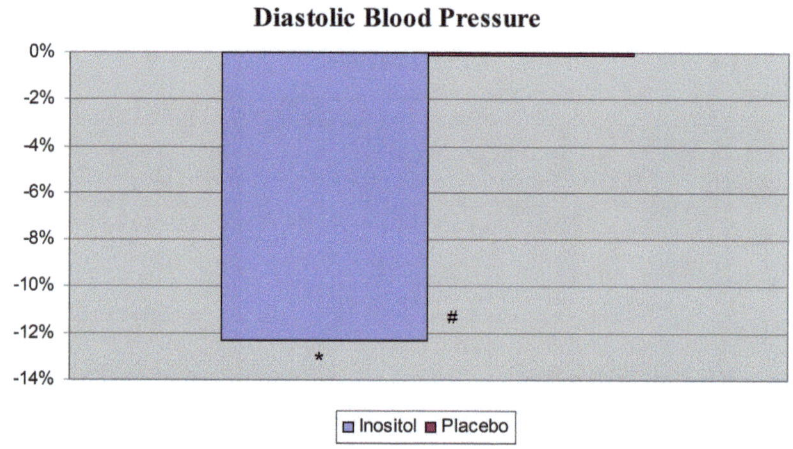

Fig. 18.8 Percentage reduction of diastolic blood pressure in myoinositol and placebo group after 6 months of treatment. The histograms show the significant statistical difference of: #Inositol versus placebo group mean values after 6 months $P<0.0001$, *Inositol group mean basal value versus 6 months $P<0.0001$. Figure was created using the results from *Giordano D et al., Menopause, 2011*

pressure, the decrease of systolic (−7 %) and diastolic (−16 %) mean values was similar to the Fontbonne et al. study [46], using metformin for 12 months in overweight people with impaired glucose tolerance. But the most important result in this study is the critical reduction of serum insulin and consequently insulin resistance (HOMA), which was about double compared to other insulin-sensitizing substances such as pioglitazone [44], rosiglitazone [45], and metformin [46]; and these drugs are, at the moment, the gold standard of therapy for patients with impaired glucose tolerance.

The recent study of Baillargeon et al. [34] might suggest a possible explanation for these results; they found that D-chiro-inositol-containing inositolphosphoglycan, a mediator of insulin action, is defective in obese women affected by polycystic ovary syndrome. Since almost all the women in our study were obese, and probably with a defective production of inositolphosphoglycan, consequently they would have benefited from taking myoinositol supplementation.

Conclusions

In conclusion, metabolic syndrome maybe one of estrogen decreased consequences in postmenopausal women. These women experience CVD events more frequently in their third age. The first approach to the syndrome must be a life-style change, including low-caloric diet and physical activity. A new chance in pharmacological treatment may be myoinositol, which is a natural supplement, capable of reducing insulin resistance and all other features of metabolic syndrome.

References

1. Rexrode KM, Carey VJ, Hennekens CH, Walters EE, Colditz JA, Stampfer MJ, et al. Abdominal adiposity and coronary heart disease in women. JAMA. 1998;280:1843–8.
2. Van Gaal LF, Wauters MA, De Leeuw IH. The beneficial effects of modest weight loss on cardiovascular risk factors. Int J Obes Relat Metab Disord. 1997;21 Suppl 1Suppl 1:S5–9.
3. Parini P, Angelin B, Rudling M. Importance of estrogens receptor in hepatic LDL receptor regulation. Arterioscler Thromb Vasc Biol. 1997;17:1800–5.
4. Amarenco P, Labreuche J, Touboul PJ. High-density lipoprotein cholesterol and risk of stroke and carotid atherosclerosis: a systematic review. Atherosclerosis. 2008;196:489–96.
5. van Lennep JE R, Westerveld HT, Erkelens DW, van der Wall EE. Risk factors for coronary heart disease: implications of gender. Cardiovasc Res. 2002;53:538–49.
6. Gaziano JM, Hennekens CH, O'Donnell CJ, Breslow JL, Buring JE. Fasting triglycerides, high-density lipoprotein, and risk of myocardial infarction. Circulation. 1997;96:2520–5.
7. Scanu AM, Lawn RM, Berg K. Lipoprotein(a) and atherosclerosis. Ann Intern Med. 1991;115:209–18.
8. Mendelsohn ME, Karas RH. Estrogen and the blood vessel wall. Curr Opin Cardiol. 1994;9:619–26.
9. Van Buren G, Yang D, Clark E. Estrogen induced uterine vasodilatation is antagonized by L-nitroarginine methyl ester, an inhibition of nitric oxide synthesis. Am J Obstet Gynecol. 1992;16:828–32.
10. Collins P, Rosano G, Jiang C, Lindsay D, Sarrel PM, Poole-Wilson PA. Cardiovascular protection by estrogen—a calcium antagonist effect? Lancet. 1993;341:1264–5.
11. Welch GN, Loscalzo J. Hyperhomocysteinemia and atherothrombosis. N Engl J Med. 1998;338:1047–8.
12. Stamler JS, Osborne JA, Jaraki O, Rabbani LE, Mullins M, Singel D, et al. Adverse vascular effects of homocisteine are modulated by endothelium-derived relaxing factor and related oxides of nitrogen. J Clin Invest. 1993;91:308–18.
13. Giltay EJ, Hoogeveen EK, Elbers JM, Gooren LJ, Asscheman H, Stehouwer CD. Effects of sex steroids on plasma total homocysteine levels; a study in transsexual males and females. J Clin Endocrinol Metab. 1998;83:550–3.
14. Hu G, Qiao Q, Tuomilehto J, Balkau B, Borch-Johnsen K, Pyorala K, et al. Prevalance of the metabolic syndrome and its relation to all-cause and cardiovascular mortality in nondiabetic European men and women. Arch Intern Med. 2004;164:1066–76.
15. Reaven GM. Banting lecture 1988. Role of insulin resistance in human disease. Diabetes. 1988;37:1595–607.
16. Expert Panel on Detection, Evaluation, and Treatment of High Blood Cholesterol in Adults. Executive summary of the third report of the national cholesterol education program (NCEP) expert panel on detection, evaluation, and treatment of high blood cholesterol in adults (adult treatment panel III). JAMA. 2001;285:2486–97.
17. Eckel RH, Grundy SM, Zimmet PZ. The metabolic syndrome. Lancet. 2005;365:1415–28.
18. Grundy SM, Cleeman JI, Daniels SR, Donato KA, Eckel RH, Franklin BA, et al. Diagnosis and management of the metabolic syndrome. An American Heart Association/National Heart, Lung, and Blood Institute. Scientific statement. Circulation. 2005;112:2735–52.
19. Grundy SM, Hansen B, Smith Jr SC, Cleeman JL, Kahn RA. American Heart Association; National Heart, Lung, and Blood Institute; American Diabetes Association. Clinical management of metabolic syndrome: report of the American Heart Association/National Heart, Lung, and Blood Institute/American Diabetes Association conference on scientific issues related to management. Circulation. 2004;109:551–6.
20. Chobanian AV, Bakris GL, Black HR, Cushman WC, Green LA, Izzo Jr JL, et al. The seventh report of the joint National Committee on Prevention, Detection, Evaluation, and Treatment of High Blood Pressure: the JNC 7 report. JAMA. 2003;289:2560–72.
21. Orozco LJ, Buchleitner AM, Gimenez-Perez G, Roquè I Figuls M, Richter B, Mauricio D. Exercise or exercise and diet for preventing type 2 diabetes mellitus. Cochrane Database Syst Rev. 2008;(3):CD003054. Review.
22. De Micheli A. Italian standards for diabetes mellitus 2007: executive summary: diabete Italia, AMD Associazione Medici Diabetologi, SID Societè Italiana di Diabetologia. Acta Diabetol. 2008;45:107–27.

23. Larner J. Multiple pathways in insulin signalling—fitting the covalent and allosteric puzzle pieces together. Endocr J. 1994;2:167–71.
24. Ortmeyer HK, Bodkin NL, Lilley K, Larner J, Hansen BC. Chiroinositol deficiency and insulin resistance. I. Urinary excretion rate of chiroinositol is directly associated with insulin resistance in spontaneously diabetic rhesus monkeys. Endocrinology. 1993;132:640–5.
25. Asplin I, Galasko G, Larner J. Chiro-inositol deficiency and insulin resistance: a comparison of the chiro-inositol- and the myo-inositol-containingcontaining insulin mediators isolated from urine, hemodialysate, and muscle of control and type II diabetic subjects. Proc Natl Acad Sci USA. 1993;90:5924–8.
26. Ortmeyer HK, Huang LC, Zhang L, Hansen BC, Larner J. Chiroinositol deficiency and insulin resistance. II. Acute effects of D-chiroinositol administration in streptozotocin-diabetic rats, normal rats given a glucose load, and spontaneously insulin-resistant rhesus monkeys. Endocrinology. 1993;132:646–51.
27. Baillargeon JP, Nestler JE. Polycystic ovary syndrome: a syndrome of ovarian hypersensitivity to insulin? J Clin Endocrinol Metab. 2006;91:22–4.
28. Baillargeon J-P, Diamanti-Kandarakis E, Ostlund Jr RE, Apridonidze T, Iuorno MJ, Nestler JE. Altered D-chiroinositol urinary clearance in women with polycystic ovary syndrome. Diabetes Care. 2006;29:300–5.
29. Baillargeon JP, Nestler JE, Ostlund REJ, Apridonidze T, Diamanti-Kandarakis E. Greek hyperinsulinemic women with or without polycystic ovary syndrome display altered inositols metabolism. Hum Reprod. 2008;23: 1439–46.
30. Nestler JE, Jakubowicz DJ, Reamer P, Gunn RD, Allan G. Ovulatory and metabolic effects of D-chiro-inositol in the polycystic ovary syndrome. N Engl J Med. 1999;340:1314–20.
31. Pak Y, Huang LC, Lilley KJ, Larner J. In vivo conversion of [3H]myoinositol to [3H]chiroinoistol in rat tissues. J Biol Chem. 1992;267:16904–10.
32. Cheang KI, Baillargeon JP, Essah PA, Ostlund Jr RE, Apridonidze T, Islam L, et al. Insulin-stimulated release of D-chiro-inositol-containing inositolphosphoglycan mediator correlates with insulin sensitivity in women with polycystic ovary syndrome. Metabolism. 2008;57:1390–7.
33. Baillargeon JP, Iuorno MJ, Jakubowicz DJ, Apridonidze T, He N, Nestler JE. Metformin therapy increases insulin-stimulated release of D-chiro-inositol-containing inositolphosphoglycan mediator in women with polycystic ovary syndrome. J Clin Endocrinol Metab. 2004;89:242–9.
34. Baillargeon J-P, Iuorno MJ, Apridonidze T, Nestler JE. Uncoupling between insulin and release of a D-chiro-inositol-containing inositolphosphoglycan mediator of insulin action in obese women with polycystic ovary syndrome. Metab Syndr Relat Disord. 2010;8:127–36.
35. Iuorno MJ, Jakubowicz DJ, Baillargeon JP, Dillon P, Gunn RD, Allan G, et al. Effects of D-*chiro*-inositol in lean women with the polycystic ovary syndrome. Endocr Pract. 2002;8:417–23.
36. Papaleo E, Unfer V, Baillargeon JP, Fusi F, Occhi F, De Santis L. Myo-inositol may improve oocyte quality in intracytoplasmic sperm injection cycles. A prospective, controlled, randomized trial. Fertil Steril. 2009;91:1750–4.
37. Papaleo E, Unfer V, Baillargeon JP, De Santis L, Fusi F, Brigante C, et al. Myo-inositol in patients with polycystic ovary syndrome: a novel method for ovulation induction. Gynecol Endocrinol. 2007;23:700–3.
38. Genazzani AD, Lanzoni C, Ricchieri F, Jasonni VM. Myo-inositol administration positively affects hyperinsulinemia and hormonal parameters in overweight patients with polycystic ovary syndrome. Gynecol Endocrinol. 2008;24:139–44.
39. Giordano D, Corrado F, Santamaria A, Quattrone S, Pintaudi B, Di Benedetto A, et al. Effects of myo-inositol supplementation in postmenopausal women with metabolic syndrome: a perspective, randomized, placebo-controlled study. Menopause. 2011;18:102–4.
40. Isomaa B, Almgren P, Tuomi T, Forsén B, Lahti K, Nissén M, et al. Cardiovascular morbidity and mortality associated with the metabolic syndrome. Diabetes Care. 2001;24:683–9.
41. Sowers JR, Epstein M, Froholich ED. Diabetes, hypertension, and cardiovascular disease. An update. Hypertension. 2001;37:1053–9.
42. Haffner SM, Miettinem H, Stern MP. The homeostasis model in the San Antonio Hearth study. Diabetes Care. 1997;20:1087–92.
43. Santamaria A, Giordano D, Corrado F, Pintaudi B, Interdonato ML, Di Vieste G, et al. One-year effect of myo-inositol supplementation in postmenopausal women with metabolic syndrome. Climacteric. 2011;15(5):490–5.
44. Gupta AK, Smith SR, Greenway L, Bray GA. Pioglitazone treatment in type 2 diabetes mellitus when combined with portion control diet modifies the metabolic syndrome. Diabetes Obes Metab. 2009;11:330–7.
45. Esposito K, Ciotola M, Carleo D, Schisano B, Saccomanno F, Sacco FC, et al. Effect of rosiglitazone on endothelial function and inflammatory markers in patients with the metabolic syndrome. Diabetes Care. 2006;29: 1071–6.
46. Fontbonne A, Diouf I, Baccara-Dinet M, Eschwege E, Charles MA. Effects of 1-year treatment with metformin on metabolic and cardiovascular risk factors in non-diabetic upper-body obese subjects with mild glucose anomalies: a post-hoc analysis of the BIGPRO1 trial. Diabetes Metab. 2009;35:385–91.

Chapter 19
Leptin and Obesity in Ovarian Dysfunction in Menopause

Patrick Rene Diel and Carmen Weigt

Key Points

- In postmenopausal women, there is an increased tendency for developing obesity and metabolic syndrome.
- The physiological key event for changes in the body composition in menopausal women is the massive loss of circulating sex steroids.
- Estrogens regulate energy expenditure via fat and glucose metabolism and movement behavior.
- Obesity in postmenopausal women is associated with a huge increase in circulating leptin.
- There is evidence for an intensive cross talk between leptin and estrogens in the regulation of ovarian function and energy balance.
- Increased leptin levels are a risk factor for the development of cancer.
- Reducing fat mass is cancer prevention.
- Strategies for the prevention and treatment of menopausal and postmenopausal obesity and the associated elevated leptin serum concentrations must target the decrease of circulating estrogen levels and the resulting changes in metabolic pathways in combination with physical inactivity.

Keywords Obesity • Energy homeostasis • Estrogens • Estrogen receptor alpha • Estrogen receptor beta • Fat metabolism • Leptin • Menopause

Abbreviations

AgRP	Agouti-related protein
BMI	Body mass index
CART	Cocaine- and amphetamine-regulated transcript
E2	17β-estradiol

P.R. Diel, Ph.D. (✉)
Department of Cellular and Molecular Sports Medicine, German Sports University Cologne,
Institute of Cardiovascular Research and Sports Medicine, Am Sportpark Müngersdorf 6,
50933 Cologne, Germany
e-mail: Diel@dshs-koein.de

C. Weigt, Dipl. Biol.
German Sports University Cologne, Am Sportpark Müngersdorf 6, 50933 Cologne, Germany

C.J.H. Martin et al. (eds.), *Nutrition and Diet in Menopause*, Nutrition and Health,
DOI 10.1007/978-1-62703-373-2_19, © Springer Science+Business Media New York 2013

ER alpha	Estrogen receptor alpha
ER beta	Estrogen receptor beta
ERKO	Estrogen receptor knockout
GnRH	Gonadotropin-releasing hormone
HDL	High-density lipoprotein
HRT	Hormone replacement therapy
IGF1	Insulin-like growth factor 1
LDL	Low-density lipoprotein
LH	Luteinizing hormone
NPY	Neuropeptid Y
OVX	Ovariectomized
PAX7	Paired box 7
POMC	Proopiomelanocortin
PPAR gamma	Peroxisome proliferator-activated receptor gamma
PPAR delta	Peroxisome proliferator-activated receptor delta
SERM	Selective estrogen receptor modulator
VLDL	Very-low-density lipoprotein
ZDF	Zucker diabetic fatty rat

Introduction

The prevalence of obesity, a major risk for chronic diseases such as type 2 diabetes, insulin resistance, dyslipidemia, hypertension, cardiovascular disease, coronary heart disease, diseases of liver and gall bladder, and certain forms of cancer, is dramatically increasing [1, 2], especially in postmenopausal women. Already in 1997, the WHO formally recognized obesity as a global epidemic [3]. In 2005, approximately 1.6 billion adults (age 15+) around the world were overweight (BMI greater than 25 kg/m^2)—at least 400 million of them were obese (BMI greater than 30 kg/m^2). And the numbers will continue to rise [1, 4]. A combination of genetic, behavioral, and environmental factors is considered to be responsible for this epidemic rapid growth of obesity and overweight over the last several decades [5, 6]. However, the main reason is thought to be a chronic imbalance of energy homeostasis due to increased consumption of high-caloric nutrition, combined with a lack of physical activity [2, 4]. Nowadays, obesity affects virtually all ages, sexes, races, and socioeconomic groups, and therefore poses a serious social and psychological problem.

Body Composition in Postmenopausal Women

In postmenopausal women, there is an increased tendency for gaining weight, but to date it remains unclear whether the menopausal transition itself leads to weight gain. During menopause, the reduced production of endogenous ovarian hormones together with physical inactivity results in a significant change in the body composition, characterized by an increase of adipose tissue and a loss of muscle mass. Postmenopausal women in average have 20 % larger fat mass than premenopausal women. With respect to health effects especially the change in fat distribution is of relevance. In premenopausal women fat is distributed in the so-called gynoid pattern (Fig. 19.1). Here we find a fat accumulation around the hips and thighs, causing a “pear-shape.” In contrast, the android pattern is characterized by an accumulation of adipose tissue mainly around the trunk and upper body, in areas such as the abdomen, chest, shoulder, and nape of neck. This pattern is also called “apple-shaped” and is more common in men than in

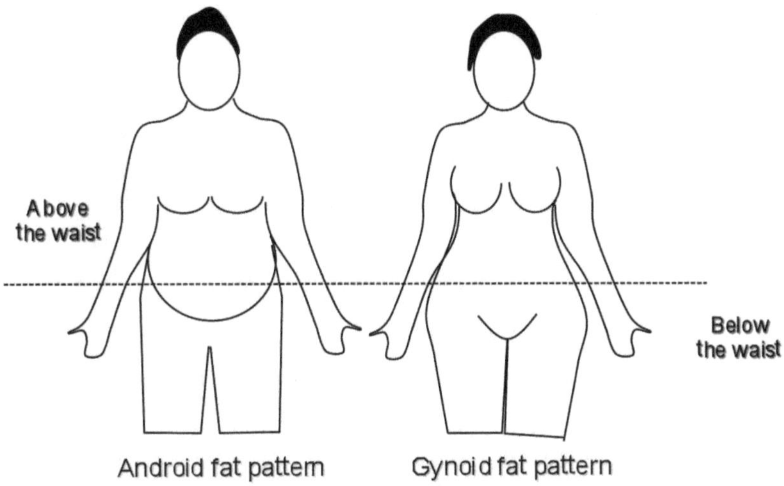

Fig. 19.1 Android and gynoid fat distribution pattern. The difference between the android (*left*, typical for men) and gynoid (*right*, typical in premenopausal women) fat distribution pattern is depicted

women. Epidemiologic studies correlate the android fat pattern with an increased risk to develop cardiovascular diseases. During menopause fat distribution becomes resembles that in men and the amount of android fat is significantly higher in postmenopausal women than in premenopausal women [7]. In contrast, muscle mass in women starts to decrease after the third decade of age, and shows an accelerated decline after the fifth decade. Studies have shown a muscle mass decline of 0.6 % per year after menopause [8].

Ovarian Dysfunction in Obesity and the Metabolic Syndrome

The physiological key event for the observed changes in the body composition in menopausal women is the massive loss of circulating sex steroids. In menopause a strong and sudden decrease of E2 and progesterone production by the ovaries occurs. In contrast, the levels of total and free testosterone, dehydroepiandrosterone sulfate and androstenedione decline more or less steadily with age. In general, circulating androgen levels seem not to be affected by ovarian dysfunction in natural menopause [9]. The major promotion of the physiological changes associated with ovaries dysfunction is neither attributed to the loss of androgenic hormone production nor to decreasing progesterone levels. Physiological changes are mainly caused by the loss of estrogens. This is confirmed by studies in rodents where ovariectomy resulted in body weight gain (Fig. 19.2) and the development of obesity, whereas treatment with E2 antagonized these effects [10, 11]. Estrogens directly influence energy homeostasis through modulation of glucose and lipid metabolism [12]. Moreover, estrogen withdrawal during menopause has significant effects on metabolism such as reduced glucose tolerance, abnormal plasma lipid composition, elevated blood pressure, increased sympathetic tone, endothelial dysfunction, and vascular inflammation. As a result disorders like hypertension, diabetes mellitus, and coronary artery disease are increasing. In combination these disorders are called metabolic syndrome, which is characterized by an increased risk of developing cardiovascular diseases and diabetes and as a consequence by premature death. Among the US population more than 43 % of the adults older than age 60 are affected by the metabolic syndrome. The percentage of women having the metabolic syndrome is higher than that of men [13], underlining the role of estrogens in the development of this metabolic disorder.

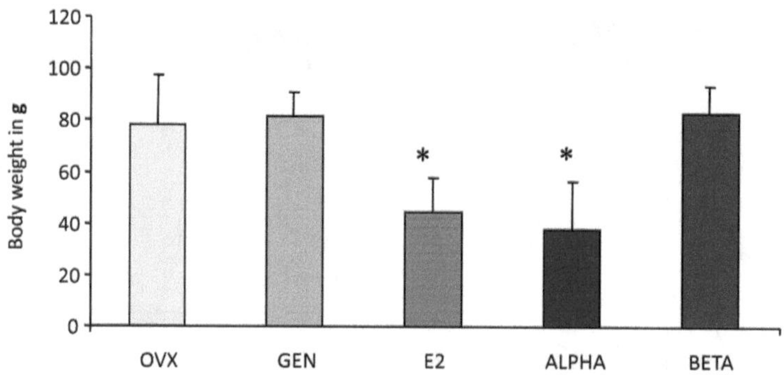

Fig. 19.2 Effect of estrogen withdrawal on body weight. Female OVX rats were treated with vehicle (control), Gen, E2, Alpha, or Beta for 3 weeks ($n=5$). Treatment with E2 and ALPHA decreased body weight gain, whereas the weight gain in animals substituted with GEN and BETA was unchanged compared to control. OVX = ovariectomized, Gen = phytoestrogen genistein, E2 = 17β-estradiol, Alpha = ER alpha specific agonist, Beta = ER beta specific agonist. Data shown are means ± SD. *Asterisk* marks values significantly different from OVX ($p \leq 0.05$), modified from Hertrampf et al. [30]

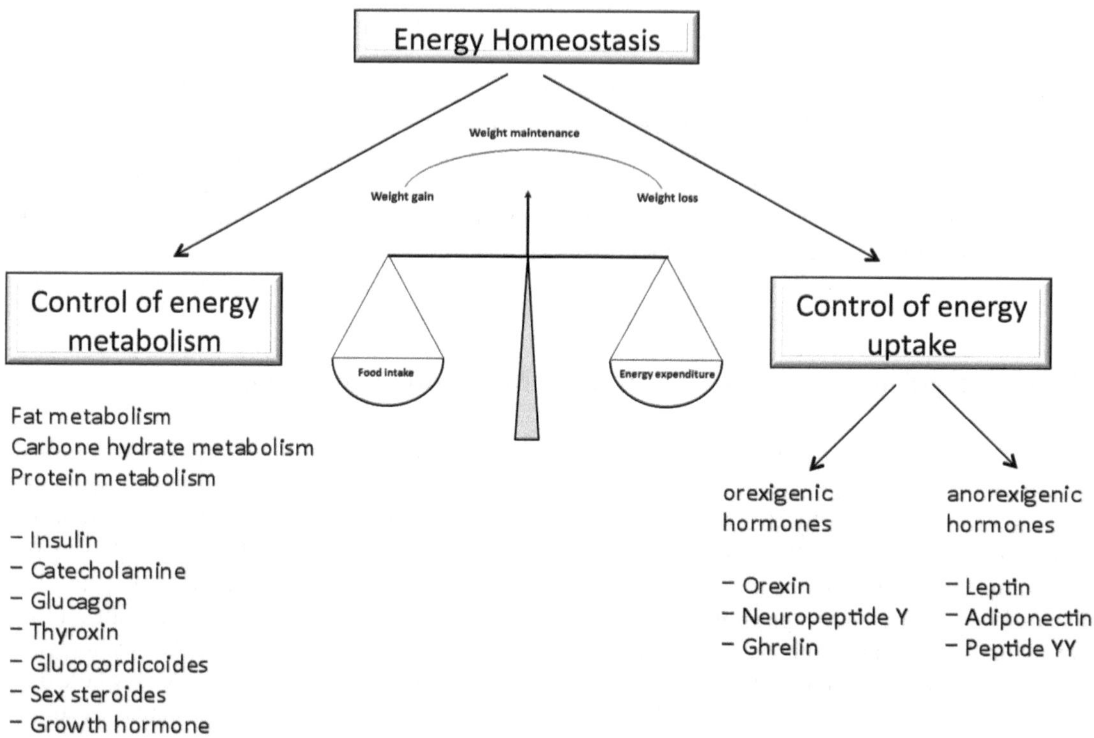

Fig. 19.3 Regulation of energy homeostasis by hormones. The model depicts the regulation of energy homeostasis through interaction between the periphery (control of energy metabolism by several hormones that are involved in fat, lipid, and protein metabolism) and the brain (control of energy uptake by orexigenic and anorexigenic hormones)

Hormones in the Regulation of Energy Homeostasis

The accumulation of excessive body fat in obesity is the result of a chronic imbalance of energy. In obesity the intake of energy exceeds their expenditure (Fig. 19.3). A balance between calorie uptake and/or increment of energy expenditure is the most effective way to avoid the development of obesity.

Strategies to reduce obesity must include either an elevation of energy expenditure and/or a suppression of energy intake. Energy metabolism but also intake of food is strictly controlled via the hypothalamus by hormones. Here we can distinguish between hormones involved in the control of energy metabolism and hormones involved in the control of food intake. Hormones involved in energy intake are for example insulin and glucagon, catecholamines and glucocorticoids, thyroxin, sex steroids, and growth hormone. Hormones controlling food uptake are divided in orexigenic hormones, that increase appetite, and in anorexigenic hormones, that suppress appetite. Appetite regulation is a highly complex process involving hypothalamic neuropeptides and peripheral signals like adipokines and gut hormones. Examples for orexigenic hormones are peptides such as ghrelin, orexin, and neuropeptide Y. High circulating concentrations of orexigenic hormones increases the hunger feeling and therefore enhances food consumption. By contrast, anorexigenic hormones include molecules like leptin and peptide YY. High circulating concentrations of anorexigenic hormones result in feeling of satiety and decrease food consumption. Interestingly, also hormones like insulin but also estrogens or androgens have been identified to function in an orexigenic as well as in an anorexigenic manner [14].

Estrogens

In females estrogens are a key player in energy metabolism. As a logical consequence the massive decline of circulating estrogens in menopausal women results in massive changes in the energy balance of the body. Estrogens are the primary female sex hormones. These steroid hormones are mainly produced by developing follicles in the ovaries, the corpus luteum, and the placenta. Smaller amounts of estrogens are also produced in the adrenal glands, the liver, the mammary gland, and the adipose tissue. Therefore, in postmenopausal women the secondary sources of estrogens are of main importance.

Cellular signaling of estrogens is mediated via two distinct ERs, ER alpha and ER beta, which belong to the nuclear receptor family of transcription factors. Both receptors are located at different chromosomal segments and have tissue and gender specific expression patterns. Like many other members of the nuclear receptor family, ERs contain of functionally distinct domains. ER alpha and ER beta differ, inter alia, considerably in the ligand binding domain, representing the key requirement for SERMs [15, 16]. Therefore, the binding affinity of the ligand as well as the cellular/nuclear context in which the ligand acts, enable a wide range of combinations to modulate a physiological response to E2 or a SERM. SERMs like Tamoxifen and Raloxifene are examples of tissue specific estrogenic activity and it is assumed that in the underlying molecular mechanism also the ER subtype plays a role [17, 18]. Other interesting compounds with affinity to ERs are plant derived. Based on their chemical structure the phytoestrogens genistein and daidzein can activate both ER subtypes, but have greater binding affinity to ER beta than to ER alpha [19].

Estrogens play an important role in many different tissue types, affecting both male and female physiology. The highest amounts of ERs are found in target tissues with reproductive functions. These target organs are the mammary gland, the ovaries, the vagina, and the uterus. In these tissues E2 stimulates cell proliferation and the biosynthesis of the progesterone receptor [20]. In the male organism ERs can be detected in the epididymis and the prostate. In recent years, studies with ERKO mice heightened the interest for novel estrogen targets in different tissues [21–23], such as the cardiovascular system, prostate, skeletal muscle, and intestinal epithelium (Fig. 19.4). In this context, investigation of ER subtype-specific actions seems to be promising and studies with ERKOs and SERMs suggest that ER beta selective compounds are useful for treating diseases like prostate cancer, autoimmune diseases, neurodegeneration, malignancies of the immune system, and colon cancer [24].

Estrogen deficiency seems to be involved in many pathologic processes like arteriosclerosis [25], osteoporosis [26], and degenerative processes in the CNS [27], whereas elevated estrogen levels are believed to support the development and promotion of tumors [28].

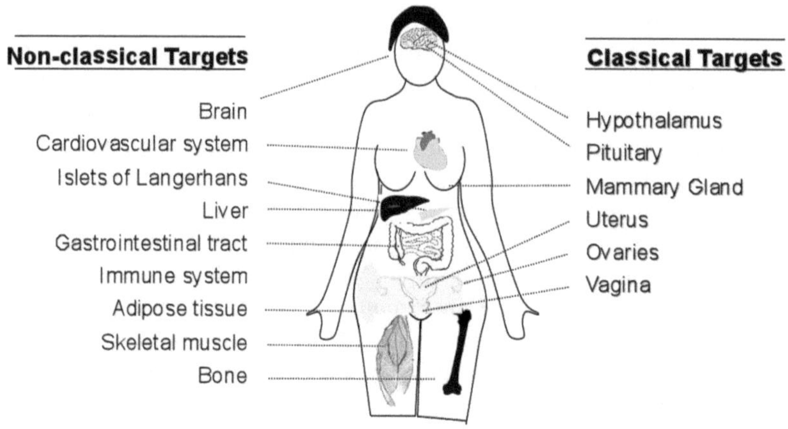

Fig. 19.4 Target tissues of estrogens in women. Estrogen-sensitive organs in women, classified into classical (tissues with reproductive function) and nonclassical (non-reproductive organs) tissues, are illustrated

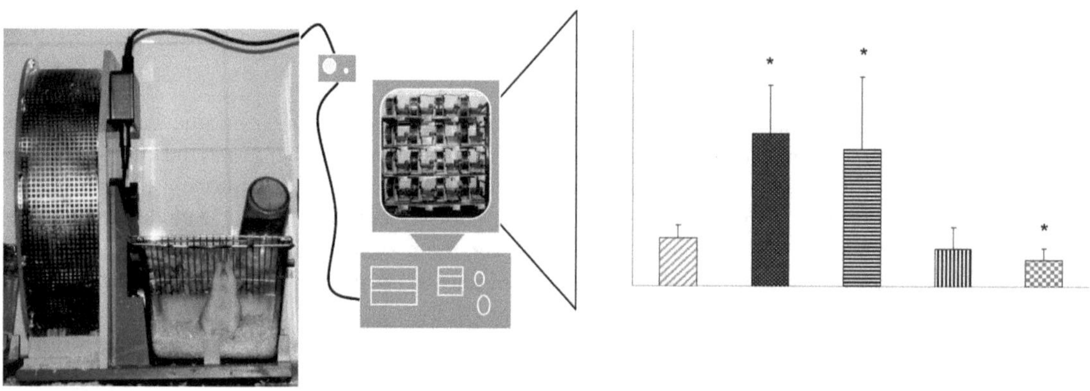

Fig. 19.5 Effect of estrogen withdrawal on movement drive. Voluntary movement activity of female rats was measured over a period of 3 weeks ($n=5$). As compared to vehicle treated OVX rats (control), movement activity of OVX rats was significant increased by treatment with E2 and Alpha, whereas substitution of Beta had no effect. Administration of Gen decreased movement activity. OVX=ovariectomized, Gen=phytoestrogen genistein, E2=17β-estradiol, Alpha=ER alpha specific agonist, Beta=ER beta specific agonist. Data shown are means±SD. *Asterisk* marks values significantly different from OVX ($\rho \leq 0.05$), modified from Hertrampf et al. [30]

Effects of Estrogens on Movement Behavior

Physical inactivity is one of the major risk factors for the development of obesity and the metabolic syndrome. Therefore, effects of estrogens on the movement behavior are an important issue with respect to the observed weight gain in postmenopausal women. It has been demonstrated that in genetically modified mice that do not express ERs [29] the movement activity is significantly reduced. Studies in OVX female rats further demonstrated that the withdrawal of estrogens in blood circulation is directly correlated to reduced physical activity [30]. Investigations with ER subtype-selective agonists [31] indicate that treatment with the ER alpha selective agonist, but not with the ER beta selective agonist significantly increased the movement activity of OVX rats (Fig. 19.5). Furthermore, this effect was antagonized by co-treatment with a pure antiestrogen [30].

Interestingly, in these investigations application of the isoflavone genistein, which is a major component of soy led to significantly decreased locomotor activity. Similar observations have been made for other phytoestrogens. For example, the isoflavone coumestrol disrupts estrogen-enhanced locomotor activity [32]. A possible mechanism could be a functional anti-estrogenic action of phytoestrogens mediated through ER beta. Such effects have been described in the paraventricular nucleus [33]. In addition, ER beta selective ligands have been shown to produce antianxiety behavior when administered systemically to OVX rats [34]. These observations are of relevance with respect to recommendations concerning the application of isoflavones for the treatment of postmenopausal complaints.

Effects of Estrogens on Fat Metabolism

Estrogens have the ability to modulate absolute fat mass and fat distribution. Effects of estrogens on serum lipid profiles are well described. The loss of ovarian function after the onset of postmenopause is associated with hypercholesteremia coupled with low HDL and high LDL and VLDL levels [35]. In animal experiments ovariectomy raises the concentrations of total cholesterol, HDL, LDL, and VLDL. Treatment with E2 and an ER alpha selective agonist led to a significant reduction of total cholesterol, LDL, and VLDL. In such animals the LDL/HDL ratio as well as the (VLDL+LDL)/HDL ratio is more favorable concerning the development of cardiovascular diseases [36]. This beneficial impact of E2 on blood lipids explains the relative cardiovascular protection of premenopausal women in comparison to women after menopause and men [37]. Effects of estrogens on blood lipids are mediated via ER alpha, which is in agreement with the observation that the liver as the most important tissue in the modulation of blood lipid composition expresses primarily the ER alpha [38].

Beside blood lipid profiles estrogens have been shown to modulate fatty acid metabolism directly. Body fat gain due to estrogen deficiency and in succession obesity seems to be associated with decreased lipolysis as well as fat oxidation [39]. In rodent models of menopause the ability to oxidate fatty acids was influenced by treatment with E2, which was indicated by a changed respiratory exchange ratio [40]. Furthermore, treatment with E2 was associated with reduced adipose tissue mass and adipocyte size and a down-regulation of lipogenic genes in adipocytes, liver, and skeletal muscle. E2 appears to promote the partitioning of free fatty acids toward oxidation by up-regulating the expression of PPAR delta and its downstream targets and also by directly and rapidly activating AMP-activated protein kinase [41].

Effects of Estrogens on Glucose Metabolism

Besides their effects on fat metabolism estrogens have also been demonstrated to be important regulators of insulin and glucose sensitivity. Obese intact female rats have a significant higher glucose tolerance than OVX animals [40]. Interestingly, both ER subtypes, the ER alpha and the ER beta appear to be involved in the modulation of glucose sensitivity. ER alpha-deficient mice revealed profound insulin resistance and impaired glucose tolerance [42], clearly indicating that the ER alpha has a protective role in metabolic disorders by improving insulin sensitivity and glucose tolerance. But even the ER beta has been demonstrated to be an important mediator of glucose sensitivity. In vitro experiments using ER beta transfected 3T3-L1 cells showed a decreased adipogenesis in comparison to control cells (untransfected cells). This observation was mediated via a negative cross talk of ER beta with PPAR gamma. Similar results were obtained from in vivo studies. Increased PPAR gamma activity was observed in gonadal fat from ER beta-deficient mice. These animals showed increased body weight gain and fat mass in the presence of improved insulin sensitivity and glucose tolerance [43]. Moreover, estrogens seem to modulate insulin resistance and glucose sensitivity systemically via effecting body composition. Studies in OVX animals provide evidence that estrogens possess anabolic activity, which is mainly mediated via ER beta. Animals treated with an ER beta selective agonist revealed relative low visceral body fat and serum leptin, but a relative high body weight comparable to untreated OVX animals. In these animals the soleus muscle mRNA expression of IGF1 and PAX7, genes involved in growth, repair and maintenance of skeletal muscle, were modulated and the soleus muscle fiber cross-sectional areas were significantly larger as compared with untreated OVX animals [36]. Additionally, ER beta specific agonists have been demonstrated to accelerate the regeneration of damaged skeletal muscles in female mice and rats and revealed anabolic activity in a classical Hershberger assay using healthy male Wistar rats [44]. These observations may result in an improved glucose tolerance, insulin sensitivity, and an enhanced utilization of glucose and lipids in the skeletal muscle of such treated animals treated. Therefore, the overall increase of muscle mass caused by the ER beta indicates to an additional important mechanism by which estrogens improve insulin sensitivity.

Leptin

In the late 1950s, in mice an obese phenotype was identified as the result of overnutrition and a decrease of energy expenditure [45]. The responsible identified gene was named *ob* (obese). From a variety of experiments it became evident that these mice were unable to produce an important circulating factor. This factor was discovered in 1994 and named leptin [46]. Leptin, a protein hormone with a size of 16 kDa (116 amino acids), is obviously a key player in regulating food intake and energy expenditure. The main sources of leptin synthesis are the adipocytes of the white adipose tissue. Leptin secretion is pulsative and follows a circadian rhythm. Highest levels are reached between midnight and early morning, whereas the lowest levels can be measured in the early to mid-afternoon. The concentration of circulating leptin in the blood stream is directly proportional to the whole body fat mass. Thus, leptin serves as an index of body energy storage. In lower levels, leptin secretion has also been identified in brown fat tissue, ovaries, skeletal muscle, stomach, epithelial cells of the mammary gland, bone marrow, pituitary gland, and liver [47]. The hormone acts on specific regions of the brain (primarily the hypothalamus) to reduce food intake and to enhance energy expenditure by modulating the expression of several neuropeptides [48, 49]. Leptin receptors have been identified in two different populations of neurons that are primarily located in the hypothalamic arcuate nucleus. The first subpopulation of neurons secretes the neuropeptides AgRP and NPY, which are suppressed by leptin. Both peptides are appetite-stimulating. The second population of neurons secretes POMC and CART, which in turn are appetite-suppressing. The secretion of theses peptides is stimulated by leptin [50].

In normal physiology the mechanism to regulate appetite and energy uptake by leptin secretion involves the total amount of body fat. High amounts of body fat correlate directly with high concentrations of circulating leptin and restrict appetite, and vice versa (Fig. 19.6).

Beside the described regulation of leptin by fat mass, different studies have identified a variety of factors, which modulate the secretion and serum concentrations of leptin in humans. Leptin levels decrease after short-term fasting. Sleep deprivation also reduces serum levels of leptin, whereas restful sleep can increase leptin. The sex hormones testosterone and E2, emotional stress as well as exercise training also influence leptin secretion. Beside of its activity as an anorexigenic hormone the numbers of physiology effects related to leptin action is steadily increasing. For example, in the cardiovascular system high levels of leptin are considered as a risk factor in the process of arteriosclerosis [51]. Furthermore, leptin is involved in fertility [52], the polycystic ovary syndrome [53], bone metabolism [54], inflammation [55], and has been described to have anti-hyperglycemic activity through improvement of insulin sensitivity in muscles and liver as well as the ability to prevent the accumulation of lipids in non-adipose tissues [56, 57].

In human reproduction, leptin levels are believed as a regulatory mechanism to prevent pregnancy in a situation of starvation and malnutrition. The ovulatory cycle is linked to energy balance and

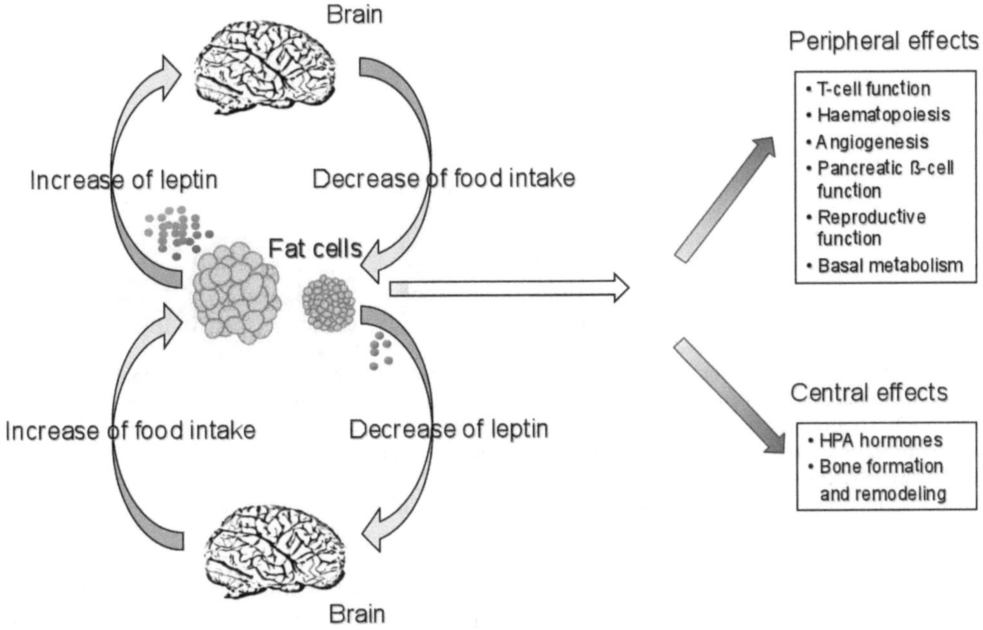

Fig. 19.6 Physiological effects of leptin. Circulating leptin, highly expressed in adipocytes, is directly proportional to the amount of fat cells and controls food intake by acting on receptors in the brain. Beside this primary function leptin has been shown to be involved in several other peripheral and central functions of the body

energy flux. A negative energy balance interfere the maturation of follicles in the ovaries and results in menstrual cycle disorders. Low leptin levels are associated with decreased fertility [58], indicating that leptin is involved in the regulation of these adaptations.

With respect to bone homeostasis leptin increases cortical bone mass. Such mechanisms indicate to an adaptation to compensate higher mechanical loading caused by an increased body weight [54]. Similar effects have been described for IGF1 to adapt bone stability to a higher muscle mass.

Of enormous physiological and pathogenic importance are the effects of leptin on the immune system and the inflammatory response. Increased leptin levels appear to function as an acute pro-inflammatory mechanism. This mechanism may prevent cellular stress induced by overeating. High caloric uptake increases the levels of insulin, leptin, and cortisol that results finally in a steady increase of fat cell size and number. Therefore, elevated fat accumulation within inner organs like liver, muscle or arteries is believed to induce inflammation in affected tissues at the cellular level [59]. Many details of the involved molecular mechanisms are still under investigation, but leptin as a powerful modulator of immune and inflammatory responses is undisputed.

Leptin, Estrogens, and Ovarian Dysfunction in Postmenopausal Women

On the one hand leptin plays a crucial role in the regulation of energy balance including energy-intensive neuroendocrine processes such as reproduction. On the other hand, gonadal sex steroids such as testosterone and E2 play a central role in the regulation of reproduction, but also contribute to the regulation of energy. High serum levels of leptin suppresses food uptake but increases energy expenditure, whereas estrogen deficiency promotes food uptake and inhibits energy expenditure. Therefore, there is evidence for an intensive cross talk between leptin and estrogens in both the regulation of ovarian func-

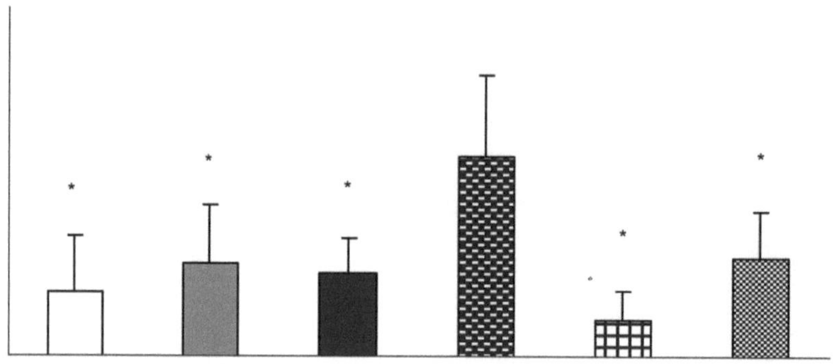

Fig. 19.7 Effects of estrogen withdrawal and physical activity on serum leptin in female rats. Female rats (SHAM and OVX) were subdivided into sedentary (no ex) and exercise training (ex) groups ($n=6$). A subset of OVX rats were treated with E2. After 6 weeks, ovariectomy without physical activity results in a significant increase of serum leptin. Treatment with E2 as well as physical activity antagonized the leptin increase, a combination of both act in an additive manner. SHAM = SHAM-operated, OVX = ovariectomized, E2 = 17β-estradiol. Data shown are means ± SEM. *Asterisk* marks values significantly different from OVX no ex ($p \leq 0.05$), modified from Zoth et al. [62]

tion and energy balance. It is well known that interruption of leptin signaling results in serious reproductive disorders. For example, leptin knockout mice display a reproductive dysfunction that can be reversed by leptin treatment. In humans leptin treatment has been shown to restore GnRH and LH secretion and pubertal development in leptin-deficient patients. Leptin pulsatility is positively and strongly correlated with LH and estrogen levels in normal cycling women. In the hypothalamus estrogen and leptin receptors are co-localized in neurons known to coordinate metabolism and gonadal function [60].

As described above, during menopause estrogen levels decrease dramatically. Taking in mind the mentioned cross talk mechanisms between leptin and estrogens it is to expect that estrogen deficiency also affects circulating leptin levels. Indeed, obese postmenopausal women have lower leptin levels when compared to premenopausal counterparts. However, estrogen administration did not significantly change serum leptin concentrations in hypo-estrogenized women. Therefore, it seems that menopause is characterized by a decreased expression of the obese gene but estrogens are unlikely the main causal factor for this observation [61].

Interestingly, in obese and OVX female rats estrogen treatment, especially in combination with physical activity, results in a decrease of circulating leptin levels. This reduction is probably not a central effect and is mainly caused by a change in body composition towards a reduced fat mass [62] (Fig. 19.7).

Leptin Resistance

Although high serum leptin concentrations suppress appetite and energy uptake it is amazing to note that obese individuals have higher leptin levels than lean individuals. Obese individuals with a high fat mass that do not respond to their extremely high levels of circulating leptin have developed the so-called leptin resistance [63]. Clinical trials have demonstrated that leptin treatment of the affected participants does not result in any weight-reducing effects. The molecular mechanisms involved in leptin resistance are still a matter of discussion and under investigation. One logical explanation could be a mutation in the leptin receptor. Animal models like the ZDF rat exactly represent this physiological situation. ZDF rats carry a mutated leptin receptor, have an extremely obese phenotype and display all physiological symptoms of a metabolic syndrome. However, in humans only few cases of obesity are due to monogenic syndromes like mutations of the leptin receptor. In the most cases leptin resistance seems to be a multifactorial phenomenon. An important aspect in obesity is the observation of an impaired transport of leptin across the blood-brain barrier. In this context, a saturation of the transporter due to extremely high leptin levels in such individuals is postulated. As a consequence the transport activity of leptin in the hypothalamus is decreased [64]. Transport of leptin into the brain is also affected by the high concentration of lipids in obese individuals. Additionally, a soluble form of the leptin receptor has been described, which also antagonizes leptin transport by inhibiting surface binding and endocytosis of leptin [65]. Like other hormones leptin signaling is subject to negative feedback regulation, which seems to be more pronounced in the obese state and associated hyperleptinemia. Targeting molecular mechanisms of leptin resistance is of basic importance for the treatment of obesity. Because of the existing link between high leptin levels and the development of cancer, especially breast cancer, such therapies should reduce not only body weight and fat mass of individuals concerned, but also the leptin production.

Leptin and Cancer Risk

The impact of obesity on the development of cardiac disease and diabetes is well known and documented, but there is also increasing evidence for a direct link between obesity and carcinogenesis. It has become apparent that especially in postmenopausal women obesity constitutes a major risk factor of developing breast cancer [66]. The underlying molecular mechanisms, which could explain the link of massive body fat to an increased risk of cancer in a variety of tissues, especially in colon and breast, are still under investigation. In this context, the increased secretion of estrogenic compounds and growth factors by the adipose tissue appears to be an important factor [67]. Further, leptin has been demonstrated to play an important role in the carcinogenesis of both the breast and the colon. Leptin and its receptor are detectable in normal and cancer mammary epithelium. The cross talk between the estrogen receptor and leptin provide a relevant mechanism, which may results in an increase of carcinogenesis in estrogen sensitive tissues [68]. In breast cancer cell lines treatment with leptin stimulates growth and DNA synthesis and seems to modulate the sensitivity of such cells towards estrogens especially to ER alpha. Leptin has also been described to increase the local estrogen synthesis in the malignant breast tissue via a stimulation of aromatase expression and appears to interfere with the action of antiestrogens in such cells. This implies that leptin may also play a role in the development of antiestrogen resistance and may also directly interfere with anticancer drugs. Beside breast cancer, in tumors of the colon an increased expression of the leptin receptor is detectable too. Like observed in breast cancer cells also colon cancer cells respond to leptin treatment with an increase of proliferation and DNA synthesis and a decreased sensitivity towards apoptotic stimuli [68]. In general, it seems that many types of cancer cells can respond to leptin as a mitogen/survival factor. Epidemiological studies measuring cancer risk in relation to obesity indicate that excess body fat can increase the risk of developing postmenopausal breast cancer, colon cancer, and endometrial cancer. Moreover, local leptin concentrations in the tumors appear to be critical for their progression. Therefore, leptin synthesis within the tumor surrounded by adipose tissue may be of great importance, especially in the breast (Fig. 19.8).

Conclusions

The decrease of circulating estrogen levels as a consequence of the ovarian dysfunction and the resulting changes in metabolic pathways in combination with physical inactivity are the major reasons for the development of obesity in postmenopausal women. Therefore, strategies for the prevention and treatment of menopausal and postmenopausal obesity and the associated elevated leptin serum concentrations must target these issues.

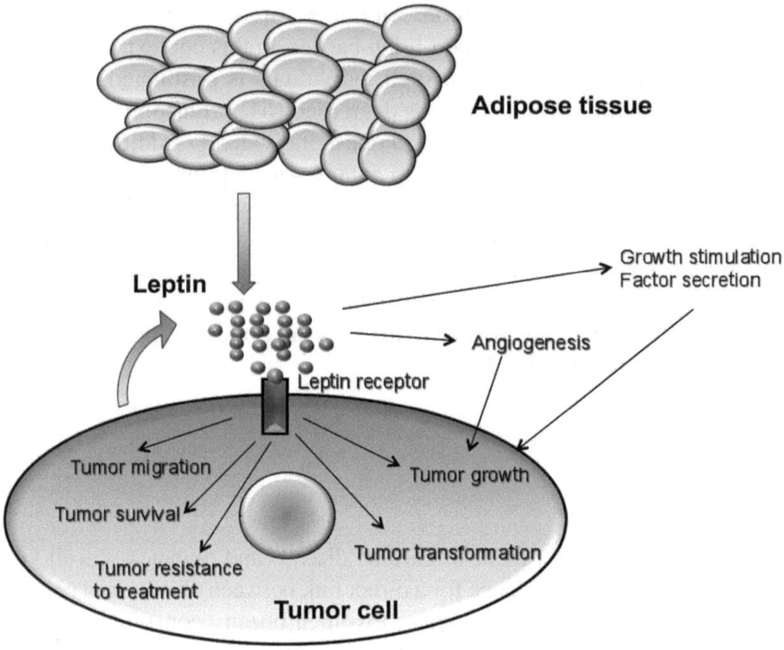

Fig. 19.8 Effects of leptin on tumor development and growth. Beside its neuroendocrine function in the brain leptin can act as a mitogen and an angiogenesis factor. Since in cancer cells leptin as well as its receptor display a significant overexpression relative to non-cancer cells leptin binding to its receptor may result in enhanced cell proliferation, growth and survival, angiogenesis, and migration

Animal experiments have revealed that treatment of OVX animals with estrogens can prevent the development of obesity and insulin resistance [69, 70]. Clinical studies also indicated that HRT prevented or reduced weight and body fat gain in postmenopausal women [71, 72]. HRT based on the idea that the treatment with estrogens and progestins may prevent physiological complaints caused by diminished circulating estrogen and progesterone.

In 2002, results from the so-called Million Women Study indicated that HRT may result in a larger incidence of breast cancer, heart attacks, and strokes [73]. As a result of these findings, the Women's Health Initiative recommended that women should take the lowest feasible dose of HRT for the shortest possible time to avoid these risks. As alternatives to HRT plant-derived compounds exerting endocrine effects are discussed. There are claims that phytoestrogens are potential alternatives to classical HRT. However, whether effects of phytoestrogens are beneficial in postmenopausal women or not is controversially discussed. The same controversy exists regarding the outcome of phytoestrogen intake in respect to breast cancer. It has been reported that the isoflavone genistein decreases food intake, body weight, adipose tissue mass, and positively affects serum lipid profiles in animals. However, the administered concentrations of phytoestrogens in these studies exceeded such dosages which can be reached by nutritional uptake. In animal studies, where the treatment with phytoestrogens results in serum concentrations comparable to such measured in the Asian population with a high nutritive uptake of phytoestrogens, no effects on the above described parameters were observed [36, 74, 75]. In contrast, there is evidence that phytoestrogens in such low doses might affect insulin sensitivity via anabolic effects on muscle mass [36, 44].

Exercise training might be a suitable alternative to HRT, especially in the treatment of obesity and the metabolic syndrome. Indeed, physical training in animals decreases fat deposition and enhances insulin sensitivity [76]. A number of studies have shown beneficial effects of exercise training in

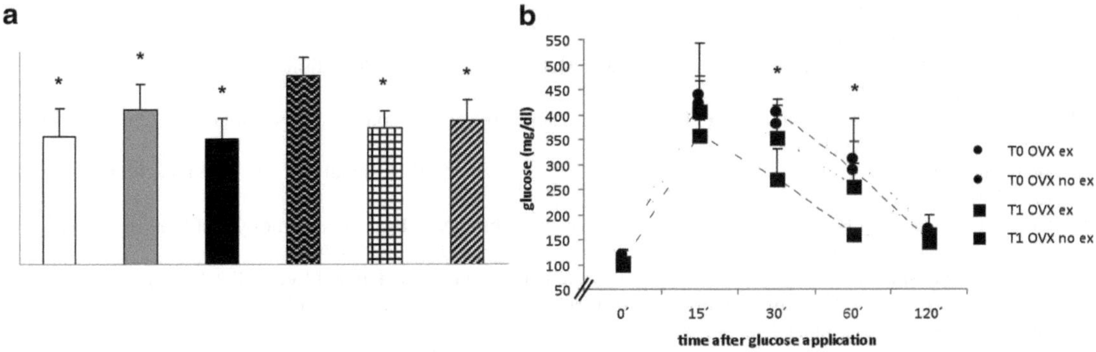

Fig. 19.9 Effects of exercise on visceral fat content and insulin sensitivity in already established obesity. Female rats (SHAM and OVX) were kept for 8 month on a high fat diet. After developing obesity, the animals were classified into sedentary (no ex) and exercise training (ex) groups ($n=5$). A subset of OVX animals were substituted with E2 for 6 weeks. After the intervention period the exercise training of obese animals resulted in a significant decrease of visceral body fat (**a**) and an increase of insulin sensitivity (**b**). SHAM = SHAM-operated, OVX = ovariectomized, E2 = 17β-estradiol, T0 = before treatment period, T1 = after treatment period. Data shown are means ± SEM. Mean values were significantly different for the following comparisons: (**a**) *asterisk* vs. OVX no ex, (**b**) *asterisk* vs. T1OVX ex at the same time point ($p \leq 0.05$), modified from Zoth et al. [40]

combination with estrogen treatment to prevent the development but also to treat established metabolic syndrome [62, 77] (Fig. 19.9).

All these data suggest that hormone treatment in combination with exercise training could be a very effective strategy to encourage the therapy of diet-induced obesity and its metabolic consequences in postmenopausal women. Taking in mind the health risks of classical HRT hormone active compounds like SERMs or nutritional uptake of phytoestrogens should be considered as alternatives.

References

1. Chan RS, Woo J. Prevention of overweight and obesity: how effective is the current public health approach. Int J Environ Res Public Health. 2010;7:765–83.
2. Newbold RR, Padilla-Banks E, Jefferson WN. Environmental estrogens and obesity. Mol Cell Endocrinol. 2009;304:84–9.
3. Caballero B. The global epidemic of obesity: an overview. Epidemiol Rev. 2007;29:1–5.
4. Low S, Chin MC, Deurenberg-Yap M. Review on epidemic of obesity. Ann Acad Med Singapore. 2009;38:57–9.
5. Comuzzie AG, Williams JT, Martin LJ, Blangero J. Searching for genes underlying normal variation in human adiposity. J Mol Med. 2001;79:57–70.
6. Goulart AC, Zee RY, Rexrode KM. Estrogen receptor 1 gene polymorphisms and decreased risk of obesity in women. Metabolism. 2009;58:759–64.
7. Ley CJ, Lees B, Stevenson JC. Sex- and menopause-associated changes in body-fat distribution. Am J Clin Nutr. 1992;55:950–4.
8. Rolland YM, Perry 3rd HM, Patrick P, Banks WA, Morley JE. Loss of appendicular muscle mass and loss of muscle strength in young postmenopausal women. J Gerontol A Biol Sci Med Sci. 2007;62:330–5.
9. Davison SL, Bell R, Donath S, Montalto JG, Davis SR. Androgen levels in adult females: changes with age, menopause, and oophorectomy. J Clin Endocrinol Metab. 2005;90:3847–53.
10. Hertrampf T, Degen GH, Kaid AA, et al. Combined effects of physical activity, dietary isoflavones and 17beta-estradiol on movement drive, body weight and bone mineral density in ovariectomized female rats. Planta Med. 2006;72:484–7.
11. Hertrampf T, Seibel J, Laudenbach U, Fritzemeier KH, Diel P. Analysis of the effects of oestrogen receptor alpha (ERalpha)- and ERbeta-selective ligands given in combination to ovariectomized rats. Br J Pharmacol. 2008;153:1432–7.

12. Ropero AB, Alonso-Magdalena P, Quesada I, Nadal A. The role of estrogen receptors in the control of energy and glucose homeostasis. Steroids. 2008;73:874–9.
13. Miranda PJ, DeFronzo RA, Califf RM, Guyton JR. Metabolic syndrome: definition, pathophysiology, and mechanisms. Am Heart J. 2005;149:33–45.
14. Eckel LA. The ovarian hormone estradiol plays a crucial role in the control of food intake in females. Physiol Behav. 2011;104:517–24.
15. Heldring N, Pike A, Andersson S, et al. Estrogen receptors: how do they signal and what are their targets. Physiol Rev. 2007;87:905–31.
16. Kuiper GG, Carlsson B, Grandien K, et al. Comparison of the ligand binding specificity and transcript tissue distribution of estrogen receptors alpha and beta. Endocrinology. 1997;138:863–70.
17. Diel P. Tissue-specific estrogenic response and molecular mechanisms. Toxicol Lett. 2002;127:217–24.
18. Ohmichi M, Tasaka K, Kurachi H, Murata Y. Molecular mechanism of action of selective estrogen receptor modulator in target tissues. Endocr J. 2005;52:161–7.
19. Kuiper GG, Lemmen JG, Carlsson B, et al. Interaction of estrogenic chemicals and phytoestrogens with estrogen receptor beta. Endocrinology. 1998;139:4252–63.
20. Horwitz KB, Koseki Y, McGuire WL. Estrogen control of progesterone receptor in human breast cancer: role of estradiol and antiestrogen. Endocrinology. 1978;103:1742–51.
21. Korach KS, Emmen JM, Walker VR, et al. Update on animal models developed for analyses of estrogen receptor biological activity. J Steroid Biochem Mol Biol. 2003;86:387–91.
22. Gustafsson JA. What pharmacologists can learn from recent advances in estrogen signalling. Trends Pharmacol Sci. 2003;24:479–85.
23. Carpenter KD, Korach KS. Potential biological functions emerging from the different estrogen receptors. Ann N Y Acad Sci. 2006;1092:361–73.
24. Koehler KF, Helguero LA, Haldosen LA, Warner M, Gustafsson JA. Reflections on the discovery and significance of estrogen receptor beta. Endocr Rev. 2005;26:465–78.
25. Henderson BE, Ross RK, Paganini-Hill A, Mack TM. Estrogen use and cardiovascular disease. Am J Obstet Gynecol. 1986;154:1181–6.
26. Turner CH, Sato M, Bryant HU. Raloxifene preserves bone strength and bone mass in ovariectomized rats. Endocrinology. 1994;135:2001–5.
27. Fillit H, Weinreb H, Cholst I, et al. Observations in a preliminary open trial of estradiol therapy for senile dementia-Alzheimer's type. Psychoneuroendocrinology. 1986;11:337–45.
28. Colditz GA. Epidemiology of breast cancer. Findings from the nurses' health study. Cancer. 1993;71:1480–9.
29. Ogawa S, Chan J, Gustafsson JA, Korach KS, Pfaff DW. Estrogen increases locomotor activity in mice through estrogen receptor alpha: specificity for the type of activity. Endocrinology. 2003;144:230–9.
30. Hertrampf T, Gruca MJ, Seibel J, Laudenbach U, Fritzemeier KH, Diel P. The bone-protective effect of the phytoestrogen genistein is mediated via ER alpha-dependent mechanisms and strongly enhanced by physical activity. Bone. 2007;40:1529–35.
31. Hillisch A, Peters O, Kosemund D, et al. Dissecting physiological roles of estrogen receptor alpha and beta with potent selective ligands from structure-based design. Mol Endocrinol. 2004;18:1599–609.
32. Garey J, Morgan MA, Frohlich J, McEwen BS, Pfaff DW. Effects of the phytoestrogen coumestrol on locomotor and fear-related behaviors in female mice. Horm Behav. 2001;40:65–76.
33. Patisaul HB, Melby M, Whitten PL, Young LJ. Genistein affects ER beta- but not ER alpha-dependent gene expression in the hypothalamus. Endocrinology. 2002;143:2189–97.
34. Walf AA, Frye CA. ERbeta-selective estrogen receptor modulators produce antianxiety behavior when administered systemically to ovariectomized rats. Neuropsychopharmacology. 2005;30:1598–609.
35. van Beek AP, de Ruijter-Heijstek FC, Erkelens DW, de Bruin TW. Menopause is associated with reduced protection from postprandial lipemia. Arterioscler Thromb Vasc Biol. 1999;19:2737–41.
36. Weigt C, Hertrampf T, Zoth N, Fritzemeier KH, Diel P. Impact of estradiol, ER subtype specific agonists and genistein on energy homeostasis in a rat model of nutrition induced obesity. Mol Cell Endocrinol. 2012;351:227–38.
37. Dubey RK, Imthurn B, Barton M, Jackson EK. Vascular consequences of menopause and hormone therapy: importance of timing of treatment and type of estrogen. Cardiovasc Res. 2005;66:295–306.
38. Matthews J, Gustafsson JA. Estrogen signaling: a subtle balance between ER alpha and ER beta. Mol Interv. 2003;3:281–92.
39. Horowitz JF, Klein S. Whole body and abdominal lipolytic sensitivity to epinephrine is suppressed in upper body obese women. Am J Physiol Endocrinol Metab. 2000;278:E1144–52.
40. Zoth N, Weigt C, Zengin S, et al. Metabolic effects of estrogen substitution in combination with targeted exercise training on the therapy of obesity in ovariectomized Wistar rats. J Steroid Biochem Mol Biol. 2012;130:64–72.
41. D'Eon TM, Souza SC, Aronovitz M, Obin MS, Fried SK, Greenberg AS. Estrogen regulation of adiposity and fuel partitioning. Evidence of genomic and non-genomic regulation of lipogenic and oxidative pathways. J Biol Chem. 2005;280:35983–91.

42. Cooke PS, Heine PA, Taylor JA, Lubahn DB. The role of estrogen and estrogen receptor-alpha in male adipose tissue. Mol Cell Endocrinol. 2001;178:147–54.
43. Foryst-Ludwig A, Clemenz M, Hohmann S, et al. Metabolic actions of estrogen receptor beta (ERbeta) are mediated by a negative cross-talk with PPARgamma. PLoS Genet. 2008;4:e1000108.
44. Velders M, Schleipen B, Fritzemeier KH, Zierau O, Diel P. Selective estrogen receptor-beta activation stimulates skeletal muscle growth and regeneration. FASEB J. 2012;26(5):1909–20. doi:10.1096/fj.11-194779.
45. Hausberger FX. Behavior of transplanted adipose tissue of hereditarily obese mice. Anat Rec. 1959;135:109–13.
46. Zhang Y, Proenca R, Maffei M, Barone M, Leopold L, Friedman JM. Positional cloning of the mouse obese gene and its human homologue. Nature. 1994;372:425–32.
47. Margetic S, Gazzola C, Pegg GG, Hill RA. Leptin: a review of its peripheral actions and interactions. Int J Obes Relat Metab Disord. 2002;26:1407–33.
48. Rosen ED, Spiegelman BM. Adipocytes as regulators of energy balance and glucose homeostasis. Nature. 2006;444:847–53.
49. Schwartz MW. Central nervous system regulation of food intake. Obesity (Silver Spring). 2006;14 Suppl 1Suppl. 1:1S–8.
50. Schwartz MW. Brain pathways controlling food intake and body weight. Exp Biol Med (Maywood). 2001;226:978–81.
51. Taleb S, Herbin O, Ait-Oufella H, et al. Defective leptin/leptin receptor signaling improves regulatory T cell immune response and protects mice from atherosclerosis. Arterioscler Thromb Vasc Biol. 2007;27:2691–8.
52. Anifandis G, Koutselini E, Louridas K, et al. Estradiol and leptin as conditional prognostic IVF markers. Reproduction. 2005;129:531–4.
53. Cervero A, Dominguez F, Horcajadas JA, Quinonero A, Pellicer A, Simon C. The role of the leptin in reproduction. Curr Opin Obstet Gynecol. 2006;18:297–303.
54. Ducy P, Amling M, Takeda S, et al. Leptin inhibits bone formation through a hypothalamic relay: a central control of bone mass. Cell. 2000;100:197–207.
55. Fantuzzi G, Faggioni R. Leptin in the regulation of immunity, inflammation, and hematopoiesis. J Leukoc Biol. 2000;68:437–46.
56. Kamohara S, Burcelin R, Halaas JL, Friedman JM, Charron MJ. Acute stimulation of glucose metabolism in mice by leptin treatment. Nature. 1997;389:374–7.
57. Minokoshi Y, Kim YB, Peroni OD, et al. Leptin stimulates fatty-acid oxidation by activating AMP-activated protein kinase. Nature. 2002;415:339–43.
58. Donato Jr J, Cravo RM, Frazao R, Elias CF. Hypothalamic sites of leptin action linking metabolism and reproduction. Neuroendocrinology. 2011;93:9–18.
59. Wabitsch M, Jensen PB, Blum WF, et al. Insulin and cortisol promote leptin production in cultured human fat cells. Diabetes. 1996;45:1435–8.
60. Gao Q, Horvath TL. Cross-talk between estrogen and leptin signaling in the hypothalamus. Am J Physiol Endocrinol Metab. 2008;294:E817–26.
61. Cento RM, Proto C, Spada RS, et al. Leptin levels in menopause: effect of estrogen replacement therapy. Horm Res. 1999;52:269–73.
62. Zoth N, Weigt C, Laudenbach-Leschowski U, Diel P. Physical activity and estrogen treatment reduce visceral body fat and serum levels of leptin in an additive manner in a diet induced animal model of obesity. J Steroid Biochem Mol Biol. 2010;122:100–5.
63. Considine RV, Sinha MK, Heiman ML, et al. Serum immunoreactive-leptin concentrations in normal-weight and obese humans. N Engl J Med. 1996;334:292–5.
64. Vila R, Adan C, Rafecas I, Fernandez-Lopez JA, Remesar X, Alemany M. Plasma leptin turnover rates in lean and obese Zucker rats. Endocrinology. 1998;139:4466–9.
65. Dardeno TA, Chou SH, Moon HS, Chamberland JP, Fiorenza CG, Mantzoros CS. Leptin in human physiology and therapeutics. Front Neuroendocrinol. 2010;31:377–93.
66. Stephenson GD, Rose DP. Breast cancer and obesity: an update. Nutr Cancer. 2003;45:1–16.
67. Ahima RS, Flier JS. Adipose tissue as an endocrine organ. Trends Endocrinol Metab. 2000;11:327–32.
68. Garofalo C, Surmacz E. Leptin and cancer. J Cell Physiol. 2006;207:12–22.
69. Bryzgalova G, Lundholm L, Portwood N, et al. Mechanisms of antidiabetogenic and body weight-lowering effects of estrogen in high-fat diet-fed mice. Am J Physiol Endocrinol Metab. 2008;295:E904–12.
70. Jones ME, Thorburn AW, Britt KL, et al. Aromatase-deficient (ArKO) mice have a phenotype of increased adiposity. Proc Natl Acad Sci U S A. 2000;97:12735–40.
71. Samaras K, Hayward CS, Sullivan D, Kelly RP, Campbell LV. Effects of postmenopausal hormone replacement therapy on central abdominal fat, glycemic control, lipid metabolism, and vascular factors in type 2 diabetes: a prospective study. Diabetes Care. 1999;22:1401–7.
72. Santen RJ, Allred DC, Ardoin SP, et al. Postmenopausal hormone therapy: an Endocrine Society scientific statement. J Clin Endocrinol Metab. 2010;95:s1–66.

73. Beral V. Breast cancer and hormone-replacement therapy in the Million Women Study. Lancet. 2003;362:419–27.
74. Naaz A, Yellayi S, Zakroczymski MA, et al. The soy isoflavone genistein decreases adipose deposition in mice. Endocrinology. 2003;144:3315–20.
75. Penza M, Montani C, Romani A, et al. Genistein affects adipose tissue deposition in a dose-dependent and gender-specific manner. Endocrinology. 2006;147:5740–51.
76. Latour MG, Shinoda M, Lavoie JM. Metabolic effects of physical training in ovariectomized and hyperestrogenic rats. J Appl Physiol. 2001;90:235–41.
77. Green JS, Stanforth PR, Rankinen T, et al. The effects of exercise training on abdominal visceral fat, body composition, and indicators of the metabolic syndrome in postmenopausal women with and without estrogen replacement therapy: the HERITAGE family study. Metabolism. 2004;53:1192–6.

Chapter 20
Fat and Fat Distribution in Menopause: Chinese Aspects

Xiaoguang Ma, Wei He, and Shankuan Zhu

Key Points

- Available studies on body fat distribution and menopause suggest that menopause is associated with an acceleration in the accumulation of abdominal adipose tissue, and most likely, intra-abdominal fat.
- This trend toward central obesity favors increased cardiovascular, cancer, and metabolic risks, and may partially mediate the increased morbidity and mortality after menopause.
- Compared with other races and ethnic groups, Asians such as Chinese, Japanese, and Singaporeans were reported to be with lower BMI but with higher percent body fat and more abdominal fat at any given level of BMI.
- Chinese women undergoing menopausal transition and postmenopausal women were associated with decreased lean mass, and increased percent body fat, trunk fat mass, and trunk–leg fat mass ratio comparing with women remained premenopausal.
- Limited evidence identified the effect of menopause on fat distribution among Chinese women; however, more research was needed to confirm the findings with longitudinal design, larger sample size, and more advanced measuring technologies.

Keywords Menopause • Fat distribution • Abdominal fat • Body composition • Central obesity • Chinese aspects

Abbreviations

WHR	Waist-to-hip ratio
SWAN	Study of women's health across the nation
WC	Waist circumference

X. Ma, M.D., M.Phil.
Department of Epidemiology and Biostatistics, Arnold School of Public Health, University of South Carolina, 800 Sumter Street, Columbia, SC 29201, USA
e-mail: ma26@email.sc.edu

W. He, M.D. • S. Zhu, M.D., Ph.D. (✉)
Obesity and Body Composition Research Center, Chronic Disease Research Institute, Zhejiang University School of Public Health, 866 Yu-hang-tang Road, Hangzhou, Zhejiang 310058, China
e-mail: hewei_1984@hotmail.com; zsk@zju.edu.cn

C.J.H. Martin et al. (eds.), *Nutrition and Diet in Menopause*, Nutrition and Health,
DOI 10.1007/978-1-62703-373-2_20, © Springer Science+Business Media New York 2013

DXA	Dual energy X-ray absorptiometry
BMI	Body mass index
CT	Computed tomography
MRI	Magnetic resonance imaging
MRS	Magnetic resonance spectroscopy
SHBG	Sex hormone binding globulin
HRT	Hormone replacement therapy

Introduction

Obesity is a medical condition in which excess body mass has accumulated to the extent that it may cause an adverse effect on health, leading to reduced life expectancy and/or increased health problems including cardiovascular disease, type 2 diabetes, cancer, osteoarthritis and so on [1]. Changes in body composition, including the amount and distribution of body fat, are important predictors of cardiovascular risk. In particular, abdominal fat accumulation is associated with increased risks for cardiovascular diseases [1, 2]. Menopause is commonly defined as the absence of menses for 12 consecutive months. Endocrine changes resulting from menopause not only lead to cessation of reproduction and accompanying symptoms in women, but also dramatically impact health in postmenopausal life. Recent studies have found that change of body composition may mediate the relationship between menopause and adverse health outcomes. The findings about effects of menopause on body composition have been inconsistent due to different study design and characteristics of target populations: some studies have observed a progressive increase in fat mass, decrease in lean mass, and a shift to a more central body fat distribution caused by menopause, but others have not, especially after controlling the effects of aging [3–5]. This chapter discusses the effects of menopause on body composition and potential behind mechanisms with particularly Chinese aspects.

Menopause and Body Composition

Two patterns of body fat distribution have been usually observed, the accumulation of fat in the central region (android or apple shape) and the accumulation of fat in the gluteo-femoral region (gynoid or pear shape). The accumulation of fat in the central region (intra-abdominal) has been linked to increased risk of cardiovascular diseases independent of overall obesity. Despite conflicting results, menopause was believed to associate with weight gain, increased fat mass and abdominal fat, and a shift to a more central, android body fat distribution.

Menopause, Body Weight and Total Body Fat

Women tended to gain weight with aging, and many women reported their weight gain started around the time of their menopause [6]. A number of studies on Caucasian middle-aged women reported an annual weight gain of about 0.5 kg or more, however there did not appear to be an independent effect of menopause on the weight gain [7, 8]. Wing et al. studied 485 US women who were initially premenopausal and followed them for 3 years during which 61 were postmenopausal, 94 were perimenopausal, and 279 were still premenopausal. However, they found the weight gain was similar in the women who remained premenopausal and those who had a natural menopause [8]. In a comparison of premenopausal and postmenopausal Caucasian women matched for age, premenopausal women actually had a higher mean body weight [5, 9]. These evidence suggest that weight gain in midlife among women per se is more consistent with a pattern of chronologic aging, and not uniquely due to the menopausal transition.

Nevertheless, body weight consists of many compartments and components, and thus weight change alone is not an adequate indicator to the underlying changes in body composition that occur during menopause [6]. Wang and colleagues found that total lean mass decreased during the menopausal transition among Danish women [4], which indicated that increases in fat mass may occur with menopause despite a lack of change or even a reduction in body weight. Toth et al. claimed that total body mass was 28 % higher and percentage fat was 17 % higher in postmenopausal than in premenopausal US women, and a similar pattern of differences in total adiposity was noted in subsamples of premenopausal and postmenopausal women matched by age [10]. A longitudinal analysis of 6-year changes in body composition among African-American and Caucasian women showed menopause was associated with substantial weight gain, significant increases in fat mass, and loss of skeletal muscle mass. The pattern of change in weight is linear, suggesting only an age effect, whereas the changes in fat mass and skeletal muscle mass were more with curvilinear pattern over time, suggesting a menopause effect [11, 12].

Menopause and Central Fat Distribution

In addition to body weight and total fat, more literature suggested that it was not just the amount of fat but also its distribution that determined the risk associated with obesity [13]. Excess abdominal fat is as great a risk factor for disease as excess body fat per se [1]. Although some studies using anthropometric measurements of abdominal fat distribution most often failed to detect an effect of the menopause transition after adjust for age [14, 15], both cross-sectional [16] and longitudinal studies [9, 17] have shown a menopause-related increase in central adiposity among Caucasians, independent of the effect of age and total body adiposity. By comparing postmenopausal with age-matched controls premenopausal US women, Poehlman et al. found that the transition to menopause was associated with an increase in the waist-to-hip ratio (WHR) and total body fat [17]. Using data from the Study of Women's Health Across the Nation (SWAN) among African-American and Caucasian women, Sowers et al. found that waist circumference (WC) continued to increase over time but the rate of increase slowed approximately 1 year after the final menstrual period, which indicated that both chronological aging and ovarian aging contribute to substantial changes in WC [12]. However, in subsequent SWAN longitudinal analyses with longer follow-up and including Japanese and Chinese women, change in waist seemed to be linear in relation to the final menstrual period [5].

The dual energy X-ray absorptiometry (DXA) provides more details information on whole-body and regional estimates of fat mass, even though this technique does not differentiate subcutaneous from intra-abdominal adipose tissue compartments [18]. Several studies have reported a shift toward abdominal fat distribution among African-Americans and Caucasians at menopause based on DXA data [12, 19–21]. Dawson-Hughes and Harris studies body composition changes across a 1-year period in 125 postmenopausal US women and found an increase in trunk fat measured by DXA. However, as there was no premenopausal comparison group in this study, it is not clear whether this change was due to menopause per se or aging [22, 23]. Gambaccianni and colleagues examined DXA measured trunk fat in a sample of premenopausal, perimenopausal, and postmenopausal Caucasian women, and found both perimenopausal and postmenopausal women had higher total and central body fat compared to premenopausal women. The effect of the menopause was further confirmed in a subgroup of women matched for age and body mass index (BMI) [24].

Menopause and Ectopic Fat

Ectopic fat is defined as excess adipose tissue in locations not classically associated with adipose tissue storage, such as visceral, heart, liver, and bone marrow [2]. Ectopic fat is an important predictor of metabolic (in particular insulin resistance) and cardiovascular disease, carrying more risk than general fat accumulation [25]. For instance, intra-abdominal visceral fat is most highly associated with increased health risks, and some studies indicate that visceral obesity may be a better predictor of morbidity and mortality related to cardiovascular diseases and type 2 diabetes than general obesity [26].

Computed tomography (CT) is current gold standard technique which can quantify both subcutaneous and intra-abdominal adipose tissue depots [27]. Toth and colleagues found that postmenopausal African-American and Caucasian women had a 49 % greater intra-abdominal and a 22 % greater abdominal subcutaneous fat area compared to premenopausal women. The menopause-related difference in intra-abdominal fat persisted after statistical adjustment for age and total body fat mass, whereas no difference in abdominal subcutaneous fat was noted [10]. Enzi et al. have reported that postmenopausal Italian women have a decreased subcutaneous-to-visceral fat ratio measured by CT scan comparing to age-matched premenopausal women [28]. Similar findings were reported by Lovejoy et al. in a longitudinal study in which they found that all African-American and Caucasian women gained subcutaneous fat over time but only those who became postmenopausal had a significant increase in visceral adipose tissue [3]. However, studies using the magnetic resonance imaging (MRI) reported no significant effect for menopause on abdominal fat accumulation. Schreiner et al. concluded that menopause did not accelerate intra-abdominal fat accumulation, though a very small sample of postmenopausal US women was examined in this study [29].

Recent findings suggested an association between bone marrow fat and bone loss, and osteoporosis has been proposed as the "obesity of bone" [30]. However, little literature was available for the change of bone marrow fat during menopause, and whether this change is associated with menopause-induced osteoporosis. Using proton (^{1}H) magnetic resonance spectroscopy (MRS), Griffith found that in females vertebral marrow fat content rose sharply between 55 and 65 years of age while in males vertebral marrow fat content rose more slowly throughout life with no sharp rise in above range of age [31]. This increased deposition in marrow fat concurs with recognized changes in extraosseous fat distribution in postmenopausal females, which suggested that the bone marrow fat deposition may be menopause-related. More studies are needed before any conclusion can be made.

In summary, there are discrepancies in previous cross-sectional studies which may be related to the methodology used for the measurement of body fat distribution. Studies using anthropometric measures (WC or WHR) more likely failed to detect the difference independent of age and total fat. DXA and CT led to the conclusion that the menopause accelerated the selective deposition of intra-abdominal fat. Available longitudinal studies supported an increase in central fat accumulation occurring with menopause.

Mechanism Behind Menopause and Body Composition

The sex hormones have been suggested to play a critical role in menopause-related changes in body fat and fat distribution. Menopause is of occurrence with decline of estrogen levels. A number of studies reported that menopause-induced hormonal changes may be associated with abdominal fat distribution. Haffer et al. found that in postmenopausal Mexican-American and non-Hispanic white women overall adiposity and an unfavorable body fat distribution are associated with decreased sex hormone binding globulin (SHBG) concentration [32]. Observational studies and clinical trials have showed the effect of hormone replacement therapy (HRT) on fat distribution [33, 34]. The HRT using among postmenopausal women was associated with prevention, attenuation, or delay of abdominal fat accumulation related to menopause [35]. Therefore, changes in fat distribution during menopausal transition may be related to the dynamics of hormone such as estrogens and SHBG.

The physiologic basis for the shifting fat distribution after menopause appears to be a decreased lipoprotein lipase activity in femoral adipocytes and a loss of the high lipolytic responsiveness of abdominal and mammary adipocytes that is observed in premenopausal women [36]. Thus, unlike premenopausal women, postmenopausal women do not preferentially deposit fat in the periphery but are equally likely to deposit fat in adipose depots in the trunk. Lindberg et al. have also shown that treatment with estrogen in postmenopausal women restores the lipoprotein lipase activity of the femoral adipocytes [37].

In contrast to the stable patterns of daily food intake observed in males of many species, in females of many species caloric intake are cyclic and correlate with phases of the menstrual or estrous cycle [23]. When estrogen is elevated and progesterone is low, female show a significant decrease in caloric intake. Furthermore, it has been reported in female rodent models, physiologic levels of estrogen within the estrus phase was inversely related to food intake [23, 38]. Given the data linking changes in estrogen levels to alterations in food intake across the menstrual cycle, it might be expected that the decrease in estrogen at menopause may cause changes in eating behavior. Unfortunately, few studies have investigated the effect of menopause on food intake. A recent study found a decrease of energy intake after the onset of menopause compared with 3–4 years before the onset, but a slightly increase were found 2 years after the menopause [3].

In addition to affecting total energy intake, cyclic fluctuations in reproductive hormones also affect preference for macronutrients, such as fat and carbohydrate. In female rodents, low levels of estradiol during the luteal phases of the cycle are associated with increased preference and intake of fat [39]. In a recent longitudinal study, after adjustment for changes in total energy intake, protein, carbohydrate seem to decline overtime and were relatively higher in the years preceding onset of menopause than those after menopause. In contrast, fat intakes were higher 2 years after menopause onset compared with menopause onset and tended to increase over time [3].

Current literature indicated that natural menopause may be associated with reduced energy expenditure during rest and physical activity, both of which could contribute to a positive energy balance and weight gain in menopausal women [23]. Women experience a gradual fall in resting metabolic rate after menopause. In a recent study, 24 h energy expenditure and sleeping energy expenditure decreased significantly with age, however, the decrease in sleeping energy expenditure was 1.5-fold greater in women who become postmenopausal compared with premenopausal controls [3]. There appear to be at least two components contribute to this change. First, it has been reported that menopausal women have slightly decreased resting metabolic rate because of the loss of fat free mass [6, 23]. Fat free mass plays a major role in RMR, and can explain 63 % variations in resting metabolic rate [40]. Furthermore, changes in fat-free mass, including a postmenopausal decline in both soft lean tissue mass and bone mass, are mainly menopause-related [4]. Second, the decreased metabolic rate in postmenopausal women may be due in part to the loss of ovarian function and luteal phase of the menstrual cycle, which can theoretically reduce energy expenditure by about 15,000–20,000 Kcal per year [6]. Cyclic variation in resting energy expenditure was found in premenopausal women. During the 14-day luteal phase following ovulation, core temperature increased, as well as 8–16 % increase in total energy expenditure measured by direct and indirect calorimetry [6, 41].

The estrogen/testosterone pathway may play an important role in the regulation of physical activity [42]. In rodents, wheel running is reduced after surgical/pharmacological gonadectomy and is increased after hormones are reinforced via capsules or injections. However, in human subject, whether the decline in hormone concentration after menopause will cause a reduction in physical activity is still unclear. Dorn et al. investigated breast cancer risk in premenopausal and postmenopausal US women with and without cancer. As a component of this analysis, the researchers asked the subjects to recall their strenuous physical activity patterns during the previous 2 years, and found a reduction in physical activity level after menopause [43]. In a recent longitudinal study, physical activity decreased 30.2 % in subjects who were initially premenopausal and then become postmenopausal during the follow-up. However, in subjects who remain menopause, it decreased even a slightly higher (38.7 %), which suggest an aging effect rather than menopause effect.

Chinese Aspects

Compared with other races and ethnic groups, Asians such as Chinese, Japanese, and Singaporeans were reported to be with lower BMI but with higher percent body fat and more abdominal fat at any given level of BMI [44–47]. Chinese women in early menopausal transition were noted with the lowest unadjusted level of serum estradiol and SHBG comparing to other ethnic groups in SWAN study. The BMI was significantly correlated with all reproductive and somatic hormones measured in the perimenopause [48]. Therefore, the effect of menopause on fat and fat distribution may be different for Chinese women.

The evidence on changes of body composition during menopausal transition was extremely limited in Asian, particularly Chinese population. Teh et al. revealed an age-related increase in abdominal fat, but they did not consider the effect of menopause in their study [49]. Including menopause effect in a cross-sectional study, Sternfeld and colleagues reported a lower lean mass and possibly higher percent body fat in perimenopausal and postmenopausal Chinese women than in those in other ethnic groups [21]. Only one longitudinal study was available to date to evaluate the changes of body composition during menopausal transition in Chinese women [50]. A total of 438 middle-aged Chinese women aged 44–55 years were recruited with 30-month follow-up in Hong Kong. After controlling age, age of menarche and education level, women undergoing menopausal transition and postmenopausal women were associated with decreased lean mass, and increased percent body fat, trunk fat mass, and trunk–leg fat mass ratio comparing with women remained premenopausal (Fig. 20.1).

More studies with longitudinal design were encouraging to examine the effect of menopause on body composition among Chinese women. No Asian studies examined intra-abdominal fat changes during menopausal transition using CT, current gold standard to measure body composition. More research was warranted in Chinese menopausal women.

Conclusion

In conclusion, careful examination of available studies on body fat distribution and menopause suggested that menopause was associated with an acceleration in the accumulation of abdominal adipose tissue, and most likely, intra-abdominal fat. This trend toward central obesity favors increased cardiovascular, cancer, and metabolic risks, and may partially mediate the increased morbidity and mortality after menopause. Limited evidence identified the effect of menopause on fat distribution among Chinese women; however, more research was needed to confirm the findings with longitudinal design, larger sample size, and more advanced measuring technologies.

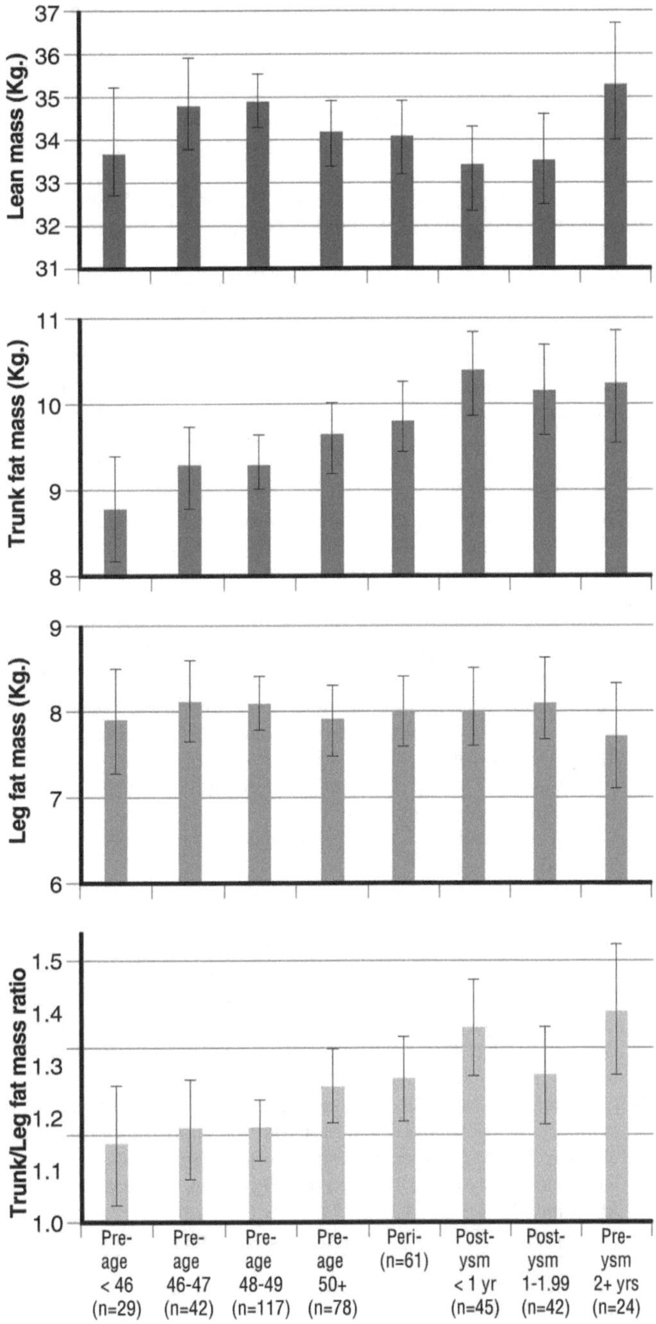

Fig. 20.1 Baseline cross-sectional body composition measurements by age-menopausal status, adjusted for body mass index (kg m^{-2}). Adapted from [50]

References

1. Consultation, W. H. O. Obesity: preventing and managing the global epidemic. World Health Organ Tech Rep Ser. 2000;894:i-xii, 1–253.
2. Britton KA, Fox CS. Ectopic fat depots and cardiovascular disease. Circulation. 2011;124(24):e837–41.
3. Lovejoy JC, Champagne CM, de Jonge L, Xie H, Smith SR. Increased visceral fat and decreased energy expenditure during the menopausal transition. Int J Obes (Lond). 2008;32(6):949–58.

4. Wang Q, Hassager C, Ravn P, Wang S, Christiansen C. Total and regional body-composition changes in early postmenopausal women: age-related or menopause-related? Am J Clin Nutr. 1994;60(6):843–8.
5. Wildman RP, Sowers MR. Adiposity and the menopausal transition. Obstet Gynecol Clin North Am. 2011;38(3):441–54.
6. Heymsfield SB, Gallagher D, Poehlman ET, Wolper C, Nonas K, Nelson D, et al. Menopausal changes in body composition and energy expenditure. Exp Gerontol. 1994;29(3–4):377–89.
7. Brown WJ, Williams L, Ford JH, Ball K, Dobson AJ. Identifying the energy gap: magnitude and determinants of 5-year weight gain in midage women. Obes Res. 2005;13(8):1431–41.
8. Wing RR, Matthews KA, Kuller LH, Meilahn EN, Plantinga PL. Weight gain at the time of menopause. Arch Intern Med. 1991;151(1):97–102.
9. Bjorkelund C, Lissner L, Andersson S, Lapidus L, Bengtsson C. Reproductive history in relation to relative weight and fat distribution. Int J Obes Relat Metab Disord. 1996;20(3):213–9.
10. Toth MJ, Tchernof A, Sites CK, Poehlman ET. Effect of menopausal status on body composition and abdominal fat distribution. Int J Obes Relat Metab Disord. 2000;24(2):226–31.
11. Sternfeld B, Dugan S. Physical activity and health during the menopausal transition. Obstet Gynecol Clin North Am. 2011;38(3):537–66.
12. Sowers M, Zheng H, Tomey K, Karvonen-Gutierrez C, Jannausch M, Li X, et al. Changes in body composition in women over six years at midlife: ovarian and chronological aging. J Clin Endocrinol Metab. 2007;92(3):895–901.
13. World Health Organization, International Association for the study of Obesity, International Obesity TaskForce. The Asia-Pacific perspective: Redefining obesity and its treatment. Sydney: Health Communications; 2000.
14. Tchernof A, Poehlman ET, Despres JP. Body fat distribution, the menopause transition, and hormone replacement therapy. Diabetes Metab. 2000;26(1):12–20.
15. Pasquali R, Casimirri F, Pascal G, Tortelli O, Morselli Labate A, Bertazzo D, et al. Influence of menopause on blood cholesterol levels in women: the role of body composition, fat distribution and hormonal milieu. Virgilio Menopause Health Group. J Intern Med Mar. 1997;241(3):195–203.
16. Zamboni M, Armellini F, Milani MP, De Marchi M, Todesco T, Robbi R, et al. Body fat distribution in pre- and post-menopausal women: metabolic and anthropometric variables and their inter-relationships. Int J Obes Relat Metab Disord. 1992;16(7):495–504.
17. Poehlman ET, Toth MJ, Gardner AW. Changes in energy balance and body composition at menopause: a controlled longitudinal study. Ann Intern Med. 1995;123(9):673–5.
18. Lee SY, Gallagher D. Assessment methods in human body composition. Curr Opin Clin Nutr Metab Care. 2008;11(5):566–72.
19. Ley CJ, Lees B, Stevenson JC. Sex- and menopause-associated changes in body-fat distribution. Am J Clin Nutr. 1992;55(5):950–4.
20. Morita Y, Iwamoto I, Mizuma N, Kuwahata T, Matsuo T, Yoshinaga M et al. Precedence of the shift of body-fat distribution over the change in body composition after menopause. J Obstet Gynaecol Res. 2006;32(5):513–6.
21. Sternfeld B, Bhat AK, Wang H, Sharp T, Quesenberry Jr CP. Menopause, physical activity, and body composition/fat distribution in midlife women. Med Sci Sports Exerc. 2005;37(7):1195–202.
22. Dawson-Hughes B, Harris S. Regional changes in body composition by time of year in healthy postmenopausal women. Am J Clin Nutr. 1992;56(2):307–13.
23. Geiselman PJ, Smith SR. Estrogen's role in the regulation of appetite and body fat. In: Kohlstadt I, editor. Scientific evidence for musculoskeletal, bariatric, and sports nutrition. Boca Raton, FL: CRC/Taylor & Francis; 2006.
24. Gambacciani M, Ciaponi M, Cappagli B, De Simone L, Orlandi R, Genazzani AR. Prospective evaluation of body weight and body fat distribution in early postmenopausal women with and without hormonal replacement therapy. Maturitas. 2001;39(2):125–32.
25. Gastaldelli A, Basta G. Ectopic fat and cardiovascular disease: what is the link? Nutr Metab Cardiovasc Dis. 2010;20(7):481–90.
26. Ibrahim MM. Subcutaneous and visceral adipose tissue: structural and functional differences. Obes Rev. 2010;11(1):11–8.
27. Toth MJ, Tchernof A, Sites CK, Poehlman ET. Menopause-related changes in body fat distribution. Ann N Y Acad Sci. 2000;904:502–6.
28. Enzi G, Gasparo M, Biondetti PR, Fiore D, Semisa M, Zurlo F. Subcutaneous and visceral fat distribution according to sex, age, and overweight, evaluated by computed tomography. Am J Clin Nutr. 1986;44(6):739–46.
29. Schreiner PJ, Terry JG, Evans GW, Hinson WH, Crouse 3rd JR, Heiss G. Sex-specific associations of magnetic resonance imaging-derived intra-abdominal and subcutaneous fat areas with conventional anthropometric indices. The atherosclerosis risk in communities study. Am J Epidemiol. 1996;144(4):335–45.
30. Rosen CJ, Bouxsein ML. Mechanisms of disease: is osteoporosis the obesity of bone? Nat Clin Pract Rheumatol. 2006;2(1):35–43.

31. Griffith JF, Yeung DK, Ma HT, Leung JC, Kwok TC, Leung PC. Bone marrow fat content in the elderly: a reversal of sex difference seen in younger subjects. J Magn Reson Imaging. 2012;36(1):225–30.
32. Haffner SM, Katz MS, Dunn JF. Increased upper body and overall adiposity is associated with decreased sex hormone binding globulin in postmenopausal women. Int J Obes. 1991;15(7):471–8.
33. Sumino H, Ichikawa S, Yoshida A, Murakami M, Kanda T, Mizunuma H et al. Effects of hormone replacement therapy on weight, abdominal fat distribution, and lipid levels in Japanese postmenopausal women. Int J Obes Relat Metab Disord. 2003;27(9):1044–51.
34. Troisi RJ, Wolf AM, Mason JE, Klingler KM, Colditz GA. Relation of body fat distribution to reproductive factors in pre- and postmenopausal women. Obes Res. 1995;3(2):143–51.
35. Gambacciani M, Ciaponi M, Cappagli B, Piaggesi L, De Simone L, Orlandi R, et al. Body weight, body fat distribution, and hormonal replacement therapy in early postmenopausal women. J Clin Endocrinol Metab. 1997;82(2):414–7.
36. Rebuffe-Scrive M, Eldh J, Hafstrom LO, Bjorntorp P. Metabolism of mammary, abdominal, and femoral adipocytes in women before and after menopause. Metabolism. 1986;35(9):792–7.
37. Lindberg UB, Crona N, Silfverstolpe G, Bjorntorp P, Rebuffe-Scrive M. Regional adipose tissue metabolism in postmenopausal women after treatment with exogenous sex steroids. Horm Metab Res. 1990;22(6):345–51.
38. Mystkowski P, Schwartz MW. Gonadal steroids and energy homeostasis in the leptin era. Nutrition. 2000;16(10):937–46.
39. Lovejoy JC. The influence of sex hormones on obesity across the female life span. J Womens Health. 1998;7(10): 1247–56.
40. Johnstone AM, Murison SD, Duncan JS, Rance KA, Speakman JR. Factors influencing variation in basal metabolic rate include fat-free mass, fat mass, age, and circulating thyroxine but not sex, circulating leptin, or triiodothyronine. Am J Clin Nutr. 2005;82(5):941–8.
41. Webb P. 24-hour energy expenditure and the menstrual cycle. Am J Clin Nutr. 1986;44(5):614–9.
42. Bowen RS, Turner MJ, Lightfoot JT. Sex hormone effects on physical activity levels: why doesn't Jane run as much as Dick? Sports Med. 2011;41(1):73–86.
43. Dorn J, Vena J, Brasure J, Freudenheim J, Graham S. Lifetime physical activity and breast cancer risk in pre- and postmenopausal women. Med Sci Sports Exerc. 2003;35(2):278–85.
44. Wang J, Thornton JC, Russell M, Burastero S, Heymsfield S, Pierson Jr RN. Asians have lower body mass index (BMI) but higher percent body fat than do whites: comparisons of anthropometric measurements. Am J Clin Nutr. 1994;60(1):23–8.
45. Wang J, Thornton JC, Burastero S, Shen J, Tanenbaum S, Heymsfield SB, et al. Comparisons for body mass index and body fat percent among Puerto Ricans, blacks, whites and Asians living in the New York City area. Obes Res. 1996;4(4):377–84.
46. Frohlich MW, Parker DS. Running gels backwards to select DNA molecules larger than a minimum size. Biotechniques. 2001;30(2):264–6.
47. Lear SA, Humphries KH, Kohli S, Birmingham CL. The use of BMI and waist circumference as surrogates of body fat differs by ethnicity. Obesity (Silver Spring). 2007;15(11):2817–24.
48. Randolph Jr JF, Sowers M, Gold EB, Mohr BA, Luborsky J, Santoro N, et al. Reproductive hormones in the early menopausal transition: relationship to ethnicity, body size, and menopausal status. J Clin Endocrinol Metab. 2003;88(4):1516–22.
49. Teh BH, Pan WH, Chen CJ. The reallocation of body fat toward the abdomen persists to very old age, while body mass index declines after middle age in Chinese. Int J Obes Relat Metab Disord. 1996;20(7):683–7.
50. Ho SC, Wu S, Chan SG, Sham A. Menopausal transition and changes of body composition: a prospective study in Chinese perimenopausal women. Int J Obes (Lond). 2010;34(8):1265–74.

Chapter 21
Nutrition and Breast Cancer in Premenopausal and Postmenopausal Women in Uruguay

Alvaro L. Ronco and Eduardo De Stéfani

Key Points

- The epidemiologic links between nutrition and breast cancer in the Uruguayan population have been thoroughly analyzed mainly through case–control studies.
- The disease seems to have differences between premenopausal and postmenopausal women concerning the possible role of diet.
- Although a Western dietary pattern was found of risk for the whole population, most of the putative protective patterns appear as useful mainly for postmenopausal breast cancer.
- Achieving a balance of dietary Ω-6/Ω-3 fatty acids and a balance of muscle/fat ratio combined with changes in the somatotype through physical exercise emerge as specific goals for which some practical interventions during early ages could lower the risk of premenopausal cancer.
- Regarding the country-specific generated evidence and despite its limitations it is fully justified from a medical and ethical viewpoint to give certain guided nutritional recommendations to women, since no adverse side effects are expected to occur.

Keywords Breast cancer • Diet • Foods • Nutrients • Anthropometry • Patterns • Menopause

Abbreviations

BC	Breast cancer
HCA	Heterocyclic amines
FFQ	Food frequency questionnaire
OR	Odds ratio
CI	Confidence interval
RR	Relative risk
PUFA	Polyunsaturated fatty acids
BMI	Body mass index

A.L. Ronco, M.D. (✉)
Oncology and Radiotherapy Unit, Pereira Rossell Women's Hospital, Bvar. Artigas 1550, Montevideo 11300, Uruguay
e-mail: alronco@gmail.com; aronco@verusbiotech.com

E. De Stéfani, M.D.
Grupo de Epidemiología, Departamento de Patología, Facultad de Medicina, Universidad de la República,
Av. Italia s/n y Las Heras, Montevideo 11600, Uruguay

C.J.H. Martin et al. (eds.), *Nutrition and Diet in Menopause*, Nutrition and Health,
DOI 10.1007/978-1-62703-373-2_21, © Springer Science+Business Media New York 2013

Introduction

Breast cancer (BC) is a major public health issue in developed societies, but its incidence has been rising in several developing countries over the past years [1]. Uruguay is among those with the highest rates in the world (Fig. 21.1) according to international data [2]. Uruguay is a South American developing country but sharing some features of developed societies, as a very high level of red meat consumption (the highest beef per capita intake in the world) [3], a high human development index (50° in the world ranking, by factors as birth rate, infant mortality, life expectancy, literacy among others) [4] and an aged population [5]. In other words, a developing country has displayed a high occurrence of a disease typical of developed countries.

During the years 1994–2011 the authors have produced more than 50 scientific works on nutrition and BC in Uruguayan women, trying to thoroughly analyze possible associations between them. Some of the studies were case–control type ones analyzing diet [6–15], lately not only carried out following conventional analysis but also factor analysis in search of nutritional patterns [16–18]. Anthropometric analyses were also performed in Uruguayan women [19–22]. Some multisite studies gave us additional information about the associations of selected foods and/or nutrients and the disease [23–29]. Recently, after a thorough review focusing on primary prevention [30], we have published the first book focusing specifically on nutrition and BC [31].

The studies were mostly performed in population admitted to public hospitals (who belong to low socioeconomic strata) coming from the whole country but we also analyzed a population sample belonging to the private healthcare system (mid-to-high socioeconomic strata) in the capital city, Montevideo, in order to cover different risk populations.

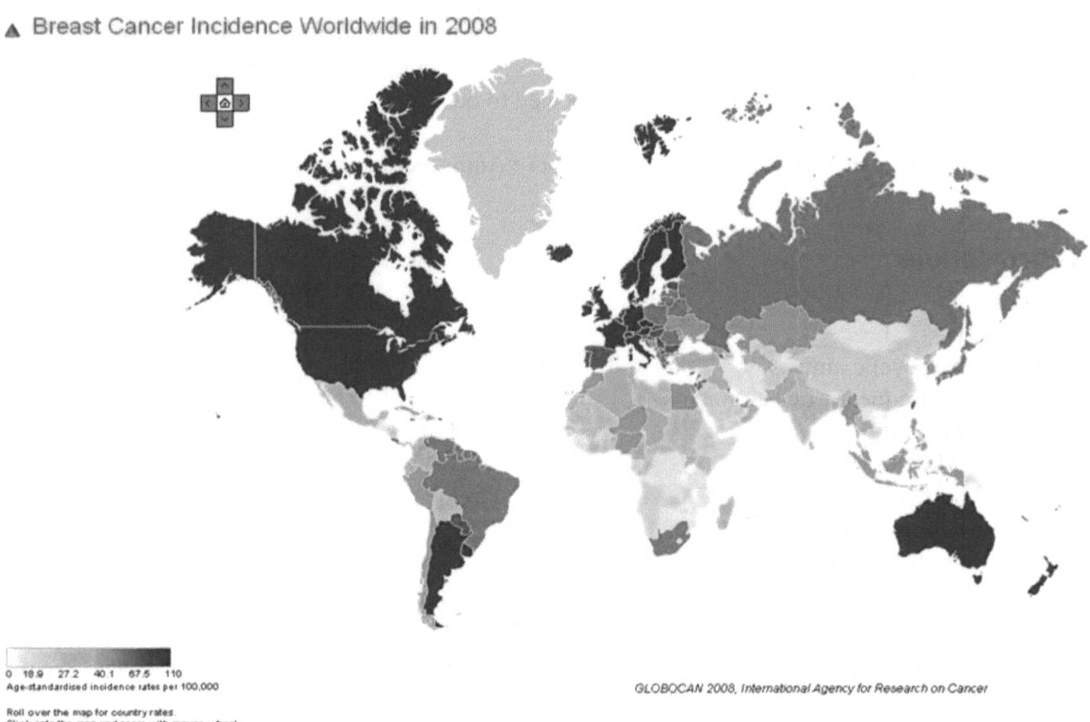

Fig. 21.1 Breast cancer incidence worldwide: age-standardized rates (world population). *Source*: Ref. [2]

General Features

Methodology

The research was carried out based on population subsets belonging to some of the two existing healthcare systems. Cases were women with certified BC with a recent diagnosis, residents in Uruguay for ten or more years and of ages between 24 and 84 years old.

(a) The public system. Patients were admitted to the major hospitals in Montevideo, the capital city of Uruguay. Controls were patients not afflicted with cancer, with nutritional, hormonal, or gynecologic diseases. The most common diseases were: bone fractures, eye disturbances, abdominal hernia, and traumas. Besides, the studies which focused on anthropometry involved control women having a recent normal mammogram (labeled as Bi-rads 1).
(b) The private system. Patients were affiliated to a medical institution, which was representative of the private healthcare system, all residents in Montevideo or neighbor locations. Of them, controls were women having a recent normal mammogram (labeled as Bi-rads 1).

Questionnaire

All patients were face-to-face interviewed with a structured questionnaire shortly after admittance to the hospitals. The questionnaire included sections on socio-demographic variables, a complete history of tobacco smoking, a complete history of alcohol drinking, a section on occupational exposures based on job titles and its duration, menstrual and reproductive variables, self reported height and weight 5 years before the interview, family history of cancer in first- and second-degree relatives and a food frequency questionnaire (FFQ) representative of the Uruguayan diet, including intake of soft drinks, coffee, tea, mate, and vitamins supplementation.

Studies at public hospitals involved a FFQ on 64 foods and at the private center on 120 foods. Each FFQ asked about food consumption 5 years prior to diagnosis in cases and prior to the interview in controls, taking into account that within a period of few years diet may be recalled with acceptable levels of misclassification. The FFQ was not validated, but was tested for reproducibility with reasonably good results [16]. The questionnaire of 120 items was a modification of the previous one, having added some details concerning selected items not only of nutritional interest but also of epidemiologic interest. Furthermore, it allowed the estimation of total energy intake of each subject. For each one of the dietary items, a serving size was estimated, based on the tables of nutrients we consulted. All dietary questions of our semiquantitative questionnaire were open-ended, in order to manage each food as a continuous variable. They were converted into servings/year, multiplying by the most adequate time units each answer deserved. We have considered this type of registration of information as the best expression of the true intake, instead of forcing answers within preexisting categories. In order to calculate daily nutrients or energy, we compiled an analysis program which made the sum of all individual values, each one obtained after multiplying the number of servings/year by the ratio nutrient content or calories of the serving/100 g of each individual food, divided by 365 days. Most typical or average servings of solid foods are within the range of 100–150 g, and fluid foods are included in a cup of 200 ml.

The distribution of all study subjects was categorized into tertiles, quartiles, or quintiles (depending on the circumstances) for each food, food group, or nutrient. Crude and adjusted Relative risks (RR) were estimated through the application of unconditional logistic regression [32]. Potential confounding factors were included in the multivariate models. They were usually: age, residence, education level, family history of BC, body mass index. In each study, other variables which could be correlated with the interest variables were also entered in the regression models. The trend after adjustment by covariates was determined by chi2 test. The 95 % confidence intervals for every RR were calculated. Most calculations were performed with the STATA® software (College State, TX).

Explored Items

The Uruguayan studies which were carried out on diet and BC have reported information about different types of meats and their preparation, heterocyclic amines, fatty foods, dairy foods, vegetables, fruits, fiber, types of fats, phytoestrogens, macronutrients, selected bioactive substances, as well about dietary patterns and their relationship with this type of cancer. Regarding the other arm of nutrition, that is, anthropometry, our studies were focused on two main aspects: fat and muscle fractions and body shape. For these studies we have applied original techniques as body composition and somatotype.

Foods

In the 1990s, a high intake of red meat was found as the main dietary risk factor for BC among Uruguayan women [6, 7]. A logistic regression model, controlling for age, residence, family history of BC in first degree relatives, parity, age at menarche, prior history of benign breast diseases, total calories, vegetables intake and fat intake estimated the ORs of the highest quartiles for total meat (OR = 2.19), red meat (OR = 2.79), and white meat (OR = 0.63), which were significant in all women and in postmenopausal ones (Table 21.1). Their *p*-values for trend were 0.03, 0.006, and 0.03 respectively. In the same way, a risk increase in high consumers of beef (OR = 4.75) and lamb (OR = 2.90) as well a risk decrease in high intake of fish (OR = 0.63) were significant among postmenopausal women. This suggested a possible accumulative effect, in which duration in addition to intensity of intake could be playing an important role, given the higher mean age of postmenopausal women compared to premenopausal ones.

As an example of risk estimates comparing premenopausal and postmenopausal women, Fig. 21.2 presents adjusted ORs for red meat intake, having linear trends for both conditions. Figure 21.3 displays the adjusted ORs for beef intake, which had the highest value among postmenopausal women. White meat intake is shown in Fig. 21.4. Trends tended to be rather similar for both menopausal statuses, but they were significant only among the postmenopausal subset.

Concerning dairy products, the significant negative associations we have described for ricotta cheese (OR = 0.45) and skimmed yoghurt (OR = 0.41), as well as the significant positive associations for gruyere cheese (OR = 1.93), whole milk (OR = 2.84), chocolate milk (OR = 2.85), total milk

Table 21.1 Dietary patterns associated to the risk of breast cancer found in Uruguayan women

Dietary pattern	Premenopausal	Postmenopausal	Heterogeneity
Fatty	1.26 (0.82–1.95)	0.82 (0.69–0.98)	0.02
Western	2.45 (1.69–3.57)	1.62 (1.40–1.88)	0.10
White meat	0.91 (0.65–1.28)	0.78 (0.68–0.89)	0.06
Prudent	1.00 (0.75–1.34)	0.71 (0.61–0.83)	0.009

Differences by menopausal status
Adjusted for age, residence, urban/rural status, education, family history of breast cancer among first degree relatives, age at menarche, parity, and total energy intake

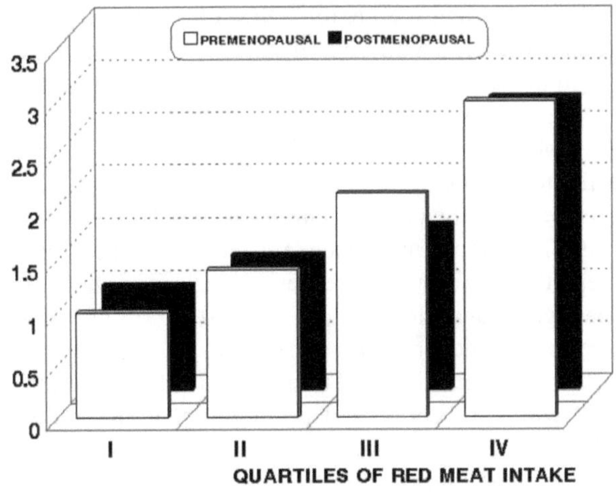

Fig. 21.2 Adjusted risk estimates for red meat intake, discriminated by menopausal status

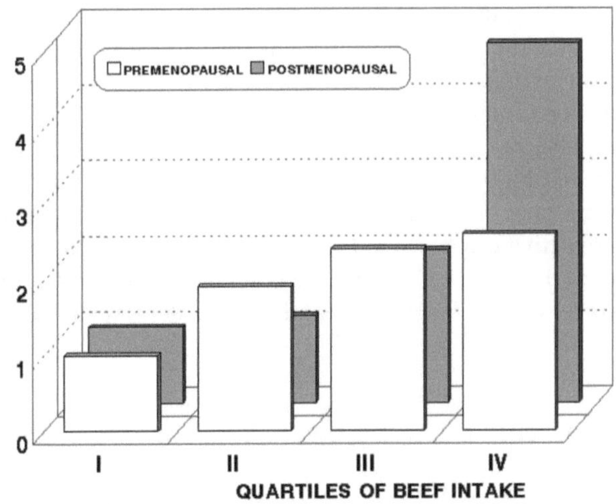

Fig. 21.3 Adjusted risk estimates for beef intake, discriminated by menopausal status

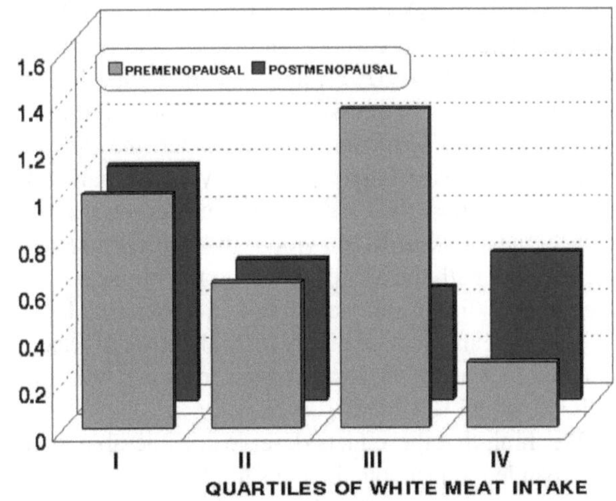

Fig. 21.4 Adjusted risk estimates for white meat intake, discriminated by menopausal status

(OR = 1.99), and ice cream (OR = 1.98) in our paper [12], were present mainly among postmenopausal women, who constituted a very large fraction of the study sample. A reanalysis of the original data allow us to state that the quoted associations were significant only among postmenopausal women.

Vegetables and fruits intake [10] displayed differences in both menopausal statuses of the subset affiliated to the public healthcare system. Considered together, they tended to reduce the risk but this was significant only among postmenopausal women (OR for the highest quartile = 0.60, 95 % CI 0.37–0.99) and not among premenopausal ones (OR for the highest quartile = 0.53, 95 % CI 0.17–1.64). Nevertheless, only cooked vegetables supported a significant protective effect for the latter (OR for the highest quartile = 0.22, 95 % CI 0.07–0.71), while only raw vegetables were significantly protective for postmenopausal women (OR for the highest quartile = 0.48, 95 % CI 0.30–0.79).

Besides, tomatoes and tomato-derived foods were found as protective. Raw tomatoes were associated with a moderate and not significant risk reduction (RR for the highest quartile = 0.62, 95 % CI 0.36–1.06), foods dressed with tomato sauce displayed a strong protective and significant effect (RR for the highest quartile = 0.30, 95 % CI 0.17–0.52). The effects were also restricted to the postmenopausal subset. Since lycopene has been one of the most protective nutrients in our research, it would explain partially the effect of total vegetables, also considering that this carotenoid is the one prevailing in tomatoes.

In addition, the highest intake of fruit was not associated with the risk of BC in premenopausal women (OR = 1.16, 95 % CI 0.40–3.36), whereas it was borderline negatively associated among postmenopausal ones (OR = 0.62, 95 % CI 0.38–1.02). Our analysis of fruit consumption among women affiliated to the private healthcare system [16], revealed that total fruits (OR for the highest tertile = 0.44, 95% CI 0.23–0.86) and citrus fruits (OR for the highest tertile = 0.27, 95 % CI 0.13–0.55) were protective but also restricted to the postmenopausal subset. Citrus fruits displayed a stronger protective effect when the regression model included a term for vitamin C (OR for the highest tertile = 0.13, 95 % CI 0.05–0.33). In nutritional epidemiology of cancer, a significant reduction of 87 %, such as in the latter, is very strong and deserves to be remarked.

Nutrients

Polyunsaturated Ω-6 and Ω-3 Fatty Acids

The analysis of polyunsaturated fatty acids (PUFA) intake in Uruguayan women [14] found that high intakes of Ω-6 PUFA were significantly and positively associated with the risk of BC (OR = 7.20 for ages <55 and OR = 4.05 for ages >= 56, comparing the highest with the lowest tertiles). The intake of Ω-3 was negatively and significantly associated among the younger half (OR = 0.20 for the highest tertile) but not significantly for the older one (OR = 0.67). The ratio Ω-6/Ω-3 was also significantly and positively associated among the younger half (OR = 5.51), but no association was detected for the older ones (OR = 1.09). Although results come from a small sample of patients belonging to the subset with highest risk in Montevideo, the evidence reinforces the preventive potential of dietary recommendations with the aim of reducing the impact of the disease. These associations are consistent with the previous findings concerning white meat intake [13].

A significant increase of risk for high intake of fried fish was observed (OR = 1.99, 95 % CI 1.02–3.88). On the other hand, the intake of not fried fish had a significant inverse association with the risk of BC (OR = 0.48, 95 % CI 0.24–0.93).

We think that these facts deserve considerable attention because recommendations probably should be expanded to promote the consumption of these white meats, but after having preparation modalities which do not imply the intake of high levels of some fats or the production of HCAs during cooking.

Apparently the protective effect of Ω-3 PUFA and the risk increase of Ω-6 PUFA would be stronger among younger women (mostly presumably premenopausal) than among the older ones (mostly presumably postmenopausal). The Ω-6 PUFA are constituents of common seed oils (corn, sunflower, soybean, for example) as well as of margarines—largely promoted as safe substitutes of butter and lard. The frying process changes some of these PUFA from Cis to the Trans chemical structure. Trans-fatty acids are not established as risk factors for BC, but they deserve to be studied more thoroughly, since fried foods are very common in Western dietary patterns. We cannot preclude the probability of a higher sensitivity among young breasts to these fatty acids, based on our findings among premenopausal women.

Vitamins and Bioactive Substances

The intake of vitamins and bioactive substances was analyzed more than a decade ago [10]. Only few items showed some association to the risk of BC among premenopausal women in our study population: vitamin C, vitamin E, quercetin, and kaempferol. The general protective effect of carotenes, for example, is restricted to postmenopausal women. Also fiber and folate intake were negatively associated with the risk of BC only among the postmenopausal subset.

Besides, total fat intake displayed a non significant increase in risk (OR for the highest quartile = 1.90, 95 % CI 0.61–5.93) among premenopausal women, but it was stronger and significant only among postmenopausal ones (OR for the highest quartile = 3.91, 95 % CI 2.36–6.49).

Nutritional Patterns

Factor analysis is considered as a powerful statistical method in search of finding dietary patterns and it has been reported as more efficient than the traditional reductionist approach [33]. This type of analysis has shed some light on the links between diet and BC, partially differing from the statements cited in the World Cancer Research Fund report [34] about the insufficiency of evidence for dietary patterns.

Regarding Diet, our analyses found four food patterns, which were entitled as follows: Fatty, Western, White meat, and Prudent. They showed differences between premenopausal and postmenopausal status, which are presented in Table 21.1.

Both subsets tend to display heterogeneity, in spite of the non significant *p*-value obtained when testing the Western pattern ($p = 0.10$). The analysis suggests that only Western pattern would be strongly positively associated with the risk of premenopausal BC, but the other patterns of this subset would not be associated. Among postmenopausal women, the risk association of Western pattern (based on meats and fats) is clear. The same applies for the putative protective association of White Meat and Prudent patterns. On the contrary, the negative association of the Fatty pattern in postmenopausal women is not clear; nevertheless, the original publication [16] displayed no association for this high-fat pattern for the whole sample. We can not preclude the relative weight of calcium from dairy foods and also the PUFA from fish, counterbalancing the risky associations of a high-fat diet.

The Factor analysis designed to study nutrients associated to the risk of BC, has lead to find three nutrient patterns in Uruguayan women. The present analysis with a larger sample allowed the authors to find a third pattern (grain-based) which was not present in the original paper [17]. Results are shown in Table 21.2.

Once again, the influence coming from the nutrients derived from animal-based diets showed no heterogeneity between subsets. The involved high fat, high cholesterol and high heterocyclic amines intake combined together increase the risk for the whole population. We had reported that this pattern involved

Table 21.2 Nutrient patterns associated to the risk of breast cancer found in Uruguayan women

Nutrient pattern	Premenopausal	Postmenopausal	Heterogeneity
Animal-based	3.40 (1.55–7.43)	2.24 (1.60–3.14)	0.90
Grain-based	1.77 (0.90–3.47)	0.99 (0.73–1.34)	0.06
Plant-based	1.27 (0.87–1.84)	0.72 (0.61–0.86)	0.003

Differences by menopausal status
Adjusted for age, residence, urban/rural status, education, family history of breast cancer in first-degree relatives, body mass index, age at menarche, parity, total energy intake, and both patterns

stronger risks among those women with a family history of BC in first degree [17]. Besides, many of the components of a prudent pattern are comprised in the plant-based patterns and it was not associated with risk among the younger subset of the sample but it was among postmenopausal women.

Undoubtedly, if most of these results were confirmed by new analyses, the possibilities of having basic recommendations for primary prevention of BC are encouraging since young women are a subgroup which is difficult to protect through nutritional guidelines. In fact, contrary to what happens to postmenopausal women, there are a few items suggesting a role of risk association or a protective association among young, premenopausal women. The rationale and numerous advantages for recommending a frequent intake of fishes that are rich sources of Ω-3 PUFA (tuna, sardines, salmon, cod, among others) as well as the supplementation through the intake of oil fish were given in a recent publication [31].

We accept that while there is no clear evidence that any specific dietary component can effectively reduce BC risk [35], the fact that several foods have convergence on a few dietary patterns—and probably beyond these latter could be even fewer nutrient patterns—is something we could probably profit from, for preventive nutritional recommendations which we have recently proposed [30].

Anthropometry

Somatotype

We investigated the possible role of physical shape in the risk of BC in 1,254 Uruguayan women, using an innovative methodology which was well known in the fitness world and athletic assessment: the somatotype [19]. It is defined as "a quantitative description of the present shape and composition of the human body" [36], a method developed by W.H. Sheldon 60 years ago [37]. This method describes three body components: (1) Endomorphy, which features the relative adiposity; (2) Mesomorphy, which features the muscular size; and (3) Ectomorphy, which features the linearity or slenderness derived from the ponderal index (height in cm divided by the cube root of weight in kg). These components differ among populations according to age, sex, and origins. For example, an extreme endomorphism has a pear-shape, with wide hips and narrow shoulders. An extreme mesomorphism is featured by wide shoulders and relatively narrow hips (edge-shaped), more typical of men than of women. And an extreme ectomorphism has narrow shoulders, chest and hips, together with thin arms and legs and reduced amount of muscle or fat.

Somatotype methodology has been scarcely used in the medical field, with examples related to cardiovascular risk [38–42], obesity [43, 44] and rarely in cancer research [45, 46]. The changes that occur in a somatotype happen during childhood to maturity and they can be modified through physical training and/or nutrition. The somatotype is expressed by a score produced by the three components, calculated from certain body measurements and specific formulas. In addition, results can be

Table 21.3 Differences of the endomorphy among premenopausal and postmenopausal Uruguayan women, associated to the risk of breast cancer

Endomorphy					
	n	Low	Mid	High	Trend
Cutpoints		≤6.0	6.1–7.5	≥7.6	
Premenopausal	725				
Cases/Controls	217/508				
Crude OR (95 % CI)		1.00 (ref)	1.20 (0.80–1.79)	1.85 (1.25–2.72)	0.002
Adjusted OR (95 % CI)		1.00 (ref)	1.68 (1.07–2.62)	4.67 (2.51–8.68)	<0.001
Postmenopausal	853				
Cases/Controls	224/629				
Crude OR (95 % CI)		1.00 (ref)	0.96 (0.64–1.43)	1.43 (0.98–2.10)	0.04
Adjusted OR (95 % CI)		1.00 (ref)	1.31 (0.83–2.08)	2.72 (1.56–4.75)	<0.001

Adjustment included age, age at menarche, parity, age at first live birth, months of breastfeeding, years between menarche and first delivery, BMI, BMI at age 18, use of oral contraceptives and family history of BC. For postmenopausal, age at menopause was included as a regression term

graphically represented through the so called somatochart, in which a point corresponds to the score previously calculated.

The study of the somatotype allowed us to quantify the proportions and shapes of the studied women. Although the global somatotype pattern for the population was a mixtured endo-mesomorphic one, women with BC displayed higher endomorphism than healthy controls. In other words, we have observed in our sample that patients with BC tended to be more "pear-shaped," regardless of their slender, medium, or obese external appearance. Besides, we did not find differences in the mesomorphism and ectomorphism. Endomorphism exhibited a dose-effect pattern, which is a strength for being a possible risk factor. Results were also slightly stronger among premenopausal women and in women with normal weight (BMI < 25 kg/m^2), although they were not statistically heterogeneous [19].

All results related to endomorphism, which are presented in Table 21.3, were obtained through a similar analysis of the master database, which currently has 1,578 analyzable patients registered. A high endomorphism was positively associated with BC risk among premenopausal women (adjusted OR = 4.67, 95 % CI 2.51–8.68, *p* value for trend <0.001) as well as among postmenopausal ones (adjusted OR = 2.72, 95 % CI 1.56–4.75, *p*-value for trend <0.001). In conclusion, high endomorphism is similar in its risk association taking into account the menopausal status of women.

From the viewpoint of somatotype, the somatochart translates the findings and represent the mean values of each subgroup. Postmenopausal women had almost the same values for BC cases and healthy controls. Healthy premenopausal women were less endomorphic and mesomorphic than postmenopausal ones. And premenopausal cases of BC were somehow in the way between the normal premenopausal and the postmenopausal ones. It seemed as if younger women with BC had acquired a body morphology which would be directed towards the one of older ones. In other words, the body shape of the former ones appeared as if it were advanced in time getting closer to those of these latter.

Body Composition

Anthropometric data were used to quantify body size and body proportions. The following body measures were determined: BMI, fat fraction, bone fraction, muscle fraction, fat weight, muscle weight, and FMR. Calculations of body measures were based on the Faulkner protocol [47] according to the anatomic four compartments method of De Rose [48].

Table 21.4 Odds ratios and 95 % confidence intervals for the fat/muscle ratio stratified by menopausal status and by BMI, associated with the risk of breast cancer

Premenopausal	Fat/muscle ratio				
Patients	*n*	I 95 % CI	II 95 % CI	III 95 % CI	IV 95 % CI
Fat/muscle ratio		≤1.01	1.02–1.46	1.47–2.20	≥2.21
All	730	1.00	2.22 (1.25–3.95)	3.29 (1.89–5.73)	4.53 (2.63–7.80)
Normal weight	335	1.00	1.42 (0.80–3.87)	3.26 (1.50–7.09)	4.94 (2.34–10.5)
Overweight	221	1.00	3.23 (0.82–12.6)	6.21 (1.79–21.5)	6.34 (1.85–21.7)
Obese	174	1.00	5.73 (1.35–24.2)	4.87 (1.19–19.9)	9.48 (2.22–40.5)
Postmenopausal					
All	854	1.00	1.20 (0.76–1.90)	1.77 (1.12–2.78)	3.18 (2.01–5.02)
Normal weight	207	1.00	1.99 (0.76–5.22)	1.92 (0.71–5.19)	4.73 (1.85–12.1)
Overweight	333	1.00	0.74 (0.30–1.81)	1.50 (0.65–3.48)	2.77 (1.22–6.26)
Obese	314	1.00	1.76 (0.85–3.64)	2.95 (1.40–6.18)	3.59 (1.61–8.00)

Adjustment included terms for age, education level, urban/rural status, family history of breast cancer in first degree, family history of breast cancer in second degree, family history of other cancers in first degree, age at menarche, age at first live birth, difference menarche—age at first live birth, number of live births, and months of breastfeeding

In our epidemiologic case–control studies which explored body composition and its possible associations with BC in a sample of almost 1,400 women [20, 22] we reported that the higher the fat fraction was, higher was the risk of the disease. At the same time, the lower the muscle fraction was, also higher was the risk of BC. The original paper did not make stratified analyses by menopausal status. Hence, we have herewith analyzed an updated database (almost 1,600 patients) in order to show results of the fat/muscle ratio, categorized into quartiles, displaying the stratified analysis. The logistic regression model included terms for: age, education, urban/rural status, family history of BC in first and second degree, family history of other cancers in first degree, age at menarche, age at first live birth, number of live births, months of breastfeeding, use of oral contraceptives and body mass index. The Table 21.4 displays the results.

Despite the menopausal status, women experience an increase of risk when the fat/muscle ratio increases, and this trend is stronger among premenopausal women. Apparently, getting a balance 1:1 of muscle/fat ratio would be a desirable goal for having a low risk. The low-risk subset (in this case, the reference category) includes every woman with a ratio up to 1, which means for example a good situation for women who practice some sports in which the fat fraction is recognized as low. The combination here arises as the best: physical activity plus low fat/muscle ratio, the former can lead to the latter. Besides, younger women display an increasing trend with the BMI: the situation is worse among obese women than among those with normal weight. Again, we can have an opposite situation as the above described: the combination of obesity and a high fat/muscle ratio. Lack of physical activity can lead to both of them. These associations, nevertheless, were not so clear among the older subset.

Conclusions

The epidemiologic nutritional studies performed in Uruguayan women found some differences in association to their risk of BC and their menopausal status (e.g., dietary patterns, anthropometric features). We should recognize once again, therefore, that the disease seems to be different for premenopausal than for postmenopausal women. Although the Western dietary pattern was found of risk for the whole population, most of the putative risk and protective patterns appeared as useful mainly for the older subset. Anyway, achieving on one hand a balance of dietary Ω-6/Ω-3 fatty acids through inclusion of fish oil supplements and substitution of seed oils by olive oil, and on the other hand achieving a balance of muscle/fat ratio combined with changes in the somatotype through physical exercise, emerge as possible practical interventions during early ages for lowering the risk for premenopausal cancer. The evaluated components found together in vegetables and fruits may have a synergistic protective effect on BC risk, as suggested by foods and nutrients patterns; the same applies, but in an opposite direction, to meats and fats combined, also expressed by such dietary patterns. Anyway, other unmeasured factors in these foods may also influence risk and this possibility must be recognized. Regarding the country-specific generated evidence and despite its limitations, we are convinced that giving certain guided nutritional recommendations to women would be fully justified from a medical and ethical viewpoint, since no adverse side effects are expected to occur. Furthermore, such recommendations would be relatively simple to promote, facing the challenge of only counting on a small available dietary background with the potential for preventing premenopausal BC.

References

1. Bray F, Mc Carron P, Parkin DM. The changing global patterns of female breast cancer incidence and mortality. Breast Cancer Res. 2004;6:229–39.
2. Ferlay J, Shin HR, Bray F, et al. GLOBOCAN 2008, Cancer incidence and mortality worldwide: IARC Cancerbase No.10. Lyon, France: International Agency for Research on Cancer. http://globocan.iarc.fr. Accessed 17 Aug 2010.
3. Matos E, Brandani A. Review on meat consumption and cancer in South America. Mutat Res. 2002;506–507:243–9.
4. United Nations Organization, Program of human development. Human development index rankings. http://hdr.undp.org/en/statistics/. Accessed 27 Apr 2010.
5. U.S. Census Bureau. International data base, http://www.census.gov/ipc/www/idb/country.php. Accessed 30 Apr 2010.
6. Ronco AL, De Stéfani E, Mendilaharsu M, Deneo-Pellegrini H. Meat, fat and the risk of breast cancer: a case-control study from Uruguay. Int J Cancer. 1996;65:328–31.
7. De Stéfani E, Ronco AL, Mendilaharsu M, Guidobono M, Deneo-Pellegrini H. Meat intake, heterocyclic amines, and risk of breast cancer: a case-control study in Uruguay. Cancer Epidemiol Biomarkers Prev. 1997;6:573–81.
8. De Stéfani E, Correa P, Ronco A, et al. Dietary fiber and risk of breast cancer. Nutr Cancer. 1997;28:14–9.
9. De Stéfani E, Deneo-Pellegrini H, Mendilaharsu M, Ronco AL. Essential fatty acids and breast cancer: a case-control study in Uruguay. Int J Cancer. 1998;76:491–4.
10. Ronco AL, De Stéfani E, Boffetta P, et al. Vegetables, fruits, and related nutrients and risk of breast cancer: a case control study in Uruguay. Nutr Cancer. 1999;35(2):111–9.
11. Ronco AL, De Stéfani E. Fitoestrógenos y riesgo de cáncer mamario: un estudio caso control. Rev Med Urug. 1999;15:94–102.
12. Ronco AL, De Stéfani E, Dáttoli R. Dairy foods and risk of breast cancer: a case-control study in Montevideo, Uruguay. Eur J Cancer Prev. 2002;11(5):457–63.
13. Ronco AL, De Stéfani E, Fabra A. White meat intake and the risk of breast cancer: a case-control study in Montevideo, Uruguay. Nutr Res. 2003;23(2):151–62.
14. Ronco A, De Stéfani E, Deneo-Pellegrini H, et al. Consumo de grasas poliinsaturadas y riesgo de cáncer de mama: un estudio caso-control. Rev Bras Nutr Clin. 2005;20 Suppl 1Suppl 1:S1–SS8 (p.12).
15. Ronco AL, De Stéfani E, Deneo-Pellegrini H. Fruit intake and risk of breast cancer: a case-control study. In: Louis PF, editor. Frontiers in breast cancer research. New York: Nova Science; 2008. p. 175–86.
16. Ronco AL, De Stefani E, Boffetta P, et al. Food patterns and risk of breast cancer: a factor analysis study in Uruguay. Int J Cancer. 2006;19(1):1672–8.
17. Ronco AL, De Stéfani E, Aune D, et al. Nutrient patterns and risk of breast cancer in Uruguay. Asian Pac J Cancer Prev. 2010;11(2):519–24.
18. Ronco AL, De Stéfani E, Deneo-Pellegrini H, et al. Dietary patterns and risk of ductal carcinoma of the breast: a factor analysis in Uruguay. Asian Pac J Cancer Prev. 2010;11(5):1187–93.
19. Ronco AL, Mendoza B, Varas X, et al. Somatotype and risk of breast cancer: a case-control study in Uruguay. Braz J Epidemiol. 2008;11(2):215–27.
20. Ronco AL, Boeing H, De Stéfani E, et al. A case-control study on fat to muscle ratio and risk of breast cancer. Nutr Cancer. 2009;61(4):466–74.
21. Ronco AL, De Stéfani E. Diabetes, overweight and risk of breast cancer: a case-control study in Uruguay. Proceedings of the II International Symposium on Breast Cancer Prevention; 2011 Oct 9–11; Rennes, France. p. 57.

22. Ronco AL, De Stéfani E. Interrelationships between body composition and somatotype and the risk of breast cancer. Proceedings of the II International Symposium on Breast Cancer Prevention; 2011 Oct 9–11; Rennes, France. p. 59.
23. De Stéfani E, Deneo-Pellegrini H, Boffetta P, et al. Dietary patterns and risk of cancer: a factor analysis in Uruguay. Int J Cancer. 2009;124(6):1391–7.
24. Aune D, De Stéfani E, Ronco AL, et al. Meat consumption and the risk of cancer: a case-control study in Uruguay. Cancer Therapy. 2009;7:174–87.
25. Aune D, De Stéfani E, Ronco AL, et al. Legume intake and the risk of cancer: a multisite case–control study in Uruguay. Cancer Causes Control. 2009;20(9):1605–15.
26. Aune D, De Stéfani E, Ronco AL, et al. Fruits, vegetables and the risk of cancer: a multisite case-control study in Uruguay. Asian Pac J Cancer Prev. 2009;20:419–28.
27. Aune D, De Stéfani E, Ronco AL, et al. Egg consumption and the risk of cancer: a multisite case-control study in Uruguay. Asian Pac J Cancer Prev. 2009;10(5):869–76.
28. De Stéfani E, Aune D, Boffetta P, et al. Salted meat consumption and the risk of cancer: a multisite case-control study in Uruguay. Asian Pac J Cancer Prev. 2009;10(5):853–7.
29. Aune D, Deneo-Pellegrini H, Ronco AL, et al. Dietary folate intake and the risk of 11 types of cancer: a case–control study in Uruguay. Ann Oncol. 2011;22(2):444–51.
30. Ronco AL, De Stéfani E, Stoll M. Hormonal and metabolic modulation through nutrition: towards a primary prevention of breast cancer. Breast. 2010;19:322–32.
31. Ronco AL, De Stéfani E. Nutritional epidemiology of breast cancer. Amsterdam: Springer; 2011.
32. Breslow NE, Day NE. (Editors) Statistical methods in cancer research. Vol. 1. The analysis of case-control studies. Lyon: IARC Sci Publ; 1980.
33. Slattery ML, Boucher KM, Caan BJ, et al. Eating patterns and risk of colon cancer. Am J Epidemiol. 1998;148:4–16.
34. World Cancer Research Fund/American Institute for Cancer Research. Food, nutrition, physical activity, and the prevention of cancer: a global perspective. Washington DC: American Institute for Cancer Research; 2007.
35. Mahoney MC, Bevers T, Linos E, Willett W. Opportunities and strategies for breast cancer prevention through risk reduction. CA Cancer J Clin. 2008;58:347–71.
36. Carter JEL, Heath BH. Somatotyping: development and applications. Cambridge: Cambridge University Press; 1990.
37. Sheldon WH. The somatotype, the morphophenotype, and the morphogenotype. Cold Spring Harb Symp Quant Biol. 1951;15:373–82.
38. Garn SM, Gertler MM, Sprague HB. Somatotype and serum-cholesterol. Circulation. 1950;2:380–91.
39. Gordon E, Tobias PV, Mendelsohn D, Seftel H, Howson A. The relationship between somatotype and serum lipids in male and female young adults. Hum Biol. 1987;59:459–65.
40. Morris RW, Jacobs ML. On the application of somatotyping to the study of constitution in disease. S Afr J Clin Sci. 1950;1:347–70.
41. Valkov J, Matev T, Hristov I. Relationship between somatotype and some risk factors for ischemic heart disease. Folia Med (Plovdiv). 1996;38:17–21.
42. Malina RM, Katzmarzyk PT, Song TMK, et al. Somatotype and cardiovascular risk factors in healthy adults. Am J Hum Biol. 1997;9:11–9.
43. Seltzer CC, Mayer J. Body build (somatotype) distinctiveness in obese women. J Am Diet Assoc. 1969;55:454–8.
44. Koleva M, Nacheva A, Boev M. Somatotype, nutrition, and obesity. Rev Environ Health. 2000;15:389–98.
45. Kolodchenko VP. Body build and soft tissue malignancies. Vopr Onkol. 2000;29:56–60.
46. Eiben OG, Buday J, Bosze P. Physique of patients with carcinoma of the female genital tract. Eur J Gynaecol Oncol. 2004;25:683–8.
47. Faulkner J. Physiology of swimming and diving. In: Falls H, editor. Exercise physiology. Baltimore: Academic; 1968.
48. De Rose EH, Pigatto E, Celi R. Kinanthropometry, physical education and sport training. Brasilia: SEED; 1984 (in Portuguese).

Chapter 22
Obesity, Nutrition, and Cancer in Menopause: European Perspectives

Krasimira Aleksandrova

Key Points

- Excess body weight increases the risk of cancer at several sites in European women, including endometrium, colon, and breast in postmenopausal women.
- The association of obesity with the risk of cancer in many developed European countries suggests that adoption of a "Western diet" characterized by high energy intake may be an underlying cause of malignancy.
- Several dietary factors that may potentially influence the accumulation of body fat include high consumption of energy-dense food, rich in total fat and red meat, and refined carbohydrate, and low in fiber, fruits, and vegetables.
- Epidemiological evidence in large European cohort studies suggests that women with diets high in energy and saturated fat such as red meat, and low in complex carbohydrates, such as cereals and whole grains, are at increased risk of cancer, particularly of colorectal cancer.
- The association of total fat intake with cancer risk is controversial and the role of different types of fat is not well understood.
- High-glycemic foods, such as refined carbohydrates, may be of relevance to breast and endometrial cancer risk, but current evidence does not support their role for colorectal cancer risk.
- Although fruits and vegetables have a strong anticarcinogenic potential, the evidence is inconclusive possibly due to the fact that the effect of specific bioactive compounds is diluted when food groups are considered as a whole in observational research studies.
- Consideration of the dietary pattern as a whole might be useful in formulating dietary recommendations for women. Replacing the "Western-style" diet with a "Mediterranean-style" diet including poultry, fish, and plant sources of protein; olive oil and other unsaturated fats; and unrefined grains and legumes might improve overall health status and potentially lower the risk of cancer.

Keywords Obesity • Body fat distribution • Obesity-related cancer • Women • Pre-menopause • Postmenopause • Europe

K. Aleksandrova, M.P.H., Ph.D. (✉)
Department of Epidemiology, German Institute of Human Nutrition Potsdam-Rehbruecke, Arthur-Scheunert-Allee 114-116, 14558 Nuthetal, Germany
e-mail: krasimira.aleksandrova@dife.de

C.J.H. Martin et al. (eds.), *Nutrition and Diet in Menopause*, Nutrition and Health,
DOI 10.1007/978-1-62703-373-2_22, © Springer Science+Business Media New York 2013

Abbreviations

BMI	Body mass index
WC	Waist circumference
WHR	Waist-to-hip ratio
HRT	Hormonal replacement therapy
EPIC	European Prospective Investigation into Cancer and Nutrition
WCRF	World Cancer Research Fund
PARs	Population attributable risks

Introduction

Cancer mortality accounts for nearly 20 % of all deaths in the European Region being the leading cause of premature death, before the age of 65 in many European countries (28 of the 53 in the Region) [1]. An estimated 2.45 million new cancer cases occur in the European Union every year [1] and the number has been increasing in the last decades with ageing of the population (Fig. 22.1a, b). Women who have been through natural menopause may be at higher risk of developing cancer because older age is one of the established risk factors for cancer. It is estimated that one in five women in Europe will get cancer before the age of 75 [1]. In terms of share of total incidence, the eight most common types of cancer among women in Europe are breast (28.2 %), colorectal (13.5 %), lung (6.8 %), uterine (5.8 %), ovary (4.4 %), stomach (3.9 %), cervical (3.6 %), and pancreatic cancer (3.1 %) [1] (Fig. 22.2). With regard to cancer mortality the most frequent cancer types are breast (17.0 %), colorectal (13.5 %), lung (11.5 %), stomach (6.3 %), and pancreatic cancer (6.2 %) [2].

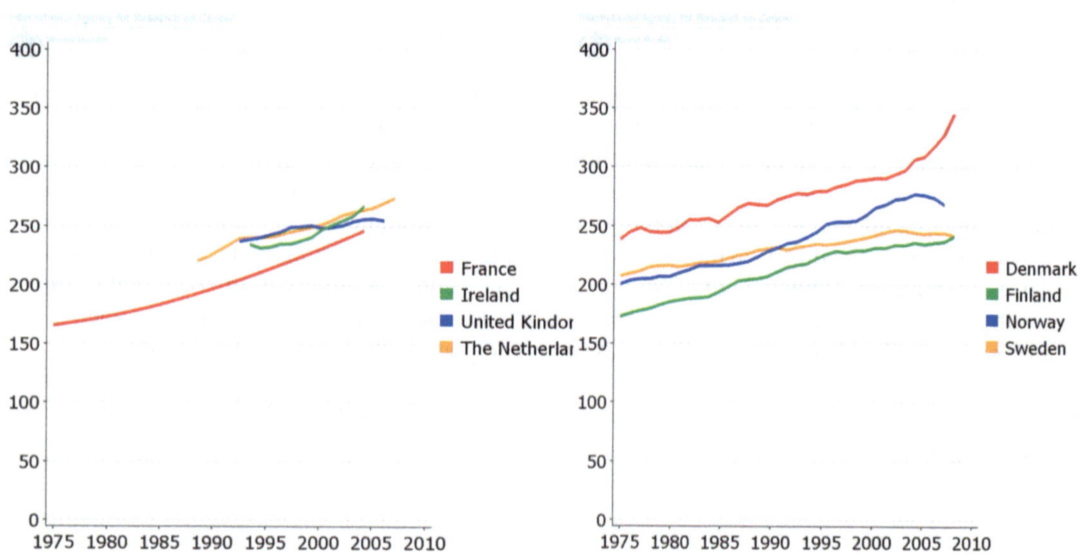

Fig. 22.1 (**a**) Trends in the incidence of breast cancer in selected countries: age-standardized rate (W) per 100,000 (France, Ireland, the United Kingdom, the Netherlands), rate (W) per 100,000, women. (**b**) Trends in the incidence of breast cancer in selected countries: age-standardized rate (W) per 100,000 (Denmark, Finland, Norway, Sweden), rate (W) per 100,000, women. From Ferlay J, Shin HR, Bray F, Forman D, Mathers C and Parkin DM. GLOBOCAN 2008, Cancer Incidence and Mortality Worldwide: IARC Cancer Base No. 10 [Internet]. Lyon, France: International Agency for Research on Cancer; 2010. Available from http://globocan.iarc.fr

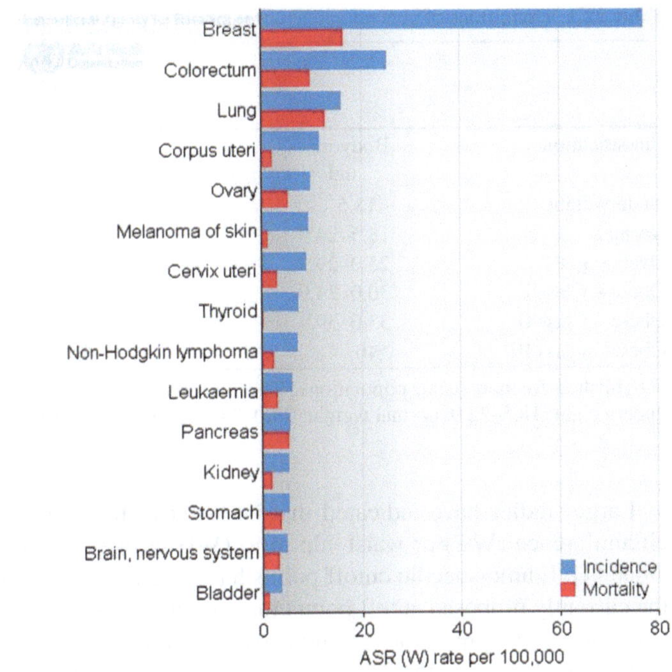

Fig. 22.2 Cancer incidence and mortality age-standardized rates in women. From Ferlay J, Shin HR, Bray F, Forman D, Mathers C and Parkin DM. GLOBOCAN 2008, Cancer Incidence and Mortality Worldwide: IARC Cancer Base No. 10 [Internet]. Lyon, France: International Agency for Research on Cancer; 2010. Available from http://globocan.iarc.fr

The burden of cancer is increasing in economically developing countries as a result of population ageing and growth as well as, increasingly, an adoption of lifestyle factors including smoking, physical inactivity, and "Westernized" diets [3]. Furthermore, growing evidence indicates that excess body weight increases the risk of cancer at several sites in women, including endometrium, colon, and breast in postmenopausal women [3]. Because obesity and diet are among the few modifiable risk factors [4], they represent an important target for cancer prevention and prognosis in both pre- and postmenopausal women.

The current review summarizes the epidemiologic evidence on the association between general and abdominal obesity, nutritional factors, and risk of cancer with a specific focus on large population-based European studies. In particular, the review outlines the perspectives for prevention in most frequent forms of obesity-related cancer in European women: breast, colorectal, and endometrial cancer.

Prevalence of Obesity in European Women

Overweight and obesity are defined as "a condition of abnormal or excessive fat accumulation in adipose tissue to the extent that health may be impaired" [5]. A standardized measure of obesity is the body mass index (BMI), calculated as weight (in kilograms) divided by height (in meters) squared. A person with a BMI of 25 or more is considered "overweight" and a person with a BMI of 30 or more is defined as "obese" [5] (Table 22.1). The prevalence of overweight and obesity is rapidly increasing in many European countries in both sexes. In the mid-1980s, 17 % of the female population in Europe had a BMI≥30 kg/m [2], whereas according to recent reports, the current prevalence of obesity in women ranges from 6.2 to 36.5 % [6]. In the 27 EU member states, obesity is more prevalent in women compared with men. According to estimates by the International Association for the Study of Obesity (2008) a total of 37 million women and 31 million men are estimated to be obese.

Table 22.1 Definitions of general and abdominal obesity[a] (based on Expert Panel, 1998) [79]

		Chronic disease risk relative to normal weight and waist circumference	
Classification	Body mass index (kg/m^2)	Men ≤102 cm Women ≤88 cm	Men >102 cm Women >88 cm
Underweight	<18.5	–	–
Normal	18.5–24.9	–	–
Overweight	25.0–29.9	Increased	High
Obese—Class I	30.0–34.9	High	Very high
Obese—Class II	35.0–39.9	Very high	Very high
Obese—Class III	≥40	Extremely high	Extremely high

[a]Established for non-Asian populations. The recently proposed classification for Asian populations is BMI < 18.5, underweight; 18.5–22.9, normal weight; 23.0–24.9, overweight; 25.0–29.9, obese class I; >30.0, obese class II [80]

Large studies have indicated that body fat distribution as determined by measurement of waist circumference (WC) or waist–hip ratio (WHR) may be a better predictor of cancer risk than BMI alone [4]. Ethnic-specific cutoff points have been suggested to better reflect chronic disease risk and the currently proposed cutoff points for European populations are 94 cm in men and 80 cm in women [7]. Data on the prevalence of indices for abdominal obesity in Europe, though, is scarce. Based on data from the European Prospective Investigation into Cancer and Nutrition (EPIC) [8], among 163,851 women, in the menopausal age of 50–64 years from nine western European countries, the mean WC levels in vary from 77.2 cm in South of France to 95.0 cm in Murcia, Spain [9].

Epidemiological Evidence Linking Obesity and Cancer in Women

The World Cancer Research Fund (WCRF) expert panel (2007) has concluded that there is sufficient scientific evidence showing that obesity is an important risk factor for the cancers of breast (in postmenopausal women), colon, endometrium (the lining of the uterus), kidney, and esophagus [4]. A recent analysis based on data from 30 European countries has estimated population attributable risks (PARs) associated with obesity in women to be 4.1 % corresponding to 43,046 incident cancer cases that potentially could have been prevented if these women were not obese [10]. Nearly 65 % of cases attributable to obesity are accounted for by three cancer types, including endometrial cancer (33,421 new cases), postmenopausal breast cancer (27,770 new cases) and colorectal cancer (23,730 new cases) [10].

Breast Cancer

Over the last two decades a number of European epidemiological studies have supported the evidence that BMI is negatively associated to premenopausal breast cancer risk and positively associated to postmenopausal breast cancer risk. For example, in the EPIC study, based on 73,542 premenopausal and 103,344 postmenopausal women, body size has been associated with breast cancer risk in postmenopausal but not premenopausal women [11]. Increased central obesity that primarily occurs during or after menopause may be a more specific marker of the metabolic consequences of obesity and a better indicator of risk than body weight itself. In the Dutch "DOM" cohort including 11,663 women, WHR has been a more specific indicator of breast cancer risk in postmenopausal women compared to

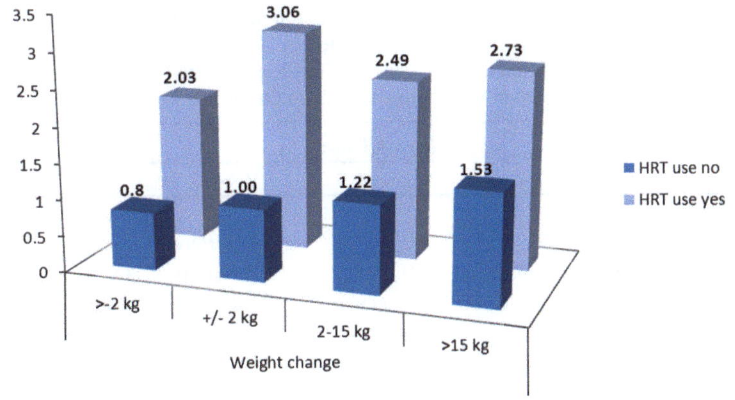

Fig. 22.3 Multivariate adjusted HR of breast cancer by weight change category and current hormonal replacement therapy (HRT) use in postmenopausal women ($n=57{,}923$), the EPIC study (adapted from Fig. 1 in Lahmann et al. (2005). British Journal of Cancer, 93:582–9. Reprinted with permission from Macmillan Publishers Ltd. Copyright (2005)

BMI [12]. Studies have shown that the association between weight change and breast cancer risk is modified by menopausal status, with higher weight gain associated with decreased risk for premenopausal women and increased risk for postmenopausal women [13]. In Europe, EPIC data has suggested large adult weight gain to be a significant predictor of breast cancer in postmenopausal women not taking exogenous hormones [14]. The interaction between percentage body fat and hormonal replacement therapy (HRT) supports the etiologic hypothesis that higher risk of breast cancer in overweight postmenopausal women may be attributed to the excess level of circulating estrogens [11, 14] (Fig. 22.3). This is a biologically plausible pathway since estrogen is also produced in fat tissue and, after menopause, when the ovaries stop producing hormones, fat tissue becomes the most important estrogen source [15].

Colorectal Cancer

Current research indicates that there is a moderate but consistently reported association between general obesity as determined by BMI and colorectal cancer incidence and mortality [16]. The relative risk associated with obesity is higher in men than in women [16]. However, abdominal obesity, as determined by WC or WHR, is similarly strongly associated with colon cancer in men and women, suggesting that in women abdominal obesity is a more important risk factor for colon cancer than general obesity [16]. Potential reasons for these differences may be sought in the different body compositions of men and women [17]. Approximately 30 % of fat in men with a normal weight can be stored in visceral area, while normal-weight women have low quantities of visceral fat. If visceral adipose tissue is primarily involved in tumorigenesis, this may explain why BMI alone may not accurately reflect colon cancer risk that is associated with abdominal fat accumulation in women. This hypothesis has been supported by findings from EPIC showing that abdominal obesity is a risk factor for colon cancer in both sexes and suggesting that fat distribution is more important than body weight or BMI for disease risk in women [17]. In this study, men and women in the highest compared with the lowest gender-specific quintile of WHR had a 50 % higher risk of developing colon cancer over a mean follow-up period of 6 years. The association of body fat accumulation and risk of colon cancer in postmenopausal women may be associated with HRT use. In the EPIC study estrogen-only and estrogen plus progestin therapy have not been significantly associated with colorectal cancer risk [18] and obesity and estrogen status have been shown to interact in influencing colon cancer risk [19]. Among postmenopausal women, the positive association of WC and WHR with risk of colon cancer has not been apparent in women who used HRT (Table 22.2). Unlike for breast cancer, estrogen appears to be protective for colon cancer for women overall [20].

Table 22.2 Relative risks (RRs) and 95 % confidence intervals (CIs) of colon cancer across quintiles of anthropometric measures in postmenopausal women stratified by hormone replacement therapy (HRT) use at baseline in the European Prospective Investigation into Cancer and Nutrition[a] (adapted from Table 6 in Pischon et al. (2006). J Natl Cancer Inst. 98(13):920–31. Reprinted with permission from Oxford University Press. Copyright (2006))

	No HRT use		HRT use	
Measure	N[b]	RR (95 % CI)	N[b]	RR (95 % CI)
BMI, kg/m^2				
<21.7	40	1 (Referent)	21	1 (Referent)
21.7–23.5	50	0.96 (0.63–1.45)	15	0.69 (0.35–1.35)
23.6–25.7	77	1.21 (0.82–1.78)	17	0.80 (0.41–1.56)
25.8–28.8	83	1.11 (0.75–1.64)	20	1.10 (0.57–2.10)
≥28.9	86	1.12 (0.75–1.67)	8	0.72 (0.31–1.70)
P_{trend}[c]		0.52		0.88
Waist circumference[d], cm				
<70.2	25	1 (Referent)	17	1 (Referent)
70.2–75.8	48	1.30 (0.80–2.11)	21	1.07 (0.55–2.06)
75.9–80.9	71	1.35 (0.85–2.14)	17	0.79 (0.39–1.57)
81.0–88.9	85	1.39 (0.88–2.19)	17	0.90 (0.44–1.83)
≥89.0	106	1.68 (1.06–2.64)	9	0.76 (0.32–1.80)
P_{trend}[c]		0.02		0.46
WHR[d]				
<0.734	27	1 (Referent)	19	1 (Referent)
0.734–0.768	40	1.02 (0.62–1.66)	19	0.79 (0.41–1.53)
0.769–0.802	75	1.55 (1.00–2.42)	11	0.46 (0.21–0.99)
0.803–0.845	85	1.51 (0.97–2.34)	14	0.69 (0.34–1.43)
≥0.846	107	1.76 (1.14–2.72)	17	0.96 (0.47–1.94)
P_{trend}[c]		0.002		0.89

[a]Relative risks derived from multivariable Cox regression models using age as the underlying time variable and stratified by center and age at recruitment with additional adjustment for smoking status (never, past, current, or unknown), education (no school degree or primary school, technical or professional school, secondary school, university degree, or unknown), alcohol consumption (continuous), physical activity (inactive, moderately inactive, moderately active, active, or missing), fiber intake (continuous), and consumption of red and processed meat (continuous), fish and shellfish (continuous), and fruits and vegetables (continuous). BMI = body mass index; WHR = waist-to-hip ratio
[b]Number of colon cancer patients
[c]P_{trend} (two-sided) across categories is based on the median anthropometric variable within quintiles as a continuous variable and was calculated using the Wald chi-square statistic
[d]Relative risks for weight, waist and hip circumference, and WHR are also adjusted for height (continuous)

Endometrial Cancer

Endometrial cancer is the most common gynecological cancer with increasing incidence worldwide [21] and in Europe [1, 22] over the last decades. Current evidence suggests that obesity as determined by BMI is strongly associated with incident endometrial cancer [23]. Among 20 different cancer types, endometrial cancer has ranked highest in terms of obesity-associated risk with a 60 % higher risk per 5 kg/m^2 increase in BMI [4]. Similar risk estimates have been obtained in a meta-analysis based on studies in European populations [23]. The risk of endometrial cancer associated with obesity has been slightly higher for postmenopausal women compared with premenopausal women and HRT use has been suggested to modify the BMI–endometrial cancer risk association, such that the risk was higher in HRT users compared to non-users [23] (Fig. 22.4). The lifetime exposure to hormones and hyperestrogenia are among the most commonly discussed putative mechanisms potentially explaining

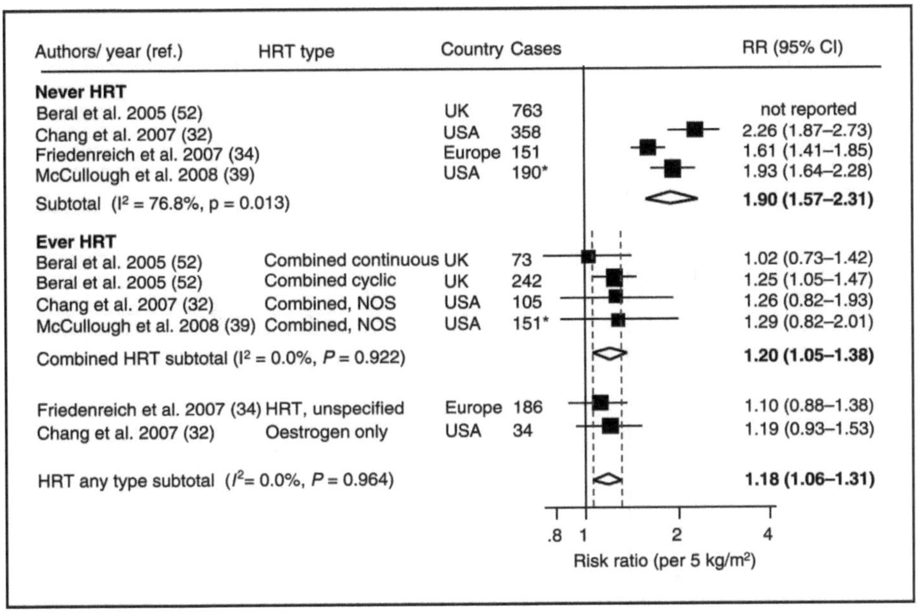

Fig. 22.4 Forest plot of the associations between 5 kg/m^2 BMI increase (linear model) and endometrial cancer risk by studies, which reported results stratified by hormone replacement therapy (HRT) use (reprinted by permission from the American Association for Cancer Research: Crosbie EJ et al. Cancer Epidemiol Biomarkers Prev. 2010;19:3119–3130)

the obesity–endometrial cancer relation. However, since there may be a residual risk associated with higher BMI among HRT users, additional independent mechanisms have been also proposed, such as hyperinsulinemia and alterations in adipokine levels (leptin, adiponectin) [23].

In summary, obesity is an important risk factor for several cancers in women, and in particular for postmenopausal breast cancer, colorectal cancer, and endometrial cancer (Table 22.3). Body fat distribution, as determined by WC or WHR, is suggested to better reflect the risk of colon cancer in women compared to general obesity measured by BMI. Further research is warranted to investigate its role in breast and endometrial cancer risk and potential interactions with exogenous hormone therapy use. Understanding molecular mechanisms that link obesity and cancer may help in developing mechanistic approaches in cancer prevention. Having into account the substantial burden of incident cancers attributable to excess weight in European women, there is a need to explore effective interventions for weight management targeted at high-risk female populations.

Obesity-Related Cancers and Nutrition

The existing association of obesity with risk of cancer in many developed European countries suggests that adoption of a "Western diet" characterized by high energy intake may be an underlying cause of malignancy [24]. Several dietary factors that may potentially influence the accumulation of body fat include high consumption of energy-dense food, rich in total fat and red meat, and refined carbohydrate, and low in fiber, fruits, and vegetables [25].

Table 22.3 General and abdominal obesity, nutritional factors, and selected cancers: Evidence for European women[a]

	Premenopausal breast cancer			Postmenopausal breast cancer			Colorectal cancer			Endometrial cancer		
	Limited	Probable	Convincing	Limited	Probable	Convincing	Limited	Probable	Convincing	Limited	Probable	Convincing
Body mass index		↓				↑			↑			↑
Waist circumference						↑			↑		↑	
Total fat				↑			↑			↑		
Saturated fat	↑			↑			↑			↑		
Monounsaturated fat				↓								
Red meat	↑			↑					↑	↑		
Processed meat				↑					↑			
Refined Carbohydrates										↑		
Glycemic index	↑			↑				↑		↑		
Glycemic load	↑			↑						↑		
Fiber					↓				↓	↓		
Fruits and vegetables				↓				↓		↓		

[a]The qualitative judgment is based on the current review on European studies in women and is in conformity with the WCRF Second Expert Panel Report [4], the WCRF/AICR. Continuous Update Project Reports for Breast Cancer (2010) [78] and Colorectal cancer (2011) [42]

Breast Cancer

Total Fat

Ecological and case–control studies have suggested a positive relation between dietary fat intake and breast cancer risk; however prospective studies, most of which involving postmenopausal women, have not supported this association [26]. Authoritative report of the WCRF has concluded that overall there is limited evidence suggesting that consumption of total fat is a cause of postmenopausal breast cancer [4]. An explanation of the null associations reported by cohort studies could be that the type of fat may be more relevant than its total amount. Fat from animal and vegetable sources differs in fatty acid composition. Animal fat is composed largely of saturated and monounsaturated fatty acids, whereas vegetable fat consists primarily of polyunsaturated, monounsaturated, and *trans*-fatty acids. For example, EPIC data has suggested that total fat is not associated with breast cancer risk, whereas there is a small but significant positive association with saturated fat intake [27]. This association has been more pronounced in postmenopausal women who have not used HRT. On the other hand, data from Mediterranean countries [28] have shown that diets rich in monounsaturated fatty acids such as olive oil are associated with lower risk of breast cancer. Although mechanistic evidence is considered as speculative, the association between fat, in particular saturated fat, and breast cancer is biologically plausible through pathways related to estrogen production and insulin resistance [27].

Carbohydrates and Glycemic Index

There is a growing recognition that breast cancer may be promoted by insulin resistance and hyperinsulinemia in the state of obesity [29]. The amount, type, and rate of digestion of dietary carbohydrate influence postprandial glycemia, insulin secretion, and average insulin concentrations [29]. Many factors influence how rapidly carbohydrates are digested and absorbed, and hence their glycemic and insulinemic effects. Concentrated sugars and refined flour products make up a large portion of the carbohydrate intake in the Western diet. One way to measure the impact of these foods on the body is through the glycemic index. The glycemic index is an indication of the blood sugar response of the body to a standardized amount of carbohydrate in a food. The glycemic load takes into account the amount of food eaten. Several large prospective studies have found no overall association between carbohydrate intake and breast cancer [30]. However, a recent meta-analysis of ten prospective cohort studies involving 15,839 cases and 577,538 participants has provided evidence that high dietary glycemic index is associated with a significantly higher risk of breast cancer [31]. Interestingly, studies in Europe have reported higher risks compared to North American studies [31]. In particular, the association between glycemic index and glycemic load and breast cancer seems to be most pronounced among women in the highest category of WC. Since WC is strongly related to hyperinsulinemia and insulin resistance, these data suggests that high-glycemic foods, such as refined carbohydrates, may be of relevance to breast cancer risk especially among women with underlying insulin resistance.

Fiber

Dietary fiber may play protective role in breast cancer through inhibition of the intestinal reabsorption of estrogens excreted by the biliary system and an increase in fecal excretion of estrogens; both mechanisms leading to lower circulating estrogen concentrations [32]. In addition, dietary fiber could play a role in modulating insulin resistance and insulin-like growth factors, which have been associated with breast cancer risk [32]. A meta-analysis of ten prospective cohort studies involving 16,848 cases and 712,195 participants has reported a significant inverse association of dietary fiber intake with risk of breast cancer [33]. The overall risk has been reduced by 11 % in a comparison of the highest with the lowest quintile of dietary fiber intake. In European studies the risk reduction has been 16 %. It is also plausible that the cancer-protective effects associated with high-fiber diet may come from components other than fiber itself. For example, a Swedish prospective study has suggested that intake of certain plant foods may be differently associated with breast cancer, such for example fiber-rich bread has been inversely associated with breast cancer incidence [34].

Fruits and Vegetables

Some epidemiological studies have suggested that diet rich in fruits, vegetables, and vegetable oil and/or selected micronutrients, such as β-carotene and vitamin E, folate, vitamin D, and calcium [35], may be protective against breast cancer risk in both premenopausal [36] and postmenopausal women [37]. However, in large European cohorts, such as EPIC, the consumption of fruits and vegetables [38], as well as dietary intake of beta-carotene, vitamin C, and vitamin E [39], has not been related to breast cancer risk. It was suggested that these inconsistent results for the associations between fruit and vegetable intake and breast cancer risk may be accounted for by heterogeneity in estrogen and progesterone receptor status of the tumors [40].

Colorectal Cancer

Total Fat and Red Meat

High energy intake coupled with low physical exercise is an adverse risk factor for colorectal cancer; however current epidemiological evidence does not support the proportion of total energy derived from total fat as a risk factor for colorectal cancer. A recent meta-analysis has suggested that dietary fat may not be associated with the increased risk of colorectal cancer [41] corresponding to the overall conclusions by the WCRF that there is limited evidence that dietary fat may be related to colorectal cancer [42]. However, according to the same report, there is convincing evidence that red meat intake, a major source of animal fat, is associated with increased risk of colon cancer [42]. EPIC data confirm these conclusions for European populations showing that colorectal cancer risk is positively associated with high consumption of red and processed meat [43, 81]. The fact that fat intake has not been associated with colon cancer suggests that other compounds may account for association with red meat consumption. For example, processing of meat may increase the presence of nitrosamine precursors in the diet and cooking methods influence the production of carcinogenic heterocyclic amines or polycyclic aromatic hydrocarbons [44]. Iron intake, which is more readily absorbed in the heme form found in red meat, may also be associated with increased risk of colorectal cancer [45].

Carbohydrates and Glycemic Index

Refined carbohydrates may act directly as a promoter of colorectal carcinogenesis, by inducing prolonged hyperglycemia and hyperinsulinemia [30, 46]. However, epidemiological evidence overall does not support the hypothesis that high carbohydrate intake, high glycemic index, and high glycemic load increase the risk of colorectal cancer in women [47]. In line with these results in EPIC, high intakes of glucose, fructose, and sucrose have not been related to colorectal cancer risk in European women [47]. Another large European cohort study, the Netherlands Cohort Study on Diet and Cancer, among 790 female colorectal cancer cases and approximately 60,000 controls followed for 11.3 years, has reported that a diet with a high glycemic load or glycemic index is not associated with a higher risk of colorectal cancer in women [48]. These findings suggest that the glycemic response to diet may not play a major role in colorectal cancer for women. While it is questionable whether glycemic load and glycemic index are adequate indicators of chronic hyperinsulinemia, future studies are needed to examine foods that closely predict insulin secretion rather than glycemic response.

Fiber

Dietary fiber may reduce the risk of colorectal cancer through several plausible mechanisms, including increased stool bulk and dilution of carcinogens in the colonic lumen, reduced transit time, and bacterial fermentation of fiber to short-chain fatty acids [49]. It is possible that part of the potential effect of fiber intake is mediated through improved weight control and reduced insulin resistance, although these may not be the main mechanisms. The potential for protection by fiber from foods in populations with current low intakes such as those living in Northern Europe has been highlighted by EPIC findings, which have suggested that an approximate doubling of total fiber intake from foods could reduce the risk of colorectal cancer by 40 % [50]. A recent meta-analysis including 25 prospective studies reported a 10 % reduction in the risk of colorectal cancer for each 10 g/day intake of total dietary fiber and cereal fiber and about a 20 % reduction for each three servings (90 g/day) of whole grain daily, and further reductions with higher intake [51]. Whole grains are a major source of several vitamins, minerals, and phytochemicals, which have anticancer properties and could plausibly influence the risk of colorectal cancer [51].

Fruits and Vegetables

Overall, epidemiological evidence has suggested that fruit and vegetable intakes are not strongly associated with colorectal cancer risk [52]. In Europe, data from EPIC provide similar results and suggest that the association of fruits and vegetables with colorectal cancer may be explained by intake of fibre. Interestingly, EPIC findings have also suggested that the association between colorectal cancer and fruit and vegetables combined and vegetables alone may be modified by smoking such that there has been an inverse association for never and former smokers and a statistically nonsignificant positive association for current smokers [53]. A possible explanation as to why large studies have not detected strong associations between fruit and vegetable intake and colorectal cancer may be that the protective effect of certain fruit or vegetable subgroups or anticarcinogenic food constituents is diluted when food groups are considered as a whole. For example, consumption of specific polyphenol-rich foods, e.g., apples, nuts, tea, and coffee, citrus fruit, and juices has been suggested to lower colorectal cancer risk [54–56].

Endometrial Cancer

Total Fat

High fat consumption may be related to endometrial cancer by increasing the levels of free estradiol and estrogen/progesterone ratio [57]. A meta-analysis combining data from two cohort studies and nine case–control studies has suggested that most fat subtypes are not associated with endometrial cancer except for total and animal fat which have been associated with a possible nonlinear decreased risk in premenopausal women [82]. Among premenopausal women, insulin provides a key stimulus to ovarian androgen synthesis and by inducing anovulation and progesterone deficiency may increase the risk of endometrial cancer [83]. Saturated fat intake may promote insulin resistance [58]. For example, a case–control study nested within EPIC found that women with elevated serum levels of C-peptide, a marker of hyperinsulinemia, have a modestly increased risk of endometrial cancer, suggesting that hyperinsulinemia may influence endometrial cancer risk [59]. Overall epidemiological evidence suggests a possible role of total fat, saturated fat, and animal fat on endometrial cancer risk; however this evidence is based mostly on case–control studies and was not confirmed by the large cohort studies [60].

Carbohydrates and Glycemic Index

High glycemic load and glycemic index diet are thought to result in high circulating insulin levels and thereby might influence the incidence of endometrial cancer [60]. Cohort studies have consistently reported that carbohydrate intake or glycemic load are positively associated with risk of endometrial cancer [60]. In Europe, the Swedish Mammography Cohort Study has reported a threefold increased risk of endometrial cancer for glycemic load among overweight women with low physical activity [61]. In EPIC, although total carbohydrates and glycemic index/load have not been with endometrial cancer overall, total carbohydrates, total dietary glycemic load, and total sugars have been associated with increased risk among postmenopausal women, particularly among never users of HRT [62].

Fiber

Estrogen exposure is a strong risk factor for endometrial cancer and since dietary fiber is related to estrogen bioavailability, lignan-rich diets may be beneficial, particularly if consumed for life [4, 63]. The epidemiological evidence on the potential protective role of dietary and circulating lignans against endometrial cancer has been controversial [64]. In Europe, a large Italian case–control study has suggested that dietary lignin intake, a cell-wall polymer, the main sources of which are green leafs and carrots, is inversely associated with endometrial cancer [65]. However, multinational European cohort studies such as EPIC have not supported the protective role of fiber in endometrial cancer risk [62].

Fruits and Vegetables

A meta-analysis based on 16 case–control studies has reported a modest inverse association of endometrial cancer with vegetable consumption, particularly for cruciferous vegetables, but not with fruit consumption [66]. However, results from large prospective studies do not support a protective role of a high intake of fruits or vegetables on the risk of endometrial cancer in older women [67].

In summary, the overall epidemiological evidence suggests that both pre- and postmenopausal women with diets high in energy and saturated fat such as red meat, and low in complex carbohydrates, such as cereals and whole grains, are at increased risk of cancer particularly of colorectal cancer (Table 22.3). The association of total fat intake and cancer risk is controversial and the role of different types of fat is not well understood. High-glycemic foods, such as refined carbohydrates, may be of relevance to breast and endometrial cancer risk, but current evidence does not support their role for colorectal cancer. Although fruits and vegetables have a strong anticarcinogenic potential, the evidence is inconclusive, possibly due to the fact that the effect of specific bioactive nutrients may be diluted when food groups are considered as a whole in observational research studies. Finally, other factors related to the individual etiological pathways of each of the different cancer types may interact with diet. For example, variations in cancer incidence can be attributed to inter-individual variation in genetic makeup that may explain the individual susceptibility to cancer. Recent research has identified gene polymorphisms that are important in apoptosis that may explain why individuals with shared environmental exposures do not always share cancer morbidity and mortality [70]. Therefore, no uniform recommendations on effective cancer-preventive diet for women can be drawn, but rather these should be cancer site specific. Further large-scale prospective studies are needed with comprehensive and precise assessment of dietary intake and with a potential to control for a variety of modifiable risk factors including lifestyle/dietary, biomarkers, and gene–diet interactions to establish the role of diet in the prevention of obesity-related cancers in women.

Implications for Prevention

Faced with the growing incidence of obesity-related cancer in Europe and around the world, scientists and medical and public health professionals are concerned with identifying effective preventive measures. Current knowledge of protective and risk factors for most common obesity-related cancers in women, such as breast, colorectal, and endometrial cancer, suggests that primary prevention by lifestyle modification in individuals should focus on weight control, alcohol intake, physical activity, and nutrition. For dietary factors, although controversy exists regarding the role of specific foods and nutrients, consideration of the dietary pattern as a whole might be useful for formulating recommendations [71]. For example, it has been estimated that up to 25 % of colorectal, 15 % of breast, and 10 % of endometrial cancers could be prevented by shifting to a healthy Mediterranean diet [72, 73] which is essentially unrelated to BMI [74]. It is characterized by high intake of vegetables, legumes, fruits and nuts, and minimally processed cereals; moderately high intake of fish; high intake of monounsaturated lipids coupled with low intake of saturated fat; low-to-moderate intake of dairies; low intake of meat products; and regular but moderate intake of alcohol (Fig. 22.5) [75, 76]. In Europe, higher adherence to Mediterranean diet has been associated with a reduction in the risk of cancer in both Mediterranean and non-Mediterranean countries [77]. Diets high in red and processed meats, saturated fats, highly refined grains and starches, and sugars may lead to a higher risk of cancer. Thus, replacing these factors with poultry, fish, and plant products as the primary sources of protein and preferring olive oil and other unsaturated fats to saturated ones, and unrefined grains and legumes as the primary sources of carbohydrates, might improve overall health status and possibly lower cancer risk. Although the role of fruits and vegetables in maintaining healthy weight and reducing cancer risk is controversial, they remain an important source of organic micronutrients such as folates, as well as a variety of phytochemicals, which may exert cancer-protective effects, therefore their intake should be still encouraged as part of the current guidance for chronic disease prevention. The potential of prevention for many supplements, including B6, remains largely uncertain; nevertheless, calcium and vitamin D supplementation is likely to be at least modestly beneficial, particularly in those with low micronutrient intakes.

Conclusions

Our understanding of the etiology of cancer has improved over the last decades. Still present knowledge has proved insufficient to allow the disease to be overcome and each year substantial number of women in Europe is being diagnosed with cancer. Maintaining healthy weight through regular physical exercises and following a balanced diet enriched with fruits, vegetables, and fiber remain the basis for cancer prevention before and after menopause. While precise anticancer mechanisms are still to be established, the expected health benefit from such lifestyle modification still might be substantial.

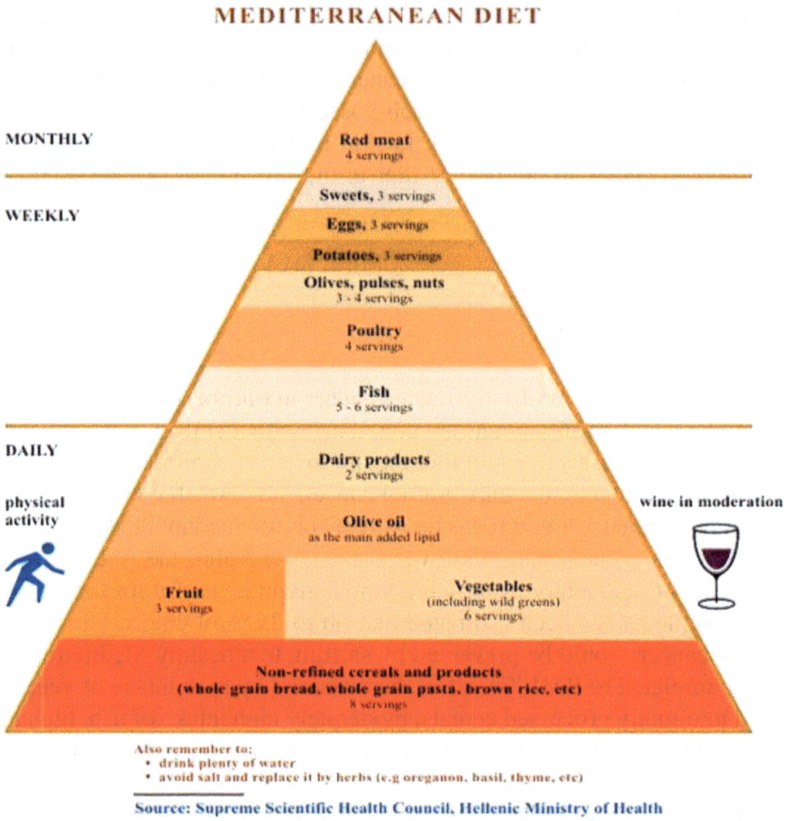

Fig. 22.5 Mediterranean diet pyramid (with permission from Prof. Antonia Trichopoulou, ref: Supreme Scientific Health Council, Ministry of Health and Welfare of Greece: dietary guidelines for adults in Greece. Archives of Hellenic Medicine. 1999;16:516-524)

References

1. Ferlay J, Shin HR, Bray F, Forman D, Mathers C, Parkin DM. Estimates of worldwide burden of cancer in 2008: GLOBOCAN 2008. Int J Cancer. 2010;127:2893–917.
2. Jemal A, Bray F, Center MM, Ferlay J, Ward E, Forman D. Global cancer statistics. CA Cancer J Clin. 2011;61:69–90.
3. Basen-Engquist K, Chang M. Obesity and cancer risk: recent review and evidence. Curr Oncol Rep. 2011;13:71–6.
4. World Cancer Research Fund/American Institute for Cancer Research. Food, nutrition, physical activity, and the prevention of cancer: a global perspective. Washington, D.C.: AICR; 2007.
5. World Health Organization. Obesity: preventing and managing the global epidemic. Report of a World Health Organization consultation. Geneva, Switzerland: World Health Organization; 2000. p. 256. WHO Obesity Technical Report Series, No. 894.
6. Berghofer A, Pischon T, Reinhold T, Apovian CM, Sharma AM, Willich SN. Obesity prevalence from a European perspective: a systematic review. BMC Public Health. 2008;8:200.
7. Alberti KG, Zimmet P, Shaw J. The metabolic syndrome–a new worldwide definition. Lancet. 2005;366:1059–62.
8. Riboli E, Hunt KJ, Slimani N, et al. European prospective investigation into cancer and nutrition (EPIC): study populations and data collection. Public Health Nutr. 2002;5:1113–24.
9. Haftenberger M, Lahmann PH, Panico S, et al. Overweight, obesity and fat distribution in 50- to 64-year-old participants in the European prospective investigation into cancer and nutrition (EPIC). Public Health Nutr. 2002;5:1147–62.

10. Renehan AG, Soerjomataram I, Tyson M, et al. Incident cancer burden attributable to excess body mass index in 30 European countries. Int J Cancer. 2010;126:692–702.
11. Lahmann PH, Hoffmann K, Allen N, et al. Body size and breast cancer risk: findings from the European prospective investigation into cancer and nutrition (EPIC). Int J Cancer. 2004;111:762–71.
12. Kaaks R, Van Noord PA, Den Tonkelaar I, Peeters PH, Riboli E, Grobbee DE. Breast-cancer incidence in relation to height, weight and body-fat distribution in the Dutch "DOM" cohort. Int J Cancer. 1998;76:647–51.
13. The International Agency for Research on Cancer (IARC): Weight Control and Physical Activity. IARC handbooks of cancer prevention. Lyon, France: IARC Press; 2002.
14. Lahmann PH, Schulz M, Hoffmann K, et al. Long-term weight change and breast cancer risk: the European prospective investigation into cancer and nutrition (EPIC). Br J Cancer. 2005;93:582–9.
15. Yoo K, Tajima K, Park S, et al. Postmenopausal obesity as a breast cancer risk factor according to estrogen and progesterone receptor status (Japan). Cancer Lett. 2001;167:57–63.
16. Aleksandrova K, Nimptsch K, Pischon T. Obesity and colorectal cancer. Front in biosci. 2013;E5:61–77.
17. Pischon T, Lahmann PH, Boeing H, et al. Body size and risk of colon and rectal cancer in the European prospective investigation into cancer and nutrition (EPIC). J Natl Cancer Inst. 2006;98:920–31.
18. Tsilidis KK, Allen NE, Key TJ, et al. Menopausal hormone therapy and risk of colorectal cancer in the European prospective investigation into cancer and nutrition. Int J Cancer. 2011;128:1881–9.
19. Slattery ML, Ballard-Barbash R, Edwards S, Caan BJ, Potter JD. Body mass index and colon cancer: an evaluation of the modifying effects of estrogen (United States). Cancer Causes Control. 2003;14:75–84.
20. Rossouw JE, Anderson GL, Prentice RL, et al. Risks and benefits of estrogen plus progestin in healthy postmenopausal women: principal results From the Women's Health Initiative randomized controlled trial. JAMA. 2002; 288:321–33.
21. Amant F, Moerman P, Neven P, Timmerman D, Van Limbergen E. Vergote I. Endometrial cancer. Lancet. 2005;366:491–505.
22. Bergstrom A, Pisani P, Tenet V, Wolk A, Adami HO. Overweight as an avoidable cause of cancer in Europe. Int J Cancer. 2001;91:421–30.
23. Crosbie EJ, Zwahlen M, Kitchener HC, Egger M, Renehan AG. Body mass index, hormone replacement therapy, and endometrial cancer risk: a meta-analysis. Cancer Epidemiol Biomarkers Prev. 2010;19:3119–30.
24. Riboli E, Norat T. Cancer prevention and diet: opportunities in Europe. Public Health Nutr. 2001;4:475–84.
25. Roberts SB, McCrory MA, Saltzman E. The influence of dietary composition on energy intake and body weight. J Am Coll Nutr. 2002;21:140S–5.
26. Alexander DD, Morimoto LM, Mink PJ, Lowe KA. Summary and meta-analysis of prospective studies of animal fat intake and breast cancer. Nutr Res Rev. 2010;23:169–79.
27. Sieri S, Krogh V, Ferrari P, et al. Dietary fat and breast cancer risk in the European prospective investigation into cancer and nutrition. Am J Clin Nutr. 2008;88:1304–12.
28. Willett WC. Specific fatty acids and risks of breast and prostate cancer: dietary intake. Am J Clin Nutr. 1997;66:1557S–63.
29. Larsson SC, Bergkvist L, Wolk A. Glycemic load, glycemic index and breast cancer risk in a prospective cohort of Swedish women. Int J Cancer. 2009;125:153–7.
30. Gnagnarella P, Gandini S, La Vecchia C, Maisonneuve P. Glycemic index, glycemic load, and cancer risk: a meta-analysis. Am J Clin Nutr. 2008;87:1793–801.
31. Dong JY, Qin LQ. Dietary glycemic index, glycemic load, and risk of breast cancer: meta-analysis of prospective cohort studies. Breast Cancer Res Treat. 2011;126:287–94.
32. Park Y, Brinton LA, Subar AF, Hollenbeck A, Schatzkin A. Dietary fiber intake and risk of breast cancer in postmenopausal women: the National Institutes of Health-AARP Diet and Health Study. Am J Clin Nutr. 2009;90: 664–71.
33. Dong JY, He K, Wang P, Qin LQ. Dietary fiber intake and risk of breast cancer: a meta-analysis of prospective cohort studies. Am J Clin Nutr. 2011;94:900–5.
34. Sonestedt E, Borgquist S, Ericson U, et al. Plant foods and oestrogen receptor alpha- and beta-defined breast cancer: observations from the Malmo Diet and Cancer cohort. Carcinogenesis. 2008;29:2203–9.
35. Chen P, Hu P, Xie D, Qin Y, Wang F, Wang H. Meta-analysis of vitamin D, calcium and the prevention of breast cancer. Breast Cancer Res Treat. 2010;121:469–77.
36. Freudenheim JL, Marshall JR, Vena JE, et al. Premenopausal breast cancer risk and intake of vegetables, fruits, and related nutrients. J Natl Cancer Inst. 1996;88:340–8.
37. Willett WC. Micronutrients and cancer risk. Am J Clin Nutr. 1994;59:1162S–5.
38. van Gils CH, Peeters PH, Bueno-de-Mesquita HB, et al. Consumption of vegetables and fruits and risk of breast cancer. JAMA. 2005;293:183–93.
39. Nagel G, Linseisen J, van Gils CH, et al. Dietary beta-carotene, vitamin C and E intake and breast cancer risk in the European prospective investigation into cancer and nutrition (EPIC). Breast Cancer Res Treat. 2010;119: 753–65.

40. Lissowska J, Gaudet MM, Brinton LA, et al. Intake of fruits, and vegetables in relation to breast cancer risk by hormone receptor status. Breast Cancer Res Treat. 2008;107:113–7.
41. Liu L, Zhuang W, Wang RQ, et al. Is dietary fat associated with the risk of colorectal cancer? A meta-analysis of 13 prospective cohort studies. Eur J Nutr. 2011;50:173–84.
42. World Cancer Research Fund and American Institute for Cancer Research. Continuous update project colorectal cancer report 2010 summary. Food, Nutrition, Physical Activity, and the Prevention of Colorectal Cancer. 2011.
43. Gonzalez CA, Riboli E. Diet and cancer prevention: contributions from the European prospective investigation into cancer and nutrition (EPIC) study. Eur J Cancer. 2010;46:2555–62.
44. Santarelli RL, Vendeuvre JL, Naud N, et al. Meat processing and colon carcinogenesis: cooked, nitrite-treated, and oxidized high-heme cured meat promotes mucin-depleted foci in rats. Cancer Prev Res (Phila). 2010;3:852–64.
45. Giovannucci E, Goldin B. The role of fat, fatty acids, and total energy intake in the etiology of human colon cancer. Am J Clin Nutr. 1997;66:1564S–71.
46. Johnson IT, Lund EK. Review article: nutrition, obesity and colorectal cancer. Aliment Pharmacol Ther. 2007;26: 161–81.
47. Michaud DS, Fuchs CS, Liu S, Willett WC, Colditz GA, Giovannucci E. Dietary glycemic load, carbohydrate, sugar, and colorectal cancer risk in men and women. Cancer Epidemiol Biomarkers Prev. 2005;14:138–47.
48. Weijenberg MP, Mullie PF, Brants HA, Heinen MM, Goldbohm RA, van den Brandt PA. Dietary glycemic load, glycemic index and colorectal cancer risk: results from the Netherlands Cohort Study. Int J Cancer. 2008;122:620–9.
49. Lipkin M, Reddy B, Newmark H, Lamprecht SA. Dietary factors in human colorectal cancer. Annu Rev Nutr. 1999;19:545–86.
50. Bingham SA, Day NE, Luben R, et al. Dietary fibre in food and protection against colorectal cancer in the European prospective investigation into cancer and nutrition (EPIC): an observational study. Lancet. 2003;361:1496–501.
51. Aune D, Chan DS, Lau R, et al. Dietary fibre, whole grains, and risk of colorectal cancer: systematic review and dose-response meta-analysis of prospective studies. BMJ. 2011;343:d6617.
52. Koushik A, Hunter DJ, Spiegelman D, et al. Fruits, vegetables, and colon cancer risk in a pooled analysis of 14 cohort studies. J Natl Cancer Inst. 2007;99:1471–83.
53. van Duijnhoven FJ, Bueno-De-Mesquita HB, Ferrari P, et al. Fruit, vegetables, and colorectal cancer risk: the European prospective investigation into cancer and nutrition. Am J Clin Nutr. 2009;89:1441–52.
54. Sun CL, Yuan JM, Koh WP, Yu MC. Green tea, black tea and colorectal cancer risk: a meta-analysis of epidemiologic studies. Carcinogenesis. 2006;27:1301–9.
55. Jenab M, Ferrari P, Slimani N, et al. Association of nut and seed intake with colorectal cancer risk in the European prospective investigation into cancer and nutrition. Cancer Epidemiol Biomarkers Prev. 2004;13:1595–603.
56. Foschi R, Pelucchi C, Dal Maso L, et al. Citrus fruit and cancer risk in a network of case-control studies. Cancer Causes Control. 2010;21:237–42.
57. Nagaoka T, Onodera H, Hayashi Y, Maekawa A. Influence of high-fat diets on the occurrence of spontaneous uterine endometrial adenocarcinomas in rats. Teratog Carcinog Mutagen. 1995;15:167–77.
58. Riccardi G, Giacco R, Rivellese AA. Dietary fat, insulin sensitivity and the metabolic syndrome. Clin Nutr. 2004;23:447–56.
59. Cust AE, Allen NE, Rinaldi S, et al. Serum levels of C-peptide, IGFBP-1 and IGFBP-2 and endometrial cancer risk; results from the European prospective investigation into cancer and nutrition. Int J Cancer. 2007;120: 2656–64.
60. Cui X, Rosner B, Willett WC, Hankinson SE. Dietary fat, fiber, and carbohydrate intake in relation to risk of endometrial cancer. Cancer Epidemiol Biomarkers Prev. 2011;20:978–89.
61. Larsson SC, Friberg E, Wolk A. Carbohydrate intake, glycemic index and glycemic load in relation to risk of endometrial cancer: a prospective study of Swedish women. Int J Cancer. 2007;120:1103–7.
62. Cust AE, Slimani N, Kaaks R, et al. Dietary carbohydrates, glycemic index, glycemic load, and endometrial cancer risk within the European prospective investigation into cancer and nutrition cohort. Am J Epidemiol. 2007;166: 912–23.
63. Adlercreutz H. Lignans and human health. Crit Rev Clin Lab Sci. 2007;44:483–525.
64. Bandera EV, Kushi LH, Moore DF, Gifkins DM, McCullough ML. Association between dietary fiber and endometrial cancer: a dose-response meta-analysis. Am J Clin Nutr. 2007;86:1730–7.
65. Bidoli E, Pelucchi C, Zucchetto A, et al. Fiber intake and endometrial cancer risk. Acta Oncol. 2010;49:441–6.
66. Bandera EV, Kushi LH, Moore DF, Gifkins DM, McCullough ML. Fruits and vegetables and endometrial cancer risk: a systematic literature review and meta-analysis. Nutr Cancer. 2007;58:6–21.
67. Kabat GC, Park Y, Hollenbeck AR, Schatzkin A, Rohan TE. Intake of fruits and vegetables, and risk of endometrial cancer in the NIH-AARP Diet and Health Study. Cancer Epidemiol. 2010;34:568–73.
68. Biel RK, Friedenreich CM, Csizmadi I, et al. Case-control study of dietary patterns and endometrial cancer risk. Nutr Cancer. 2011;63:673–86.

69. van Lonkhuijzen L, Kirsh VA, Kreiger N, Rohan TE. Endometrial cancer and meat consumption: a case-cohort study. Eur J Cancer Prev. 2011;20:334–9.
70. Gene-environment interaction in site-specific cancers. In: Samuel Wilson, Lovell Jones, Christine Couseens, and Kathi Hanna, editors. Cancer and the environment: Gene-environment interactions (roundtable on environment, health sciences, research and medicine). Washington DC: National Academy Press; 2000. p. 46–60.
71. Chan AT, Giovannucci EL. Primary prevention of colorectal cancer. Gastroenterology. 2010;138:2029–43.e10.
72. Bonaccio M, Iacoviello L, de Gaetano G, Moli-Sani Investigators. The Mediterranean diet: the reasons for a success. Thromb Res. 2012;129(3):401–4.
73. Trichopoulou A, Lagiou P, Kuper H, Trichopoulos D. Cancer and Mediterranean dietary traditions. Cancer Epidemiol Biomarkers Prev. 2000;9:869–73.
74. Trichopoulou A, Naska A, Orfanos P, Trichopoulos D. Mediterranean diet in relation to body mass index and waist-to-hip ratio: the Greek European prospective investigation into cancer and nutrition study. Am J Clin Nutr. 2005;82:935–40.
75. Couto E, Boffetta P, Lagiou P, et al. Mediterranean dietary pattern and cancer risk in the EPIC cohort. Br J Cancer. 2011;104:1493–9.
76. Trichopoulou A, Bamia C, Lagiou P, Trichopoulos D. Conformity to traditional Mediterranean diet and breast cancer risk in the Greek EPIC (European prospective investigation into cancer and nutrition) cohort. Am J Clin Nutr. 2010;92:620–5.
77. Cade JE, Taylor EF, Burley VJ, Greenwood DC. Does the Mediterranean dietary pattern or the healthy diet index influence the risk of breast cancer in a large British cohort of women? Eur J Clin Nutr. 2011;65:920–8.
78. American Institute for Cancer Research. Continuous update project breast cancer report 2010 summary. Food, Nutrition, Physical Activity, and the Prevention of Colorectal Cancer. 2011.
79. National Heart, Lung, and Blood Institute Obesity Education Initiative. Clinical guidelines on the identification, evaluation, and treatment of overweight and obesity in adults: The Evidence Report. NIH Publication No. 98-4083. National Institutes of Health, Bethesda (1998).
80. WHO expert consultation. Appropriate body-mass index for Asian populations and its implications for policy and intervention strategies. Lancet 2004;363:157–163.
81. Norat T, Bingham S, Ferrari P, Slimani N, Jenab M, Mazuir M, et al. Meat, fish, and colorectal cancer risk: the European Prospective Investigation into cancer and nutrition. Natl Cancer Inst. 2005 Jun 15;97(12):906–16.
82. Bandera EV, Kushi LH, Moore DF, Gifkins DM, McCullough ML. Dietary lipids and endometrial cancer: the current epidemiologic evidence.Cancer Causes Control. 2007 Sep;18(7):687–703.
83. Kaaks R, Lukanova A, Kurzer MS. Obesity, endogenous hormones, and endometrial cancer risk: a synthetic review. Cancer Epidemiol Biomarkers Prev. 2002;11:1531–43.

Chapter 23
Vitamin D and the Menopause: A Focus on Apoptosis in Cancer

Henk R. Franke

Key Points

- The advice of supplementation of vitamin D_3 of the different Nutritional Health Boards across the globe is too low; at least 5,000 IE daily should be taken by postmenopausal women.
- Adequate vitamin D_3 supplementation decreases the incidence and mortality of breast cancer in postmenopausal women.
- Vitamin D is an excellent candidate for the treatment of breast cancer because it induces apoptosis of breast cancer stem cells, while it does not affect normal breast stem cells.
- There are no signs of toxicity with a vitamin D intake of less than 30,000 IU/day and a serum level of 25OHD below 500 nmol/L.
- The ultimate personalized targeted drug use in combination with vitamin D will be the future for the treatment of breast cancer in postmenopausal women.

Keywords Vitamin D • Cancer stem cells • Apoptosis • Proliferation • Lab-on-a-chip

Abbreviations

25OHD	25-Hydroxyvitamin D_3
1,25-$(OH)_2D_3$	1,25-dihydroxyvitamin D_3
CI	Confidence interval
DINOMIT	Disjunction, Initiation, Natural selection, Overgrowth, Metastasis, Involution, and Transition
MRI	Magnetic resonance image
DNA	Deoxyribonucleic acid
G 0 phase	Resting phase in the cell cycle
A/P ratio	Apoptosis-to-proliferation ratio
SEM	Standard error of the mean

H.R. Franke, M.D., Ph.D. (✉)
Department of Obstetrics and Gynecology, Medisch Spectrum Twente Hospital Group,
P.O. Box 50000, 7500 KA, Enschede, The Netherlands
e-mail: h.franke@mst.nl; hrfranke@home.nl

C.J.H. Martin et al. (eds.), *Nutrition and Diet in Menopause*, Nutrition and Health,
DOI 10.1007/978-1-62703-373-2_23, © Springer Science+Business Media New York 2013

Introduction

For over 500 million years phyto- and zooplankton have been producing vitamin D. Vitamin D is a prohormone which is mainly produced in the skin after sun exposure (UVB radiation). During the postmenopausal period the skin becomes thinner and is less able to synthesize vitamin D after sun exposure. However it is also ingested through fortified dairy foods and cereals, fatty fish, multivitamins, and calcium/vitamin D supplements. Vitamin D becomes active after a two-step metabolization process. The first conversion step takes place in the liver, where the major circulating metabolite, 25-hydroxyvitamin D_3 (25OHD), is formed. The second step takes place in the kidney where the biologically active, 1,25-dihydroxyvitamin D_3, 1,25-$(OH)_2D_3$, is produced. The latter interacts with the vitamin D receptor to regulate proliferation and apoptosis (programmed cell death) in a variety of tissues, including the mammary gland [1].

Association

It became increasingly obvious that people living in areas with an elevated degree of solar UVB radiation presented lower cancer mortality rates [2]. In a randomized controlled trial of postmenopausal women the supplementation of 1,100 IU/day of vitamin D_3 plus 1,450 mg/day calcium led to a statistical significant 60 % decrease of all invasive cancer incidence (relative risk 0.40, 95 % CI 0.20–0.82, $p<0.03$) [3]. A pooled analysis of two breast cancer studies demonstrated that women with a serum 25OHD level >95 nmol/L in comparison with those with 25OHD <38 nmol/L displayed a 58 % lower risk of breast cancer (odds ratio 0.42, 95 % CI 0.31–0.55, p trend <0.02) [4].

Influence of Vitamin D on Cancer Pathogenesis

Garland et al. proposed the DINOMIT model in order to explain the transition from benign to malignant tissue and the influence of vitamin D on this process [5]. The acronym stands for Disjunction, Initiation, Natural selection, Overgrowth, Metastasis, Involution, and Transition: in short the description of the phases and the influence of an adequate serum level of 25OHD of 100–150 nmol/L on all the different steps.

- In the first phase of disjunction the loss of adherence between the epithelial cells appears within, for instance breast tissue. The decrease of E-cadherin synthesis, an intercellular adherence protein, plays a pivotal role in this process. There is an up-regulation of E-cadherins and intercellular junctions if adequate levels of 25OHD are present.
- In the initiation phase the alteration of the DNA molecules during replication has been demonstrated. As in the disjunction phase mature cells are driven to a postmitotic status by the influence of an adequate vitamin D supplementation.
- During natural selection the most aggressive and dividing cells become dominant and these selected group of cells expands towards the basement membrane. The presence of a sufficient serum level of 25OHD prevents mitosis of mature cells and therefore mitotic cloning is inhibited.
- In the overgrowth phase these highly proliferative cells invade the basement membrane and is the last step within the original organ. Here high enough levels of tissue 25OHD stops the overgrowth within the actual organ.
- If metastasis occurs the boundaries of the organ are trespassed. The tumor cells will ultimately spread to remote organs such as lymphatic nodes, liver, lungs, and finally the brain. These metastases

can invade the blood vessels of these organs and the patient will ultimately die of hemorrhage. Possibly the seasonal increase of serum 25OHD level can induce a temporary arrest of the growth of the metastases of different cancer types. A study from Norway revealed that the highest incidence of breast cancer with intact vitamin D receptors was discovered during wintertime [6]. The hypothesis of the influence of vitamin D states that it reduces proliferation and induces tight junctions between the malignant cells.

- Involution only takes place when the serum 25OHD levels are similar compared to the serum levels found during summer time and it accounts for the mitotic arrest of the malignant cells in the metastases and the original tumor.
- Transition from an acute state to a chronic disease occurs if a sufficient 25OHD level is present in the tissue. This phenomenon is also very neatly described in patients with brain tumors from France [7]. The authors suggest that longtime and highly dosed supplementation of the vitamin D metabolite, 1-apha-hydroxycholecalciferol, induced a blockade of the tumoral extension, a decrease of the gadolinium-enhanced area, and a shrinkage of the lesion. It is labeled redifferentiation. MRIs conducted on the brain demonstrated a return of the lesion, which developed after surgery, to the normal MRI image of brain tissue. Evidence suggests that if you want to achieve this last state you have to be prepared to take high doses of vitamin D supplementation during the rest of your life.

A possible explanation of the influence of vitamin D on the division of malignant cells is the down-regulation of telomerase [8]. Telomeres are single-strand DNA pieces located at the end of the chromosomes. Normal cells have a finite capacity to replicate due to the shortening of the telomeres after every cell division. Normal cells demise after 40 to 60 cell divisions; however malignant cells are immortal because they produce the enzyme telomerase which obviates the shortening of the telomeres [9]. Others have also described the antitumor activity of vitamin D such as inhibiting proliferation, stimulating cell differentiation, and inducing apoptosis in malignant cells [10].

Stem Cells

Because breast cancer is the most prevalent cancer in postmenopausal women, worldwide every year 460,000 women die of breast cancer, the role of vitamin D on normal breast stem cells and breast cancer stem cells will be explained [11, 12]. Stem cells in normal breast tissue are responsible for renewal and repair of aged and damaged tissue. The stem cells are immortal and divide asymmetrically producing two daughter cells; one of those cells is a new stem cell, and the other a progenitor cell, which will produce normal differentiated cells. They only represent a small fraction in the breast, are mainly quiescent (in the G_0 phase of the cell cycle), slowly proliferate, and have a long life span. Cancer stem cells have similar capacities as normal stem cells. Cancer stem cells probably originate from normal stem cells which are changed by genetic and epigenetic influences [13]. The importance of cancer stem cells is well documented in animal research of solid tumors. Many thousands of differentiated tumors cells need to be injected in animals to produce tumors; however as few as 20–50 cancer stem cells are sufficient to produce the same tumor [14]. Chemotherapy drugs kill differentiated breast cancer cells because they replicate; however breast cancer stem cells slowly proliferate. Furthermore, they also can efflux chemotherapeutic agents which make them resistant to conventional chemotherapy compared with differentiated cancer cells. If the cancer stem cells survive after chemotherapy they are able to produce metastases. Therefore, it is imperative that not only the differentiated breast cancer cells are killed but the breast cancer stem cells as well. Vitamin D demonstrated to be a candidate as an anticancer drug in in vitro research [15]. Further elucidation will be given in the part of the in vitro proof.

In Vitro Proof

In the laboratories of the Medisch Spectrum Twente Hospital Group and the University of Twente we performed in vitro research on breast cancer cells [16]. Human estrogen receptor-positive breast cells (MCF-7) were grown in the appropriate medium and the vitamin D metabolite $1\alpha,25(OH)_2D_3$ was added in a dose of 100 nM and 10 μM during 24, 48, 72, and 96 h. The MCF-7 cells express the vitamin D receptor. Proliferation and apoptosis were measured and the corresponding apoptosis-to-proliferation (A/P) ratio was calculated. An A/P ratio more than one means induction of apoptosis, whereas an A/P ratio less than one means stimulation of proliferation. After 96 h and with a concentration of 10 μM $1\alpha,25(OH)_2D_3$ there was a statistical significant increase of apoptosis of the MCF-7 cells (Fig. 23.1). We were able to identify, isolate, propagate, and characterize breast cancer stem cells from breast cancer cell lines and breast tumor tissue. The human breast cancer cell lines we used were the MCF-7 and the estrogen receptor-negative MDA-MB 231 cells. The number of breast cancer stem cells in human breast tumor tissue ($n=3$) was <0.5 % and in the breast cancer cell lines ($n=5$) was <5 %. From the MCF-7 cell line we isolated the cancer stem cells and these were cultured under non-adherent conditions in stem cell medium to form mammospheres (Fig. 23.2). These mammospheres express the estrogen (40 %), progesterone (20 %), and vitamin D (range 30–90 %) receptors [17].

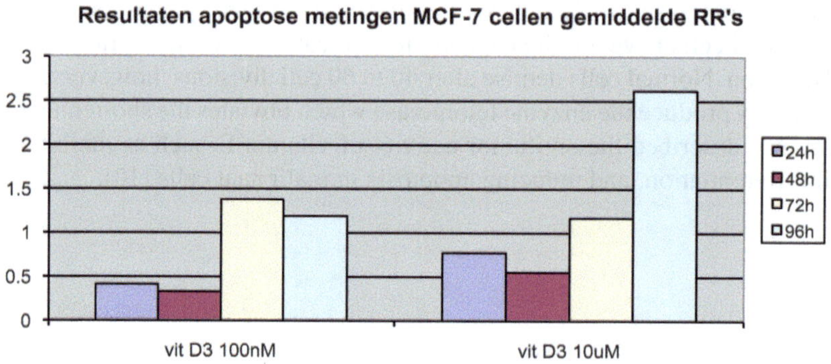

Fig. 23.1 Apoptosis-to-proliferation ratios of MCF-7 cells incubated with $1\alpha,25(OH)_2D_3$ in two doses and during four time periods. Data are represented as mean ± standard error of the mean (SEM). Permission granted by Wolters Kluwer Health. Sophie Veldhuis, Floor Wolbers, Olivier Brouckaert, et al. Cancer prevalence in osteoporotic women with low serum vitamin D levels. Menopause. 2011; 18 (3)

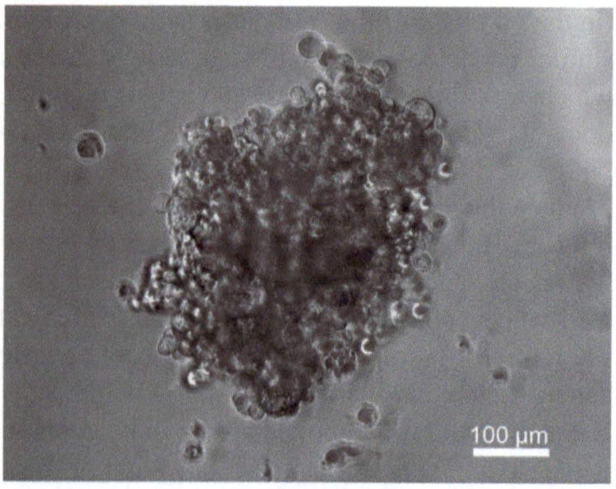

Fig. 23.2 Light microscopy picture of a mammosphere of the MCF-7 cell line cultured for 14 days under stem cell conditions

Vitamin D Supplementation and Toxicity

A serum level of 25OHD higher than 70 nmol/L would be sufficient if one only considers the treatment of postmenopausal osteoporotic patients. However this is not the optimal concentration if cancer prevention is targeted [18]. The American vitamin D council recommends the intake of at least 5,000 IU daily, especially during the postmenopausal period, because older people tend to stay at home more frequently and the intake of dietary products is lower compared with younger adults [19]. There are no signs of toxicity with a vitamin D intake of less than 30,000 IU/day and a serum level of 25OHD below 500 nmol/L [20].

Future

We will initiate a prospective randomized controlled trial in patients with a primary operable breast cancer. The intervention group will be supplemented with vitamin D in a dose of 40,000 IU/day and the control group will receive a placebo. Each group consists of 55 patients. Supplementation starts after the breast cancer diagnosis is communicated with the patient and will be continued until surgery is performed. Maximum duration of treatment is 5 weeks. The primary objective is the influence of vitamin D on the immunomarker Ki67; a proliferation marker; and caspase 3, an apoptosis marker. Furthermore, the vitamin D, estrogen, progesterone, and Her2Neu receptor status will be determined. These will be performed in the biopsy specimen and in the tumor resection specimen. In both specimens the A/P ratios will be calculated. The hypothesis is that in the resection specimen the A/P ratio will be higher in the intervention group compared with the biopsy specimen. In the control group there will probably be no difference between the biopsy and the resection specimen. A new tool in the in vitro research is the lab-on-a-chip technology. The lab-on-a-chip is a device that can perform laboratory functions on a single chip of only several millimeters in size. These microfluidic devices can be used as an "apoptosis chip" because with only a limited number of cells, acquired from a fine needle biopsy of a suspected breast cancer lump, tests can be performed. As in bacterial tests, where antibiotics are tested on the specimen, the malignant cells are analyzed with different drugs and vitamin D. The apoptosis process, which takes only a couple of hours, can be measured and eventually the most active drug can be given to the patient, the ultimate personalized targeted drug therapy. Figure 23.3 demonstrates an example of a lab-on-a-chip device.

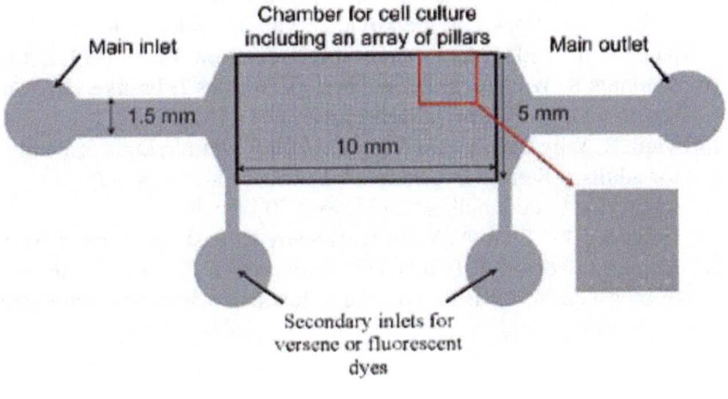

Fig. 23.3 Schematic drawing of the microfluidic "apoptosis chip"

Conclusions

Presently the medical breast cancer therapy in postmenopausal women consists of chemo- and hormone therapy which has limited rates of success. Often this approach to breast cancer treatment is referred to as "trial and error" or "one size fits all." However we strive to personalize treatment by using the most active drug in inducing apoptosis in the breast cancer cells. Breast cancer stem cells are a promising target of medical therapy because these cells need to be eradicated in order to provide long-term disease-free survival. Vitamin D is an excellent candidate for the treatment of breast cancer stem cells and differentiated breast cancer cells because it does not affect normal cells and induces apoptosis in breast cancer (stem) cells.

References

1. Hollick MF. Evolution and function of vitamin D. Recent Results Cancer Res. 2003;164:3–28.
2. Grant WB, Garland CF. The association of solar ultraviolet B (UVB) with reducing risk of cancer: multifactorial ecologic analysis of geographic variation in age-adjusted cancer mortality rates. Anticancer Res. 2006;4A:2687–99.
3. Lappe JM, Travers-Gustafson D, Davies KM, Recker RR, Heaney RP. Vitamin D and calcium supplementation reduces cancer risk: results of a randomized trial. Am J Clin Nutr. 2007;85:1586–91.
4. Garland CF, Gorham ED, Mohr S, et al. Vitamin D and prevention of breast cancer: pooled analysis. J Steroid Biochem Mol Biol. 2007;103:708–11.
5. Garland CF, Gorham ED, Mohr SB, Garland FC. Vitamin D for cancer prevention: global perspective. Ann Epidemiol. 2009;7:468–83.
6. Porojnicu AC, Lagunova Z, Robsahm TE, Berg JP, Dahlback A, Moan J. Changes in risk of death from breast cancer with season and latitude: sun exposure and breast cancer survival in Norway. Breast Cancer Res Treat. 2007;102:323–8.
7. Trouillas P, Honnorat J, Bret P, Jouvet A, Gerard JP. Redifferentation therapy in brain tumors: long-lasting complete regression of glioblastomas and an anaplastic astrocytoma under long term 1-alpha-hydroxycholecalciferol. J Neurooncol. 2001;51:57–66.
8. Jiang F, Bao J, Li P, Nicosia SV, Bai W. Induction of ovarian cancer cell apoptosis by 1,25-dihydroxyvitamin D3 through the down-regulation of telomerase. J Biol Chem. 2004;279:53213–21.
9. Hayflick L. The illusion of cell immortality. Br J Cancer. 2000;83:841–6.
10. Colston KW, Hansen CM. Mechanisms implicated in the growth regulatory effects of vitamin D in breast cancer. Endocr Relat Cancer. 2002;9:45–59.
11. Ferlay J, Shin HR, Bray F, Forman D, Mathers C, Parkin DM. Estimates of worldwide burden of cancer in 2008: GLOBOCAN 2008. Int J Cancer. 2010;127:2893–917.
12. Kakarala M, Wicha MS. Cancer stem cells: implications for cancer treatment and prevention. Cancer J. 2007;5:271–5.
13. Soltysova A, Altanerova V, Altaner C. Cancer stem cells. Neoplasma. 2005;52:435–40.
14. Dalerba P, Cho RW, Clarke MF. Cancer stem cells: model and concepts. Ann Rev Med. 2007;58:267–84.
15. Bijlsma MF, Spek CA, Zivkovic D, van de Water S, Rezaee F, Peppelenbosch MP. Repression of smoothened by patched-dependent (pro-)vitamin D3 secretion. PLoS Biol. 2006;4:1397–410.
16. Veldhuis S, Wolbers F, Brouckaert O, Vermes I, Franke HR. Cancer prevalence in osteoporotic women with low serum vitamin D levels. Menopause. 2011;18:319–22.
17. Vieth R. Why the optimal requirement for vitamin D_3 is probably much higher than what is officially recommended for adults. J Steroid Biochem Mol Biol. 2004;89–90:575–9.
18. www.vitamindcouncil.org. Accessed 20 Dec 2011.
19. Hathcock JN, Shao A, Vieth R, Heaney R. Risk assessment for vitamin D. Am J Clin Nutr. 2007;85:6–18.
20. Komen J, Wolbers F, Franke HR, Andersson H, Vermes I, van den Berg A. Viability analysis and apoptosis induction of breast cancer cells in a microfluidic device: effect of cytostatic drugs. Biomed Microdevices. 2008;5:727–37.

Chapter 24
Gynecological Malignancies and Diet in Menopause: From the Biological and Epidemiological Viewpoints

Kiyoshi Ito, Hironobu Sasano, and Nobuo Yaegashi

Key Points

- Dietary patterns can be associated with development of endometrial carcinoma in postmenopausal women.
- Daily isoflavone intake may be associated with a reduced risk of endometrial cancer development in postmenopausal women.
- Moderate degrees of daily coffee consumption may be associated with a reduced risk of endometrial cancer development in postmenopausal women.
- Protective roles of a daily high intake of vegetable or fruit in endometrial cancer development in postmenopausal women are reasonably considered dubious.
- Possible roles of daily dietary patterns in endometrial cancer risk in menopausal women will be discussed from the standpoints of estrogenic actions.
- No associations between dietary patterns and risks of ovarian cancer development have been detected in postmenopausal women.

Keywords Endometrial cancer • Dairy product • Isoflavones • Coffee • In situ estrogen metabolism • Ovarian cancer

Abbreviations

17β-HSD	17β-Hydroxysteroid dehydrogenase
STS	Steroid sulfatase

K. Ito, M.D., Ph.D. (✉)
Department of Disaster Obstetrics and Gynecology, International Research Institute of Disaster Science (IRIDeS), Tohoku University,
1-1 Seiryo-machi, Aoba-ku, Sendai, Japan
e-mail: kito@med.tohoku.ac.jp

H. Sasano, M.D., Ph.D.
Department of Pathology, Tohoku University Graduate School of Medicine, 2-1 Seiryo-machi, Aoba-ku, Sendai, Japan
e-mail: hsasano@patholo2.med.tohoku.ac.jp

N. Yaegashi, M.D., Ph.D.
Department of Obstetrics and Gynecology, Tohoku University Graduate School of Medicine,
1-1 Seiryo-machi, Aoba-ku, Sendai, Japan
e-mail: yaegashi@med.tohoku.ac.jp

C.J.H. Martin et al. (eds.), *Nutrition and Diet in Menopause*, Nutrition and Health,
DOI 10.1007/978-1-62703-373-2_24, © Springer Science+Business Media New York 2013

EST	Estrogen sulfotransferase
DHT	5α-dihydrotestosterone
ER	Estrogen receptor
AR	Androgen receptor
FDA	Food and Drug Administration
USDA	United States Department of Agriculture

Introduction

This section reviews the literature and summarizes the evidence on associations between gynecological malignancies, especially endometrial and ovarian cancers, and dietary patterns in menopausal women. Potential influence of dietary patterns on development of other gynecological malignancies (e.g., cervix, vagina, and vulva) has not been fully examined and therefore is not included in this mini review.

Endometrial Cancer

Endometrial cancer is one of the most common female pelvic malignancies in developed countries, and its incidence has recently increased in countries like Japan [1]. Important risk factors for endometrial cancer include obesity, postmenopausal unopposed estrogen use, and nulliparity regardless of ethnic or racial backgrounds. Among all human malignancies, increasing body mass index (BMI) is associated most strongly with endometrial cancer incidence and death, although predominantly in Western countries and not necessarily verified in Japan [2]. Obesity-driven type II diabetes and hypertension have also been associated with increased risk of endometrial cancer, especially endometrioid endometrial carcinoma. Obesity is certainly an established and strong risk factor for endometrial cancer in Japan and Western countries but the roles of individual dietary patterns, which are obviously different between Japan and Western countries, for instance, have not been necessarily well studied. Daily dietary patterns certainly play a pivotal role in the etiology of certain human malignancies but it is also true that there has been limited evidence with regard to the correlation between dietary patterns and risks of endometrial cancer development, especially in postmenopausal population in individual countries or societies.

Meat

The excellent systemic literature review and meta-analysis was published in 2007 [3], based on case–control data. Results suggested an increased risk of endometrial cancer development with meat consumption, particularly with red meat. Random effects dose–response summary estimates for the seven case–control studies evaluating meat consumption were 1.26 (95 % CI: 1.03–1.54) per 100 g/day of total meat and 1.51 (95 % CI: 1.19–1.93) per 100 g/day of red meat per serving. This meta-analysis included one cohort study [4] of 23,000 postmenopausal women who have been followed for 7 years. Relative risks for the intermediate and extreme terciles compared to the lowest tercile for total and red meat intake were 1.0 and 1.1, respectively, and no significant associations were detected between the amounts of total and red meat consumption and endometrial cancer risk.

After the publication of this excellent meta-analysis study, three studies [5–7] have independently evaluated the cumulative amounts of meat consumption and endometrial cancer risk until February 2012

Table 24.1 Recenvt case–control and cohort studies evaluating meat intake

Reference cases/control	Country or cohort size	Median age or total cohort	Cases/ controls	Type of study	Exposure	Contrast	OR (95 % CI)	P value
Bravi et al. [5] (2009)	Italy	60/61	454/908	Hospital-based cc	Red meat	>2 vs. <1 serving/week	2.07 (1.29–3.33)	0.002
Kabat et al. [6] (2008)	Canada	50.0/48.0	426/34,148	Cohort	Red meat	>48.49 vs. <108.99 g/day	0.86 (0.61–1.22)	0.75
Lonkhuijzen et al. [7] (2011)	Canada	58.9/59.2	107/1,830	Case–cohort	Red meat	>22.09 vs. <52.15 g/day	1.62 (0.86–3.08)	0.13

Studies evaluating meat intake, published from 2007 to February 2012, are summarized
This table is unpublished
CC case–control, *OR* odds ratio, *CI* confidence interval, *vs.* versus

(Table 24.1). One of these studies [5] was a hospital-based case–control study enrolling 454 endometrial cancer patients as compared with 908 control women. This study from Italy did indicate that a significant increment in the risks of endometrial cancer development was detected in those consuming significant red meat, with relative risk of 2.07 (95 % CI: 1.29–3.33) for an increment of 1 serving per day. However, a large cohort study of Canadian women [6] demonstrated no significant association between the risk of endometrial cancer development and consumption of red meat (relative risk = 0.86, 95 % CI: 0.61–1.22, for high vs. low intake; P trend = 0.75) or all meat (relative risk = 0.83, 95 % CI: 0.60–1.15, for high vs. low intake; P trend = 0.14). Recent case–cohort study of Canadian women (107 cases and 1,830 subcohort members) [7] also demonstrated that the risk of endometrial cancer development was increased for women who consumed more red meat (relative risk = 1.62, 95 % CI: 0.86–3.08, for high vs. low intake; P trend = 0.13) and all meat (relative risk = 1.50, 95 % CI: 0.78–2.89, for high vs. low intake; P trend = 0.14), though multivariable-adjusted estimates were not statistically significant. The results of these several case–control and case–cohort studies did at least suggest that relatively high red meat consumption may be associated with the risk of endometrial cancer development at least in Western countries or Caucasian population. However, it is also true that published cohort studies were very few, and they showed no association between meat consumption and endometrial cancer risk. In addition, the great majority of those examined were Caucasian in these published studies. Therefore, it requires further studies, particularly prospective cohort studies and more importantly those involving Asian, Arab, African, and Hispanic populations who are expected to grow more in number and to develop much higher number of endometrial malignancy in very near future.

Fish

Previously published results of meta-analysis [3] did indicate that a nonsignificant increment in the risk of endometrial cancer development was indeed significantly associated with increased consumption of fish or other seafood. Random effects dose–response summary estimate for case–control studies evaluating fish consumption was 1.04 (95 % CI: 0.55–1.98) per 100 g/day of fish per serving. In addition, results of recent case–cohort study of Canadian women [7] also reported the similar results as above. In conclusion, there has been no evidence for the association between fish consumption and risk of endometrial cancer development in pre- and postmenopausal women at this juncture. However, it obviously requires more studies involving fish- or seafood-consuming populations in order to draw definitive conclusions.

Table 24.2 Recent cohort studies evaluating vegetable or fruit intake

Reference or cohort size	Country or total cohort	Age	Cases/controls	Type of study	Exposure	Contrast	OR (95 % CI)	P value
McCullough et al. [11] 2007	The United States	50–74	435/41,400	Cohort	Vegetables	>2.6 vs. <1.0 servings/day	1.21 (0.89–1.65)	0.24
					Fruits	>2.7 vs. <0.9 servings/day	1.24 (0.90–1.70)	0.30
Kabat et al. [12] 2010	The United States	50–71	1,142/1,12,088	Cohort	Vegetables	>1.67 vs. <0.74 servings/day	1.09 (0.90–1.33)	0.55
					Fruits	>1.91 vs. <0.61 servings/day	1.30 (1.04–1.61)	0.05

Studies evaluating vegetable or fruit intake, published from 2007 to February 2012, are summarized
This table is unpublished
OR odds ratio, *CI* confidence interval, *vs.* versus

Milk and Dairy Product

Previously published epidemiological studies [3], examining associations of milk and dairy intake with the risk of endometrial cancer, were relatively few and results reported have been inconsistent.

Recently, large prospective cohort studies were published in 2011 [8]. A study of 68,019 American women who were enrolled in Nurses' Health Study (NHS) evaluated the incidence of endometrial cancer with relation to milk and dairy consumption. A total of 669 women with endometrial cancer were identified during 26 years of follow-up. Participants were 34–59 years of age at enrollment. Marginally significant association was detected between the amounts of daily intake of milk and endometrial cancer risk. The significantly positive association between the amounts of daily intake and endometrial cancer risk was detected only among the postmenopausal women (relative risk comparing 3 or more svg/day versus <1 svg/day = 1.41, 95 % CI: 1.01–1.98; *P* for trend = 0.02) and was apparent only among those who were not currently using postmenopausal hormone replacement (relative risk = 1.58, 95 % CI: 1.05–2.36; *P* for trend = 0.003). Results of this particular study did suggest that dairy product is indeed associated with an increased risk of endometrial cancer development in postmenopausal American women who are not using estrogen-containing hormones.

Fruits and Vegetables

The systematic literature review and meta-analysis published in 2007 [9], based on case–control data, suggested a modest inverse association with vegetable consumption, especially for cruciferous vegetables. The random effects summary estimates comparing high categories with low categories of intake published until 2007 were 0.71 (95 % CI: 0.55–0.91) for total vegetables, 0.85 (95 % CI: 0.74–0.97) for cruciferous vegetables, and 0.97 (95 % CI: 0.92–1.02) for total fruits. Only one prospective cohort study [10] was included in this meta-analysis. This study demonstrated no clear patterns of endometrial cancer development risks associated with fruit and vegetable consumption.

After the publication of this meta-analysis study, two cohort studies [11, 12] from the United States evaluated the daily amounts of vegetable and fruit consumption and endometrial cancer development risks until February 2012 (Table 24.2). One is a large prospective cohort study [11] enrolling 41,400 American postmenopausal women within which 435 women developed endometrial cancer during 10 years of follow-up. Participants were 50–74 years of age at enrollment. Results of this study indicated that neither total vegetable consumption (highest vs. lowest quintile: relative risk = 1.21, 95 % CI: 0.89–1.65; *P* = 0.24) nor total fruit consumption (relative risk = 1.24, 95 % CI: 0.90–1.70; *P* = 0.30) was associated with the risks of endometrial cancer development in multivariate models. Another is an even larger prospective cohort study [12] involving 112,088 women within which 1,142 women developed endometrial cancer during 8 years of follow-up. Participants were 50–71 years of age at the time of enrollment of this particular study. Results of this study indicated that relative risks for the highest compared to the lowest quintile of total vegetable and total fruit consumption were 1.09 (95 % CI: 0.90–1.33; $P=0.55$) and 1.30 (95 % CI: 1.04–1.61; $P=0.05$), respectively. There was no inverse association detected among intake of any of 13 botanical groupings of vegetables and fruits. Results of these two cohort studies above do not necessarily support an inverse association between vegetable or fruit consumption and endometrial cancer risk in postmenopausal women, which has been suggested by various media or health moguls. Therefore, protective roles of a high intake of vegetable or fruit on the risk of endometrial cancer in postmenopausal women are by no means supported by scientific evidence at least at this juncture.

Isoflavones

Isoflavones, which are a class of phytochemicals, are abundant in soybeans and have the abilities to bind to estrogen receptor (ER) [13]. Health benefits of isoflavones through Tofu or other soybean products have appeared almost every day in the media, especially in the United States. However, a careful literature review did reveal that well-executed epidemiological studies evaluating associations of dietary soy or isoflavone intake with the risk of endometrial cancer development are surprisingly very few at least at this juncture.

The meta-analysis study published in 2009 [14], based on three case–control data, indicated that relative risk for the highest compared to the lowest quintile of soy intake was 0.70 (95 % CI: 0.57–0.86). However, it is also true that data from prospective studies are enormously deficient particularly with regard to a potential influence of isoflavone and soy intake on prospective development of endometrial cancer, although one large prospective cohort study [11] enrolling 41,400 American postmenopausal women during 10 years of follow-up demonstrated that no significant association was detected between higher legume intake and endometrial cancer risk, although the significance of other isoflavone products was not necessarily mentioned in this particular study.

Since this meta-analysis study was published, one case–control study from the State of New Jersey, the United States [15], demonstrated the correlation between isoflavone intake and endometrial cancer development risks until February 2012. This is a population-based case–control study enrolling 424 endometrial cancer cases as compared with 398 control women. Results of this particular American study did suggest a decreased endometrial cancer risk in lean women taking isoflavones, which also promoted the regular exercise with everyday consumption of tofu or other soybean products at least in the US women.

Recently, the North American Menopause Society/Utian Translational Science Symposium on Soy and Soy Isoflavones was held in 2010 [16]. This interesting symposium appeared to reach the consensus statement that daily soy food consumption was associated with lower risk of endometrial cancer development at least in the United States based upon the results of observational studies.

Very recently, a large prospective cohort study was published in 2012 [17]. The study of 46,027 American nonhysterectomized postmenopausal women who were enrolled in Multiethnic Cohort (MEC) study evaluated the incidence of endometrial cancer in relation to dietary intake. A total of 489 women developed endometrial cancer during the median follow-up period of 13.6 years. Interestingly, a reduced risk of endometrial cancer development was associated with total amounts of isoflavone, daidzein, and genistein intake. Relative risk for the highest compared to the lowest quintile of total isoflavone intake was 0.66 (95 % CI: 0.47–0.91). However, it is also important to note that there was no significant association between endometrial cancer development risk and the amounts of consumption of legumes, soy, tofu, or genistein in contrast to other published studies above. The data in this study did suggest that an estimated 26.7 % (95 % CI: 5.3–45.8 %) of endometrial caners may have been prevented, providing all American women in this cohort study were to have increased their total isoflavone consumption to the level of those in the highest quintile (>7.82 mg per 1,000 kcal/day). Results of these data above, based on several case–control and one cohort studies, reasonably indicated that isoflavone consumption is indeed associated with a reduced risk of endometrial cancer development, at least in postmenopausal American women. However, it obviously requires further studies such as which forms of isoflavone intake, for instance more tofu, soy milk, or even daily supplement, could confer these putative beneficial effects of prevention of endometrial cancer development upon not only American but also other postmenopausal women in the world.

Tea

Health benefits of tea, especially green tea, have been also promoted in the media or others especially in the United States. In a very recently published meta-analysis, Butler et al. [18] suggested a decreased risk of endometrial cancer development with green tea consumption. They reported that based upon case–control studies, there was a significantly inverse correlation between the total amounts of green tea intake and cumulative risks of endometrial cancer development (relative risk=0.78, 95 % CI: 0.62–0.98). We also previously reported [19] case–control study of 152 Japanese endometrial cancer cases, limited to particular histological type of endometrioid endometrial adenocarcinoma which is considered to be estrogen-dependent cancer, as compared with 285 control Japanese women. We did detect a significant inverse association between total amounts of Japanese green tea or Ryoku-cha consumption and risks of endometrial cancer development in a dose–response relationship. What is to be noted is that this significant inverse correlation which we firstly demonstrated was consistently detected both in pre- and postmenopausal Japanese women.

However, it is also true that the results of cohort study have not been consistent with those of case–control studies. A large population-based prospective cohort study [20] enrolling 53,724 Japanese women within which 117 women developed endometrial cancer during 15 years of follow-up was conducted in Japan. In the multivariate analysis of this particular Japanese study, relative risks for endometrial cancer development in women who have consumed Japanese green tea of 1–2 cups/day, 3–4 cups/day, and 5 or more cups/day compared with <4 days/week were 1.04 (95 % CI: 0.62–1.74), 0.79 (95 % CI: 0.47–1.35), and 0.75 (95 % CI: 0.44–1.30) (*P* for trend=0.22), respectively. Green tea consumption was therefore not significantly associated with a decreased risk of endometrial cancer development in the country like Japan whose population consumed more green teas than in any other countries of the world. Therefore, there appears to be no clear evidence of protective role of green tea consumption on the risks of endometrial cancer development in postmenopausal women but the discrepancy in terms of protective effects of green teas upon endometrial cancer development may be due to the ethnical or racial differences between Japanese and others reported in the study of Butler et al. above. Therefore, further studies enrolling the subjects other than Japanese are required to verify this hypothesis. In addition, it will be more important to study which ingredients or components of green tea, especially Ryoku-cha, could confer the potential benefits, if any, upon the postmenopausal women in terms of prevention of development of endometrial cancer.

Black tea is consumed more in the world than green tea but there has been no consistent evidence of association between black tea intake and endometrial cancer development risks [18, 21]. A prospective cohort study [22] of postmenopausal women in the State of Iowa, the United States, also reported no inverse association between black tea intake and endometrial cancer development.

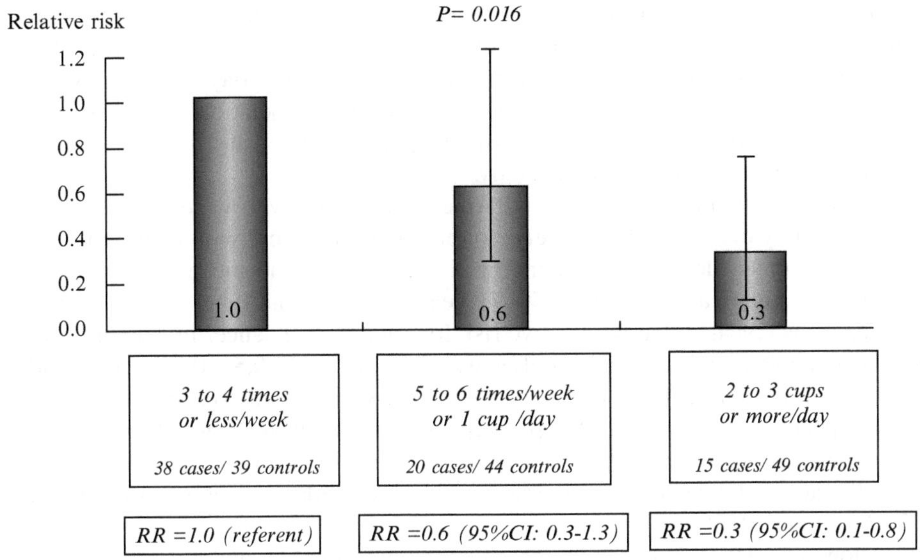

Fig. 24.1 Relative risk of endometrioid endometrial adenocarcinoma according to coffee intake in postmenopausal women (multivariate-adjusted relative risk). Multivariate-adjusted relative risk was adjusted for age, residence, education, body mass index (kg/m^2), smoking status, number of pregnancies, use of oral contraceptives, past history of diabetes mellitus, and total calorie intake. There was a significantly inverse dose–response association between coffee intake and the risk of endometrial cancer in postmenopausal women. This legend is unpublished and made from our data (Koizumi T, et al. Eur J Cancer Prev. 2008;17:358–63 [25]). *RR* relative risk, *CI* confidence interval

Coffee

Coffee is consumed far more abundantly and widely than tea in the world and this tendency has become recently more pronounced in all over the world due to the global dissemination of American-style fast food coffee shops. Therefore, it has increasingly become important to study the correlation between the amount of daily coffee consumption and potential risks of diseases, in particular, malignancy. Coffee consumption has been indeed reported to be associated with various types of cancer in epidemiological studies [23]. In an excellent meta-analysis of observational studies published up to October 2011 by Je et al. [24], it was suggested that increased coffee consumption is associated with a reduced risk of endometrial cancer development. Based on ten case–control studies, there was a significantly inverse association between the amounts of coffee intake and risks of endometrial cancer development (relative risk=0.69, 95 % CI: 0.55–0.87) in this meta-analysis. We also previously reported in [25] case–control study of 107 Japanese endometrial cancer cases that a significant inverse association was detected between the amounts of coffee consumption and risks of endometrial cancer development in a dose–response relationship in Japanese women in which the amount of coffee intake was enormously less than in American women. Interesting this association was detected in postmenopausal women, but not in premenopausal women (Fig. 24.1). Results of meta-analysis above [24] also demonstrated that based on the results of six different or independent cohort studies, there was a significantly inverse association between the amounts of coffee intake and risks of endometrial cancer development (relative risk=0.70, 95 % CI: 0.55–0.80).

Recently, two large prospective cohort studies [26, 27], which are included in this meta-analysis, have been published in 2011. One study [26] enrolling 67,470 American women in NHS evaluated the incidence of endometrial cancer with relation to the amounts of coffee intake. A total of 672 women developed endometrial cancer during 26 years of follow-up. Participants were 34–59 years of age at the time of enrollment in this study. Results of multivariate analysis revealed that the relative risk for endometrial cancer development in women who drank 4 or more cups/day compared with <1 cup/day was 0.75 (95 % CI: 0.57–0.97; *P* for trend = 0.02). The inverse associations with 4 or more cups/day was more pronounced among obese women, postmenopausal women, and those without current postmenopausal hormone use in this American study.

Another study [27] also involving 226,732 American women who were enrolled in NIH-AARP Diet and Health Study evaluated the incidence of endometrial cancer with relation to coffee intake. A total of 1,486 women developed endometrial cancer during the mean follow-up of 9.3 years. Participants in this American study were 50–71 years of age at the time of enrollment. Results of multivariate analysis revealed that the relative risk for endometrial cancer in women who drank 4 or more cups/day compared with no cups of coffee was 0.64 (95 % CI: 0.51–0.80; *P* for trend = 0.0004). The correlation of the amounts of daily coffee intake with endometrial cancer incidence varied significantly depending upon whether the participants were under the hormone replacement or not. Significant association was only detected among those who have never used postmenopausal hormone replacement therapy (relative risk comparing 4 or more cups/day versus no cups = 0.54, 95 % CI: 0.41–0.72; *P* for trend = 0.0005).

In conclusion, association between increased coffee consumption and a reduced risk of endometrial cancer is consistently detected for both case–control and cohort studies, especially in postmenopausal American women. These results suggest possible protective roles of a high intake of coffee on the risks of endometrial cancer development at least in American postmenopausal women. However, it is also important to know which components or ingredients of coffee these women have consumed on the daily basis could contribute to these remarkable protective effects of American coffee upon endometrial cancer development.

Possible Roles of Diet in Endometrial Cancer Risk at Menopausal Women: From the Viewpoint of Estrogen

Estrogen regulates a wide range of physiological responses in a variety of target tissues. It is well recognized that estrogen plays an important role in the development and progression of endometrial cancer [1]. Results of previous clinical, biological, and epidemiological studies have all demonstrated that excessive and/or prolonged exposure to estrogens not opposed by progesterone is considered to increase the potential risks of endometrial cancer development, especially that of the endometrioid type [1, 28]. However, the great majority of endometrial cancers arise during the postmenopausal period when ovaries cease to be functional. Therefore, exogenous estrogen or other sex steroid hormone taken from diets may influence and play some roles in endometrial tissue more sensitively in postmenopausal women compared to premenopausal women.

Recently, a focus has been given to the importance of in situ or intratumoral estrogen metabolism or biosynthesis, including both synthesis and degradation, in the development and progression of various human estrogen-dependent neoplasms, including breast and endometrial carcinoma [28]. Numerous studies have demonstrated that human endometrial cancer tissue contained the enzyme systems required for local biosynthesis of estrogen (Fig. 24.2). Among these enzymes, aromatase, 17β-hydroxysteroid dehydrogenases (17β-HSD), and steroid sulfatase (STS) are three principal enzymes involved in the formation of biologically active estrogen, estradiol (E2). Estrogen-dependent neoplasms such as breast and endometrioid endometrial carcinoma, in which in situ conversions from serum androgens to biologically active estrogens occur, could be considered "intracrine" tissues [28].

The possible cascade of local production of sex steroids in endometrial carcinoma is illustrated in Fig. 24.3. Androgens as substrates are generally supplied from the circulation. Androstenedione and

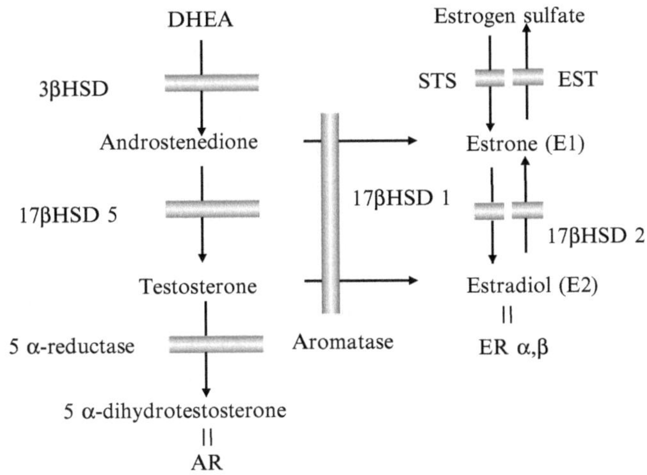

Fig. 24.2 Schema representing the production and/or metabolism of sex steroids in human tissues. Human endometrial cancer tissue contained the enzyme systems required for local biosynthesis of estrogen. Among these enzymes, aromatase, 17β-HSD, and STS are three principal enzymes involved in the formation of estradiol. This legend is unpublished. *17β-HSD* 17β-hydroxysteroid dehydrogenase, *STS* steroid sulfatase, *EST* estrogen sulfotransferase, *ER* estrogen receptor, *AR* androgen receptor, *DHEA* dehydroepiandrosterone

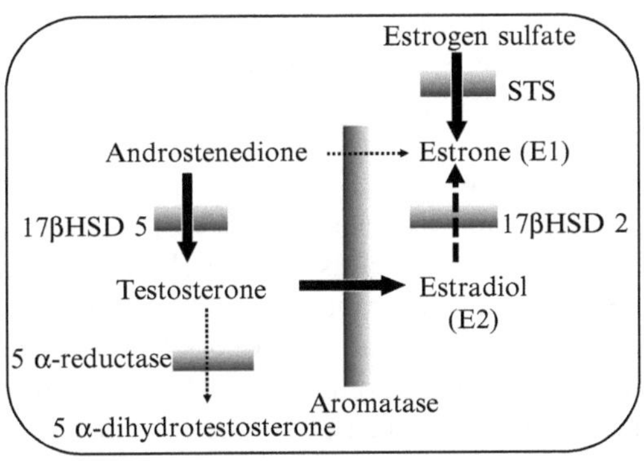

Fig. 24.3 Schema of intratumoral estrogen metabolism and synthesis in endometrial cancer. Testosterone is locally produced by 17β-HSD type 5. In addition, estradiol is locally produced by aromatase and binds to ER in the cancer cells. On the other hand, 17β-HSD type 2 expression was decreased through normal endometrium, hyperplasia, and finally cancer accordingly. 17β-HSD type 1 was not expressed in normal endometrium and its disorders. Moreover, STS overexpression was detected in endometrial cancer cells. This legend is unpublished and made from our data (Ito K, et al. Mol Cell Endocrinol. 2006;248:136–40 [29]) (Utsunomiya H, et al. J Clin Endocrinol Metab 2001;86:3436–43 [30]) (Utsunomiya H, et al. Clin Cancer Res. 2004;10:5850–6 [31]). *17β-HSD* 17β-hydroxysteroid dehydrogenase, *STS* steroid sulfatase

testosterone are both converted into E1 and E2 by aromatase located in stromal cells in cases of human endometrial carcinoma, respectively. 17β-HSD types 1 and 2, which are expressed predominantly in parenchymal or carcinoma cells, catalyze the reversible conversion of E1 and E2. 17β-HSD type 1 is not detectable and 17β-HSD type 2 and 5 are essential for the maintenance of E2 concentrations in human endometrial cancer tissues. Testosterone is produced by 17β-HSD type 5 (conversion mainly from androstenedione to testosterone). In addition, E2 is produced by aromatase (converting mainly from testosterone to E2 in the cases of endometrial malignancies compared to breast cancer). Both 17β-HSD type 5 and aromatase have been reported to be overexpressed in human endometrial cancers [29]. However, 17β-HSD type 2 expression is decreased through normal endometrium (secretory phase), hyperplasia, and finally cancer accordingly [30]. STS hydrolyzes circulating inactive estrogen sulfate to active estrogen, whereas estrogen sulfotransferase (EST) sulfonates active estrogen to estrogen sulfate. In endometrioid endometrial cancer, STS expression was detected in carcinoma cells, whereas that of STS was not detected in normal endometrium. In addition, EST expression is decreased through normal endometrium (secretory phase) to cancer [31].

From the viewpoint of estrogen action, several possible roles and mechanism of diet in endometrial cancer risk at menopausal women have been hypothesized. As we summarized above, daily dietary patterns which could play an important role in endometrial cancer risk based upon results of various epidemiological studies correspond to daily product, isoflavones, and coffee. Total and red meat consumption, which has been proposed as promoting the risks of endometrial cancer development by some, was actually by no means associated with increased risks of endometrial cancer development at least in American postmenopausal women.

Domesticated animal foods such as pork or beef, especially red meat, are well known to contain E2 which is the most potent estrogenic substance and its metabolites naturally or as a result of added substances contained in the feed or fodder/forage. In addition, the administration of exogenous sex steroids admixed with feed or fodder/forage has been widely used as a common agriculture practice in the United States to promote the growth of cattle in the more proficient fashion [3]. For instance, at least in red meat, E2 and E1 levels of American beef with FDA or USDA approval were significantly higher than those of Japanese beef or Wagyu even including Shimofuri Wagyu, respectively [32]. However, it is also important to note that E2 and E1 are not physiologically active when taken orally, since those sex steroids are completely metabolized and inactivated in liver. Therefore, high E1 or E2 levels contained in these US beef meat have been considered to be not significant in terms of potential health effects upon the consumers regardless of the amounts of E1 or E2 contained.

However, it is also true that new mechanistic insights into the potential effects of various substances contained in the diets upon the development of human endometrial cancer have been considered based upon the concept of this "intracrinology." For instance, dairy product is well known to contain estrogens mainly in the form of estrogen sulfate, a biologically inactive form of estrogen [8]. Estrogen sulfate, a hydrophilic substance which is taken orally and entered into the body, may play pivotal roles as the substance for local biosynthesis of active estrogen, because the enzyme STS, which can convert estrogen sulfate to biologically active estrogen, is indeed overexpressed in endometrial malignant tissues in postmenopausal women [31]. Therefore, the amounts of estrogen sulfate contained in the dairy products could influence the process of at least estrogen-dependent human endometrial cancer, endometrioid endometrial carcinoma.

In addition to estrogen sulfate in the dairy products, the potential beneficial roles of isoflavones may be also explained by this intracrine mechanism. The cellular actions of estrogen are mediated through ER, which is composed of two subtypes, ERa and ERb. ER is expressed in the great majority of endometrial cancer [28]. Isoflavones can possess a high binding affinity for both ERa and ERb, and therefore may act as estrogen-antagonist and limit the proliferative effects of endogenous estrogen [13]. Other potential mechanism of isoflavones is also considered through their putative important roles in in situ estrogen metabolism based on the results of various reported laboratory studies. Isoflavones were reported to stimulate 17β-HSD type 2, which contributes to the regulation of "intracrine" estrogen levels in normal human endometrium and that disruption of the control mechanism of intratissue estrogen levels may be also related to the development of endometrial malignancy [30, 33]. Furthermore, isoflavones were demonstrated to inhibit the activities of 17β-HSD type 5, which is considered one of the key enzymes for determining tissue estrogen concentration [29, 34].

As reported above, protective role of coffee intake on the risk of endometrial cancer in postmenopausal women is consistently detected in the above-mentioned epidemiological studies. Results of our study [25] limited the endometrial cancer cases to histological type of endometrioid endometrial adenocarcinoma, which is considered to be estrogen-dependent carcinoma, and detected a significant inverse association in postmenopausal women. Coffee is known to contain isoflavones, and therefore the hypothesis of isoflavones and endometrial cancer may also apply to that of coffee intake. In addition, increased coffee consumption is associated with increased blood levels of sex hormone-binding globulin (SHBG) in postmenopausal women [35]. SHBG is known to bind estradiol, and reduce the level of biologically active estrogen. Low blood levels of SHBG were also reported to be associated with increased endometrial cancer risk [36].

Further investigations are obviously required to clarify the biological mechanisms of the correlation between diet and endometrial cancer development in menopausal women, especially from the viewpoint of estrogen metabolism and actions.

Ovarian Cancer

It is well known that familial ovarian cancer is responsible for approximately 10 % of ovarian cancer cases, and pregnancy, oral contraceptives, and tubal ligation are the protective factors for ovarian cancer. However, the possible roles of diet in ovarian cancer have remained controversial. For example, red meat consumption [37] and coffee intake [23] were not associated with ovarian cancer risks in recent meta-analysis studies.

On the other hand, epidemiological studies, which examined associations of isoflavone intake with the risk of ovarian cancer, are very few and inconsistent. Results of the 2009 meta-analysis [14] indicated that relative risk for the highest compared to the lowest quintile of soy intake was 0.52 (95 % CI: 0.42–0.67). However, recent data from prospective cohort study [38] in Sweden did not necessarily support this conclusion with regard to an influence of dietary phytoestrogen intake.

The 2011 meta-analysis of tea consumption [18], based on four case–control studies, indicated that there was a significantly inverse association between green tea intake and ovarian cancer risk (relative risk=0.66, 95 % CI: 0.54–0.80). However, there was no prospective study indicated until 2012. In black tea, no association was observed from this meta-analysis [18].

In conclusion, there has been no high-quality scientific evidence which supports the association between diet and ovarian cancer risks at this juncture.

Conclusion

In gynecological malignancy of postmenopausal women, some types of diets may influence the incidence of endometrial cancer (Table 24.3). Diets which may play protective roles in endometrial cancer risk based upon the results of previous epidemiological studies include isoflavones and coffee. Dairy products may be also associated with an increased risk of endometrial cancer development in postmenopausal women who are not using estrogen-containing hormones as a replacement. There has been, however, no consistent evidence on the association between meat, fish, vegetable, and fruit consumption and risks of endometrial cancer development in postmenopausal women. In addition, there appears to be no clear evidence of protective roles of tea consumption in endometrial cancer development.

In ovarian cancer, there has been no high-quality scientific evidence which resolves the association between diet and ovarian cancer risk. Further investigation should be necessary to clarify the possible roles of diet in gynecological malignancy arising in menopausal women from the biological and epidemiological viewpoints.

Table 24.3 Dietary risk factors for endometrial cancer in postmenopausal women

Factors possibly increasing the risk
Milk and dairy products
Factors possibly decreasing the risk
Isoflavones
Coffee
Factors with an unknown effect (published data are inconsistent)
Meat
Fish
Vegetables
Fruits
Green and black tea

Dietary patterns can be associated with development of endometrial carcinoma in postmenopausal women
This table is unpublished

References

1. Amant F, Moerman P, Neven P, Timmerman D, Van Limbergen E, Vergote I. Endometrial cancer. Lancet. 2005; 366:491–505.
2. Schmandt RE, Iglesias DA, Co NN, Lu KH. Understanding obesity and endometrial cancer risk: opportunities for prevention. Am J Obstet Gynecol. 2011;205:518–25.
3. Bandera EV, Kushi LH, Moore DF, Gifkins DM, McCullough ML. Consumption of animal foods and endometrial cancer risk: a systematic literature review and meta-analysis. Cancer Causes Control. 2007;18:967–88.
4. Zheng W, Kushi LH, Potter JD, Sellers TA, Doyle TJ, Bostick RM, et al. Dietary intake of energy and animal foods and endometrial cancer incidence. The Iowa women's health study. Am J Epidemiol. 1995;142:388–94.
5. Bravi F, Scotti L, Bosetti C, Zucchetto A, Talamini R, Montella M, et al. Food groups and endometrial cancer risk: a case-control study from Italy. Am J Obstet Gynecol. 2009;200:293.e1–7.
6. Kabat GC, Miller AB, Jain M, Rohan TE. Dietary iron and haem iron intake and risk of endometrial cancer: a prospective cohort study. Br J Cancer. 2008;98:194–8.
7. van Lonkhuijzen L, Kirsh VA, Kreiger N, Rohan TE. Endometrial cancer and meat consumption: a case-cohort study. Eur J Cancer Prev. 2011;20:334–9.
8. Ganmaa D, Cui X, Feskanich D, Hankinson SE, Willett WC. Milk, dairy intake and risk of endometrial cancer: a 26-year follow-up. Int J Cancer. 2012;130:2664–71.
9. Bandera EV, Kushi LH, Moore DF, Gifkins DM, McCullough ML. Fruits and vegetables and endometrial cancer risk: a systematic literature review and meta-analysis. Nutr Cancer. 2007;58:6–21.
10. Terry P, Baron JA, Weiderpass E, Yuen J, Lichtenstein P, Nyrén O. Lifestyle and endometrial cancer risk: a cohort study from the Swedish Twin Registry. Int J Cancer. 1999;82:38–42.
11. McCullough ML, Bandera EV, Patel R, Patel AV, Gansler T, Kushi LH, et al. A prospective study of fruits, vegetables, and risk of endometrial cancer. Am J Epidemiol. 2007;166:902–11.
12. Kabat GC, Park Y, Hollenbeck AR, Schatzkin A, Rohan TE. Intake of fruits and vegetables, and risk of endometrial cancer in the NIH-AARP Diet and Health Study. Cancer Epidemiol. 2010;34:568–73.
13. Cederroth CR, Nef S. Soy, phytoestrogens and metabolism: a review. Mol Cell Endocrinol. 2009;304:30–42.
14. Myung SK, Ju W, Choi HJ, Kim SC, Korean Meta-Analysis (KORMA) Study Group. Soy intake and risk of endocrine-related gynaecological cancer: a meta-analysis. BJOG. 2009;116:1697–705.
15. Bandera EV, Williams MG, Sima C, Bayuga S, Pulick K, Wilcox H, et al. Phytoestrogen consumption and endometrial cancer risk: a population-based case-control study in New Jersey. Cancer Causes Control. 2009;20: 1117–27.
16. North American Menopause Society. The role of soy isoflavones in menopausal health: report of The North American Menopause Society/Wulf H. Utian Translational Science Symposium in Chicago, IL (October 2010). Menopause. 2011;18:732–53.
17. Ollberding NJ, Lim U, Wilkens LR, Setiawan VW, Shvetsov YB, Henderson BE, et al. Legume, soy, tofu, and isoflavone intake and endometrial cancer risk in postmenopausal women in the multiethnic cohort study. J Natl Cancer Inst. 2012;104:67–76.

18. Butler LM, Wu AH. Green and black tea in relation to gynecologic cancers. Mol Nutr Food Res. 2011;55:931–40.
19. Kakuta Y, Nakaya N, Nagase S, Fujita M, Koizumi T, Okamura C, et al. Case-control study of green tea consumption and the risk of endometrial endometrioid adenocarcinoma. Cancer Causes Control. 2009;20:617–24.
20. Shimazu T, Inoue M, Sasazuki S, Iwasaki M, Kurahashi N, Yamaji T, et al. Coffee consumption and risk of endometrial cancer: a prospective study in Japan. Int J Cancer. 2008;123:2406–10.
21. Tang NP, Li H, Qiu YL, Zhou GM, Ma J. Tea consumption and risk of endometrial cancer: a metaanalysis. Am J Obstet Gynecol. 2009;201:605.e1–8.
22. Zheng W, Doyle TJ, Kushi LH, Sellers TA, Hong CP, Folsom AR. Tea consumption and cancer incidence in a prospective cohort study of postmenopausal women. Am J Epidemiol. 1996;144:175–82.
23. Arab L. Epidemiologic evidence on coffee and cancer. Nutr Cancer. 2010;62:271–83.
24. Je Y, Giovannucci E. Coffee consumption and risk of endometrial cancer: findings from a large up-to-date meta-analysis. Int J Cancer. 2012;131:1700–10.
25. Koizumi T, Nakaya N, Okamura C, Sato Y, Shimazu T, Nagase S, et al. Case-control study of coffee consumption and the risk of endometrial endometrioid adenocarcinoma. Eur J Cancer Prev. 2008;17:358–63.
26. Je Y, Hankinson SE, Tworoger SS, DeVivo I, Giovannucci E. A prospective cohort study of coffee consumption and risk of endometrial cancer over a 26-year follow-up. Cancer Epidemiol Biomarkers Prev. 2011;20:2487–95.
27. Gunter MJ, Schaub JA, Xue X, Freedman ND, Gaudet MM, Rohan TE, et al. A prospective investigation of coffee drinking and endometrial cancer incidence. Int J Cancer. 2012;131:E530–6.
28. Ito K. Hormone replacement therapy and cancers: the biological roles of Oestrogen and progestin in tumorigenesis are different between the endometrium and breast. Tohoku J Exp Med. 2007;212:1–12.
29. Ito K, Utsunomiya H, Suzuki T, Saitou S, Akahira J, Okamura K, et al. 17Beta-hydroxysteroid dehydrogenases in human endometrium and its disorders. Mol Cell Endocrinol. 2006;248:136–40.
30. Utsunomiya H, Suzuki T, Kaneko C, Takeyama J, Nakamura J, Kimura K, et al. The analyses of 17beta-hydroxysteroid dehydrogenase isozymes in human endometrial hyperplasia and carcinoma. J Clin Endocrinol Metab. 2001;86:3436–43.
31. Utsunomiya H, Ito K, Suzuki T, Kitamura T, Kaneko C, Nakata T, et al. Steroid sulfatase and Oestrogen sulfotransferase in human endometrial carcinoma. Clin Cancer Res. 2004;10:5850–6.
32. Handa Y, Fujita H, Honma S, Minakami H, Kishi R. Oestrogen concentrations in beef and human hormone-dependent cancers. Ann Oncol. 2009;20:1610–1.
33. Brueggemeier RW, Gu X, Mobley JA, Joomprabutra S, Bhat AS, Whetstone JL. Effects of phytoestrogens and synthetic combinatorial libraries on aromatase, Oestrogen biosynthesis, and metabolism. Ann N Y Acad Sci. 2001;948:51–66.
34. Skarydová L, Zivná L, Xiong G, Maser E, Wsól V. AKR1C3 as a potential target for the inhibitory effect of dietary flavonoids. Chem Biol Interact. 2009;178:138–44.
35. Goto A, Song Y, Chen BH, Manson JE, Buring JE, Liu S. Coffee and caffeine consumption in relation to sex hormone-binding globulin and risk of type 2 diabetes in postmenopausal women. Diabetes. 2011;60:269–75.
36. Lukanova A, Lundin E, Micheli A, Arslan A, Ferrari P, Rinaldi S, et al. Circulating levels of sex steroid hormones and risk of endometrial cancer in postmenopausal women. Int J Cancer. 2004;108:425–32.
37. Wallin A, Orsini N, Wolk A. Red and processed meat consumption and risk of ovarian cancer: a dose-response meta-analysis of prospective studies. Br J Cancer. 2011;104:1196–201.
38. Hedelin M, Löf M, Andersson TM, Adlercreutz H, Weiderpass E. Dietary phytoestrogens and the risk of ovarian cancer in the women's lifestyle and health cohort study. Cancer Epidemiol Biomarkers Prev. 2011;20:308–17.

Part IV
Psychological Aspects and Cognitive Function

Chapter 25
The Psychology of the Menopause: The Experiences During the Transition and Individual Conceptualization of Menopause

Eleonora Bielawska-Batorowicz

Key Points

- The bio-psycho-socio-cultural perspective is applied in recent studies on menopausal transition.
- Studies conducted around the world indicate that there is no universal pattern of menopausal transition.
- Women with more negative attitudes towards menopause report more menopausal symptoms.
- There is no demonstrated pattern of an adverse independent effect of the menopausal transition on mood symptoms.
- Natural menopause does not lead to measurable change in cognition.
- Social reactions to the hot flush are either positive or neutral.

Keywords Menopause • Psychological symptoms • Depression • Individual conceptualization of menopause • Hot flush • Cognitive model • Cognitive behavioral therapy

Abbreviation

CBT Cognitive behavioral therapy

Introduction

The discussions on stages of menopausal transition resulted in the proposals presented by WHO Scientific Group [1] and Stages of Reproductive Aging Workshop (STRAW) [2]. These groups of experts worked out the precise terminology and classification of years around menopause. As the final menstrual period with 12 consecutive months of amenorrhea, menopause is one of the two major events (the other one is menarche) that define female reproductive activity and reproductive health [2]. Although the medical model has dominated research on menopause for a long period of time, the idea that hormonal mechanism might not be sufficient to explain the prevalence, intensity, and variety of

E. Bielawska-Batorowicz, M.Sc., Ph.D. (✉)
Institute of Psychology, University of Łódź, Smugowa 10/12, 91-433 Łódź, Poland
e-mail: psychologia@uni.lodz.pl

C.J.H. Martin et al. (eds.), *Nutrition and Diet in Menopause*, Nutrition and Health,
DOI 10.1007/978-1-62703-373-2_25,

menopausal symptoms, as well as women's experiences around the menopause, has been put forward. The concept of menopause as a cultural, sociological, and psychological phenomenon [3–5] provided a new perspective that resulted in some interesting and fruitful analyses. Therefore the bio-psycho-socio-cultural perspective becomes applied more and more often in recent studies on menopausal transition. Thus analyses of the menopause and changes related to it are conducted within a broader framework that incorporates cultural, social, and psychological factors. Such approach is advocated in the recent reviews [6, 7], where reproductive events are examined and their psychological or even psychopathological aspects are discussed. With the increased average life expectancy women live a substantial part of their lives after the menopause. Therefore the knowledge on different aspects of menopausal transition is important not only for better understanding of this phenomenon but also for better health and social policies.

The aim of this chapter is to give account of the selected psychological aspects of the menopausal transition and early postmenopause. The following issues are discussed: (1) characteristics of menopausal symptoms, including psychological symptoms; (2) the psychological correlates of intensity of menopausal symptoms; (3) the individual conceptualization of menopause and how it is related to women's menopausal experiences; and (4) psychological interventions during the menopausal transition.

What Women Experience Around Menopause: The Characteristics of Menopausal Symptoms

Vasomotor Symptoms

The bulk of research has addressed the characteristics and prevalence of menopausal symptoms [1, 8–10], as well as their correlates and predisposing factors. Studies conducted in different parts of the world indicate that experiences of women vary, and that there is no universal pattern of menopausal transition. Although it is considered that vasomotor symptoms, like hot flushes and night sweats, are the most typical for the transition, their reported prevalence is not the same in all studies. Data in Table 25.1 illustrate the disparity in frequency of such symptoms in women around the world.

As it can be seen from figures presented in Table 25.1, hot flushes and night sweats are on average more often experienced by those living in North America and Europe, and less so by women from Africa and Latin America. Nevertheless the symptoms are highly prevalent, first of all in the perimenopausal stage. Data analyzed by Freeman and Sherif [8] indicate that vasomotor symptoms might

Table 25.1 The prevalence of vasomotor symptoms during the menopausal transition around the world

The continent	Number of studies available	Percentage of perimenopausal women reporting vasomotor symptoms (range across all studies)
Europe	10	31–73
North America	10	18–79
Latin America	6	0–68
Asia	23	13–79
The Middle East	4	42–68
Africa	2	23–57
Australia	6	44–80

The table shows the percentages of women from different continents who actually experience hot flushes while becoming menopausal

Source: Based on data presented in Freeman and Sherif [8] review

be experienced also by women in postmenopausal stage, however much less often. There is also some evidence that sensations resembling vasomotor symptoms are reported by men of 45–55 years of age [11]. Studies [12] conducted in the same country that had included women of different race/ethnicity pointed to a disparity in hot flush frequency. Thus it can be assumed that besides the hormonal change and geographical region, there are other factors that impact on menopausal symptoms. Cultural background, lifestyle, attitudes towards menopause, and aging might be the most plausible determinants.

In the recent review of menopausal discomforts reported by women from different countries Sievert [10] indicates that hot flushes neither are the most common complaint nor are they reported as the most frequent symptom. In some studies analyzed by this author [10] hot flushes were not listed at all among the top four complaints, and in others they were listed on further positions. Only in one study hot flushes were listed as the most frequent problem. The complaints that used to come before hot flushes included aches/stiff joints, shoulder stiffness, headache, lack of energy, tiredness, nervousness, forgetfulness, and depression. Women had not at all listed hot flushes among their major complaints in some of the studies done in Australia, Hong Kong, Indonesia, Japan, Mexico, the Philippines, and the United States.

Psychological Symptoms

The list of symptoms experienced by menopausal women, as indicated in several reviews [1, 6, 13–15], includes psychological symptoms, like moodiness, irritability, depression, and impairment of cognitive functions such as memory and concentration. In particular, the issue of depression attracts a lot of attention.

Mood disturbances around menopause are considered as "reproductive subtype of depression" [16] and thus linked to hormonal changes associated not only with menopausal transition but also with premenstrual and postpartum phases. Studies analyzed by Ferguson et al. [14] indicate that perimenopausal women are at greater risk of depressive symptoms in comparison with their premenopausal counterparts. Some earlier reviews [17, 18] and studies [19, 20] provide contradictory evidence for the link between menopause and depression. While Maartens et al. [20] show that transition from pre- to perimenopause and from peri- to postmenopause increases significantly the depressive scores, Dennerstein et al. [19] claim a different pattern—participants in their study have expressed lower depressive symptomatology with the time passing. Avis [18] and Nicol-Smith [17] stress that there is no enough evidence to claim that the onset of menopausal transition increases the risk of depression or that during postmenopause women are more depressed than earlier in their life. However, both earlier [21] and recent studies [22–24] indicate the relationship between depression and other menopausal symptoms, i.e., women with intense vasomotor symptoms are more likely to experience depression. That is in line with the domino effect hypothesis of menopausal depression. According to its assumptions, it is not the hormonal changes alone, as it is claimed in the biochemical (direct effect) hypothesis, but the menopausal symptoms associated with these changes that increase the risk of depressive mood. As presented in Fig. 25.1 vasomotor symptoms, which are the effects of hormonal changes around the menopause, increase the likelihood that women who experience them, both during the day and at night, do not sleep well and do not get enough rest. Such sleep deprivation increases their risk of the development of irritability and depressive symptoms [18].

In contrast with both biochemical and domino effect hypotheses are the concepts that link menopausal depressive symptoms with social and psychological factors in women's lives. The plausible associations and effects are presented in Fig. 25.2. The diagram summarizes the assumptions that depressive symptoms might occur more often in those who experience more intense and frequent vasomotor symptoms, more stressful life events, and express negative attitudes towards menopause and aging. Some recent [25, 28] and earlier studies [19, 26] confirm such assumptions.

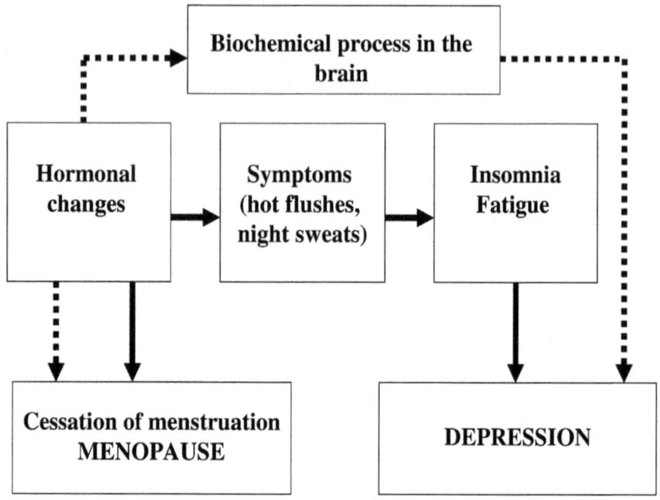

Fig. 25.1 Two mechanisms explaining the onset of depressive symptoms around the menopause—the biochemical/direct effect hypothesis (in *dotted line*) and the domino hypothesis (in *solid line*). The diagram shows how the depressive symptoms during the menopausal transition develop, i.e., either through the hormonal changes that affect the brain or through the reaction to the intense vasomotor symptoms. *Source*: Unpublished

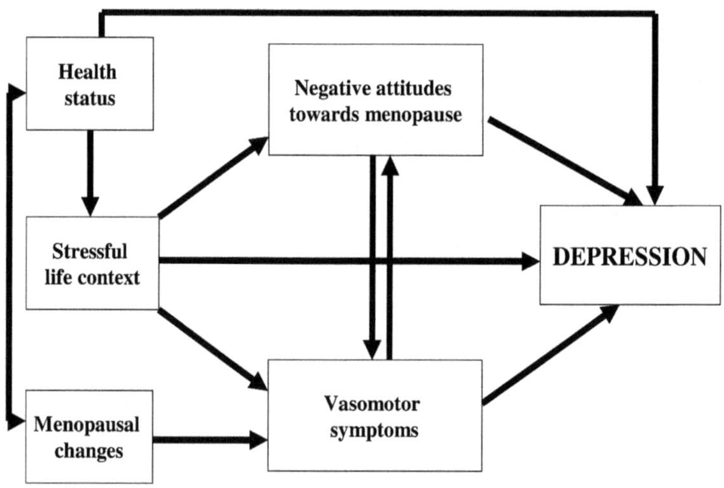

Fig. 25.2 Psychological, social, and hormonal determinants of menopausal depression. The diagram shows that depression during menopause is linked not only to hormonal changes but also to women's life situation and their attitudes towards menopause. *Source*: Based on ideas presented by Bielawska-Batorowicz [25], Woods and Mitchell [26], Greene [27]

The menopausal susceptibility to depression is more often confirmed in clinical and cross-sectional studies. When the possible correlates of mood during the menopausal transition are controlled for and mood is assessed prospectively, then the pattern is less clear. The recent review of community-based prospective cohort studies performed by Vesco et al. [29] provides arguments against the idea of menopause—depression link. The studies analyzed in the review were conducted in the period of 1966–2007 and identified by searches of Medline and PsychInfo databases. The selection of studies was based on several criteria such as the following: the subjects were women undergoing menopausal transition, their mood was evaluated prospectively at least twice, menopausal stage was included in a statistical model determining its relationship with mood symptoms, and the sample exceeded 100 menopausal women and was community based. The samples of nine studies that met the inclusion criteria varied from 226 women in the Melbourne Women's Midlife Health Project to 8,623 women in the Australian Longitudinal Study on Women's Health (ALSWH). All the studies included in total above 19,000 participants from countries such as the United States, Australia, Canada, the United Kingdom, and the Netherlands. The follow-up varied from 2 to 8 years, and mood was assessed at intervals of several months till 2 years. The analyses of results of all these studies revealed that in five of them no association between depression and menopausal transition was found, in three studies

Table 25.2 Menopausal women's complaints related to memory and concentration problems

Problems related to	Examples
Memory	Difficulties in recalling names, phone numbers
	Forgetting reasons for a particular behavior, localization of items in home/office
	Forgetting nonroutine events/appointments
	Need for memory aids (e.g., notes, lists, calendars)
	Forgetting contents of books/films/stories but not the emotional reactions
	More time necessary to think when asked questions
	Difficulty in recalling exact words when they are needed
Concentration	Difficulty with concentration
	Concentration requires much more effort
	Increased distractibility
	Listening but not attending
	Loosing track of conversation, of read text

The table shows examples of memory and concentration problems often reported by menopausal women
Source: Based on data presented by Warga [30] and Mitchell and Woods [31]

women in the menopausal transition period were more likely to be depressed, while in one study the well-being of participants increased from the early to late menopausal stage. Thus the authors of the review conclude that "there is no demonstrated pattern of an adverse independent influence of the menopausal transition on mood symptoms in mid-life women" [29].

Some other psychological symptoms recorded during menopausal transition that attract attention of both researchers and lay audience are related to cognition. Cognitive symptoms reported by menopausal women can be analyzed from their subjective perspective, when worsening of cognitive functions is recorded, and objectively, when appropriate measures are used to assess the cognitive decline. These two types of approaches may lead to different conclusions. Among the most often reported ones, there are complaints related to memory and concentration. Table 25.2, based on findings provided by Warga [30] and Mitchell and Woods [31], gives the examples of such complaints.

Subjective changes in memory and concentration are quite prevalent. Problems with worse memory were reported by 81 % of participants in Schaafsma et al. study [32] and by 62 % in Mitchell and Woods study [31]. The 72 % of Australian participants [32] reported attention problems, and the spontaneous recall of such problems was more typical for perimenopausal women in comparison with their pre- and postmenopausal counterparts. The study conducted in Brazil [33] confirmed the greater incidence of memory slips in women 5 years after the menopause in comparison with premenopausal and late postmenopausal counterparts. Their complaints were more often related to prospective than to retrospective memory. It is interesting to note that when asked about an explanation of their memory and/or concentration problems women attributed them more often to the burden of stress and the process of aging [31] than to hormonal changes and physical health. Thus the hormonal changes around menopause are not considered by women as the most important mechanism for their cognitive problems. The review of studies with objective measures for cognitive functions and hormone levels indicates that "natural menopause does not lead to measurable change in midlife cognition" [34]. This review indicates also that some memory problems should be attributed rather to mood than to menopausal hormonal changes.

There is some evidence though that subjective complaints and objective measures of cognitive functioning are related. It was found [32] that women who reported less memory problems had better scores on immediate verbal memory tasks, and those who reported less attention problems had better scores on reaction time tasks. The subjective cognitive problems were also associated with vasomotor symptoms, i.e., those with more frequent hot flushes had higher incidence of spontaneous reporting of such problems. Thus one can observe the coincidence and interdependence of different types of menopausal symptoms.

Nonhormonal Determinants of Menopausal Symptoms and Experiences

The analyses conducted in the previous section provide support for the view that menopausal women's experiences might have nonhormonal determinants. In this section issues related to menopausal experiences such as attitudes towards menopause and aging, women's self-esteem, and psychological individual differences are discussed in more details.

The research conducted in cross-cultural framework [35, 36] indicates that women in different cultures do not experience and perceive the menopausal transition in the same way. A set of beliefs—typical for a particular culture—might influence the perception and experience of menopause. These beliefs are related not only to the size and shape of the body, its inner structure, and functions but also to women's social roles and to aging members of the society. Thus it can be assumed that in cultures where getting older brings some positive changes for the position of females within a society and alleviates some previously imposed restrictions, women's perception of menopause might be more positive and the experienced symptoms less intense. Data from a variety of studies and reviews confirm the cultural differences in the perception of menopause and also the impact of increased social status linked to aging on lower intensity of menopausal symptoms [5, 35–37]. Thus the differences in the prevalence of vasomotor symptoms presented in Table 25.1 might, at least partly, be attributed to cultural and social contexts.

The recent review of studies that looked at the impact of individual attitudes on menopausal symptoms [38] provided clear evidence that those with more negative attitudes reported more symptoms, which was confirmed both in cross-sectional and prospective studies. This gives an additional support for the relationships proposed in Fig. 25.2, where negative attitudes and vasomotor symptoms are not only linked to depression but also interrelated.

Attitudes towards menopause are related to age. It was found that younger women expressed more negative attitudes than older ones, especially those in the postmenopausal phase [38]. The socially constructed image of menopause, particularly in Western cultures, includes negative elements related to women's emotional instability, cognitive decline, loss of sexual attractiveness, and symptoms that bring a lot of burden to everyday life. Such image might be accepted, shared within families, and transmitted to other family members or even another generation. Thus going through the process of transition and experiencing it may result in getting new—usually less negative—perspective on menopause. Lack of personal experience and the socially constructed image of menopause may explain as well why men's attitudes are always more negative than those of women [38], and why more positive views on menopause are held by those men whose partners express such views [38].

Research findings indicate also that menopause-related experiences are linked to several psychological characteristics. One of such characteristics is self-esteem. It was found that women with lower self-esteem, who usually evaluated themselves in more negative terms, reported more symptoms and described them as more distressing [5, 39]. The physical self was particularly strongly related to symptoms reporting. Low scores on scales used to evaluate one's physical self were identified as significant predictors of more intense psychological and vasomotor symptoms [39].

Another psychological characteristic worth discussing in the context of menopausal transition is neuroticism. The personality dimension of neuroticism is often analyzed in the health context. Persons with high level of neuroticism are more sensitive to their bodily signals and more often attribute such signals to illness or its treatment. Such persons also provide more elaborated descriptions of their symptoms and they usually evaluate their present health status much worse than those with low level of neuroticism [40]. Thus, both the sensitivity to signals from inside one's body and the way they are interpreted may increase the tendency to concentrate on symptoms and to report them. The same mechanism may explain women's tendency to attribute any symptoms and sensations to menopause. A series of studies confirmed such assumptions and indicated an increased incidence of menopausal symptoms, first of all hot flushes and night sweats, among women with high anxiety scores [5] and high neuroticism scores [41–43]. It is worth noting that a high level of neuroticism was found also in these women who denied going through the menopausal transition and considered pregnancy as the only explanation for the lack of menstruation they had experienced for several weeks [44]. High level of neuroticism can predict hormonal therapy use as indicated by the results of Loekkegaard et al. [45] study. This effect becomes nonsignificant, though, when corrected for body mass index (BMI) and current smoking.

Another individual psychological characteristic that may affect ways symptoms are experienced is temperament, particularly one of its traits, i.e., emotional reactivity. The relationships between temperament and health were conceptualized as temperamental risk factor [46]. According to this theoretical approach temperament either increases the risk of ill health or coincides with it. In particular, those with high level of emotional reactivity can either develop and practice behaviors that increase the risk of ill health or concentrate more than others on bodily sensations. In both cases the increased use of medical consultations is observed. During the menopausal transition high emotional reactivity might lead to greater incidence of symptoms both experienced and reported by women. That was confirmed in some studies conducted both with users and nonusers of hormonal therapy [43]. In both groups women with high level of emotional reactivity reported more intense and more frequent menopausal symptoms.

The research results thus indicate that there are some psychological characteristics that predispose women to experience intense symptoms during the menopausal transition. Some of these features are related to personality and temperament, and include traits such as neuroticism and emotional reactivity that are strong biological determinants. Others, like attitudes towards menopause, are acquired during the growing-up within a particular social and cultural milieu. These two types of determinants create a unique composition of characteristics that together with the hormonal changes describe individual experience and evaluation of menopausal transition and its effects.

The analyses of menopausal transition become more informative when psychological characteristics of an individual are included. They have to consider also a broader context of lifetime events and women's developmental trajectories. Such conclusion comes from results of the longitudinal project with a participation of a cohort of women followed since their birth in 1946. Their psychological symptoms were recorded over a period of 6 years when the group was 47–52 years old [47]. The findings indicate that psychological distress was not affected by the concurrent menopausal status. The perimenopausal participants did not report more symptoms when compared with premenopausal counterparts with similar level of life stress. Thus there are rather events occurring across lifetime, psychological characteristics such as high level of neuroticism, and previous mental and physical health problems, and not only menopause, that impact on women's well-being in midlife.

Individual Conceptualization of Menopause

The issue of menopausal experiences should be discussed within the perspective of an individual. The increased interest in such analyses of menopause is documented in the literature [4, 5, 48]. Thus the focus is not only on hormonal changes, a woman's health and possible health-related outcomes, but also on perception, expectations, and individual decisions related to menopause. Therefore it can be assumed that factors which determine the course of the transition should include one more factor, i.e., how a woman conceptualizes the menopause. This conceptualization of menopause together with biological processes, including hormonal changes, affects the way menopause is experienced. These relationships are presented in Fig. 25.3.

As it can be seen in Fig. 25.3, the crucial role for the way menopause is experienced is given to individual appraisal of menopause. The appraisal is based on knowledge and beliefs about menopause, both related to the course, outcomes, and more general consequences of menopausal transition. Thus more positive or more negative appraisals can be formed.

The knowledge and beliefs are both related to social and to cultural context. It is the social and cultural milieu where the beliefs are created and, at the same time, the evidence-based knowledge on

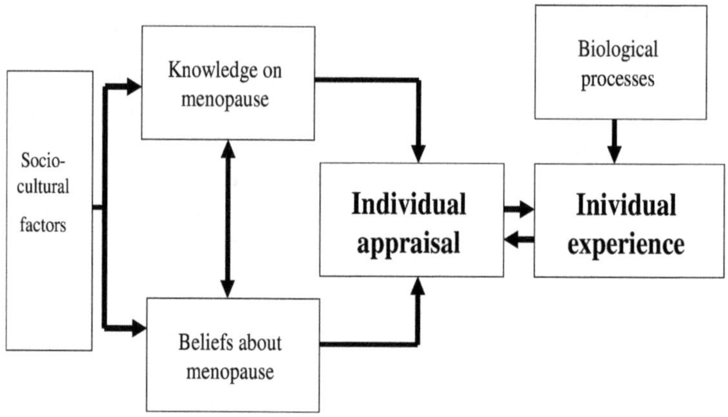

Fig. 25.3 Individual conceptualization of menopause and its impact on how menopause is experienced. The diagram shows that a woman's menopausal experience depends on her appraisal of menopause, i.e., her knowledge and beliefs developed within the particular sociocultural context. It also indicates that menopausal experiences might change the appraisal. *Source*: Unpublished

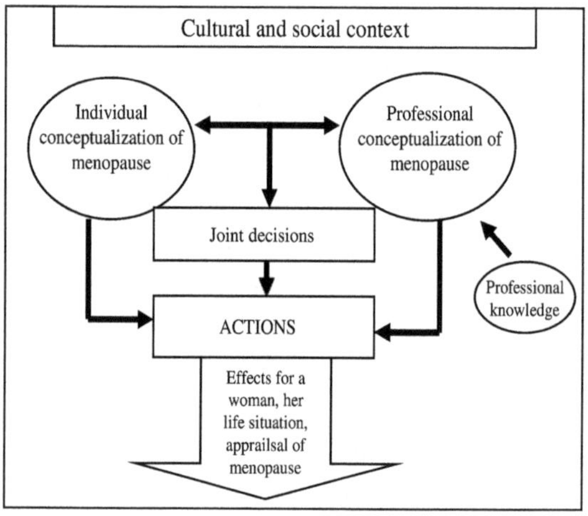

Fig. 25.4 "Two perspectives—one system": Professional and individual conceptualization of menopause. The diagram indicates that women's conceptualization of menopause should be considered during doctor–patient consultation for menopausal problems as the individual appraisal might affect the woman's decisions and actions. *Source*: Unpublished

menopause is provided. Each woman assimilates elements from both sources and uses them to form her own view on menopause or her own attitude—appraisal as named here. As indicated in the review of studies [38] on relationships between attitudes towards menopause and symptoms, women with more negative attitudes report more symptoms. Thus appraisal affects the experience, which in turn might impact on actions that are taken by women—for example searching a medical consultation for the symptoms and pursuing hormonal therapy. In Fig. 25.3 the appraisal–experience relationship is reciprocal. It is plausible that actual experiences while in the transitional period change the appraisal. Findings related to age differences in views on menopause [38] illustrate that mechanism.

A woman's conceptualization of menopause is confronted with the professional, knowledge-based conceptualization. Both are activated during the medical consultation for menopausal symptoms. In patient–doctor interaction information is shared and decisions are made. In the menopause-related context such decisions concern actions that can be taken to deal with symptoms experienced by a woman. These actions should be agreed upon and accepted by a woman. These actions are also influenced by sociocultural factors, for example by the quality of medical services, access to modern medication, and approach to management of menopause that is typical for a certain society. The effects of actions which have been agreed upon and implemented should be considered by both the patient and her doctor. All these links are presented in Fig. 25.4.

Within the approach proposed here, all actions taken within the framework of medical consultation for menopausal symptoms, hormonal therapy being one of those, have narrow and wide effects. These actions can alleviate the symptoms, which is considered as their narrow effect. By alleviating the symptoms these actions can also change the way a woman functions in her environment. Such change might bring about a new perception of menopause, which in turn might be considered as a wide effect leading to modification of individual appraisal and menopause-related beliefs. Research findings indicate that biological factors are not enough to understand individuals' experiences during menopausal transition [5] and definitely not enough to understand individual conceptualization of menopause. When this conceptualization is not taken into consideration by professionals, then the doctor–patient interaction and cooperation might be jeopardized. If the prescribed actions are not in concordance with the individual conceptualization of menopause, their effects may be very weak, as the patient, who recently started to be regarded as the subject in the menopause-related decision-making process [48], might decide not to take any of the prescribed actions.

The discrepancy between individual and professional views on menopause is interestingly illustrated by the results of the European Menopause Survey 2005 [49], a study conducted in seven countries: Belgium, France, Germany, the Netherlands, Spain, Switzerland, and the United Kingdom, with over 4,000 women examined. Although majority of the study population reported experiencing menopausal symptoms (severe ones in 63 % of the participants), and agreed that severe symptoms should be treated and hormonal treatment could alleviate the symptoms, the current use of hormonal therapy for these symptoms was 20 % on average in all the seven countries. At the same time the professional medical societies in these countries recommended administration of hormonal therapy for severe menopausal symptoms. What is more, nearly 60 % of the participants did not take any treatment at that time. Women knew about the benefits of medication, such as symptom alleviation and improvement of well-being and quality of life, but at the same time they considered risk related to hormonal treatment. The risk–benefit balance influenced their decisions about medication. When confronted with the option of hormonal treatment for their symptoms, women from the study decided not to pursue such therapy, mainly due to the increased risk of cancer. Even if doctors advised hormonal compounds, 57 % of women who had decided to alleviate their symptoms would not feel confident to use hormones, and would prefer other nonhormonal treatment.

Psychological Intervention During Menopausal Transition

Previous analyses indicate the need for multifactorial approach to women's experiences of the menopause as there are more factors that influence the menopausal transition than the hormonal changes alone. There is a substantial knowledge within health psychology on nonbiological factors related to the onset of illness, success of treatment, behavioral risk for particular health problems, and role of personality, personal resources, and social support in health and disease. Psychological theories are called upon in a variety of programs aimed at promotion of healthy lifestyle and at treatment. The search through the literature indicates that these hold true for management of menopausal transition, as well. Cognitive behavioral framework is often used in the analyses of menopausal symptoms, and the same approach is applied in interventions designed to decrease the incidence and severity of symptoms.

An interesting theoretical conceptualization of vasomotor symptoms was recently provided by Hunter and Mann [50], who proposed a cognitive model of hot flushes and night sweats. According to the assumptions of this model, hot flushes and night sweats are related to four types of determinants. The first type is the information input, which points to the relationship between the withdrawal of estrogen and central thermoregulation. The second one—the detection and attribution—refers to the processes by which physiological event is perceived as a hot flush and/or night sweat. The third type is the cognitive appraisal, which includes interpretations of hot flushes that might be considered difficult, disturbing, etc. The fourth one—behavior—describes strategies that either ameliorate or exacerbate vasomotor symptoms. The model describes the sequence of events and also points to the factors that affect hot flush/night sweat sensations. Thus estrogen withdrawal related to menopausal status changes the thermoneutral zone and thus even small variation in temperature triggers thermoregulatory mechanisms and sweating occurs, which is perceived as a hot flush. Whether such sensation is perceived as the hot flush, and how often it is perceived this way, can be affected by selective attention and focus on the body. As indicated earlier in this chapter, neuroticism may increase the incidence of hot flushes. Such relationship between negative affectivity and hot flush detection is envisaged in the cognitive model as well. The perceived hot flush could be rated as a severe one and, if so, would initiate help-seeking or other behavior. The model indicates that hot flush and night sweat ratings can be strongly affected by beliefs related to menopause and its symptoms. The model considers some additional factors that affect this input–detection/attribution–appraisal–behavior sequence. These include such external or internal triggers as hot drinks, spicy food, stress in the input phase, depressed mood, anxiety, and negative affectivity in the detection/attribution and appraisal phases [50].

The cognitive model of menopausal hot flushes and night sweats serves as a theoretical base for intervention, namely, cognitive behavioral therapy (CBT) for menopausal symptoms [51, 52]. In patients whose symptoms followed breast cancer treatment, group CBT reduced frequency of hot flushes and night sweats, and such effects were maintained 3 months after the intervention [51]. A significant reduction in negative beliefs about the menopause was observed as well.

The cognitive approach to menopause and intervention based on it assume that beliefs and automatic thoughts related to the menopause are important for frequency and severity of symptoms. The contents of such beliefs might refer to ways the symptoms are controlled by women and are perceived in social situations by other persons. Some studies indicate that the severity of experienced and reported symptoms is related to the perceived control over them. Thus, those who believe in little control over symptoms report more severe and frequent hot flushes [53, 54]. Such evaluation of hot flushes may also be accompanied by another set of beliefs, i.e., a variety of catastrophic thoughts indicating the negative interpretation of symptoms and their negative effects on women [55]. The belief that other persons would react negatively to menopausal symptoms might be a source of distress for women, and thus might increase the experienced severity of hot flushes, and prompt the avoidance of social situations. The issue whether other persons do perceive a hot flush negatively and react to a person experiencing it in a negative way has been addressed in the study with 25–45-year-old men and women [56]. Perceptions of the hot flush were measured by a scenario describing a situation at work and a female colleague 45–55 years of age whose face was redder than usual and who started to sweat. Although the sample had more negative views on menopause than perimenopausal women, the reactions to the hot flush were either positive or neutral. Only 10 % of participants stated that they would feel uncomfortable during the interaction. The symptoms described in the scenario were more often attributed to emotions (red face) or health problems (sweating) than to hormonal changes. Despite such findings that question negative beliefs of menopausal women, severe hot flushes are often considered very embarrassing and such perception underlies the search for remedies.

Conclusions

Hormonal changes that are the biological base of the cessation of menstruation are only one of the several factors that influence the menopausal transition. Although withdrawal of estrogen triggers vasomotor symptoms, the way they are experienced is shaped by social, cultural, and psychological factors. Some psychological characteristics, e.g., the level of neuroticism or an individual's attitude towards menopause and aging, can affect the peri- and postmenopausal period. Methodologically sound studies conducted with the community-based samples indicate that the effects of menopausal transition are not that negative as expected or foreseen both by women and men. Nevertheless, there is a lot of strongly held beliefs concerning the negative effects of menopause. As social cognitions proved to be important for individual appraisal of menopause, they should be recognized and considered as the target for intervention. The way an individual woman conceptualizes menopause might affect what she experiences during the transition, and what she does to deal with her symptoms. As women are more aware of factors that affect health, they become more active agents in the decision processes related to their health, including menopause and its management, and more prone to get involved in health-related behaviors that affect their well-being and quality of life.

References

1. World Health Organization Scientific Group. Research on the menopause in the 1990s. WHO Technical Report Series 866. Geneva: WHO; 1996.
2. Soules MR, Sherman S, Parrott E, Rebar R, Santoro N, Utian W, et al. Stages of reproductive aging workshop (STRAW). J Womens Health Gend Based Med. 2001;10:843–8.
3. Formanek R, editor. The meanings of menopause. Historical, medical and clinical perspectives. Hillsdale, NJ: The Analytic Press; 1990.
4. Komesaroff P, Rothfield P, Daly J, editors. Reinterpreting menopause. Cultural and philosophical issues. New York: Routledge; 1997.
5. Hunter M, Rendall M. Bio-psycho-socio-cultural perspectives on menopause. Best Pract Res Clin Obstet Gynecol. 2007;21:261–74.
6. World Health Organization. Mental health aspects of women's reproductive health. A global review of the literature. Geneva: WHO Press; 2009.
7. Soares CN, Warren M, editors. The menopausal transition. Interface between gynecology and psychiatry. Basel: Karger; 2009.
8. Freeman EW, Sherif K. Prevalence of hot flushes and night sweats around the world: a systematic review. Climacteric. 2007;10:197–214.
9. Ziv-Gal A, Flaws JA. Factors that may influence the experience of hot flushes by healthy middle-aged women. J Womens Health. 2010;19:1905–14.
10. Sievert LL. Menopause: a biocultural perspective. Piscataway, NJ: Rutgers University Press; 2006.
11. Bielawska-Batorowicz E. Wyst powanie objawów uznawanych za typowe dla menopauzy u kobiet i m czyzn w wieku 45-55 lat. Przegl Menopauz. 2005;4(1):53–60.
12. Gold EB, Sternfeld B, Kelsey JL, Brown C, Mouton C, Reame N, et al. Relation of demographic and lifestyle factors to symptoms in a multi-racial/ethnic population of women 40–55 years of age. Am J Epidemiol. 2000; 152:463–73.
13. Pinkerton JAV, Stovall DW. Reproductive aging, menopause and health outcomes. Ann N Y Acad Sci. 2010; 1204:169–78.
14. Ferguson SK, Soares CN, Harlow BL. Depression during the perimenopausal transition: what have we learned from epidemiological studies? In: Soares CN, Warren M, editors. The menopausal transition. Interface between gynecology and psychiatry. Basel: Karger; 2009. p. 66–76.
15. Sherwin BB. Estrogen and cognitive functioning in women: lessons we have learned. Behav Neurosci. 2012;126:123–7.
16. Payne JL, Teitelbaum Palmer J, Joffe H. A reproductive subtype of depression: conceptualizing models and moving towards etiology. Harv Rev Psychiatry. 2009;17:72–86.
17. Nicol-Smith L. Causality, menopause, and depression: a critical review of the literature. BMJ. 1996;16:1229–32.
18. Avis NE. Depression during the menopausal transition. Psychol Women Quart. 2003;27:91–100.
19. Dennerstein L, Lehert P, Burger H, Dudley E. Mood and the menopausal transition. J Nerv Ment Dis. 1999;187:685–91.
20. Maartens LWF, Knottnerus JA, Pop VJ. Menopausal transition and increased depressive symptomatology. A community based prospective study. Maturitas. 2002;42:195–200.
21. Hunter M, Bettersby R, Whitehead M. Relationships between psychological symptoms, somatic complaints and menopausal status. Maturitas. 1986;8:217–28.
22. Wojnar M, Drózdz W, Araszkiewicz A, Szymanski W, Nawacka-Pawlaczyk D, Urbanski R, et al. Assessment and prevalence of depression in women 45–55 years of age visiting gynecological clinics in Poland. Arch Womens Ment Health. 2003;6:193–201.
23. Reed SD, Ludman EJ, Newton KM, Grothaus LC, LaCroix AZ, Nekhlyudov L. Depressive symptoms and menopausal burden in the midlife. Maturitas. 2009;62:306–10.

24. Brown JP, Gallicchio L, Flaws JA, Tracy JK. Relations among menopausal symptoms, sleep disturbance and depressive symptoms in midlife. Maturitas. 2009;62:184–9.
25. Bielawska-Batorowicz E. Stres, objawy i przekonania dotycz ce menopauzy a obni ony nastrój u kobiet wieku 45-55 lat. Próba weryfikacji zmodyfikowanego psychospołecznego modelu depresji w okresie okołomenopauzalnym. Przegl Menopauz. 2006;5:68–74.
26. Woods NF, Mitchell ES. Pathways to depressed mood for midlife women: observations from the Seattle Midlife Women's Health Study. Res Nurs Health. 1997;20:119–29.
27. Greene JG. The psychosocial vulnerability model of the menopause. In: Aso T, Yanaihara T, Fujimoto S, editors. The menopause at the millenium. The proceedings of the 9th international menopause society world congress on the menopause. New York: The Parthenon Publishing Group; 2000. p. 536–9.
28. Lipinska-Szałek A, Sobczuk A, Pertynski T, Stetkiewicz T, Szymczak W. Wpływ czynników biologicznych i psychospołecznych na psychiczne aspekty okresu okołomenopauzalnego. Przegl Menopauz. 2003;2(6):55–61.
29. Vesco KK, Haney EM, Humphrey L, Fu R, Nelson HD. Influence of menopause on mood: a systematic review of cohort studies. Climacteric. 2007;10:448–65.
30. Warga CL. Menopause and the mind. New York: Free; 1999.
31. Mitchell ES, Woods NF. Midlife women's attributions about perceived memory changes: observation from the Seattle Midlife Women's Health Study. J Womens Health Gend Based Med. 2001;10:351–62.
32. Schaafsma M, Homewood J, Taylor A. Subjective cognitive complaints at menopause associated with declines in performance of verbal memory and attentional processes. Climacteric. 2010;13:84–98.
33. Piauilino DC, Bueno OFA, Tufik S, Bittencourt LR, Santos-Silva R, Hachul H. The prospective and retrospective memory questionnaire: a population-based random sampling study. Memory. 2010;18:413–26.
34. Henderson VW. Action of estrogens in the aging brain: dementia and cognitive aging. Biochim Biophys Acta. 2010;1800(10):1077–83.
35. Berger G. Menopause and culture. London: Pluto; 1999.
36. Bitzer J, Alder J. Cultural and ethnic influences on the menopause transition. In: Soares CN, Warren M, editors. The menopausal transition. Interface between gynecology and psychiatry. Basel: Karger; 2009. p. 41–9.
37. Rice PL. Pog laus, tsis coj khaub ncaws lawm: the meaning of menopause in Hmong women. J Reprod Infant Psychol. 1995;13:79–92.
38. Ayers B, Forshaw M, Hunter MS. The impact of attitudes towards menopause on women's symptom experience: a systematic review. Maturitas. 2010;65:28–36.
39. Shu BC, Luh WM, Li SM, Lu SY. Self-concept and menopause among mid-life women: a survey in southern Taiwan. Maturitas. 2007;57:132–8.
40. Williams PG. Personality and illness behavior. In: Vollrath ME, editor. Handbook of personality and health. Chichester: Wiley; 2006. p. 137–56.
41. Bosworth HB, Bastian LA, Rimer BK, Siegler IC. Coping styles and personality domains related to menopausal stress. Womens Health Issues. 2003;13:32–8.
42. Elavsky S, McAuley E. Personality, menopausal symptoms, and physical activity outcomes. Pers Indivd Dif. 2009;46:123–8.
43. Bielawska-Batorowicz E. Temperament, osobowość i styl radzenia sobie ze stresem a cz sto i intensywno objawów menopauzalnych. Przegl d Menopauzalny. 2007;6(2):70–6.
44. Pramataroff V, Leppert K, Strauss B. Denial of climacteric – a pilot study of a common clinical phenomenon. J Psychosom Obstet Gynecol. 2007;28:135–9.
45. Loekkegaard E, Eplov LF, Køster A, Garde K. Description of women's personality traits and psychological vulnerability prior to choosing hormone replacement therapy. Arch Womens Ment Health. 2002;5:23–31.
46. Strelau J. Temperament jako regulator zachowania z perspektywy półwiecza bada . Gda sk: Gda skie Wydawnictwo Psychologiczne; 2006.
47. Kuh D, Hardy R, Rodgers B, Wadsworth MEJ. Lifetime risk factors for women's psychological distress in midlife. Soc Sci Med. 2002;55:1957–73.
48. Murtagh MJ, Hepworth J. Narrative review of changing medical and feminist perspectives on menopause: from femininity and aging to risk and choice. Psychol Health Med. 2005;10:276–90.
49. Genazzani AR, Schneider HPG, Panay N, Nijland EA. The European menopause survey 2005: women's perceptions on the menopause and postmenopausal hormone therapy. Gynecol Endocrinol. 2006;22:369–75.
50. Hunter MS, Mann E. A cognitive model of menopausal hot flushes and night sweats. J Psychosom Res. 2010;69:491–501.
51. Hunter MS, Coventry S, Hamed H, Fentiman I, Grunfeld EA. Evaluation of a group cognitive behavioural intervention for women suffering from menopausal symptoms following breast cancer. Psychooncology. 2009;18:560–3.
52. Mann E, Smith M, Hellier J, Hunter MS. A randomized controlled trial of a cognitive behavioural intervention for women who have menopausal symptoms following breast cancer treatment (MENOS 1): trial protocol. BMC Cancer. 2011;11:44. doi:10.1186/1471-2407-11-44.

53. Chedraui P, Pèrez-López FR, Aguirre W, Calle A, Hidalgo L, Leon-Leon P. Perceived control over menopausal hot flushes in mid-aged women. Gynecol Endocrinol. 2010;26:607–11.
54. Pimenta F, Leal I, Maroco J, Ramos C. Perceived control, lifestyle, health, socio-demographic factors and menopause: impact on hot flashes and night sweats. Maturitas. 2011;69:338–42.
55. Reynolds F. Relationships between catastrophic thoughts, perceived control and distress during menopausal hot flushes: exploring the correlates of a questionnaire measure. Maturitas. 2000;36:113–22.
56. Smith MJ, Mann E, Mirza A, Hunter MS. Men and women's perceptions of hot flushes within social situations: are menopausal women's negative beliefs valid? Maturitas. 2011;69:57–62.

Chapter 26
Cognitive Decline in Menopause

Cristina Larroy and Rosa Vera

Key Points

- Cognitive decline in menopause affects episodic memory and executive functions.
- These domains are postulated to be vulnerable to and modulated by exposure to endogenous and exogenous estrogens.
- The significant amount of research that studies the relationship between estrogens and the cognitive performance in menopausal women has not produced consistent results in the last two decades.
- Further investigation taking into account different aspects as cultural items, type of menopause (natural or surgical), type of impairment in the cognitive functioning, etc. is needed to finally answer the questions regarding the role of estrogens and hormone replacement therapy on cognition.

Keywords Cognitive decline • Menopause • Estrogen • Hormone therapy • Cognitive performance

Abbreviations

THR	Therapy of hormone replacement
HT	Hormone therapy
RT	Reaction time
ET	Estrogen replacement
ETR	Estrogen replacement therapy
WHS	Women's Health Study
MT	Menopausal transition

C. Larroy (✉)
Faculty of Psychology, Department of Clinical Psychology,
Universidad Complutense de Madrid, Pozuelo de Alarcon, 28223 Madrid, Spain
e-mail: clarroyg@ucm.es

R. Vera
Legal and Forensic Psychology, Vertices Psicólogos,
Avda. Lazarejo, 106, Las Rozas, 28232 Madrid, Spain
e-mail: rosa.vera@verticespsicologos.es

C.J.H. Martin et al. (eds.), *Nutrition and Diet in Menopause*, Nutrition and Health,
DOI 10.1007/978-1-62703-373-2_26, © Springer Science+Business Media New York 2013

Introduction

Menopause is the permanent cessation of menstruation due to the depletion of ovarian follicular activity, a depletion that is part of the natural aging process in women.

It usually begins between 45 and 55 years of age. At least 50 % of menopausal women suffer from symptoms that are either irritating or very irritating to them, which implicate around 135,000 people per year in Spain. However, information about menopause, its associated symptoms, causes, and effects is very poor. Currently, 61 % of menopausal women do not know that symptoms such as osteoporosis, vascular diseases, or dysphoric states are related to menopause [1].

According to data provided by the European Commission [2], by the year 2050, it is expected that 30 % of Europeans—one in three Europeans—will be over 65 years of age, of which 11 % of these will be over 80 years of age [2]. The percentage of the female population between 45 and 60 years continues increasing gradually. The expected longevity of the population is also increasing (see Table 26.1 and Fig. 26.1).

The increased expected longevity results in women spending almost a third of their lives in a postmenopausal stage. Hence, we are talking about a very important and universally relevant problem due to the amount of people affected and the duration of time involved. The climacteric period is associated with symptoms producing long-term consequences on the health of women, not only at a physical level like hot flushes, alterations in the genitourinary system, skin problems, osteoporosis, cardiopathy, obesity, hypertension, headache, back pain, constipations, and so on but also at a psychological level like tension, irritability, anxiety, sadness, concentration problems, lack of self-confidence, sleep changes, libido changes, and memory problems.

The term "menopause" literally signifies a woman's last natural menstruation and menopause is diagnosed following a year without menstrual flow. However, usually it is used in an incorrect way to

Table 26.1 Evolution and projection * of life expectancy at birth, 1980–2020

	Male	Female	Difference
1980	72.5	78.6	6.1
1985	73.3	79.7	6.4
1990	73.4	80.5	7.1
1995	74.5	81.7	7.2
2000	76.1	82.8	6.7
2005	77.0	83.5	6.5
2010*	78.2	84.6	6.4
2015*	79.2	85.4	6.2
2020*	80.0	86.1	6.1

Source: INE. Instituto Nacional de Estadística España

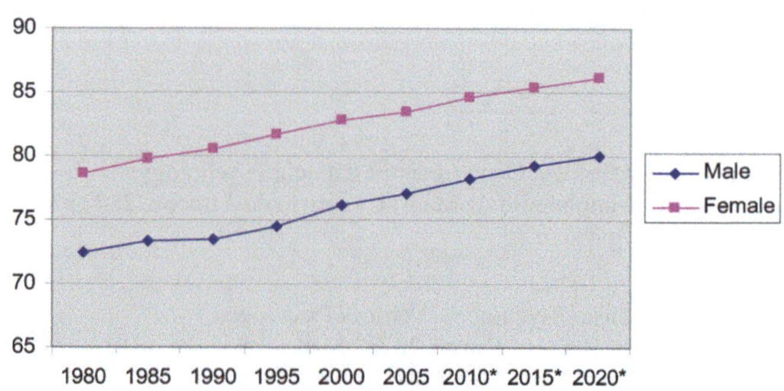

Fig. 26.1 Graphic evolution and projection * of life expectancy at birth, 1980–2020*. *Source*: INE. Instituto Nacional de Estadística España. Public data, no permission required

Table 26.2 Symptoms associated with menopause [3]

Physical symptoms	Psychological symptoms
*Hot flushes	*Burden
*Genitourinary abnormalities	*Tension
*Vaginal atrophy	*Irritability
*Urethra and bladder disorders	*Anxiety
*Skin alterations	*Sadness
*Osteoporosis	*Concentration disorders
*Ischemic heart disease	*Self-esteem problems
*Obesity	*Memory loss
*Hypertension	*Sleep disorders
*Headache, back, neck troubles	*Loss of libido
*Varicose veins	
*Tingling	

Source: Larroy, C. (2004). *Trastornos específicos de la mujer*. Madrid: Síntesis©
With permission of author

refer to the years prior and immediately following this last period [1]. The symptomatology most frequently associated with menopause is summarized in Table 26.2 [3]. Symptoms are considered primary (like hot flushes) or secondary (like anxiety or insomnia).

According to data provided [4], over half of women have mood disorders and almost 7 % of women suffer from these symptoms severely.

The traditional biomedical perspective posits that a "menopausal syndrome" is characterized by hot flashes, severe headaches, weight gain, vaginal atrophy, loss of firmness to the chest area, coldness in one's extremities, irritability, depression, and sleep disorders [5]. Nevertheless, they suggested that the researchers were not able to demonstrate the normative existence of a menopausal syndrome.

Symptoms usually do not co-occur in all menopausal women and no symptoms are consistently more frequent in postmenopausal women than in premenopausal women of a similar age. The only consistent symptoms associated with menopause include vasomotor symptoms (hot flashes, night sweats)—although these are more common in women with surgical intervention than in women with natural menopause—and vaginal changes (vaginal dryness, for example). These and other symptoms tend to occur more frequently in pre-menopause than when there is a complete cessation of menstruation. That occurs even in the case of hot flashes, which is apparently the most common symptom associated with women in this period of their lives. The underlying mechanisms are very complex due to the influence of endogenous hormones, which can vary both the frequency and intensity of hot flashes. They also can be influenced by psychological factors and may further be mediated by cultural variables.

Despite a growing body of interdisciplinary literature on menopause, there remains a dearth of comparative information regarding how women from differing socioeconomic status think about menopause, talk about it, and experience reproductive aging [6]. Sixty-one menopausal women of varied ethnic groups and or varied socioeconomic status in a Midwestern state in the USA were asked about the different meanings and experiences of menopause. The sample was as heterogeneous as possible in terms of socioeconomic and cultural factors. Women answered questions about their experiences of menopause (signs, symptoms, duration of experience, general feelings …), about external influences (what they had heard about menopause from their gynecologists, friends, family, etc.), how they experienced menopause in the context of family and work, and how the social context (socioeconomic status and ethnicity) impacts on menopause. They also provided information about the relationship between menopause and aging and the changes in their body. African American women and Chicanas, particularly working-class women, viewed menopause as a positive experience, whereas many middle-class white American women expressed more negative feelings. African American women were more likely than European Americans to talk about menopause only with same-ethnicity and/or same-sex friends. The researchers affirmed that, in this study, commonalities among women by gender and differences among women by ethnicity and socioeconomic status are exposed. The presence of ethnic differences underscores the need for more comparative studies on reproductive aging both in the USA and abroad [7].

Clearly, culture differentially influences how women experience symptoms related to menopause, both physical and psychological, in different parts of the world. Women perceive and live this experience differently, depending on their personal characteristics, psychosocial context, etc. Nevertheless, there are certain changes that can be classified as "universal."

Despite all the scientific research that has been conducted, it is still difficult to determine whether symptoms are due to the menopausal transition, due to the effects of age, or possibly due to an interaction between both factors. There is clear evidence that the decrease in estrogens causes vasomotor symptoms, urogenital atrophy, and bone loss, but the remaining symptoms may not be related to menopause and may be caused by psychological and/or cultural factors. According to research, women who perceive menopause to be either a positive or a neutral stage in life and who do not perceive it as a disease are more likely to experience the onset of menopause as a relief (36.6 %) and not as a loss (9 %). The perception of menopause status seems to depend on cultural factors and on personal or vicarious experiences. Negative attitudes (beliefs and expectations) before menopause could determine the frequency and severity of physical and psychological symptoms [8].

Cognitive Decline

Menopause has been associated with an increased risk of dementia and a growing body of research has studied the effects of reproductive senescence in cognitive function. However, menopause-related research does not paint a clear picture. This may be due to methodological limitations as many studies do not implement a randomized and a double-blind procedure and instead use heterogeneous samples (including variability in the combination of surgically and naturally menopausal women) with variability in the cognitive tests administered to participants and variability in the hormone treatment regimen, or they do not mention the etiology of menopause.

Nevertheless, it is postulated that the decline in sex steroids is an important factor in the production of different disorders, including mood and cognitive disorders (e.g., cognitive impairment). Studies suggest that ovarian hormone loss, which is associated with menopause, has deleterious consequences on cognition and hormone therapy (HT) could mitigate these effects [9].

Cognitive aging particularly affects episodic memory and executive functions, and these domains are postulated to be vulnerable to and modulated by exposure to endogenous and exogenous estrogens [10].

Compelling evidence from studies using humans, nonhuman primates, and rodents suggests that ovarian sex-steroid hormones can have rapid and profound effects on memory, attention, executive functions, and regions of the brain that mediate these processes, such as the hippocampus and prefrontal cortex. This seems to be crucial to determine how ovarian hormones, especially estrogens, modulate the physiology of the hippocampus and prefrontal cortex, and this is further crucial to the debate regarding the effects of reproductive aging and hormone treatment on cognitive function [11].

Declining estrogen levels during the menopause period, resulting in a number of changes throughout the body, have an impact at different levels [12, 13].

The brain is an organ with a large number of estrogenic receptors. Concerning the action of gonadal steroids in the central nervous system (more than 90 % of the estrogenic receptors are outside of the sexual organs), there is a high number of gonadal steroids in the brain [14]. Estrogens may influence cognitive function in different ways. Administration of estrogen increases cerebral and cerebellar blood flow, increases glucose metabolism, and enhances cholinergic activity, which is fundamental for learning and memory [15].

Since there are specific estrogen receptors in the central nervous system, it is hypothesized that the lack of these receptors causes mental and behavioral disorders during menopause. However, the mechanism by which estrogenic deficiency causes changes in cognitive and affective functions is not well known.

Estrogens may influence cognitive function in different ways. Estrogens have multiple neuroprotective effects including stimulating the production of dendrites, stimulating synaptogenesis, increasing the concentration of acetylcholine transferase in cholinergic neurons, increasing the activation of neurotrophins, and activating the mechanism of amyloidogenesis—this mechanism stimulates the processing of the non-precursor protein amiloide, resulting in increased activity of the &-secretase and protection from damage and cell death induced by oxidative stress [16].

The Use of THR for the Cognitive Decline in Menopause

Different authors posit a decrement in cognitive performance following menopause [17]. These authors, trying to prove that, designed a study, in which a battery of motor and cognitive tests was administered to 24 premenopausal women (21–47 years old) and 33 postmenopausal women (41–59 years old) to examine whether the aging over time process in some cognitive functions differed. In some cognitive tests, including driving simulation, reaction time (RT), and some visuospatial tests, there was a significant acceleration in the deterioration of functioning following menopause. The researchers suggest that this acceleration might be associated with a lack of gonadal hormones or other reproduction-related factors that may play a protective role against age-related deterioration in some cognitive functions in women.

The growing interest in studying the influence of sex hormones on cognitive performance has focused attention on hormone replacement therapy (HRT) [18]. The question is whether HT will impact every woman as she enters reproductive senescence. These findings have wide implications for future research and treatments for optimizing HT for menopausal women.

The pros and cons of estrogen therapy in postmenopausal women continue to be a major topic of debate in women's health. Much of this debate focuses on the potential benefits vs. harm of estrogen therapy on the brain and the risks for cognitive impairment associated with aging and Alzheimer's disease. Many animal and human studies suggest that estrogens can have significant beneficial effects on brain aging and cognition and, further, reduce the risk of Alzheimer's-related dementia; however, others disagree. Important discoveries have been made, and hypotheses have emerged that may explain some of the inconsistencies.

Many researchers have carried out different studies or meta-analyses on the possible effect of HRT on cognitive performance. The potential long-term benefit of estrogen replacement therapy (ET) in preventing osteoporosis and heart disease has been reasonably well established. However, the favorable effects of ET on cognitive function and on the prevention of dementia in the elderly are not well established and there is a need to revitalize this area of clinical research.

The use of estrogen replacement therapy has been associated in several studies with a lower risk of Alzheimer's and lower risk of deterioration of cognitive performance in postmenopausal women. This is a controversial issue since other studies have shown that estrogen therapy is not only useful in limiting the progression of Alzheimer's disease but that therapy applied after 65 years can even be harmful (IWH study). Nevertheless, results are quite different regarding the application of HT as a method to improve cognitive function following menopause.

This chapter presents a review of several studies on the use of external estrogens on cognition. Divergent results found in recent years are described below.

Studies that defend the use of HRT to improve cognitive performance following menopause agree that the effects are not universal and may depend on several factors, including woman's age, type of menopause (natural vs. surgical), cultural factors, etc. [19].

Neuro-protective effects of estrogens have been demonstrated consistently in cellular and animal studies; conversely, findings from studies using human participants remain inconsistent. Researchers reviewing the studies conducted in this field concluded that evidence suggests that estrogens may have beneficial, neutral, or even detrimental effects on the brain depending on the age at the time of treatment, type of menopause (natural vs. medically or surgically induced), or stage of menopause. The comparison of women who underwent bilateral oophorectomy with a control group of women provided evidence for a sizeable neuro-protective effect of estrogens for women less than 50 years of age. Several case–control studies and cohort studies also showed neuro-protective effects in women who received estrogen treatment (ET) in the early postmenopausal stage (most commonly 50–60 years of age). The majority of women in these observational studies had undergone natural menopause and were treated for the relief of menopausal symptoms. However, recent clinical trials by the Women's Health Initiative (WHI Study) showed that women who initiated ET alone or in combination with a progestin in the late postmenopausal stage (65–79 years of age) experienced an increased risk of dementia and cognitive decline, regardless of the type of menopause. Hence, researchers hypothesize that the neuroprotective effects of estrogens depend on the age at the time of administration, type of menopause, and stage of menopause. Therefore, women who underwent bilateral oophorectomy before the onset of menopause or women who experienced premature or early natural menopause should be considered for hormonal treatment if they are approximately before the age of 51 years. Other researchers have also defended this position [20, 21].

In line with these findings, other researchers [9] suggest that HT may be helpful in alleviating cognitive decline in women with surgical menopause but not in women who experience natural menopause. Hence, these beneficial effects are only evident after surgical menopause.

From a sample of 3,130 women who had a natural menopause [22], it was concluded that current HT was associated with better performance in certain cognitive domains but that these associations depended on the duration and type of treatment used. They found no evidence that HT initiated close to the onset of menopause had a beneficial effect on cognitive function in later life.

Regarding the effects of HT on neural systems, several researchers [23] base their investigation on a theory, which posits that estrogens influence cognition by activating and inactivating different neural systems. In particular, this review describes findings that estrogens bias strategies that an individual selects to solve certain cognitive and behavioral tasks, thereby regulating what an individual learns and not merely how much an individual learns. In other words, rather than acting to enhance all cognitive functions, estrogens might act quite specifically to enhance some cognitive domains and to impair others. Thus, the risks and benefits of HRT need to be weighed more broadly to include the possibility that only some aspects of cognition may be sensitive to improvement by estrogen.

Estrogen therapy may also have important neurochemical effects, direct effects on the vasculature of the body, and effects on the production of free radicals, which can be toxic to neurons [24].

Similarly, it has been found that the activation of estrogens in the hippocampus resulted in memory improvements [25]. Results suggest that the positive effect of ET may be in part produced through modulation in frontal lobe functioning under difficult task conditions. Moreover, the cholinergic hypothesis posits that the beneficial effects of estrogens on brain aging and cognition are related to interactions with cholinergic projections [26].

Researches on the cholinergic hypothesis, specifically, evidence that the beneficial effects of estrogens on brain aging and cognition are related to interactions with cholinergic projections emanating from the basal forebrain [27]. Cholinergic projections play an important role in learning and attentional processes, and their function is known to decline with advanced age and in association with Alzheimer's disease. Evidence suggests that many of the effects of estrogens on neural plasticity, on neural function, and on cognitive performance are related to or rely upon interactions with these cholinergic projections. However, studies also suggest that the effectiveness of estrogen therapy decreases with age and time after loss of ovarian function. They propose a model in which deficits in basal forebrain cholinergic function contribute to age-related changes in the response to estrogen therapy. Based on this model, they propose that cholinergic enhancing drugs, used in combination with an appropriate estrogen-containing drug regimen, may be a viable therapeutic strategy for use in older postmenopausal women with early evidence of mild cognitive decline.

By contrast, a meta-analysis [28] was conducted to critically examine how different aspects of memory functions have been evaluated in research related to menopause. Twenty articles on menopause and cognitive functioning published between 1991 and 2000 were reviewed. All studies included in the meta-analysis used groups with healthy women without dementia and evaluated specific aspects of cognitive functioning using standardized tests rather relying on self-reports of perceived functioning. All of the measures used to assess attention and concentration, verbal memory, learning and verbal expression, visual memory, concept formation, and reasoning were also reviewed. Findings from the different studies assessing attention and concentration demonstrate inconsistent results regarding hormone levels or menopausal status. Although five measures of verbal learning and memory have been considered, no unequivocal results have been reported for any one measure. Only one study found significant differences in measures of verbal expression between hormone therapy users and nonusers. In addition, no strong association between the level of estrogens and visual memory was identified in the studies reviewed. This analysis demonstrates that a wide variety of tests have been used, but a clear effect of exogenous hormone therapy on memory has not been found. It is suggested that verbal memory, visual memory, concept formation, and reasoning should be simultaneously investigated in future research, and that covariate measures of attention and concentration, verbal expression, and reasoning should also be included.

Observations that estrogens may affect verbal fluency and memory are further supported by studies of transsexuals. Sex change male-to-female transsexuals who were given estrogens performed better on short-term verbal memory tasks, but not on spatial ability tasks, compared to those who did not receive estrogens. Researchers concluded that estrogen treatment in sex change for male-to-female transsexuals has no influence on sex-typed aspect of cognition or memory [29].

It is believed that estrogen therapy is beneficial for cognitive functioning; nevertheless, there is no evidence to support the hypothesis that estrogen therapy protects women from the risk of developing Alzheimer's disease [30]. Similar conclusion: Clinical trial evidence suggests that therapy does not improve dementia symptoms in women with Alzheimer's disease and that estrogen-containing hormone therapy initiated after approximately 65 years of age increases the risk of dementia [31].

In order to examine how menopausal symptoms and estrogen therapy induced symptom relief and influenced cognition in early menopause, a cross-sectional study of 37 healthy, recently postmenopausal women with diverse menopausal symptoms was carried out [32]. Women were categorized as having low ($n=20$) or high symptoms ($n=17$) based on a validated symptom questionnaire. They completed mood and sleep questionnaires and underwent cognitive testing, including verbal memory tests, visual memory tests, emotional memory tests, and verbal fluency tests. Thirty-two of these women completed a second part of the study. Fourteen participants were randomly assigned to receive ET and 18 participants were randomly assigned to receive a placebo for 8 weeks. Before treatment and at 4 and 8 weeks, women completed the same measures as in the first part of the study. Results revealed that menopausal symptoms do not impair cognition. ET does not improve cognition despite alleviating symptoms and improving sleep in recently naturally menopausal women with diverse menopausal symptoms.

Working with 101 breast cancer patients and using 12 different cognitive tests [33], it has been found that the antiestrogen treatment with tamoxifen did not affect cognition and that hormonal changes did not appear to contribute to cognitive deficits in these patients during the first year following diagnosis. Antiestrogen treatment did not affect cognition, and the effects of induced menopause were more likely to be favorable. However, the possibility that some cognitive decline occurred in individual patients could not be excluded.

A four years longitudinal study of 2,362 participants from the Study of Women's Health Across the Nation was conducted to investigate on three domains: processing speed, verbal memory, and working memory in two periods [34]. They concluded that perimenopause was associated with a decrement in cognitive performance, characterized by women not being able to learn as well as they had during premenopause. Improvement rebounded to premenopausal levels in postmenopausal women, suggesting that menopause transition-related cognitive difficulties might be time limited. Hormone initiation prior to the final menstrual period had a beneficial effect whereas initiation after the final menstrual period had a detrimental effect on cognitive performance.

In healthy middle-aged and older participants (without the presence of dementia), the effects of estrogens on cognition can be tested through associations between serum concentrations of estrogens and estradiol. Several studies that evaluated associations between estrogen levels and cognitive performance on neuropsychological tests of episodic memory or executive functions, such as working memory (seven studies), were reviewed [10]. The results of clinical placebo-controlled trials of hormone therapy were also reviewed with objective measures in these cognitive functions (eight studies). Results were considered separately for the middle-aged women and for those in later years (age ≥ 65 years). There were no consistent associations between endogenous estrogen concentrations in serum and features of episodic memory or executive middle-aged women with natural menopause or in women after menopause. The results of clinical trials do not suggest a substantial impact of exogenous estrogens on episodic memory or executive functions. A quantitative synthesis of results from clinical trials supported the conclusion of no effect. There seems to be, according to these researchers, no benefit from the short-term exogenous hormones on cognition, yet their conclusions are clouded by the small number of studies that has been as yet conducted, the imprecise estimates of exposure to long-term estrogens, and the narrow range of neuropsychological tests implemented.

A recent study was conducted to investigate changes in the levels of cognitive symptoms (forgetting and difficulty concentrating) during the menopausal transition (MT) stages and during early postmenopause, including examining the effect of age [35]. Participants provided data during the late reproductive stage, early and late MT stages, or postmenopause ($n = 292$) stage, including menstrual calendars for staging the MT, annual health questionnaires examining social factors, morning urine samples assayed for gonadal hormones, and health diaries to rate symptoms completed several times each year. Patterns of cognitive symptoms were related to age, MT-related factors, symptoms, health-related factors, stress-related factors, and social factors with as many as 6,811 observations. The best predictors of forgetfulness when analyzed as individual covariates and in the multivariate model were age, hot flushes, anxiety, depressed mood, perceived stress, perceived health, and a history of sexual abuse. The researchers' conclusions were that menopausal transition-related factors were not significantly associated with difficulty concentrating or forgetfulness. Examining the influence of women's ages and the context in which they experience the menopausal transition would be helpful in understanding women's experiences of cognitive symptoms.

Table 26.3 presents a list of the studies reviewed, depending on the results of ERT in improving cognitive functioning.

Tables 26.4 and 26.5 present a summary of the conclusions of the studies reviewed.

Conclusions

As it can be concluded, there is still much to investigate regarding the debate on whether estrogen therapy following menopause may result in improved cognitive function in women. This discussion is based on extensive research on animals and in cell culture data showing that estrogens can positively influence the process of brain aging. Observational data also show a reduced risk of dementia by half in women who were administered estrogens around the time of menopause. However, the treatment trials have shown long-term negative effects of estrogen therapy in older women.

Although some studies and research seem to demonstrate the influence of estrogens in organizing and activating effects on brain structures and function, the significant amount of research that studies the relationship between estrogens and the cognitive performance in menopausal women has not produced consistent results in the last two decades.

Table 26.3 Summary of the studies reviewed about ERT's effectiveness

ERT's effectiveness: Yes	ERT's effectiveness: No
Halbreich et al. [17]	Miles et al. (2006) [38]
Dumas et al. (2006) [26]	Leblanc et al. [32]
Scherwin and Henry (2008) [21]	Hemerlink et al. [33]
Ryan et al. [22]	Henderson (2009) [31]
Acosta [9]	Talboom et al. (2010) [39]
Dumas et al. [26]	Hogervorst and Bandelow (2010) [40]
Gibbs [27]	Henderson and Popat [10]
Dumas et al. (2010) [26]	
Daniel and Bohacek [20]	
Picazo et al. (2011) [37]	
Rocca et al. [19]	

Created for this study, no permission required

Table 26.4 Authors defending the use of ERT to improve cognitive functioning

Halbreich et al. [17]	Gonadal hormones and other reproduction-related factors may play a protective role against age-related deterioration in some cognitive functions in menopausal status
Dumas et al. [26]	Estrogen interactions with brain cholinergic systems may underlie the positive effects of estrogen in aging
Sherwin and Henry [21]	Estrogen treatment will protect aspects of cognition in older women only when treatment is initiated soon after the menopause
Ryan et al. [22]	Hormone therapy is associated with better performance in certain cognitive domains, depending on the duration and type of treatment used
Acosta [9]	The effects of ERT are only beneficial in surgical menopause
Dumas et al. [26]	Increase in frontal activation on memory tasks after estrogen treatment
Gibbs [27]	Cholinergic enhancing drugs with estrogen-containing drug regimen may be a viable therapeutic strategy in older postmenopausal women with early evidence of mild cognitive decline
Daniel and Bohacek [20]	Positive effects on the central nervous system if estrogen administration has been initiated within a critical time period following the loss of ovarian function
Picazo et al. [37]	Effect of estrogens on cognitive deterioration depends on the frame-time after cessation of ovarian function. Other factors related with cognition and influenced by estrogens: cholinergic central transmission, spinogenesis and synaptogenesis at hippocampus, and classical genomic and rapid non-genomic effects
Rocca et al. [19]	Neuro-protective effects of estrogen depend on the age at the time of administration, type of menopause, and stage of menopause

Created for this study, no permission required

Different studies have used a wide range of general cognitive measures of memory, measures of verbal skills, measures of visual skills, measures of attention skills, measures of concentration skills, and measures of verbal comprehension and showed no significant differences between the groups being compared when controlling for age and level of education, etc. These findings challenge beliefs about the usefulness of estrogen supplementation as a protective factor against cognitive decline in women at the climacteric stage [36].

Several investigations, which concluded that hormone treatment is effective, have important limitations: errors such as labelling as homogeneous samples groups containing both middle-aged and older women, the incorrect measurement of sociocultural factors and socioeconomic status (this influences the use or nonuse of estrogen), not considering whether menopause is natural or surgical, not considering whether women have ever used HRT, study design problems or studies containing very small sample sizes, with a lack of attention to measurement tests used, failure to consider cultural differences between the selected women, etc. Some of the research that reject the effect of estrogen therapy in improving the cognitive aspects also have these same limitations.

Table 26.5 Authors denying the use of ERT to improve cognitive functioning

Miles et al. [38]	After estrogen treatment, few changes in memory or cognition were observed, and changes that were observed were not consistent across study designs
LeBlanc et al. [32]	ERT improves menopausal symptoms and sleep but does not improve cognition in naturally menopausal women
Hemerlink et al. [33]	Hormonal changes did not appear to contribute to cognitive compromise in patients with breast cancer during the first year after diagnosis. Antiestrogen treatment did not affect cognition
Henderson [31]	There is no strong indication of short-term cognitive benefit of hormone use after natural menopause, but clinical trial data are sparse
Talboom et al. [39]	Women's Health Initiative Study found that conjugated equine estrogens (the most commonly prescribed HT) do not benefit cognition
Hogervorst and Bandelow [40]	More negative effects were seen in longer studies, where positive effects were mainly seen in short-term studies (<4 months). Treatment with combined estrogens and progestagens also negatively affected the outcomes
Henderson and Popat [10]	No consistent associations between endogenous serum estrogen concentrations and episodic memory or executive functions in naturally menopausal midlife women or in older postmenopausal women

Created for this study, no permission required

As other authors do, we think that several important clinical questions need to be answered in order to clarify the role of estrogens (endogenous and exogenous) in its relationship with the cognitive and affective dysfunctions associated with menopausal transition and senile dementia. Questions as follows: Should ERT be used for menopausal women with only cognitive complaints or affective dysfunction? Does long-term ERT prevent cognitive decline in later life? Does ERT improve cognitive performance in healthy women if initiated at the time of menopause? Can ERT improve cognition and affective functions in postmenopausal women with senile dementia? Does ERT prevent the progression of Alzheimer's disease in menopausal women? Do different types of THR provoke different effects in cognition?

Thus, further investigation taking into account all these aspects is needed to finally answer these questions regarding the role of ET on cognition.

References

1. Master W, Johnson V, Kolodny RC. La sexualidad humana. Barcelona: Grijalbo; 1987.
2. Comisión Europea. Green paper "Confronting demographic change: a new solidarity between generations". 2002. Disponible en http://europa.eu.int-lex/lex/LexUriServ/site/en/com/2005/com2005_0094en04.pdf
3. Larroy C. Trastornos específicos de la mujer. Madrid: Síntesis; 2004.
4. Hurtado F, Donat F, Poveda C, Rubio C, Ull N. Mujer y climaterio: un estudio para la mejora de la calidad de vida. Cuad Med Psicosom Psiquiatr Enlace. 1999;51/52:49–68.
5. Stanton A, Lobel M, Sears S, Stein De Luca R. Psychosocial aspects of selected issues in women's reproductive health: current status and future directions. J Consult Clin Psychol. 2002;70(3):751–70.
6. Gold EB, Sternfeld B, Kelsey JL, Brown C, Mouton C, Reame N, et al. Relation of demographic and lifestyle factors to symptoms in a multi-racial/ethnic population of women 40–55 years of age. Am J Epidemiol. 1999;152(5):463–73.
7. Dillaway H, Byrnes M, Miller S, Rehan S. Talking "amon us": how women from different racial-ethnic groups define and discuss menopause. Health Care Women Int. 2008;29:766–81.
8. Delgado A, Sánchez MC, Galindo I, Pérez C, Duque MJ. Actitudes de las mujeres ante la menopausia y variables predoctoras. Aten Primaria. 2001;27(1):27–41.
9. Acosta JI. Etiology of menopause impacts cognition. DAI B Sci Eng. 2010;70(11-B):7258.
10. Henderson VW, Popat RA. Effects of endogenous and exogenous estrogen exposures in midlife and late-life women on episodic memory and executive functions. Neuroscience. 2011;191(12):129–38.
11. Boulware MI, Kent BA, Frick KM. The impact of age-related ovarian hormone loss on cognitive and neural function. Curr Top Behav Neurosci. 2012;10:165–84.

12. Romeu A, Juliá M. Fisiología de la Menopausia. In: Sánchez-Cánovas J, editor. Menopausia y Salud. Barcelona: Ariel; 1996.
13. Carnicer C, Castro OP, Paublete MC. Aspectos básicos de la fisiología del climaterio. Psiquiatria.com: Interpsiquis 2002.
14. Leal Cercós C, Crespo HM. Introducción. In: Cercós L, editor. Trastornos depresivos en la mujer. Barcelona: Masson; 1999.
15. Bochino S. Aspectos psiconeuroendócrinos de la perimenopausia, menopausia y climaterio. Revista Psiquiátrica Urug. 2005;70(1):66–79.
16. González CO. Aspectos psiconeuroendocrinos del climaterio. In: Jadresic A, Ojeda C, Pérez G, editors. Psiconeuroendocrinología. Santiago: Mediterráneo; 2000.
17. Halbreich U, Lumley LA, Palter S, Manning C, Gengo F, Joe SH. Possible acceleration of age effects on cognition following menopause. J Psychiatr Res. 1995;29(3):153–63.
18. Genazzani AR, Spinetti A, Gallo R, Bernardi F. Menopause and the central nervous system: intervention options. Maturitas. 1999;31(2):103–10.
19. Rocca WA, Grossardt BR, Shuster LT. Oophorectomy, menopause, estrogen treatment, and cognitive aging: clinical evidence for a window of opportunity. Brain Res. 2011;1379:188–98.
20. Daniel JM, Bohacek J. The critical period hypothesis of estrogen effects on cognition: insights from basic research. Biochim Byophys Acta. 2010;1800(10):1068–76.
21. Sherwin BB, Henry JF. Brain aging modulates the neuroprotective effects of estrogen on selective aspects of cognition in women: a critical review. Front Neuroendocrinol. 2008;29(1):88–113.
22. Ryan J, Carriere I, Scali J, Dartigues JF, Tzourio C, Poncet M, et al. Characteristics of hormone therapy, cognitive function, and dementia: the prospective 3C Study. Neurology. 2009;73(21):1729–37.
23. Korol DL, Manning CA. Effects of estrogen on cognition: implications for menopause. In: Carroll ME, Overmier JB, editors. Animal research and human health: advancing human welfare through behavioural science. Washington, DC: American Psychological Association; 2001. p. 305–22.
24. Fillit H. Future therapeutic developments of estrogen use. J Clin Pharmacol. 1995;35(9 Suppl):25S–8.
25. Frick JM, Fernández SM, Harburger LL. A new approach to understanding the molecular mechanisms through wich estrogens affect cognition. Biochim Byophys Acta. 2010;1800(10):1045–55.
26. Dumas JA, Kutz AM, Naylor MR, Jonhson JV, Newhouse PA. Increased memory load-related frontal activation after estradiol treatment in postmenopausal women. Horm Behav. 2010;58(5):929–35.
27. Gibbs RB. Estrogen therapy and cognition: a review of the cholinergic hypothesis. Endocr Rev. 2010;31(2):224–53.
28. Rice K, Morse C. Measuring cognition in menopause research: a review of test use. Climacteric. 2003;6(1):2–22.
29. Miles C, Green R, Sanders G, Hines M. Estrogen and memory in a transsexual population. Horm Behav. 1998;34:199–208.
30. Tinelli A, Menis T, Brotto F, Tinelli R, Tinelli FG. Depression, menopause and hormonal replacement therapy (HRT). Minerva Ginecol. 2003;55(3):221–31.
31. Henderson VW. Action of estrogens in the aging brain: dementia and cognitive aging. Biochim Biophys Acta. 2009;18020(10):1077–83.
32. Leblanc ES, Neiss MB, Carello PE, Samuels MH, Janowsky JS. Hot Flashes and estrogen therapy do not influence cognition in early menopausal women. Menopause. 2007;14(2):191–202.
33. Hemerlink K, Henschel V, Untch M, Bauerfeind I, Lux MP, Munzel K. Short-term effects of treatment induced hormonal changes on cognitive function in breast cancer patients. Cancer. 2008;113(9):2431–9.
34. Greendale GA, Huang MH, Wight RG, Lutters C, Avis N, Johnston J, et al. Effects of the menopause transition and hormone use on cognitive performance in midlife women. Neurology. 2009;72(21):1850–1857.
35. Mitchell ES, Woods NF. Cognitive symptoms during the menopausal transition and early postmenopause. Climacteric. 2011;14(2):252–61.
36. Morse CA, Rice K. Memory after menopause: preliminary considerations of hormone influence on cognitive functioning. Arch Womens Ment Health. 2005;8:155–62.
37. Picazo O, Espinosa-Raya J, Jimenez-Trejo F, Suarez J. Current Topics in Medicinal Chemistry Volume 11, 2011;13:1742–49(8).
38. Miles C, Green R, Hines M. Estrogen treatment effects on cognition, memory and mood in male-to-female transsexuals. Hormones and Behavior (2006) xxx–xxx. www.sciencidirect.com.
39. Talboom JS, Engler-Chiurazzi EB, Whiteaker P, Simard AR, Lukas R, Acosta JI, et al. A component of Premarin((R)) enhances multiple cognitive functions and influences nicotinic receptor expression. Horm Behav. 2010;58(5):917–28.
40. Hogervorst E, Bandelow S. Sex steroids to maintain cognitive function in women after the menopause: A meta-analyses of treatment trials. Maturitas. 2010;66(1):56–71.

[illegible]

Chapter 27
An Overview of Menopausal Dietary Supplements and Cognition

Yuri N. Clement

Key Points

- Cognitive decline in menopause: Many women complain about memory loss and cognitive deficits during the menopausal transition and after menopause.
- Estrogens in cognitive function: Estrogens play a key role in memory and cognition, and hormone replacement therapy once thought to improve mental function, may actually have a negative impact.
- Risks with HRT: Clinical evidence shows increased health risks associated with long-term hormone replacement therapy and many menopausal women are resorting to dietary supplements to alleviate symptoms, including memory loss and cognitive decline.
- Role for phytoestrogens: Supplements containing phytoestrogens (isoflavones), abundant in soy and red clover, are commonly used as "natural" hormone replacement.
- Clinical evidence on dietary supplements: Twelve randomized, placebo-controlled clinical trials were identified which assessed the effect of six different dietary supplements on the performance of various tests of memory and cognitive function in postmenopausal women.
- Soy and isoflavone supplements: Nine out of the twelve RCTs assessed the effect of soy and isoflavone supplements on mental function in menopausal women.
- Study flaws: Most studies had several methodological shortfalls which limit the conclusions drawn.
- Suggestive results: Five studies suggest that supplementation with isoflavones, soy and *Gingko biloba* significantly improved performance on various tests of memory and cognitive function.
- Conclusions: The current clinical evidence does not support the use of dietary supplements, including soy, isoflavones, red clover, gingko, ginseng, or black cohosh for the amelioration of memory loss and cognitive decline in menopause.

Keywords Memory loss • Cognitive decline • Soy • Isoflavones • Black cohosh • Red clover • *Gingko biloba* • Black cohosh

Y.N. Clement, B.Sc., Ph.D. (✉)
Faculty of Medical Sciences, Pharmacology Unit, The University of the West Indies,
St. Augustine, Trinidad and Tobago
e-mail: Yuri.Clement@sta.uwi.edu; yuriclem@yahoo.com

C.J.H. Martin et al. (eds.), *Nutrition and Diet in Menopause*, Nutrition and Health,
DOI 10.1007/978-1-62703-373-2_27, © Springer Science+Business Media New York 2013

Abbreviations

ERβ	Estrogen receptor beta
HRT	Hormone replacement therapy
RCT	Randomized controlled trial
ITT	Intention-to-treat analysis
CEE/MPA	Conjugated equine estrogens plus medroxyprogesterone acetate

Introduction

A significant number of postmenopausal women complain of memory loss and cognitive decline [1] and it has been proposed that the dramatic fall in sex hormones during this life stage may be responsible for such changes [2]. It has also been suggested that the performance at various mental tasks may be influenced, not only by the precipitous fall in hormone levels during menopause, but by the cumulative lifetime exposure to estrogens [3]. Estrogens, in addition to their role in regulating reproductive function, play a substantial role in memory and cognitive function and influence verbal fluency, verbal memory, episodic memory, focussing attention, speed of information processing, planning, and mental flexibility (Fig. 27.1). In vitro and in vivo studies have shown that estrogens modulate central neurotransmitters by regulating hippocampal neurogenesis and long-term potentiation; these are important physiological events in the creation of episodic memory [4]. Additionally, several in vitro and in vivo studies have demonstrated that estrogens activate ERβ which leads to the transcriptional up-regulation of protective genes [5].

In a small cross-sectional study, which included 63 premenopausal, perimenopausal, and postmenopausal women, Portin and colleagues [6] showed that low levels of endogenous estrogens had no effect on any aspect of memory. However, the levels of estrogens were directly related to performance at cognitive tests such as sustained attention, attention suppression and reaction time. Other researchers have postulated that total endogenous levels of estrogens may not accurately predict

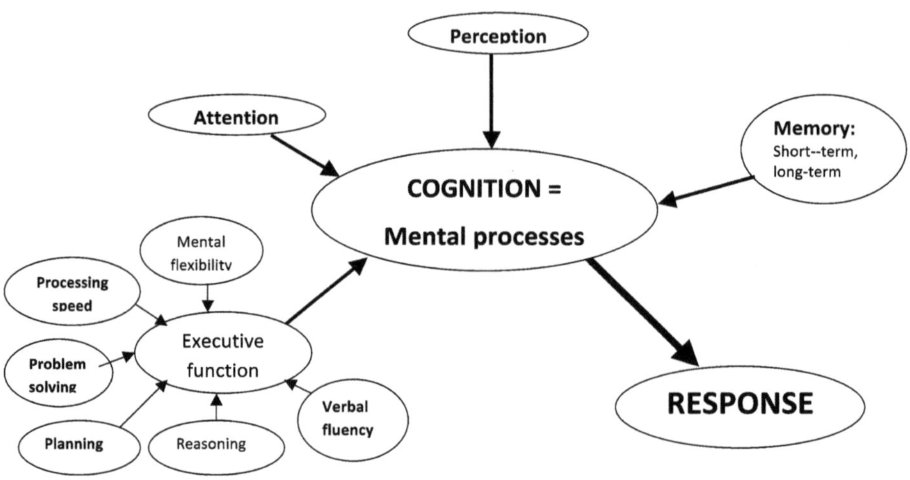

Fig. 27.1 Schematic representation of components of cognition. The cognitive response is dependent of numerous factors, which include multiple aspects of memory, executive function, perception and attention. The interplay between these factors would determine cognitive function and it is thought that changes in estrogen levels during the menopause affect various aspects of cognition

the concentrations of these hormones that are centrally available to affect cognitive function. In a prospective study, which included 425 elderly women (over 65 years old) and conducted over a 6-year period, it was shown that performance at memory and cognitive tasks were three times lower in women with lower levels of non-protein-bound and bioavailable estradiol [7]. In contrast, the results from the Rancho Bernardo study, which included 343 postmenopausal women with median age of 70 years, showed otherwise. In this study higher levels of endogenous estrone and bioavailable estradiol were associated with an almost doubled likelihood of decline in a standardized category fluency test over a 4-year period (this test measured cognitive flexibility and executive function) [8]. Further conflicting results by Herlitz and colleagues [9] demonstrated that the stage of menopause or estrogens levels did not affect performance at memory and cognitive function tasks, but it was not clear whether non-protein-bound or free estrogens levels were measured in this study.

A small study, which included 189 women, demonstrated that stage of menopause did not affect attention, verbal fluency or memory; however, women in late menopause performed worse at higher order cognitive function tests, such as planning and mental flexibility [10]. More recently, a large prospective study which included 1,903 women followed over 6 years measured various aspects of cognitive function and correlated performance on standardized tests to depressive and anxiety symptoms during various phases of premenopause, perimenopause, and postmenopause [11]. The authors reported that no learning occurred following repeated exposure to cognitive tests during late perimenopause, and this did not correlate with either depressive or anxiety symptoms. Additionally, high-level depressive symptoms had a small, but significant, negative impact on processing speed. Likewise, anxiety negatively affected episodic memory and attention which subsequently altered learning. Other investigators have also attributed these menopausal-related changes in memory and cognitive function to heightened anxiety and depression associated with this mid-life transition [4]. Another study showed that cognitive decline is progressive over the menopause, with processing speed and working memory being the most affected parameters [12].

Effect of Hormone Replacement Therapy on Cognition

Hormone replacement therapy (HRT) was used successfully for many years to treat vasomotor symptoms and it was also thought to provide neuroprotection and consequently preserve memory and cognition. However, the clinical evidence is inconsistent as some studies suggest preservation [13], whereas others demonstrate deleterious effects on cognitive function [14]. Other authors have suggested that these differences may be influenced by menopause type (natural versus surgical), hormone replacement type (estrogen-only versus estrogen/progesterone), or menopause stage (early versus late) [15]. However, a meta-analysis by Lethaby and colleague [16], with a total of 10,114 women from six RCTs, showed that long-term HRT did not arrest menopause-associated cognitive decline.

Reports of increased HRT-associated risks of breast cancer, stroke, and venous thrombosis [17] have sparked an interest in dietary supplements as alternative hormone replacement for the alleviation of menopausal symptoms, including the amelioration of memory loss and cognitive decline [18].

Dietary Supplements in Menopause

Many dietary supplements are available which have been recommended for the treatment of menopausal symptoms, including the management of memory loss and cognitive decline. Some of the more popular supplements include soy (*Glycine max* L.), red clover (*Trifolium pratense* L.), black cohosh (*Actaea racemosa* L; *Cimicifuga racemosa* [L.] Nutt.), evening primrose seed oil (*Oenothera biennis* L.), dong quai (*Angelica sinensis* L.), ginseng (*Panax ginseng* C.A. Mey), and *Gingko biloba* [19].

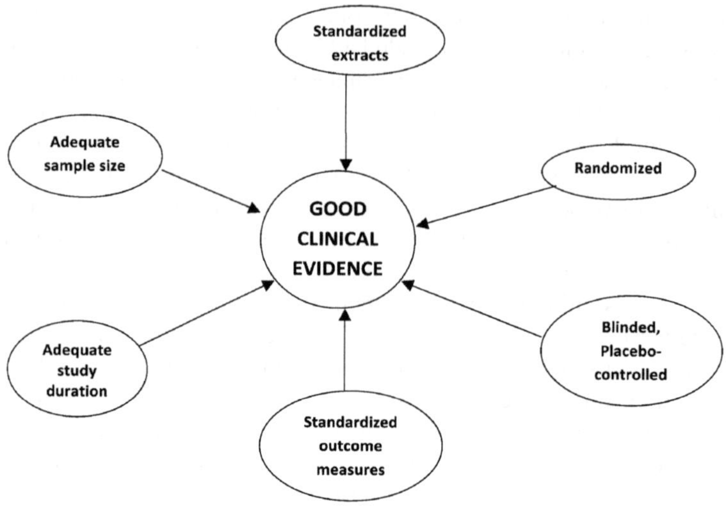

Fig. 27.2 Selection criteria for clinical studies. Although many clinical studies are conducted, the gold standard for good clinical evidence come from double-blind, placebo-controlled clinical trials. These studies must have sufficient sample size, of adequate duration and use standardized outcome assessments

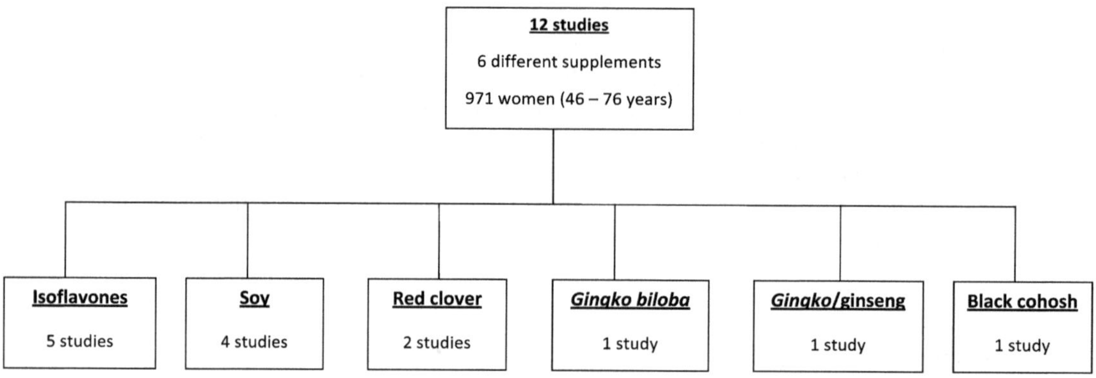

Fig. 27.3 List of included studies. These studies satisfied all the selection criteria which would provide good clinical evidence, i.e., double-blind, placebo-controlled clinical trials

A literature search of electronic databases was undertaken using key words such as herbal preparation, herbal medicine, phytomedicine, *Gingko biloba*, dietary supplement, soy, isoflavones, phytoestrogen, red clover, black cohosh, cognitive, memory loss, menopause, and randomized clinical trial. Studies considered for discussion here were all randomized, placebo-controlled trials which lasted for at least 6 weeks using validated instruments to assess performance at memory and cognitive function tasks (Fig. 27.2).

The results of the search of the electronic databases showed that 12 RCTs were conducted which investigated the effect of soy, isoflavone, Gingko, ginseng, red clover, and black cohosh supplementation compared with placebo or HRT and lasted between 6 weeks and 12 months (Fig. 27.3). Most of the studies were conducted in either the USA [20–23] or the UK [24–27]; the other studies were done in the Netherlands [28], Italy [29], Australia [30], and China [31].

There were a total of 971 postmenopausal women in these trial and the details are presented in Table 27.1. Women included in these studies were between 46 and 76 years of age (early to late menopause), had either natural or surgical menopause, not currently on HRT and with varying severity of vasomotor symptoms. Most of the studies were of parallel design and compared dietary supplement with either placebo or HRT. However, two trials utilized a crossover design, in which women were first randomly divided into two groups to receive either dietary supplement or placebo for 6 months,

Table 27.1 Summary of included clinical trials of herbal supplements for cognition in menopause

Supplement, authors, year	Participants, study design and age range	Treatment, dose and study duration	Treatment assignment/ completers	Cognitive tests performed—*outcome measures*	Main findings	Conclusions and comments
Soy, Kreijkamp-Kaspers et al. (2004) [36]	Sample size, 202 Double-blind, placebo-controlled Age, 60–75 years	Soy protein (99 mg isoflavones)/day vs. placebo. Duration, 12 months	88 women in soy protein group and 87 in placebo group had baseline and at least 1 post-intervention analysis, respectively. There was 24 % dropout with 75 women in soy group and 78 in placebo completing all intervention analyses, respectively.	Mini-Mental State Examination Rey Auditory Verbal Learning Test – *Verbal episodic memory* Doors Test – *Visual memory* Digit Span Test – *Short-term memory, working memory, verbal fluency* Boston Verbal Competency – *Verbal competence,Semantic retrieval* Digit Symbol Substitution Test – *Cognitive and perceptual speed* Trailmaking Test A1, A2 and B – *Complex attention and flexibility* Dutch Adult Reading Test – *Verbal intelligence quotient*	For memory tests, the soy group performed marginally better than placebo-treated women; however, this was not statistically significant. There were no differences between treatment groups for the more complex cognitive tasks which required concentration and visual attention. Depression did not influence performance at cognitive tasks.	Supplementation with soy over the long term had no significant effect on any aspect of memory or complex cognitive functioning in postmenopausal women 60 years and older. *Most of women in this study were postmenopausal for at least 18 years. Study duration was long-term and sample size sufficiently large to detect treatment effect. Methodological quality was moderate. There was significant attrition due to adverse effects, but intention-to-treat analysis was performed.*

(continued)

Table 27.1 (continued)

Supplement, authors, year	Participants, study design and age range	Treatment, dose and study duration	Treatment assignment/ completers	Cognitive tests performed—*outcome measures*	Main findings	Conclusions and comments
Soy, Duffy et al. (2003) [24]	Sample size, 36 Double-blind, placebo-controlled trial. Age, 50–60 years	Soy supplement (60 mg isoflavones/day) vs. placebo Duration, 12 weeks	18 in soy supplement group and 15 in placebo group completed study.	Weschler Memory Test – *Immediate memory* Delayed Matching To Sample Test – *Short-term memory* Long-term episodic memory Category generation Frontal lobe function – *Test of rule learning and reversal, Planning ability* Paced Auditory Serial Addition Test – *Sustained attention*	Dietary soy supplement resulted in significant improvements in both short-term and long-term episodic memory. Soy improved the ability to learn rule reversal, planning ability and sustained attention.	Soy isoflavones (60 mg/day) over 12 weeks improved many aspects of cognitive functioning in postmenopausal women. *Sample size and study duration may have been inadequate to establish treatment effect.* *Methodological quality was poor with inadequate reporting of sequence generation, allocation concealment and outcome assessor blinding. Although 12 out of 33 women (or 36%) did not complete the rule learning and reversal test the authors reported that soy had a statistically significant effect.*
Soy, Basaria et al. (2009) [20]	Sample size, 93 Double-blind, placebo-controlled trial. Age range (46–76 years)	Soy milk (160 mg isoflavones) vs. cow's milk (placebo) Duration, 12 weeks	38 in soy milk group and 46 in placebo group completed study.	National Adult Reading Test – *Intelligence scale* Cube Comparisons Test – *3-Dimensional spatial ability* Identical Pictures Test – *Matching ability* Verbal Fluency Test – *Executive function* Trial Making Test: Parts A & B – *Visuomotor skills and executive function* Groove Pegboard Test – *Psychomotor speed*	Improvements were observed in both groups from baseline to 12 weeks, but there were no differences between groups for any of the cognitive tests.	A relatively high intake of soy isoflavones (160 mg/day) over a 12-week period had no significant beneficial effects on any measured aspect of cognition in this study. *On average, most women in this study were postmenopausal for about 6 years. Study duration of 12 weeks may have been inadequate to determine treatment effect.*

Soy/isoflavone, Fournier et al. (2007) [21]	Sample size, 79 Double-blind, placebo-controlled trial. Age range, 48–65 years (Mild and moderate vasomotor symptoms)	Three treatment groups: Cow's milk/placebo vs. Soy milk (72 mg/day isoflavones)/placebo vs. Cow's milk/isoflavones (70 mg/day) Duration, 16 weeks	27 women in cow's milk/placebo group, 25 women in soy milk (72 mg/day isoflavones)/placebo group and 27 women in cow's milk/isoflavones (70 mg/day) group were initially randomized.	Stroop Task – *Selective attention* Digit Ordering – *Verbal working memory* Color Matching – *Spatial Working Memory* Benton Visual Retention Test – *Visual-spatial, short-term memory recall* Visual Pattern Recognition – *Visual long-term memory* Forward Digit Span – *Verbal memory span* Corsi Block-Tapping – *Spatial, memory span*	Neither dietary nor supplement isoflavones had any significant effect on selective attention measures compared with placebo. Also, dietary soy and supplement did not improve performance on any of the memory tests.	"… consumption of isoflavones in supplement or dietary (soy milk) … did not have an appreciable effect on attention or memory in healthy post-menopausal women." *On average, most women in this study were postmenopausal for about 8 years. Data set incomplete for Color Matching test due to video recording device errors.* *A small sample size and short intervention period may have contributed to some of the insignificant results. Adequate blinding was observed only in the two treatment arms were participants were treated with soy milk and isoflavone capsules (active interventions).*

(continued)

Table 27.1 (continued)

Supplement, authors, year	Participants, study design and age range	Treatment, dose and study duration	Treatment assignment/ completers	Cognitive tests performed—*outcome measures*	Main findings	Conclusions and comments
Isoflavone, Ho et al. (2007) [31]	Sample size, 191 Double-blind, placebo-controlled trial Age range, 55–76 years	Isoflavone (80 mg/day) vs. placebo Duration, 6 months	85 women in isoflavone group and 91 women in placebo group completed the study.	Hong Kong List Learning Test – *Learning and memory* Rey-Osterrieth Complex Figure Test/Wechsler Memory Scale-Revised – *Visuospatial constructional ability and visual memory* Trail Making Test – *Executive function* Verbal Fluency Test – *Language ability* Digit Span Test – *Attention and concentration* Digit Vigilance Test – *Immediate verbal recall* Finger Tapping Test – *Simple motor speed* Boston Naming Test – *Picture naming*	There were no significant differences in the changes in memory and cognitive tests at the follow-up between the treatment and placebo groups.	Soy isoflavones at 80 mg/day over 6 months did not produce any improvement in either memory or cognitive function in generally healthy and asymptomatic Chinese postmenopausal women. *The methodological quality of the study was adequate with sufficient sample size, blinding and intention-to-treat analysis. The study was probably limited by its relatively short duration and the fact that dietary isoflavone intake in Asian populations is relatively high. This habitual intake of soy may have a protective effect on cognitive function and memory, even in the placebo group, and thus may have reflected in the overall outcome.*

Isoflavone Kritz-Silverstein et al., 2003 [22]	Sample size, 56 Double-blind, placebo controlled trial. Age range, 55–74 years	Isoflavone (110 mg/day) vs. placebo Duration, 6 months	28 women initially assigned to each treatment group. 26 women in isoflavone group and 27 women in placebo group completed the study.	Trials A & Trials B – *Visuomotor tracking and attention* Category Fluency – *Verbal memory* Logical Memory and Recall – *Immediate and delayed verbal memory*	Although isoflavone treatment produce improvements in all but one test (Trials A), positive change was only statistically significant for verbal memory.	In this relatively small study which lasted 6 months, isoflavone supplementation (110 mg/day) produced increases in performance on memory and cognitive test, with statistically significant changes in verbal memory. *No sample size estimation was done.*
Isoflavone File et al., 2005 [25]	Sample size, 50 Double-blind, placebo-controlled trial Age range, 51–66 years	Isoflavone (60 mg/day) vs. placebo Duration, 6 weeks	25 in isoflavone (60 mg/day) group and 25 in placebo group initially randomized.	Delayed Matching To Sample Test – *Short-term nonverbal memory* Weschler Memory Scale – *Short-term and long-term verbal memory* IDED Test – *Mental flexibility* Stocking of Cambridge Test – *Planning ability* Paced Auditory Serial Addition Test – *Sustained attention*	Soy supplementation caused significant improvements in short-term nonverbal memory, mental flexibility and planning.	This small study of short duration showed that soy supplementation (60 mg isoflavones) significantly improved short-term memory and frontal lobe function. *There are some methodological deficiencies as sample size estimation was not done and study duration was short. A large number of participants (44 %) were not able to complete the IDED test which measured mental flexibility, yet the authors concluded that soy significantly improved this aspect of cognitive function.*

(continued)

Table 27.1 (continued)

Supplement, authors, year	Participants, study design and age range	Treatment, dose and study duration	Treatment assignment/ completers	Cognitive tests performed—*outcome measures*	Main findings	Conclusions and comments
Isoflavone Casini et al., 2006 [29]	Sample size, 78 Double-blind, placebo-controlled, cross-over trail Age range, approx. 50 years	Isoflavone (60 mg/day) vs. placebo Duration, 6 months per phase (1 month washout)	39 women initially assigned to each treatment group. 38 women in each group completed both phases of the study.	Digit Symbol Test – *Psychomotor performance* Digit Span Test – *Immediate auditory attention, Mental flexibility* Visual Scanning Test – *Distractibility, visual inattentiveness*	Isoflavone supplementation produced significant improvements in performance of the Digit Symbol Test and Digit Span Test.	The use of isoflavone (60 mg/day) supplements over a 6-month period produced a significant improvement in cognitive function in postmenopausal women. *No sample size estimation was done. Is may be possible that practice effects may have affected cognitive testing in both arms in the crossover design.*
Gingko biloba Elsabagh et al., 2005 [26]	Sample size, 96 Double-blind, placebo-controlled trial. Age range, 51–67 years	*Gingko biloba* (120 mg/day) vs. placebo. Duration, 6 weeks	48 women initially assigned to each treatment group. 45 women in gingko group and 42 women in placebo group completed study. *Stage +1* (*≤5 years postmenopausal*) 25 in placebo group 18 in gingko group *Stage +2* (*>5 years postmenopausal*) 17 in placebo group 27 in gingko group	Paced Auditory Serial Addition Test – *Sustained attention* Weschler Memory Scale-Revised – *Immediate and delayed recall* Delayed Matching-to-Sample Test – *Short-term, nonverbal memory* Picture Recall – *Long-term memory* Category generation Stocking of Cambridge Task – *Spatial planning ability* Intra/Extra Dimensional Shift Task – *Mental flexibility*	Gingko supplementation did not improve memory, sustained attention or planning ability. However, improvement of mental flexibility limited to older women with longer duration of menopause.	The authors found that improvement in mental flexibility was restricted to older women who were more cognitively impaired, and this may indicate a threshold of cognitive ability at which gingko is effective after chronic treatment periods. *No sample size estimation was done and the study period was relatively short.*

Gingko/ginseng Hartley et al., 2004 [27]	Sample size, 70 Double-blind, placebo-controlled trial. Age range, 51–66 years	Capsule containing gingko (120 mg)/ginseng (200 mg) per day vs. placebo. Duration, 12 weeks	27 women in the intervention group and 30 women in placebo group completed the study.	Paced Serial Attention Test – *Sustained attention* Weschler Memory Scale-Revised—*Immediate and delayed recall* Delayed Matching-To-Sample Test – *Short-term, nonverbal memory* Picture Recall – *Long-term episodic memory* Category generation Frontal lobe function – *Test of rule learning and reversal, Planning ability*	Supplementation with the gingko/ginseng combination did not improve performance on any of the episodic memory or cognitive tests.	The combination supplement did not improve memory or cognition over the 12-week period in these postmenopausal women. *There was no justification of the sample size used and about 20 % of participants dropped out of the study without sufficient explanation.*
Red clover Howes et al., 2004 [30]	Sample size, 30 Double-blind, placebo-controlled, cross-over trail Age range, >60 years	Red clover (57 mg isoflavones/day) vs. placebo Duration, 6 months per phase (1 month washout)	15 women entered each phase to receive either red clover or placebo group. 14 women from each group completed the study.	Weschler Memory Scale Revised—*Immediate auditory attention, Working memory, Word association memory, Verbal memory, Visual memory, Visual-spatial intelligence, Processing Speed, Verbal Reasoning* Trial A & Trial B Tests – *Processing speed, Prefrontal lobe function* Boston Naming Test – *Word naming* Controlled Oral Word Association – *Verbal fluency*	Generally, there were no notable differences in memory and cognitive tests between women taking red clover isoflavones compared to those taking placebo when results were adjusted for multiple comparisons.	Although red clover isoflavones appeared to be associated with a small improvement in the visual-spatial intelligence test and a slightly worse performance in the immediate auditory attention test, compared with placebo, these results did not reach statistical significance when adjusted for multiple comparisons. *There is no justification for the sample size. It is possible that practice effects on the memory and cognitive tests may have affected performance in both arms in this crossover design.*

(continued)

Table 27.1 (continued)

Supplement, authors, year	Participants, study design and age range	Treatment, dose and study duration	Treatment assignment/ completers	Cognitive tests performed—*outcome measures*	Main findings	Conclusions and comments
Red clover/ Black cohosh Maki et al., 2009 [23]	Sample size, 66 (all women had natural menopause, with ≥35 weekly hot flushes) Double-blind, placebo-controlled trial. Age range, 44–66 years	CEE(0.625 mg)/ MPA(2.5 mg)/ day vs. red clover (120 mg/day) vs. black cohosh (128 mg/day) vs. placebo Duration, 12 months	17 women in CEE/ MPA group, 17 women in placebo group, 14 in red clover (120 mg/day) group and 18 in black cohosh (128 mg/day) group completed the study.	California Verbal Learning Test (modified) – *Short- and long-delay recall* Weschler Memory Scale – *Immediate and delay recall* Benton Visual Retention Test – *Short-term memory* Modified Card Rotation Test – *Visuospatial ability* Letter Fluency Test – *Verbal fluency* Digit Span Forward and Backward – *Attention and working memory* Brief Test of Attention-Modified – *Auditory attention* Finding As Test – *Visuoperceptual speed*	Supplementation with either red clover or black cohosh over 12 months had no significant impact on the performance on any memory or cognitive tests.	Red clover and black cohosh supplements had no beneficial effects on any aspect of memory or cognitive function. *There is no justification for the sample size.*

Details of each study are provided to include dosage, duration, the range of cognitive tests used, and the results obtained. Conclusions of the studies were extracted from the original publications and commentaries (*in italics*) on study design, which may impact on the results and conclusions, are provided by the author

following by a 1-month washout period, before being switched to the alternative treatment for a further 6 months [29, 30]. One small trial had four treatment arms: CEE/MPA (HRT), red clover, black cohosh, and placebo [23]. A wide array of memory and cognitive tests were used; however, the most commonly assessed outcomes were episodic memory, visual memory, visuospatial memory, sustained attention, planning ability, mental flexibility, and frontal lobe function.

Effect of Soy Isoflavone Supplementation on Memory Loss and Cognitive Function

The chemical structure of phytoestrogens (isoflavones found in soy), such as genistein and daidzein, closely resembles estradiol and it has been postulated that these compounds mimic the actions of endogenous estrogens. It has been suggested that these isoflavones act as "natural" hormone replacements in menopause which could reduce vasomotor symptoms, such as hot flashes and night sweats, as well as improve memory and cognitive function [32]. At high physiological concentrations phytoestrogens have similar affinity to estrogen receptors, particularly ER-β. It has been proposed that the similarity in receptor interaction would translate to transcriptional modulation that would enhance memory and cognitive function.

Dietary intake of soy isoflavones is relatively high in Asian countries [33] and some researchers have postulated that this may explain the lower reported frequency and severity of menopausal symptoms in these populations [34]. However, two epidemiological studies which included postmenopausal Asian [35] and Dutch [36] women showed that there was no relationship between long-term dietary intake of isoflavones and performance at cognitive tests. It was suggested by these authors that isoflavone plasma levels following normal dietary intake may not be sufficiently high to illicit a biological response. However, it was shown that higher dietary intake of lignans was associated with better performance at tests which assessed executive function, processing capacity and speed [36]. Unfortunately, there were no RCTs which assessed the effect of lignans supplementation on memory and cognitive function.

Soy and isoflavones were the most commonly investigated dietary supplements, with 9 out of the 12 clinical trials identified assessing the effect of these supplements on various aspects of memory and cognitive function. These studies lasted for 12, 16 weeks or 12 months and women were given between 60 and 160 mg/day as a standardized supplement or soy protein/milk.

Four studies, with a total of 344 women, assessed whether soy (isoflavone supplement, protein or milk) had any beneficial effect on performance on memory and cognitive tests in postmenopausal women [20, 21, 24, 28]. Only one out of these four studies [24] showed that the daily consumption of soy supplement (containing 60 mg isoflavones over 12 weeks) improved several aspects of memory and cognitive function including long-term recall of pictures, mental flexibility, planning and sustained attention in postmenopausal women between 50 and 60 years of age. It should be noted that this study had the shortest duration (12 weeks) and the smallest sample size (33 women).

Five studies, with a total of 414 women and lasting for either 6 weeks or 6 months, assessed the performance of postmenopausal women on memory and cognition tests following supplementation with standardized isoflavones [21, 22, 25, 29, 31]. Three out of these five studies demonstrated that daily supplementation with isoflavones (60 or 110 mg) caused statistically significant improvements in numerous aspects of recall, including verbal memory, short-term nonverbal memory and backwards memory. Additionally, these studies showed that isoflavone supplementation improved various domains of cognitive function, such as mental flexibility, planning, psychomotor performance and immediate auditory attention.

It should be noted that the two studies with the largest sample sizes (with 175 and 176 women), longer duration (lasting 6 months and 1 year) and most comprehensive battery of memory and cognitive tests did not demonstrate any benefit of soy or isoflavone supplementation on outcome measures [28, 31].

Effect of Other Dietary Supplements on Memory and Cognitive Function

Red clover is another popular supplement used to alleviate menopausal symptoms. It is also abundant in phytoestrogens (isoflavones) such as biochanin A and formononetin, with lower levels of daidzein and genistein, also found in soy. It has been postulated that red clover isoflavones would have "natural" estrogenic activity to reduce menopause-associated symptoms, including the improvement of memory and cognitive function.

Two studies investigated the effect of red clover supplementation on mental function [23, 30]. Although both studies ran for 12 months, they had relatively small sample sizes, with one study 30 women were included in a cross-over design [30] and the other had four treatment arms with the red clover arm having just 14 participants [23]. In the study with the cross-over design, all women had a natural menopause with frequent vasomotor symptoms. In these two studies, it was shown that supplementation with red clover (57 or 120 mg isoflavones per day) given over 6 months or 1 year did not improve performance on a battery of memory and cognitive tests.

Gingko biloba is another commonly used herb thought to prevent age-related decline in memory and cognitive function. The leaves of the herb contain several flavonoid glycosides and terpenoids, such as ginkgolides and bilobalides, which are reputed to have physiological action which preserves function. Elsabagh and colleagues [26] conducted a trial in which women at early and late menopause were grouped and randomly given *Gingko* supplement (120 mg/day) or placebo for 6 weeks. The authors demonstrated that there were no improvements in the performance in any of memory and cognitive tests in women in the early stages of menopause. However, the study indicated that for women in the menopause for more than 5 years, supplementation over 6 weeks significantly improved performance at cognitive tests which assessed mental flexibility. The short duration of the study should be noted, and it is not known whether improvement in function would have persisted had the study period been extended.

Interestingly, another study used a proprietary preparation containing a mixture of *Gingko biloba* (120 mg) and ginseng (200 mg) which was given to women twice daily for 12 weeks [27]. Unlike the study by Elsabagh and colleagues [26], supplementation in this trial over a longer period did not produce any significant improvement in sustained attention, episodic memory, or frontal lobe function.

Black cohosh does not contain phytoestrogens, but compounds which interact with the human μ-opiate and serotonin receptors. Consequently, it is thought that black cohosh would not have any major effects in modulating menopause-associated memory loss and cognitive decline. Maki and colleagues [23] assessed the effect of black cohosh (128 mg/day) over 12 months as one of four treatment arms. In this study 18 women were treated with black cohosh and supplementation did not improve performance on any of the memory or cognitive function tests.

Methodological Quality of Clinical Trials

Most of the included RCTs had methodological shortfalls, such as inadequate sample size, unclear reporting of the generation of the randomized sequence, allocation concealment, and lack of intention-to-treat analysis in trials with dropouts (Table 27.2).

A trial of good methodological quality must have an adequate sample size with sufficient statistical power to detect significant differences between intervention groups. Trials with small sample sizes are at risk of overestimating the effects of interventions, which could lead to misleading conclusions. Seven studies [21–23, 25–27, 29] did not adequately report how the sample sizes were estimated. The authors of one study simply assumed that the sample size was more than enough to detect effects of acute and short-term treatment, although they provided no statistical justification for the sample size [27]. In another study, the authors acknowledged that the small sample size and short intervention

Table 27.2 Methodological quality assessment of included studies

First author, year	Adequate sequence generation	Allocation concealment	Patient blinding	Care provider blinding	Outcome assessor blinding	Incomplete outcome data	Dropout reported, with reasons	ITT done	Comparable groups at baseline	Quality of clinical evidence
Kreijkamp-Kaspers, 2004 [36]	+	+	+	+	?	+	+	+	+	Good
Duffy, 2003 [24]	?	?	+	+	?	+	+	–	+	Fair
Basaria, 2009 [20]	+	?	+	+	?	–	+	–	+	Fair
Fournier, 2007 [21]	?	?	?	?	?	+	?	–	+	Poor
Ho, 2007 [31]	+	+	+	+	+	+	+	+	+	Excellent
Kritz-Silverstein, 2003 [22]	+	?	+	+	?	–	+	–	+	Fair
File, 2005 [25]	?	?	+	+	?	+	–	–	+	Fair
Casini, 2006 [29]	?	?	+	+	?	+	+	?	+	Fair
Elsabagh, 2005 [26]	?	?	+	+	?	–	+	–	+	Fair
Hartley, 2004 [27]	?	?	+	+	?	?	+	–	+	Fair
Howes, 2004 [30]	+	+	+	+	?	?	+	?	+	Good
Maki, 2009 [23]	+	?	+	+	?	–	+	–	+	Fair

The quality of the clinical evidence is dependent on adequate methodological design which would provide unbiased data. The Cochrane Collaboration tool assesses the various parameters which would determine whether a clinical study satisfied the rigorous requirements needed to provide good clinical evidence. Following assessment the methodological design of each study is rated as excellent, good, fair or poor

Yes = +; No = –; Unclear = ?, ITT = intention-to-treat analysis

duration may have adversely affected the outcome [21]. It is interesting to note that four out of the five studies which showed significant benefits of supplementation had no statistical basis for the sample sizes used [22, 25, 26, 29].

Only six out of the 12 RCTS, reported an adequate method used to generate the random sequence [20, 22, 23, 28, 30, 31]. Fournier and colleagues [21] first matched women by age and IQ, and then randomized them to one of three interventions; but no method was described with regard to the manner in which the randomization sequence was generated.

Only three studies adequately reported on the method used treatment allocation concealment [28, 30, 31]. In those studies, women were given an envelope or bottle labelled with a randomized number (corresponding to the treatment group) containing capsules of dietary supplements or identical placebo. To further ensure concealment, labelled envelopes and bottles were prepared by personnel not directly involved in the conduct of the trial. This process of allocation concealment was more likely to ensure that complete blinding occurred for both participants and care providers. The absence of such allocation concealment increases the likelihood that the blinding process becomes compromised during the course of the trial, and ultimately affecting the measurement of the outcomes. Only one study reported that outcome assessors, who were distinct from the care providers, were also blinded to treatment allocation [31].

Most studies had participants, who, for whatever reason, did not complete the study as intended. One study did not report the reasons for dropout of participants [21], and only two studies performed intention-to-treat (ITT) analysis to account for attrition [28, 31]. Only one study reported that all randomized participants were retained for the entire duration of the trial and that all outcome data were available for analysis [25]. In another study it was unclear whether there were any dropouts, but inspection of the results revealed that the data was incomplete for some cognitive tasks for all treatment groups [21]. In all of the other studies attrition rates were given, however in some studies the treatment group [23, 27] or the reasons for attrition [22, 29] were not stated. Despite the sometimes high level of dropout in most studies, only two RCTs performed an intention-to-treat analysis [28, 31].

Although most trials presented the results for all outcome measures, only four RCTs clearly reported outcome data for all initially randomized participants [20, 22, 23, 26]. In two trials, although significant numbers of participants (over 40 %) did not complete frontal lobe function tests the authors concluded that dietary supplementation produced statistically significant improvements in this aspect of cognitive function [24, 25].

These methodological shortfalls would inadvertently affect the validity of the findings and their clinical implications. Albeit, only one study [31] was of sufficiently high methodological quality, with adequate reporting of sequence generation, blinding of participants, care providers and outcome assessors, allocation concealment, attrition and ITT analysis. This trial showed that 6-month supplementation with isoflavone (80 mg/day) did not improve performance at memory or cognitive function tests in Chinese postmenopausal women.

Conclusion

Besides experiencing varying vasomotor symptoms, many menopausal women also complain of deficits in memory and cognitive function. Although HRT has been used successfully to treat vasomotor symptoms, some studies have shown that it actually worsens mental function. Additionally, recent findings show that long-term use of HRT is strongly correlated to increased risks of breast cancer and stroke. Consequently, many women are now exploring the use of "natural" alternatives, including dietary supplements which they deem to be safe and efficacious. Many dietary supplements for the treatment of menopausal symptoms are available and this chapter critically examined the clinical evidence provided by randomized placebo-controlled clinical trials with regard to improvement in memory and cognitive function.

Twelve randomized controlled trials were identified which evaluated six different dietary supplements including soy, isoflavones, *Gingko biloba*, a *Gingko biloba*–ginseng mixture, red clover, and black cohosh. Trials had varying sample sizes, supplement doses and duration of treatment. Several different validated tests were used to assess memory and cognitive function. Five trials suggest that supplementation with isoflavones, soy, and *Gingko biloba* improved various aspects of memory and cognition. However, most of the trials with positive results had small sample sizes and several methodological shortfalls. The larger, well-designed studies did not report any significant benefit with supplementation. Overall, the current clinical evidence fails to demonstrate any beneficial effect of dietary supplementation on memory and cognition in menopause.

References

1. Sullivan Mitchell E, Fugate WN. Midlife women's attributions about perceived memory changes: observations from the Seattle Midlife Women's Health Study. J Womens Health Gend Based Med. 2001;10(4):351–62.
2. Halbreich U, Lumley LA, Palter S, Manning C, Gengo F, Joe SH. Possible acceleration of age effects on cognition following menopause. J Psychiatr Res. 1995;29(3):153–63.
3. Smith CA, McCleary CA, Murdock GA, Wilshire TW, Buckwalter DK, Bretsky P, et al. Lifelong estrogen exposure and cognitive performance in elderly women. Brain Cogn. 1999;39:203–18.
4. Henderson VW. Cognitive changes after menopause: influence of estrogen. Clin Obstet Gynecol. 2008;51(3): 618–26.
5. Markou A, Duka T, Prelevic GM. Estrogens and brain function. Hormones. 2005;4(1):9–17.
6. Portin R, Polo-Kantola P, Polo O, Koskinen T, Revonsuo A, Irjala K, et al. Serum estrogen level, attention, memory and other cognitive functions in middle-aged women. Climacteric. 1999;2(2):115–23.
7. Yaffe K, Lui LY, Grady D, Cauley J, Kramer J, Cummings SR. Cognitive decline in women in relation to non-protein-bound oestradiol concentrations. Lancet. 2000;356(9231):708–12.
8. Laughlin GA, Kritz-Silverstein D. Higher endogenous estrogens predict four year decline in verbal fluency in post-menopausal women: the Rancho Bernardo Study. Clin Endocrinol (Oxf). 2010;72(1):99–106.
9. Herlitz A, Thilers P, Habib R. Endogenous estrogen is not associated with cognitive performance before, during or after menopause. Menopause. 2007;14(3 Pt 1):425–31.
10. Elsabagh S, Hartley DE, File SE. Cognitive function in late versus early postmenopausal stage. Maturitas. 2007;56:84–93.
11. Greendale GA, Wight RG, Huang MH, Avis N, Gold EB, Joffe H, et al. Menopause-associated symptoms and cognitive performance: results for the study of Women's Health across the Nation. Am J Epidemiol. 2010;171: 1214–24.
12. Schaafsma M, Homewood J, Taylor A. Subjective cognitive complaints at menopause associated with declines in performance of verbal memory and attentional processes. Climacteric. 2010;13(1):84–98.
13. Ryan J, Carriere I, Scali J, Dartigues JF, Tzourio C, Poncet M, et al. Characteristics of hormone therapy, cognitive function, and dementia: the prospective 3C Study. Neurology. 2009;73(21):1729–37.
14. Khoo SK, O'Neill S, Byrne G, King R, Travens C, Tripcony L. Postmenopausal hormone therapy and cognition: effects of timing and treatment type. Climacteric. 2010;13(3):259–64.
15. Daniel JM, Bohacek J. The critical period hypothesis of estrogen effects in cognition: insights from basic research. Biochim Biophys Acta. 2010;1800(10):1068–76.
16. Lethaby A, Hogervorst E, Richards M, Yesufu A, Yaffe K. Hormone replacement therapy for cognitive function in postmenopausal women. Cochrane Database Syst Rev. 2008;23(1):CD003122.
17. Dietel M. Hormone replacement therapy (HRT), breast cancer and tumor pathology. Maturitas. 2010;65(3):183–9.
18. Borrelli F, Ernst E. Alternative and complementary therapies for the menopause. Maturitas. 2010;66(4):333–43.
19. Low DT. Menopause: a review of botanical dietary supplements. Am J Med. 2005;118(Suppl 12B):98–108.
20. Basaria S, Wisniewski A, Dupree K, Bruno T, Song MY, Yao F, et al. Effect of high-dose isoflavones on cognition, quality of life, androgens, and lipoprotein in post-menopausal women. J Endocrinol Invest. 2009; 32(2):150–5.
21. Fournier LR, Ryan Borchers TA, Robison LM, Wiediger M, Park JS, Chew BP, et al. The effects of soy milk and isoflavone supplements on cognitive performance in healthy, postmenopausal women. J Nutr Health Aging. 2007;11(2):155–64.

22. Kritz-Silverstein D, Von Mühlen D, Barrett-Connor E, Bressel MA. Isoflavones and cognitive function in older women: the SOy and Postmenopausal Health In Aging (SOPHIA) Study. Menopause. 2003;10(3):196–202.
23. Maki PM, Rubin LH, Fornelli D, Drogos L, Banuvar S, Shulman LP, et al. Effects of botanicals and combined hormone therapy on cognition in postmenopausal women. Menopause. 2009;16(6):1167–77.
24. Duffy R, Wiseman H, File SE. Improved cognitive function in postmenopausal women after 12 weeks of consumption of a soya extract containing isoflavones. Pharmacol Biochem Behav. 2003;75:721–9.
25. File SE, Hartley DE, Elsabagh S, Duffy R, Wiseman H. Cognitive improvement after 6 weeks of soy supplements in postmenopausal women is limited to frontal lobe function. Menopause. 2005;12(2):193–201.
26. Elsabagh S, Hartley DE, File SE. Limited cognitive benefits in Stage +2 postmenopausal women after 6 weeks of treatment with Ginkgo biloba. J Psychopharmacol. 2005;19(2):173–81.
27. Hartley DE, Elsabagh S, File SE. Gincosan (a combination of Ginkgo biloba and Panax ginseng): the effects on mood and cognition of 6 and 12 weeks' treatment in post-menopausal women. Nutr Neurosci. 2004;7(5–6):325–33.
28. Kreijkamp-Kaspers S, Kok L, Grobbee DE, de Haan EH, Aleman A, van der Schouw YT. Dietary phytoesreogen intake and cognitive function in older women. J Gerontol A Biol Sci Med Sci. 2007;62(5):556–62.
29. Casini ML, Marelli G, Papaleo E, Ferrari A, D'Ambrosio F, Unfer V. Psychological assessment of the effects of treatment with phytoestrogens on postmenopausal women: a randomized, double-blind, crossover, placebo-controlled study. Fertil Steril. 2006;85(4):972–8.
30. Howes JB, Bray K, Lorenz L, Smerdely P, Howes LG. The effects of dietary supplementation with isoflavones from red clover on cognitive function in postmenopausal women. Climacteric. 2004;7(1):70–7.
31. Ho SC, Chan ASY, Ho YP, So EK, Sham A, Zee B, et al. Effects of soy isoflavone supplementation on cognitive function in Chinese postmenopausal women: a double-blind, randomized controlled trial. Menopause. 2007;14(3):489–99.
32. Belcher SM, Zsarnovszky A. Estrogenic actions in the brain: estrogen, phytoestrogens, and rapid intracellular signalling mechanisms. J Pharmacol Exp Ther. 2001;299(2):408–14.
33. Adlercreutz H, Hämäläinen E, Gorbach S, Goldin B. Dietary phyto-oestrogens and the menopause in Japan. Lancet. 1992;339(8803):1233.
34. Ho SC, Chan SG, Yip YB, Cheng A, Yi Q, Chan C. Menopausal symptoms and symptom clustering in Chinese women. Maturitas. 1999;33(3):219–27.
35. Haung MH, Luetters C, Buckwalter GJ, Seeman TE, Gold EB, Sternfeld B, et al. Dietary genistein intake and cognitive performance in a multiethnic cohort of midlife women. Menopause. 2006;13(4):621–30.
36. Kreijkamp-Kaspers S, Kok L, Grobbee DE, de Haan EH, Aleman A, Lampe JW, et al. Effect of soy protein containing isoflavones on cognitive function, bone mineral density, and plasma lipids in post-menopausal women: a randomized controlled trial. JAMA. 2004;292(1):65–74.

Chapter 28
Black Cohosh for the Menopausal Transition: Issues of Safety and Efficacy

Gail B. Mahady

Key Points

- Black cohosh is an alternative therapy used for the management of menopausal symptoms by perimenopausal and postmenopausal women.
- Data from the clinical trials are, at best, conflicted with many older clinical trials of poor quality showing beneficial effects in reducing vasomotor symptoms and the Kupperman Index.
- However, the most recent, rigorous National Institutes of Health funded clinical studies have failed to note any benefit in reducing hot flashes and in fact have show that black cohosh alone, or in combination with soy may actually be worse than placebo.
- The published clinical data for black cohosh has shown few adverse events, including the most recent trials. In particular, there was no evidence for hepatotoxicity of black cohosh during the 12-month intervention.
- However, there are now well over 75 case reports of hepatotoxicity associated with the ingestion of black cohosh products. While reviews of these data have not completely proven causality, this combined with the conflicting data for efficacy from the clinical indicates that at this point in time black cohosh cannot be recommended for management of the menopausal transition.

Keywords Black cohosh • Climacteric • Hepatoxicity • Hot flashes • Menopause • Vasomotor symptoms

Abbreviations

BMI	Body mass index
CAM	Complementary and alternative medicine
CE	Conjugated estrogen
CEE	Conjugated equine estrogens
FSH	Follicle stimulating hormone
HALT	Herbal alternatives for menopause
HAMA	Hamilton anxiety rating scale

G.B. Mahady, Ph.C., Ph.D. (✉)
Department of Pharmacy Practice, PAHO/WHO Collaborating Centre for Traditional Medicine,
College of Pharmacy, University of Illinois, Rm 122, 833S. Wood Street, MC 886, Chicago, IL 60612, USA
e-mail: mahady@uic.edu

C.J.H. Martin et al. (eds.), *Nutrition and Diet in Menopause*, Nutrition and Health,
DOI 10.1007/978-1-62703-373-2_28, © Springer Science+Business Media New York 2013

HT	Hormone therapy
KI	Kupperman index
LH	Luteinizing hormone
MPA	Medroxyprogesterone acetate
MRS	Menopause rating scale
NIH	National Institutes of Health
RCT	Randomized controlled clinical trial
SDS	Self-assessment depression scale
USP-NF	United States Pharmacopeia–National Formulary
WHI	Women's health initiative

Introduction

According to the World Health Organization the elderly make up the fastest-growing segment of the world population, and women make up the majority of the aging populations in all countries [1]. Accordingly, by the year 2025 the number of people over the age of 65 years of age will reach >800 M (10 % of the total population), of which 60 % will be women [2]. By the year 2030 there will be more than 60 million postmenopausal women in the USA and approximately 1.2 billion postmenopausal women worldwide [1–3]. Understanding the onset of this transition, as well as the development of novel therapeutic alternatives for the treatment of menopause related symptoms has become increasingly important, particularly in light of twenty-first century age demographics. Women in developed countries will spend approximately one third of their lives in the postmenopausal state [4].

Menopause is defined as the point in time following 12 consecutive months of amenorrhea and occurs in response to normal physiologic changes in the hypothalamic–pituitary–ovarian axis [2, 3]. The menopausal transition (climacteric) starts with the perimenopausal period that usually occurs 2–8 years prior to the last menstrual period, and for the last 12 months of amenorrhea preceding menopause. During this period, fewer ovarian follicles develop in each menstrual cycle [3]. In addition, during the perimenopausal period the ovaries produce less estradiol, progesterone, and androgens, resulting in irregular menstrual cycles, heavier or lighter flow, periods of amenorrhea, and worsening or newly developing premenstrual symptoms. Eventually, ovarian follicle production stops, and menstruation ceases. The postmenopausal period refers to the first 5 years or so following menopause when hormonal fluctuations are still present [3].

Since menopause is a major physiological and psychological event in the lives of all women, how women respond to and cope with the menopausal transition depends on a variety of factors including cultural and socioeconomic status, level of education, degree of physical symptoms, and attitudes toward treatment. Since menopause is associated with negative social meanings in Western culture, many women have very negative opinions about the menopausal transition which may impact overall mental and physical health [5]. In fact, a recent study suggests that women with more negative attitudes towards menopause in general report more symptoms during the menopausal transition [6]. In the United States, most women experience menopause by the age of 51, and between 55 and 82 % of women will experience vasomotor symptoms (hot flashes) or other symptoms such as depression, mood swings, sleep disorders, vaginal dryness, and joint pain [7, 8]. While most women experience symptoms acutely for only the first 4–5 years, approximately 10 % will have severe symptoms that may persist for more than 10 years [9]. Between 10 and 25 % of women will suffer such severe symptoms that they will seek treatment from their health care provider [9, 10]. Interestingly, several studies have found significant correlations between race/ethnicity and the prevalence of menopausal symptoms and hormone levels [11, 12]. The Study of Women's Health Across the Nation was one of the largest multiethnic studies focused on the relationship of socio-demographic and lifestyle factors on menopausal symptoms experienced by women in the United States [12]. The study involved 12,425 women of African-American, Japanese, Chinese, Hispanic, and Caucasian descent, and the results suggested that ethnicity serves as a significant predictor for the prevalence of menopausal symptoms. Over 50 % of late perimenopausal women surveyed reported hot flashes or night sweats, with Hispanic and African American women reporting the most frequent hot flashes and night sweats. Additionally, Hispanic women reported experiencing urine leakage, vaginal dryness, and heart palpitations most frequently, whereas Japanese and Chinese women reported fewer symptoms in general with the exception of heart palpitations and forgetfulness [12].

The menopausal transition is associated with an increased risk of chronic diseases such as osteoporosis, cardiovascular disease, Alzheimer's disease, and lower urogenital dysfunction that can significantly impact the quality of life for women [13, 14]. A good example is osteoporosis, which is a progressive disease with important clinical implications because osteoporosis-related hip fractures are a great source of disability and mortality [14]. Data from the United States indicates that by the age of 60–70, *only* one in nine Caucasian women have normal bone mineral density. After the age of 80, about 70 % of women have osteoporosis [15]. The incidence of osteoporosis is 80 % higher in women than in men and approximately 15 % of Caucasian women over the age of 50 will experience an osteoporosis-related hip fracture during their lifetime [15, 16]. In addition to chronic diseases, the relationship between the perceived change in the quality of life and the menopausal transition, with regard to physical health, psychosomatic status, and personal life appears to be altered [17–19]. One study has demonstrated that the menopausal transition is significantly associated with a decrease in perceived physical health and psychosomatic status [17]. Approximately 79–83 % of women reported that their physical health or energy levels had decreased over the previous year. Forty-one percent of women reported an increase in psychosomatic stress by the age of 48 years that increased to 47 % by the age of 54 years. However, it is interesting to note that women with two or more children reported an improvement in psychosomatic domain and personal life, while only physical inactivity was a significant risk factor for declining physical health [17].

For many years hormone therapy (HT) was widely regarded as standard of care for the management of menopausal symptoms and recommended for the prevention of cardiovascular disease irrespective of age, especially for high-risk women such as those with existing coronary heart disease [4, 9]. Many clinical trials reported that HT (estrogen alone or estrogen plus progestin) was the most effective therapy for hot flashes and sleep disturbances, reducing symptoms by 80–90 %, while other therapies such as vitamins, clonidine, and antidepressants reduce symptoms by approximately 30–60 % [4, 9, 17]. Other observed additional benefits included decreased vaginal dryness, stress incontinence, urinary tract infections, and increased skin elasticity and thickness. Now, HT is no longer the first choice due to significant concerns about safety and efficacy [4, 9, 17]. The Women's Health Initiative, one of several studies exploring the risks and benefits of HT use in postmenopausal women, displaced the common belief of the protective effects provided by HT (29). Data generated from this randomized trial showed an increased risk of heart disease (29 %), breast cancer (26 %), and events such as strokes (41 %) in women using HT. However, HT demonstrated a protective effect against colon cancer (37 %) and hip fractures (34 %), secondary to osteoporosis [20]. The WHI results, in combination with clinical contraindications and generalized fear of HT, have left many women with the opinion that HT is inadequate or inappropriate for the treatment of menopausal symptoms [20].

Thus, many women have turned to complementary and alternative medicine (CAM) such as herbal therapies as replacement for HT to treat menopausal symptoms. While there are many such CAM available for use by women such as soy, red clover, and black cohosh, it is black cohosh that has been the most extensively investigated with well over 30 clinical trials.

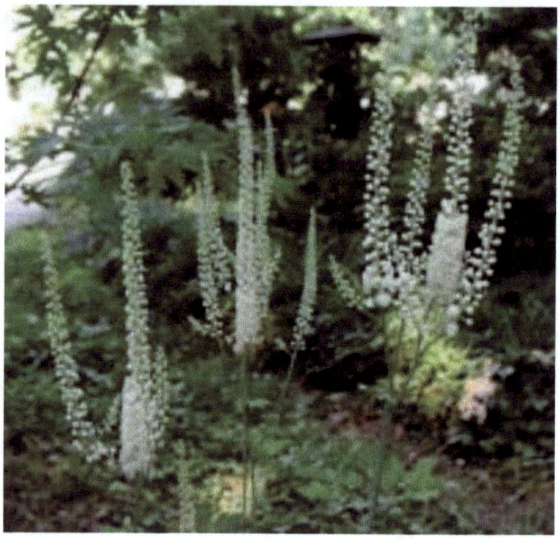

Fig. 28.1 *Actea racemosa* L. [syn. *Cimicifuga racemosa* (L.) Nutt., Ranunculaceae]

Black Cohosh History and Background

Black cohosh, known scientifically as *Actaea racemosa* L. [syn. *Cimicifuga racemosa* (L.) Nutt., Ranunculaceae] (Fig. 28.1), is a coarse perennial woodland herb with large compound leaves, and a thick, knotted rhizome (root) system native to North America [21]. There are numerous other vernacular (common) names for this plant, including black snakeroot, black root, bugbane, rattle root, rattle top, rattle squawroot, snake root, and rattleweed [22]. Historically, black cohosh rhizomes (roots) were routinely used as medicine by the Native American Indians, including the Penobscot, Winnebago, and Dakota, for the treatment of coughs, colds, constipation, fatigue, and rheumatism, as well as to increase breast milk production [23, 24]. In 1832, a tincture of black cohosh rhizome was used for the treatment of pain and inflammation associated with endometriosis, rheumatism, neuralgia, and dysmenorrhea [24]. A fluidextract of black cohosh was official in the United States National Formulary for over 100 years from 1840 to 1946. Black cohosh appeared in the first edition of the United States Dispensatory in 1833 and remained through 1955 for a total of 122 years [25]. In 2001, both the rhizome and the dry rhizome extract of black cohosh were proposed once again for inclusion in the dietary supplements section of the United States Pharmacopeia–National Formulary (USP–NF) and the monograph became official in the Second Supplement to USP 30–NF 25 (2007) [26]. Black cohosh is currently also monographed as Rhizoma Cimicifugae Racemosae in the WHO monographs [22] and as Black Cohosh in the British Herbal Pharmacopeia.

Chemistry

The major chemical constituents of black cohosh are the triterpene glycosides principally beta-xylopyranosides and alpha-arabinopyranosides [22, 26]. The aglycones are mostly derived from acteol and cimigenol. A cyclopropane ring is a common feature of these compounds, which are structurally related to cycloartenol. One of the triterpene glycosides, 23-epi-26-deoxyactein (formerly 27-deoxyactein; Fig. 28.2), is the constituent usually selected for standardization of commercial black cohosh products because of its abundance in roots and rhizomes. Other constituents present in the rhizome include tannins, resin, fatty acids, starch, sugars, and aromatic acids including ferulic acid,

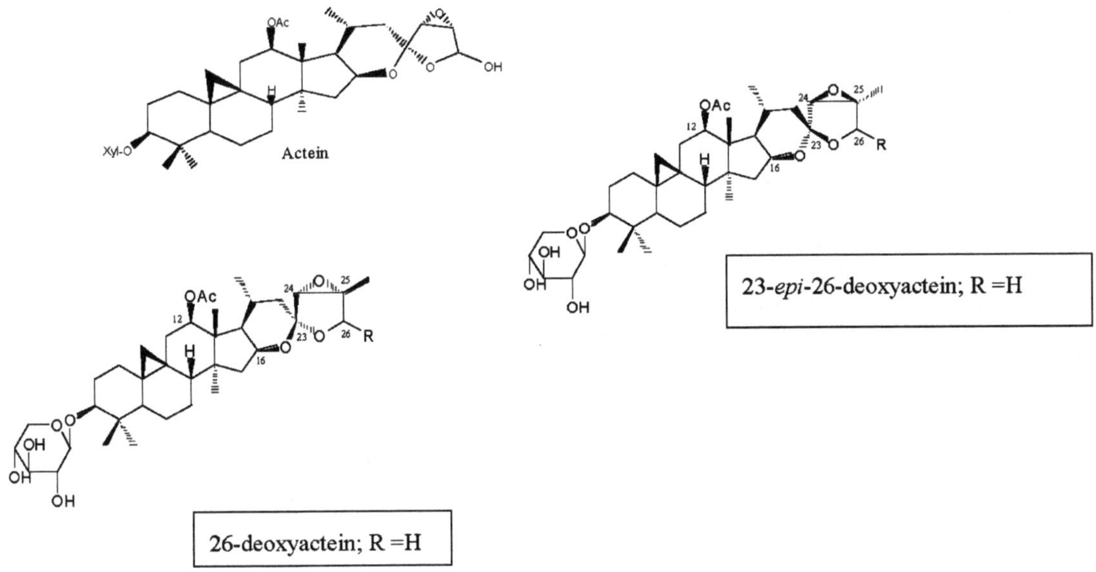

Fig. 28.2 Structures of actein and its derivatives present in black cohosh rhizomes

Fig. 28.3 The structures of the fukinolic and cimicifugic acids isolated from black cohosh rhizomes

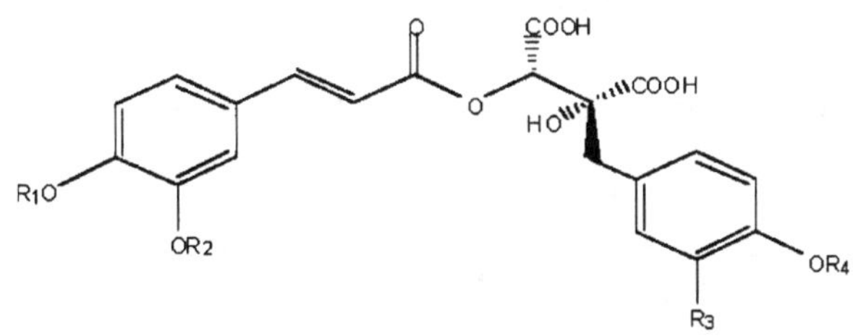

Cimicifugic acid A: R_1 =H, R_2=Me, R_3=OH, R_4=H
Cimicifugic acid B: R_1 =Me, R_2=H, R_3=OH, R_4=H
Fukinolic acid: R_1 = R_2=H, R_3=OH, R_4=H

isoferulic acid, caffeic acid, and fukinolic and cimicifugic acids (Fig. 28.3). Dietary supplements of black cohosh may be adulterated or substituted with other species *of Actaea*, especially the American species *Actaea podocarpa* (syn. *Cimicifuga americana*; yellow cohosh) because of the similarity of the underground parts. A number of Asian species of Actaea may also be marketed as black cohosh. These include *A. cimicifuga* (syn. *Cimicifuga foetida*), *A. dahurica* (syn. *C. dahurica*), and *A. heracleifolia* (syn. *C. heracleifolia*). *Cimicifuga dahurica* is also sold under the name "sheng ma," and it is frequently referred to as "black cohosh." Black cohosh may also be adulterated or substituted with blue cohosh, *Caulophyllum thalictroides*.

Black Cohosh Clinical Trials

The standardized extracts and other commercial products of black cohosh are prepared from the dried rhizomes and roots of the plant [22, 37, 38]. Remifemin® is a commercially available black cohosh product that is a dried 40 % (also 60 %) isopropanol extract of the roots and rhizomes. The extract is standardized to contain 1 mg of total triterpenes calculated as 27-deoxyactein (now known as 26-deoxyactein) per 20 mg of extract. In addition, Klimadynon®/Menofem®, (CR BNO 1055) is another commercially available product, the extracts are aqueous ethanol extracts; however, the exact composition is proprietary.

In terms of alternative medicines for the management of menopause, black cohosh has a large number of published clinical trials [29–50]. Prior to 2003, there were at least 25 published reports detailing observational and case studies of black cohosh for the treatment of various gynecological ailments including menopause [27, 28]. Since 2003, another nine studies have been performed [29–31, 44–50]. Since 1982, approximately 16 clinical trials have assessed the efficacy of the most commonly used standardized black cohosh extract, a 40 % isopropyl alcohol or a 60 % ethanol extract of the roots and rhizomes (both known as Remifemin®) for the symptomatic treatment of climacteric symptoms such as anxiety, hot flushes, profuse sweating, insomnia, and vaginal atrophy [32–44]. Of the 16 trials, at least 10 were randomized controlled or comparison trials [33–35, 37, 40, 42, 43, 46, 47, 49] and the other studies were uncontrolled. Two clinical trials have assessed the safety and efficacy of the black cohosh product CR BNO 1055 (Klimadynon®/Menofem®) [43, 44]. More recently the NIH funded clinical trials have tested a number of black cohosh products including one from Pure World (Hackensack, NJ, USA). All these studies reported no benefit for menopause [29–31].

National Institutes of Health Funded Clinical Trials Performed in the United States

The most recent NIH funded randomized controlled clinical trial evaluated the safety and efficacy of black cohosh and red clover (*Trifolium pratense* L.) for the relief of menopausal symptoms [29]. The study assessed the effectiveness and safety of an ethanolic extract of black cohosh roots/rhizomes and an ethanolic extract of the aerial parts of red clover in a 12 month, randomized, 4-armed, double-blinded, placebo-controlled trial with 0.625 mg conjugated equine estrogens (CEE)/2.5 mg medroxyprogesterone acetate (MPA; Prempro™; Wyeth Pharmaceuticals, Philadelphia, PA) as the positive control. Only menopausal women with an intact uterus were recruited for the trial, thus requiring the use of an estrogen/progestin regimen for the positive control group. The primary outcome was a reduction in vasomotor symptoms, and the sample size calculation was based on clinical outcomes from prior research studies. The study was powered only to compare each botanical product and positive control with placebo, but not to each other. In addition to the primary outcome, secondary outcomes measures included safety assessments, relief of somatic symptoms including insomnia, joint pain, sleep and fatigue, mood changes (depression and anxiety), sexual dysfunction (vaginal dryness, dyspareunia, libido, anorgasmia), and health related quality of life. Validated instruments used to evaluate secondary outcome measures included the Greene Climacteric Scale (somatic symptoms and quality of life), Pittsburgh Sleep Quality Index, the Positive and Negative Affect Schedule, and the Kupperman Index. The results of this NIH funded study showed that only the positive control, CEE/MPA, produced a significant reduction in hot flushes as compared with the placebo group. Reductions in vasomotor symptoms over the 12-month study period for the 4 study groups were as follows: the CEE/MPA group had a 94 % reduction in vasomotor symptoms (71 vasomotor symptoms per week at baseline to 5 at follow-up), with the placebo group showing the next greatest reduction in vasomotor symptoms (63 %; from 52 to 19). The red clover group showed a 57 % reduction in hot flashes (from 58 to 25), and the black cohosh group had the smallest reduction in vasomotor symptoms, 34 % (from 65 to 43) [29]. With regard to secondary outcomes, red clover subjects showed a reduction in anxiety over the 12-month study compared to placebo. While no other beneficial secondary outcomes were observed in the study, save for the reduction of anxiety among red clover users, it is important to recognize that the study was not powered to properly evaluate these diverse secondary clinical outcomes.

There was no increased incidence of safety issues for either of the botanical study groups, with no anticoagulant effect being observed in the subjects in the red clover group and no hepatotoxicity observed among subjects in the black cohosh group. In addition, there was no evidence of an adverse effect on breast tissue or endometrial thickness for either botanical preparation [29]. This study was a rigorous, well designed and executed trial with few dropouts, excellent patient compliance and using a chemically and biologically standardized black cohosh extract. However, this was an extract developed by the University of Illinois at Chicago Botanical Center that had no previous clinical data for efficacy, and had no track record in terms of other black cohosh products test in clinical trials. Thus, it is difficult to compare this trial with trials of other products. The study used a 75 % ethanol extract of black cohosh, but there were few details of the product, the dosage form used, and dosing regime, and there were no details of the matching placebo in the publication. Furthermore, a pharmacokinetic study by the same group of the product (presumably used in the clinical trial) showed that the half-life of the black cohosh extract was very short [31]. The pharmacokinetic study used of one of its most abundant triterpene glycosides, 23-epi-26-deoxyactein as the marker compound. Single doses of black cohosh extract containing 1.4, 2.8, or 5.6 mg of 23-epi-26-deoxyactein were administered to 15 healthy, menopausal women. Serial blood samples and 24-h urine samples were obtained; blood chemistry, hormonal levels, and 23-epi-26-deoxyactein levels were determined. Pharmacokinetic analyses of 23-epi-26-deoxyactein in sera indicated that the maximum concentration and area under the curve increased proportionately with dosage, but that the half-life was ~2 h for all dosages [31]. One NIH funded study for black cohosh was performed at Columbia University and was completed, but has yet to be published. This study also used the Pure World extract and found no benefit to black cohosh extracts for the management of menopausal symptoms (Kronenberg F, personal communication 2008).

The second US study (Herbal Alternatives for Menopause, HALT) was a 12-month, randomized, double-blind, placebo-controlled trial conducted from May 2001 to September 2004 and was also funded by the NIH [30]. The HALT trial was designed to investigate the effects of three naturopathic approaches for vasomotor symptom relief and HT compared with placebo. The trial involved 351 women (ages 45–55 years) with two or more vasomotor symptoms per day. Of the 351 subjects, 52 % of the women were in perimenopausal (≥1 skipped menses within the preceding 12 months) and 48 % were postmenopausal (no bleeding within 12 months, or follicle-stimulating hormone (FSH) level >20 IU/mL if patient had undergone hysterectomy without bilateral oophorectomy); and 2 or more vasomotor symptoms per day over 2 weeks (≥6 moderate to severe symptoms). The outcomes measured included the rate and intensity of vasomotor symptoms (1 = mild to 3 = severe), and the Wiklund Vasomotor Symptom Subscale. The patients were randomized to receive (1) Black cohosh extract, 160 mg daily; (2) multibotanical with black cohosh, 200 mg daily, and 9 other ingredients; (3) multibotanical plus dietary soy counseling; (4) CEE, 0.625 mg daily, with or without medroxyprogesterone acetate, 2.5 mg daily; or (5) placebo. The black cohosh (Pure World, Inc., Hackensack, New Jersey) and the multibotanical, ProGyne, (Progena Professional Formulations, Albuquerque, New Mexico) were encapsulated to study specifications. The results of this study showed that the daily vasomotor symptoms, symptom intensity, and the Wiklund Vasomotor Symptom Subscale score did not differ between the herbal interventions and placebo at 3, 6, or 12 months or for the average over all the follow-up time points ($P>0.05$ for all comparisons). However, at 12 months, the vasomotor symptom intensity was significantly worse with the multibotanical plus soy intervention than with placebo ($P=0.016$). The difference in vasomotor symptoms per day between placebo and any of the herbal treatments at any time point was less than 1 symptom per day; for the average over all the follow-up time points, the difference was less than 0.55 symptoms per day (40). The difference for HT versus placebo was –4.06 vasomotor symptoms per day for the average over all the follow-up time points (95 % CI, –5.93 to –2.19 symptoms per day; $P<0.001$) [30]. This study was a robust, RCT but again used a product that had never been tested in clinical trial and therefore cannot be compared with the trials for other products.

Randomized Clinical Trials Performed in Europe

The therapeutic effects of the black cohosh extract CR BNO 1055 (Klimadynon®/Menofem®) were assessed in 62 postmenopausal women to determine its effects on symptoms, bone metabolism, and endometrial thickness, and compared with those of conjugated estrogens (CE) and placebo [43]. Postmenopausal women, 40–60 years of age, were included if they met the criteria of body mass index (BMI) <30, last menstrual bleeding at least 6 months ago, i.e., perimenopausal women with postmenopausal hormone values (17β-estradiol ≤40 pg/ml, FSH ≥25 mU/ml) at all visits, at least three hot flushes per day (as documented in a diary), menopause rating scale (MRS) items 1–6, sum of scores ≥1.7 at visits 1 and 2, MRS item 1 (hot flushes) ≥0.3 at visits 1 and 2. The women were included in the double-blind, randomized, placebo- and conjugated estrogen (CE)-controlled study, and treated either with CR BNO 1055 (daily dose corresponding to 40 mg herbal drug, $n=20$), 0.6 mg CE ($n=22$), or matching placebo ($n=20$), for 3 months. The outcomes measured included menopausal symptoms that were assessed by the menopause rating scale (MRS, 10 symptoms) and a diary. Levels of CrossLaps (marker of bone degradation) were determined by ELECSYS system and bone-specific alkaline phosphatase (marker of bone formation) by an enzymatic assay. Endometrial thickness was measured via transvaginal ultrasound; vaginal cytology was also studied. The primary efficacy criterion and secondary variables were measured by the change from baseline to end point. Analysis of the results of the study showed that the total scores in all 10 MRS items were similar for the black cohosh product and CE, and but were not quite statistical significant ($P=0.0506$; 0.0513). CR BNO 1055 had no effect on endometrial thickness, which was significantly increased by treatment with CE. Vaginal superficial cells were increased after treatment with CE ($P=0.0001$), and were slightly increased after treatment with CR BNO 1055, but this was not statistically significant as compared with placebo ($P=0.0542$). Bone turnover after 12 weeks was reduced in both the black cohosh arm and the CE arm, these data were statistically significant ($P=0.0136$; 0.0138). While this was one of the better clinical trials for black cohosh, the study still suffered from a number of problems. First 97 patients were initially randomized with one of the inclusion criteria being no menstrual bleeding for at least 6 months ago (normally 12 months, so these patients may be considered perimenopausal); however, 35 patients were eventually excluded from the final analyses due to masked ovulary or unovulatory cycles and BMI>30. Thus, the dropout rate was very high and may have impacted the final outcome data. In addition, the baseline characteristics of the patients are noted as being comparable in all treatment groups; however, no actual data are given or statistical analysis is shown. Furthermore, the study suffers from the lack of an adequate description of the black cohosh extract and the placebo, as well as a short 12-week treatment period. Finally, the study conclusions are somewhat deceptive. While it is true that CR BNO 1055 gave similar results to low dose CE (0.6 mg/day), with the exception of bone turnover, none of these results were statistically significant ($P>0.05$) as compared with placebo, including the data for CE [43]. So technically neither the low dose CE nor the CR BNO 1055 extract reduced symptoms in menopausal women in this study.

A 12-week randomized, double-blind, placebo-controlled trial compared the efficacy of Remifemin® with that of conjugated estrogens or placebo for the treatment of menopausal symptoms and vaginal atrophy [37]. Eighty women, between the ages of 45 and 58 years old, were treated with 8 mg/day of the extract (corresponding to 48–140 mg of the dried herb), or 0.625 mg/day of conjugated estrogens, or placebo. The primary outcomes were measured included the Kupperman Index (KI) for menopausal symptoms, the Hamilton Anxiety Rating Scale (HAMA), and the vaginal maturity index. After 12 weeks of treatment, all groups showed improvements. However, a significant decrease in the Kupperman Index (34–14) was observed in the group treated with Remifemin® ($P<0.001$), indicating an improvement in menopausal symptoms. In addition, there was a significant decrease in the HAMA scale ($P<0.001$) indicating a reduction in anxiety; as well as a significant improvement in the proliferative status of the vaginal epithelium ($P<0.01$), suggesting a possible estrogenic effect of

Remifemin®. Minor estrogenic-like adverse events were reported including headache, weight gain, mastalgia and leg heaviness in the group treated with the extract. The primary criticisms of this study include the lack of effect of the low dose estrogen (0.625 mg), which was reported to be less effective than placebo, and the short treatment period of 12 weeks [37].

A randomized comparison study assessed the efficacy of Remifemin® for the treatment of menopausal symptoms, induced by hysterectomy [34]. Sixty women under the age of 40, who had undergone a partial hysterectomy and retained one ovary, were treated with estriol (1 mg/day), conjugated estrogens (1.25 mg/day), an estrogen–progesterone sequence therapy (2 mg estradiol and 1 mg norethindrone acetate) or Remifemin® (8 mg/day, corresponding to 49–140 mg of dried herb) for six months. The results of each treatment were determined at 4, 8, 12, and 24 weeks, and outcomes were measured using a modified KI, as well as the serum concentrations of FSH and luteinizing hormone (LH). The results showed a statistically significant decrease in menopausal symptoms in all treatment groups ($P=0.01$), as verified by reductions in a modified KI. Conjugated estrogens or estrogen–progesterone combinations appeared to be slightly more effective than the Remifemin®; however, no statistically significant difference between the three treatment groups was observed. Serum levels of LH and FSH did not change in any of the treatment groups [34]. The major flaws of this trial were the lack of inclusion of a placebo group, and the lack of change in FSH of LH levels in those patients treated with estrogen or the estrogen/progesterone combination. In addition, no treatment resulted in a decrease in the KI below 15 points [34].

A controlled comparison trial, involving 60 women between the ages of 45 and 60 years, assessed the efficacy of the Remifemin® to that of conjugated estrogens or diazepam for the treatment of climacteric symptoms [40]. The outcomes measured included a modified Kupperman menopausal index (mKI) comprised of the following symptoms: hot flushes, nocturnal sweating, nervousness, headache and palpitations. Assessment of changes in the vaginal epithelium proliferation was also performed. Psychological symptoms were measured using the HAMA and self-assessment depression scale (SDS). The patients were treated with 80 drops of a 60 % ethanol extract of Remifemin®, or 0.625 mg conjugated estrogens or 2 mg diazepam for a period of 12 weeks. All three forms of therapy reduced the mKI, HAMA and SDS. A reduction in atrophic changes in the vaginal mucosa was also observed in the groups treated with Remifemin® or conjugated estrogens. Treatment with the Remifemin® was reported to produce the best improvements in all measures; however, no actual data are given. In addition, this study did not use a placebo arm [40].

A randomized, double-blind parallel-group clinical trial involving 152 perimenopausal and postmenopausal women with climacteric symptoms compared the effects of two different doses of Remifemin® (corresponding to 39 mg drug versus 127 mg drug/day) over 6 months [35]. A decrease in the Kupperman-Menopause Index (beginning value 31) was observed after two weeks in both treatment groups. Both dosage levels had similar therapeutic safety and efficacy. After 6 months of treatment, the number of responders ($KI<15$) was approximately 90 %. No effects on the levels of LH, FSH, sex hormone binding globulin, prolactin, estradiol, and vaginal cytology parameters were observed. Unfortunately, again neither placebo nor comparison drug was used in this investigation [35]. Details of some further 2003–2006 positive European studies for black cohosh are presented in Table 28.1. Overall the clinical trials published in Europe have been positive; however, these studies were not as rigorous as the studies performed in the USA and there were numerous methodological flaws in many of the trials.

Adverse Events and Safety of Black Cohosh Extracts

Data from the clinical trials and post-marketing surveillance studies have generally found very few serious adverse events associated with the ingestion of black cohosh extracts (Table 28.2). A multicenter, post-marketing surveillance study involving 629 women with menopausal symptoms assessed

Table 28.1 Overview of some of the positive clinical trials since 2003 and product information for black cohosh extracts for the treatment of menopausal symptoms

Clinical trial	*N*	Population	Control	Treatment	Black cohosh product specifications	Outcomes measured	Results
Wuttke et al. (2003)	62	Postmenopausal women	Conjugated estrogens (CE) (0.6 mg/day); or placebo for 12 weeks	CR BNO 1055 Klimadyon/Menofem (40 mg/day) for 12 weeks	Dried aqueous/ethanolic extract (58 %, v/v) of the black cohosh rhizome, with a drug to extract ratio of 6–9:1. Standardized to isoferulic acid (determined by HPLC) at 50–110 µg/100 mg extract	Menopause rating scale (MRS)	Statistically significant reduction in MRS score; however, reduction in hot flashes (item 1 on MRS) did not differ significantly between groups. Beneficial effect on bone metabolism and vaginal cytology reported in both CE and CR BNO groups. CR BNO had no effect on endometrial thickness, which was increased by CE
Frei-Kleiner et al. (2005)	122	Perimenopausal and postmenopausal women	Matching placebo for 12 weeks	CR-99, 42 mg/day for 12 weeks	60 % Ethanol extract; 29–55 mg with an average of 42 mg crude drug	Hot flashes, Kupperman Index, MRS	Weekly weighted score of hot flashes or Kupperman Index showed no superiority of the tested black cohosh extract compared to placebo. Analysis of a subgroup of patients with a Kupperman Index ≥20 showed a significant reduction in this index ($P<0.018$), with a decrease of 47 and 21 % was observed in the black cohosh and placebo group, respectively. The weekly weighted scores of hot flashes ($P<0.052$) and the menopause rating scale ($P<0.009$) showed statistically significant results in the subgroup
Nappi et al. (2005)	64	Postmenopausal women	Low dose (25 µg) transdermal estradiol (TTSE2) for 12 weeks	Remifemin 40 mg/day for 12 weeks	40 % Aqueous isopropanol extract of black cohosh rhizomes (20 mg/tablet)	Hot flash diaries, Green's climacteric scale, Symptom rating scale for anxiety and depression	Both CR and low-dose TTSE2 significantly reduced the number of hot flushes per day ($P<0.001$) and vasomotor symptoms ($P<0.001$), starting at the first month of treatment. An identical effect was evident also for both anxiety ($P<0.001$) and depression ($P<0.001$) that were significantly reduced following 3 months of both CR and low-dose TTSE2

Osmers et al. (2005)	304	Postmenopausal women	Matching placebo for 12 weeks	Remifemin 40 mg/day for 12 weeks	40 % Aqueous isopropanol extract of black cohosh rhizomes (20 mg/tablet)	menopause rating scale (MRS)	The Remifemin extract was more effective than placebo ($P<0.001$). The effect size was 0.03–0.05 MRS units, which is similar to recent hormone replacement therapy study results (0.036 Menopause rating scale units). Women in the early climacteric phase benefited more than in the late phase. The hot flush sub-score was the most effective measure of the extract's activity
Uebelhack et al. (2006)	301	Postmenopausal women	Matching placebo for 16 weeks	Remifemin 40 mg/day plus St. John's wort for 16 weeks	40 % Aqueous isopropanol extract of black cohosh rhizomes (20 mg/tablet) plus 70 mg St. John's wort	Menopause rating scale (MRS) and Hamilton depression rating scale	Treatment decreased the menopause rating scale by 50 % (0.46±0.13 to 0.23±0.13) as compared with 19.6 % (0.46±0.14 to 0.37±0.15) in the placebo group. The Hamilton depression rating scale total score decreased 41.8 % in the treatment group (18.9±2.2 to 11.0±3.8 points), and 12.7 % in the placebo group (18.9±2.1 to 16.5±4.3). Treatment with Remifemin plus St. John's wort was significantly ($P<0.001$) superior to placebo in both measures
Verhoeven et al. (2005)	124	Perimenopausal women	Olive oil containing matching placebo	Soy extract 125 mg plus 1,500 mg evening primrose oil, 100 mg black cohosh extract, 200 mg calcium, vitamin D, and vitamin E	100 mg black cohosh extract providing 8 mg deoxyactein	Modified Kupperman Index, Green's Climacteric scale, visual analogue scale	At weeks 6 and 12, all scores in both groups had improved as compared with baseline, though the overall difference in scores between the groups was not statistically significant. Olive oil was not a good choice for a placebo as it is not physiologically inert

Table 28.2 Adverse events rate and discontinuation rates for clinical trials 1982–2001

Author, year	Number of Remifemin menopause-treated subjects	Study duration	Study population	Remifemin menopause dose	Discontinuation rastes (reason for discontinuation)	Adverse events observed N (%)
		Double-blind studies				
Stoll (1988)	26	12 Weeks	Women aged 40–56 with menopausal complaints	2 Tablets, twice a day	1 (Protocol noncompliance)	3 Weight gain (11.54 %), 1 stimulation (3.85 %), 1 myodynia (3.85 %), 7 not specified (26.92 %)
Nesselhut and Liske (1999)	40	12 Weeks	Women with menopausal symptoms	Variable	0	0
Liske et al. (2002)	152	12/24 Weeks	Women aged 43–60 with menopausal complaints	Tablets: 127.3 and 39.0 mg, herbal drug daily	3 (Adverse events); 8 (lack of efficacy); 2 (protocol noncompliance); 1 (administrative); 5 (other)	5 Gastrointestinal (3.3 %), 3 CNS (3.3 %), 5 breast/genital (3.3 %) and 2 other (2.63 %)
Jacobson et al. (2001)	69	8 Weeks	Women with breast cancer	I tablet twice daily with meals	0	0
		Open studies				
Stolze (1982)	629	8 Weeks	Women with menopausal symptoms	40 Drops of liquid, twice a day	No discontinuation reported	44 Nonspecific
Daiber (1983)	36	12 Weeks	Women with contraindications to hormone therapy	40 Drops of liquid, twice a day	4 Mild gastrointestinal	0
Vorberg (1984)	50	12 Weeks	Women with contraindications to hormone the rapy	40 Drops of liquid, twice a day	0	0
Warnecke (1985)	19	12 Weeks	Women aged 45–60, with irregular or no bleeding and menopausal symptoms	40 Drops of liquid, twice a day	1 (Lack of efficacy)	Not specified
Petho (1987)	50	6 Months	Women previously treated with hormones for menopausal symptoms	2 Tablets, twice a day	0	0

the efficacy of an ethanol extract of black cohosh (dose of 40 drops twice daily of Remifemin® over 8 weeks of treatment [40]). Only 7 % of the patients reported adverse events such as nausea, vomiting, headaches, and dizziness. These symptoms however were short-lived and none required discontinuation of therapy [40]. In another post-marketing study, administration of Remifemin® to 40 menopausal women (dose of 136 mg per day for 3 months—normal dose is 40–80 mg/day) did not significantly change endometrial status, vaginal cytology, or reproductive hormones from baseline [41]. In one of the most recent studies, no significant differences between the black cohosh treatments and placebo for any of the assessed safety parameters including breast and endometrial safety, liver enzymes, complete blood count, or lipid profiles were noted and there was no evidence for hepatotoxicity of black cohosh during the 12-month intervention [29]. However, there have been numerous case reports suggesting that administration of black cohosh extracts may be associated with increased incidence of hepatoxicity, in the form of severe acute hepatitis and fulminant liver failure [51, 52]. A report from the United States Pharmacopeia analyzed information from human clinical case reports, adverse event reports, animal pharmacological and toxicological data, pertaining to liver damage associated with black cohosh ingestion. Data were obtained from many sources, including the European Medicines Agency, Health Canada, the Australian Therapeutic Goods Administration, and the US Food and Drug Administration. In this study, 30 reports that associated the use of black cohosh products with liver damage were analyzed. All the reports of liver damage were assigned possible causality, and none were assigned probable or certain causality. The report concluded that the link between liver damage reports and black cohosh was weak and not of "certain" causality. However, there were many weaknesses in the adverse event reporting including incomplete case information and unknown products, confounding variables such as use of alcohol and other concurrent medications, and preexisting risk factors [51]. However, considering the serious nature of the adverse events, the report concluded that hepatotoxicity was possible and could not be ruled out [51]. Subsequent reviews on the subject have refuted the hepatoxicity potential of black cohosh and suggested that data from 69 reports was insufficient to support the concept of hepatotoxicity in a "primarily suspected causal relationship" for black cohosh [52–54]. However, at this point in time there are ~75 case reports of hepatotoxicity associated with the ingestion of black cohosh containing supplements. Due to the difficulty in proving direct causality for hepatotoxic agents in general, coupled with the inability to prove that black cohosh is not responsible for the reported cases of hepatotoxicity, it seems prudent on the part of health care professionals to err on the side of caution as far as safety is concerned with black cohosh. In the UK, the Committee on Herbal Medicinal Products of the European Medical Agency issued a public statement in 2006 advising patients to stop taking black cohosh products and consult their doctor immediately if they develop signs and symptoms suggestive of liver injury. A similar recommendation was made by British Medicines and Health products Regulatory Agency, the Therapeutic Goods Administration in Australia and the Canadian Natural Health Product Directorate (Table 28.3).

Conclusion

Black cohosh has been used historically as an herbal remedy and is currently advocated as an alternative therapy for menopausal symptoms. Review of the published randomized clinical trials, suggests that treatment with a standardized black cohosh extract may be of some benefit for treating the symptoms of menopause. However, the majority of these studies are limited by poor methodology. Data from the newer RCTs are negative and do not support the use of black cohosh in menopausal women. There also appears to be of little benefit for black cohosh in perimenopausal women as well. Thus, considering the lack of sufficient clinical data supporting its use in the management of the menopausal transition, and the potential for serious adverse events especially in women using other concomitant medications and alcohol the use of black cohosh by perimenopausal and postmenopausal women cannot be recommended.

Table 28.3 Proposed caution and warning labels for black cohosh products from regulatory agencies around the world

1. Proposed USP caution labels for black cohosh products (2008): "Caution: In rare cases black cohosh has been reported to affect the liver. Discontinue use and consult a healthcare professional if you have a liver disorder or if you develop symptoms of liver trouble, such as abdominal pain, dark urine or jaundice." This labeling statement is not mandatory but voluntary (62)
2. European Medicines Agency (EMEA) and the Committee on Herbal Medicinal Products (HMPC) advice to patients concerning black cohosh products (2006): "Patients should stop taking *Cimicifugae racemosae rhizoma* (Black Cohosh, root) and consult their doctor immediately if they develop signs and symptoms suggestive of liver injury (tiredness, loss of appetite, yellowing of the skin and eyes or severe upper stomach pain with nausea and vomiting or dark urine)." www.ema.europa.eu/docs/en_GB/document_library/Public_statement/2009/12/WC500016766.pdf
3. Health Canada advise to concerning black cohosh products (2006): Consumers should exercise caution in the use of products containing black cohosh, and consult a health care practitioner if they have concerns about its use. Consumers should discontinue the use of products containing black cohosh and consult a physician if they have unusual fatigue, weakness, loss of appetite, or if they develop symptoms suggestive of liver injury such as yellowing of the skin or whites of the eyes, dark urine, or abdominal pain. In 2010 the Health Canada Web site reported another 6 cases of potential hepatoxicity associated with the use of product containing black cohosh—-www.hc-sc.gc.ca/dhp-mps/medeff/bulletin/carn-bcei_v20n1-eng.php
4. The Australian Therapeutic Goods Administration (TGA) in 2006 decided that medicines containing black cohosh (*Actaea racemosa* syn. *Cimicifuga racemosa*) should be labeled with the following statement: "Warning: Black cohosh may harm the liver in some individuals. Use under the supervision of a healthcare professional." Products containing black cohosh were required to contain this warning label. http://www.tga.gov.au/cm/blkcohosh.htm

References

1. Anon. In: WHO Annual Report 2001, Geneva, Switzerland, World Health Organization Publications Office, 2003.
2. Houmard BS, Seifer DB. Predicting the onset of menopause. In: Seifer DB, Kennard EA, editors, Menopause, endocrinology and management. Totowa, NJ: Humana Press; 1999. p. 1–20.
3. World Health Organization Scientific Group. Research on the menopause. In: WHO Technical Report Ser. 670, Geneva, Switzerland: World Health Organization Publications Office; 1981.
4. Rice VM. Strategies and issues of managing menopause-related symptoms in diverse populations: ethnic and racial diversity. Am J Med. 2005;118:142S–7.
5. Smith MJ, Mann E, Mirza A, Hunter MS. Men and women's perceptions of hot flushes within social situations: are menopausal women's negative beliefs valid? Maturitas. 2011;69:57–62.
6. Ayers B, Forshaw M, Hunter MS. The impact of attitudes towards the menopause on women's symptom experience: a systematic review. Maturitas. 2010;65:28–36.
7. Freedman RR. Physiology of hot flashes. Am J Hum Biol. 2001;13:453–64.
8. Gold EB, Sternfeld B, Kelsey JL, Brown C, Mouton C, Reame N et al. Relation of demographic and lifestyle factors to symptoms in a multi-racial/ethic population of women 40–55 years of age. Am J Epidemol. 2000;152:463–73.
9. Grodstein F, Stampler MJ, Colditz GA, Willet WC, Manson JE, Joffe M et al. Postmenopausal hormone therapy and mortality. New Eng J Med. 1997;336:1769–75.
10. Avis NE, Stellato R, Crawford S, Johannes C, Longcope C. Is there a menopausal syndrome? Menopausal status and symptoms across racial/ethnic groups. Soc Sci Med. 2001;52:345–56.
11. Avis NE, Ory M, Matthews KA, Schocken M, Bromberger J, Colvin A. Health-related quality of life in a multiethnic sample of middle aged women: Study of Women's Health Across the Nation (SWAN). Med Care. 2003; 41:1262–76.
12. Palacios S, Sanchez-Borrego R, Forteza A. The importance of preventative health care in post-menopausal women. Maturitus. 2006;52S:S53–60.
13. National Osteoporosis Foundation. Disease Facts. http://www.nof.org/osteoporosis/diseasefacts.htm. Accessed 7 Nov 2011.
14. Stevenson JC, Cust MP, Ganger KF, Hillard TC, Lees B, Whitehead MI. Effects of transdermal versus oral hormone replacement therapy on bone density in spine and proximal femur in postmenopausal women. Lancet. 1990; 336:265–9.
15. Mishra G, Kuh D. Perceived change in quality of life during menopause. Soc Sci Med. 2006;62:93–102.

16. Avis NE, Crawford SL, McKinlay SM. Psychosocial, behavioral, and health factors related to menopause symptomology. J Wom Health. 1997;3:103–20.
17. Schwingl PJ, Hulka BA, Harlow SD. Risk factors of menopausal hot flashes. Obstet Gynecol. 1994;84:29–34.
18. Beyene Y. Cultural significance and physiological manifestations of menopause: a biocultural analysis. Cult Med Psychiatr. 1986;10:47–71.
19. Stewart DE. Menopause in highland Guatemala Mayan women. Maturitas. 2002;43:11–9.
20. Writing Group for the Women's Health Initiative Investigators. Risks and benefits of estrogen plus progestin in health of postmenopausal women. JAMA. 2002;288:321–33.
21. Compton JA, Culham A, Jury SL. Reclassification of *Actaea* to include *Cimicifuga* and *Soulica* (Ranunculaceae) phylogeny inferred from morphology, nrDNA, ITS and cpDNA trnL-F sequence variation. Taxon. 1998;47:593–635.
22. Mahady GB, Fong HHS, Farnsworth NR. Rhizoma Cimicifugae Racemosae. In: WHO Monographs on selected medicinal plants. Vol II. Geneva, Switzerland: World Health Organization; 2002. p. 55–65.
23. Brinker F. Review of Macrotys (black cohosh). Eclectic Med J. 1996;2:2–4.
24. Foster S. Black cohosh: *Cimicifuga racemosa*. A literature review. Herbalgram. 1999;45:35–49.
25. Mahady GB, Fabricant D, Chadwick LR, Dietz B. Black Coshosh: an alternative therapy for menopause? Nutr Clin Care. 2002;5:282–9.
26. United States Pharmacopoeia. USP 34-NF (2030) Supplemental Information for Articles of Botanical Origin. Supplemental Information and General Guidance Protocols: Black Cohosh Rockville, MD: USP; 2011.
27. Soni KK, Lawal TO, Locklear TD, Mahady GB. Black cohosh for menopause: safety and efficacy issues and future perspectives. Drug Information J. 2011;45:37–44.
28. Mahady GB, Huang Y, Doyle BJ, Locklear TD. Black cohosh (*Actaea racemosa*) for the mitigation of menopausal symptoms: recent developments in clinical safety and efficacy. J Wom Health. 2006;2:773–83.
29. Geller SE, Shulman LP, van Breemen RB, Banuvar S, Zhou Y, Epstein G, et al. Safety and efficacy of black cohosh and red clover for the management of vasomotor symptoms: a randomized controlled trial. Menopause. 2009;16: 1156–66.
30. Newton K, Reed S, LaCroix A, Grothaus L, Ehrlich K, Guiltinan J. Treatment of vasomotor symptoms of menopause with black cohosh, multibotanicals, soy, hormone therapy, or placebo: a randomized trial. Ann Intern Med. 2006;145:869–79.
31. van Breemen RB, Liang W, Banuvar S, Shulman LP, Pang Y, Tao Y, et al. Pharmacokinetics of 23-epi-26-deoxyactein in women after oral administration of a standardized extract of black cohosh. Clin Pharmacol Ther. 2010;8:219–25.
32. Daiber W. Klimakterische Beschwerden: ohne Hormone zum Erfolg. Ärztliche Praxis. 1983;35:1946–7.
33. Düker EM. Effects of extracts from *Cimicifuga racemosa* on gonadotropin release in menopausal women and ovariectomized rats. Planta Medica. 1991;57:424–7.
34. Lehmann-Willenbrock E, Riedel HH. Klinische und endokrinologische Untersuchungen zur Therapie ovarieller Ausfallerscheinungen nach Hysterektomie unter Belassung der Adnexe. Zentralblatt Gynäkologie. 1988;110: 611–8.
35. Liske E, Hanggi W, Henneicke-von Zepelin HH, Boblitz N, Wiistenberg P, Rahlfs VW. Physiological investigation of a unique extract of black cohosh (Cimicifugae racemosae rhizome): a 6-month clinical study demonstrates no systemic estrogenic effect. J Wom Health Gender-Based Med. 2002;11:163–74.
36. Pethö A. Klimakterische Beschwerden. Umstellung einer Hormonbehandlung auf ein pflanzliches Gynäkologikum möglich? Ärztliche. Praxis. 1987;38:1551–3.
37. Stoll W. Phytopharmakon beeinflußt atrophisches Vaginalepithel Doppelblindversuch Cimicifuga vs Östrogenpraparat. Therapeutikon. 1987;1:7–15.
38. Stolze H. Der andere Weg, klimakterische Beschwerden zu behandeln. Gyne. 1982;1:14–6.
39. Vorberg G. Therapie klimakterischer Beschwerden. Zeitschrift für Allgemeinmedizin. 1984;60:626–9.
40. Warnecke G. Influencing menopausal symptoms with a phytotherapeutic agent. Die Medizinische Welt. 1985;36: 871–4.
41. Nesselhut T, Liske E. Pharmacological measures in postmenopausal women with an isopropanolic aqueous extract of Cimifugae racemosae rhizomae (abstract). Menopause. 1999;6:331.
42. Jacobson JS, Troxel AB, Evans J, Klaus L, Vahdat L, Kinne D, et al. Randomized trial of black cohosh for the treatment of hot flashes among women with a history of breast cancer. J Clin Oncol. 2001;19:2739–45.
43. Wuttke W, Seidlova-Wuttke D, Gorkow C. The Cimicifuga preparation BNO 1055 vs. conjugated estrogens in a double-blind placebo-controlled study: effects on menopause symptoms and bone markers. Maturitas. 2003;44 Suppl 1Suppl 1:S67–77.
44. Munoz GH, Pluchine S. *Cimicifuga racemosa* for the treatment of hot flashes in women surviving breast cancer. Maturitas. 2003;44 Suppl 1Suppl 1:S59–65.
45. Frei-Kleiner S, Schaffner W, Rahlfs VW, Bodmer Ch, Birkhäuser M. *Cimicifuga racemosa* dried ethanolic extract in menopausal disorders: a double-blind placebo-controlled clinical trial. Maturitas. 2005;51:397–404.
46. Nappi RE, Malavasi B, Brundu B, Facchinetti F. Efficacy of *Cimicifuga racemosa* on climacteric complaints: a randomized study versus low-dose transdermal estradiol. Gynecol Endocrinol. 2005;20:30–5.

47. Osmers R, Friede M, Liske E, Schnitker J, Freudenstein J, Henneicke-von Zepelin HH. Efficacy and safety of isopropanolic black cohosh extract for climacteric symptoms. Obstet Gynecol. 2005;105:1074–83.
48. Pockaj BA, Loprinzi CL, Sloan JA, Novotny PJ, Barton DL, Hagenmaier A, et al. Pilot evaluation of black cohosh for the treatment of hot flashes in women. Cancer Invest. 2004;22:515–21.
49. Uebelhack R, Blohmer JU, Graubaum HJ, Busch R, Gruenwald J, Wernecke KD. Black cohosh and St. John's wort for climacteric complaints: a randomized trial. Obstet Gynecol. 2005;107:247–55.
50. Verhoeven MO, van der Mooren MJ, van de Weijer PH, Verdegem PJ, van der Burgt LM, Kenemans P. Effect of a combination of isoflavones and *Actaea racemosa* Linnaeus on climacteric symptoms in healthy symptomatic perimenopausal women: a 12-week randomized, placebo-controlled, double-blind study. Menopause. 2005;12: 412–20.
51. Mahady GB, Low Dog T, Barrett ML, Chavez ML, Gardiner P, Ko R, et al. United States Pharmacopeia review of the black cohosh case reports of hepatotoxicity. Menopause. 2008;15:628–38.
52. Teschke R. Black cohosh and suspected hepatotoxicity: inconsistencies, confounding variables, and prospective use of a diagnostic causality algorithm. A critical review. Menopause. 2010;17:426–40.
53. Teschke R, Schwarzenboeck A, Schmidt-Taenzer W, Wolff A, Hennermann KH. Herb induced liver injury presumably caused by black cohosh: a survey of initially purported cases and herbal quality specifications. Ann Hepatol. 2011;10:249–59.
54. Teschke R, Schmidt-Taenzer W, Wolff A. Spontaneous reports of assumed herbal hepatotoxicity by black cohosh: is the liver-unspecific Naranjo scale precise enough to ascertain causality? Pharmacoepidemiol Drug Saf. 2011;20:567–82.

Part V
Preclinical Studies: Implications for Human Health

Chapter 29
Animal Models of Menopausal Metabolism

Jameela Banu and Gabriel Fernandes

Key Points

- Estrogen loss during and after menopause increases the risk of developing several diseases.
- This chapter describes the available animal models for studying the manifestation of the diseases as well as characterizing therapies.
- Alzheimer's disease: Transgenic mouse models with selective single or multiple mutations
- Cardiovascular disease: Knockout mouse models, rabbit, and large animals
- Osteopororsis: Ovariectomized rodent and large animal models, knockout mouse
- Metabolic syndrome: Pancreatectomy models, transgenic and knockout mouse models, dietary interventions, spontaneous mutant rodents.

Keywords Menopause • Estrogen loss • Alzheimer's • Cardiovascular disease • Osteoporosis • Metabolic syndrome

Abbreviations

AD	Alzheimer's disease
APP	Amyloid precursor proteins
FORKO	Follicle stimulating hormone receptor knockout
CVD	Cardiovascular disease
ApoE	Apolipiprotein E
LDLR	Low density lipoprotein receptor
CETP	Cholesteryl ester transfer protein

J. Banu, M.Sc., Ph.D. (✉)
Coordinated Program in Dietetics and Department of Biology, University of Texas - Pan American
and Division of Clinical Immunology and Rheumatology, Department of Medicine and Medical Research Division,
Edinburg Regional Academic Health Center, University of Texas Health Science Center,
1201 W University Dr, TX 78539-2999, USA
e-mail: banuj@utpa.edu

G. Fernandes, M.Sc., Ph.D.
Division of Clinical Immunology and Rheumatology, Department of Medicine, University of Texas
Health Science Center, 7703, Floyd Curl Dr, San Antonio, TX 78229, USA
e-mail: Fernandes@uthscsa.edu

C.J.H. Martin et al. (eds.), *Nutrition and Diet in Menopause*, Nutrition and Health,
DOI 10.1007/978-1-62703-373-2_29, © Springer Science+Business Media New York 2013

SAMP6	Senescence accelerated mouse prone 6
OPG	Osteoprotegrin
HSV-TK	Herpes simplex thymidine kinase
GK	Goto Kakizaki
WOKW	Wistar Ottawa Karlsburg W

Introduction

Menopause is a physiological condition that ends the reproductive phase in women. This happens between the ages of 45 and 60 and there is individual variation in the onset of menopause. The major change is the sudden drop in estrogen levels. Estrogen is important for normal functioning of several organs including brain, heart, bone, and pancreas apart from maintaining the female reproductive system physically and metabolically. Loss of estrogen is implicated in various disease conditions like Alzheimer's, cardiovascular disease (CVD), metabolic syndrome (MS), and osteoporosis. As menopause occurs, estrogen loss together with age factor accelerates the onset and progression of certain diseases or at the least puts postmenopausal women at higher risk of developing these diseases.

In order to have successful treatment and prevention strategies, and to understand the mechanism behind the manifestation of the disease animal models are commonly used. Animal models are inevitable for biomedical research as they not only help in identifying successful treatment options but also help in determining any side effects the treatment agents may cause. Animal models are developed for a specific disease such that it has close phenotypic and physiological characteristics, in addition to the manifestation of the disease as in humans. Animal models that simulate diseases occurring in humans can be developed by several different approaches including chemical treatments, dietary interventions, surgery and genetic manipulations. In this chapter, we have listed animal models available to study the diseases that occur in postmenopausal women like Alzheimer's, atherosclerosis, metabolic syndrome, and osteoporosis.

Alzheimer's Disease

Alzheimer's is a disease that occurs in the elderly, it is a progressive neurodegenerative disease that slowly but steadily decreases the memory of these patients. Although this is an age related disease occurring in both men and women, there is evidence that estrogen decreases proteins like b-amyloid peptides [1] and loss of estrogen increases the formation of these peptides that may lead to the onset of Alzheimer's disease (AD) [1]. One of the important reasons for neurodegeneration in AD is the formation of plaques by these proteins that result from the processing of amyloid precursor proteins (APP) [2]. A few transgenic mice have been developed to study AD, most of them are a result of overexpressing APP gene. The first transgenic mouse model developed is the PDAPP mice [3] which overexpressed human APP transgene containing the Indiana mutation and controlled by platelet derived growth factor b promoter and have spatial learning memory deficits which increases with age [4]. Older mice showed significant synaptic loss. Hsiao et al. [5] developed the Tg-2576 mice which overexpressed human APP transgene with the Swedish mutation and hamster prion protein promoter. With age, these mice developed plaques similar to those found in AD patients and are also the most widely studied AD mouse models. APP23 mice are a single mutation derived transgene and showed

Table 29.1 Mice available for research in Alzheimer's disease

Mice	Characteristics	References
PDAPP	Overexpress APP Indiana mutation	[3]
Tg-2576	Overexpress APP Swedish mutation	[5]
APP23	Single mutation in APP gene	[2]
APPDutch	Single mutation in APP gene	[6]
APP/PSI	Double mutation	[7]
Tg-CRND8	Multiple mutation	[2]
Tg-SwD1	Dutch, Iowa, Swedish mutations	[9]
hAPP-Arc	Artic mutation	[10]
TgArcSwe	Artic and Swedish mutation	[11, 12]
APP_{si}/PSI	APP and Presenillin-1	[13, 14]
APP/PSikt	Knock-in mutation	[15]
5xFAD	Swedish, Florida, London familial Alzheimer's disease	[16, 17]
TAPP	Tau mutation	[2]
3xTg-AD	Tau mutation	[20]
FORKO	Follicle stimulating hormone knockout	[21]

independent reduction in spatial memory [2]. APPDutch mice were developed with a single mutation and it shows extensive vascular deposition of peptides [6]. Double mutant mice APP/PSI were also developed and these mice showed decreased spatial memory [7].

Other transgenic models were developed using multiple mutations to improve some of the existing models. Tg-CRND8 was generated to express multiple mutations of human APP gene. They develop neuropathology very early (3 months) and have spatial learning impairment at 6 months [2]; however, neurodegeneration was absent [8]. A triple mutant transgene, Tg-SWD1, was generated with Dutch, Iowa, and Swedish mutations in the human APP gene which expressed impaired spatial learning and memory beginning at 3 months of age [9]. The multiple transgene hAPP-Arc mice exhibited plaque deposits [10] while another multiple mutant, Tg-ArcSwe mice had age-related decrease in spatial memory even before plaque formation [11, 12]. APP_{SI}/PSI transgenic mice, showed changes with age, plaque deposition from 3 months of age and develop age-related synaptic loss [13, 14]. So far, APP/PSiKT mice generated from knock-in mutation have shown the extreme neurological changes from 2.5 months of age [15]. Severe neuronal pathology was generated in a multiple mutant 5xFAD mice which showed decreased spatial memory tasks beginning at 4 months of age [16, 17].

Another protein that is implicated in AD is Tau, which is abundant in the neurons and stabilizes microtubules [18]. Tau mutations have been used to generate transgenic mice like TAPP mice which exhibited neurofibrillary tangles and plaques from 8 months of age [2]. A multiple mutant 3xTg—AD mice was generated and age-related changes occurred in Tau which impaired spatial memory from young age [19, 20].

The most relevant model that simulates estrogen imbalance is the follicle stimulating hormone receptor knockout (FORKO) mice [21] which exhibit changes in the central nervous system (biochemically and morphologically) [22, 23]. They also develop metabolic syndrome [24].

So far, research related to AD has been dependent on transgenic mice that were developed based on proteins that regulate the manifestation of the disease (Table 29.1). Unfortunately, a single model cannot be picked as 'The Model' for AD, as each of these models express different symptoms of the disease except for decrease in spatial memory. However, development of these transgenic mice has facilitated in understanding AD and when they are crossbred have given some enlightenment into the disease.

Cardiovascular Disease

It is very well established that menopausal women are at high risk of developing cardiovascular disease CVD. CVD is referred to any disease of the heart, arteries, and veins which includes atherosclerosis. Atherosclerosis is a disease of the arteries where the arterial wall accumulates fat or salt deposits in the smooth muscle fibers narrowing the arterial lumen, reducing the amount of oxidized blood flow to various tissues eventually leading to heart attacks, stroke and inflammation. Estrogen is a cardioprotective agent and it modulates the inflammatory responses in atherosclerosis [25].

Animal models to study atherosclerosis were developed with dietary modifications or genetic manipulation [26]. One very widely used animal model to study atherosclerosis is the apolipoprotein E null (ApoE–/–) mice. ApoE is a protein that mediates the transport of dietary cholesterol and triglycerides into cells [27]. This protein is implicated in AD as well. ApoE–/– mice spontaneously develop hypercholesterolemia with regular diet, show artherosclerotic lesions with histopathological progression as in humans [28]. These mice have been widely used to study dietary and drug interventions [29–34] and understanding the disease itself [34–37]. Mice that lack the low density lipoprotein receptor gene (LDL–/–) were generated and these mice also develop hypercholesterolemia and atherosclerosis under normal diet conditions [38]. When crossbred with ApoE–/– mice, the double knockout mice (LDR–/–apoE–/–) develop severe atherosclerosis. However, they do not respond to drug treatments very well. Several transgenic mice with mutations in ApoE gene (apoE3Leiden (E3L)) were generated and these also simulate the human disease condition at varying degrees [39, 40]. Recently, E3L/cholesteryl ester transfer protein (CETP) is a more promising mouse model to study the effects of drugs for atherosclerosis [41, 42]. Invasive procedures like surgical exclusion of the arteries have also been carried out in mice [43–45].

Rabbits have been used to study atherosclerosis for a long time as the development of the disease is very similar to that seen in humans and have been successfully used to identify drugs and understand their mechanism of action [46, 47]. Recently, a rabbit model has been developed to study inflammation associated atherosclerosis [48] and plaques in vascular injuries [49].

In addition to rodents and rabbit models, large animals have also been developed to study cardiovascular diseases. Open chest models for induction of myocardial infarction have been established in pigs [50, 51] using catheterization and coronary intervention techniques. Pigs are also used to study atherosclerosis [52]. Correction procedures using various kinds of stents have been widely studied in pigs as well [53, 54]. Sheep and dogs also have been used in CVD related research mainly dealing with treatment strategies [55, 56].

Perhaps the most understanding about CVD in menopausal women comes from Cynomolgus monkeys. These animals have elucidated the effects of estrogen on arteries. It is reported that postmenopausal physiology is a determinant for postmenopausal atherosclerosis [57].

Many animal models have been used to study CVD from rodents to nonhuman primates (Table 29.2). Although a single model cannot be recommended, mice and monkeys have elucidated the mechanistic side of the disease while pigs have served best for therapeutic purposes.

Table 29.2 Animal models for cardiovascular diseases

Animal model	Characteristics/studies	References
$ApoE^{-/-}$	Apolipoprotein E knockout/hypercholestrolemia	[27]
$LDL^{-/-}$	Low density lipoprotein receptor knockout/hypercholesterolemia, atherosclerosis	[38]
ApoE3Leiden (E3L)	apoE3leiden variant/fatty liver, atherosclerosis	[40, 41]
CETP	E3L/cholesteryl ester transfer protein	[41, 42]
Rabbits	Atherosclerosis, drug interventions	[46, 47]
Pigs	Stents, myocardial infarction, atherosclerosis	[50, 51]
Sheep	Heart failure	[56]
Dogs	Heart failure	[55]
Monkeys	Estrogen and cardiovascular system	[57]

Osteoporosis

One of the major medical conditions which menopausal and postmenopausal women face is osteoporosis. In this disease there is excessive bone loss leading to thinning of bones making them susceptible to fractures with minor trauma. Living conditions of individuals with fractures are severely compromised. As estrogen plays a major role in maintaining bones, sudden decrease in estrogen levels, during and after menopause, initiates excessive bone resorption resulting in loss of bone.

The most common animal model used in osteoporosis research is the ovariectomized rat model [58, 59]. Surgical removal of the ovaries simulates menopause by decreasing estrogen levels and initiating bone loss. In the ovariectomized rat model, different bone sites lose bone at different rates as seen in humans. A significant amount of bone is lost in the proximal tibial metaphysis (below the knee joint), 14 days after surgery [59, 60]; in the femoral neck (where femur attaches to the hip bone), 30 days after surgery [61]; and in the lumbar vertebrae, 60 days after surgery [62]. A characteristic feature after ovariectomy is the loss of cancellous bone first, followed by loss of cortical bone much later (between 90 and 120 days) [63, 64]. The rat model is also the FDA approved model to study any interventions for osteoporosis [65]. In addition to rats, ovariectomized mice are also used in osteoporosis research to characterize therapeutic agents. Rats and mice are commonly used for treatment interventions in osteoporotic research, which includes hormones (estrogen supplementation, growth hormone, parathyroid hormone, calcitonin, and vitamin D) [66–69], nutritional supplements (calcium, fatty acids) [70–74], natural and synthetic bioactive compounds (selective estrogen receptor modulators, bispohsphonates, statins) [75–78] and alternative medicines (herbs and herbal compounds) [79–84]. Further, bones of certain transgenic mice such as Senescence accelerated mouse prone 6 (SAMP6) have been characterized to have accelerated aging process. These mice have low bone mass, increased bone resorption, and decreased bone formation, and get spontaneous leg fractures [85] and are used to study fracture healing [86]. Another transgenic mouse model, is the osteoprotegrin (OPG) deficient mice. OPG is a glycoprotein that affects bone metabolism. Overexpression of OPG leads to prevention of bone loss while knocking out the expression of OPG causes severe bone loss [87]. Moreover, OPG–/– mice do not have trabecular bone, so may not be good models for postmenopausal bone loss. Overexpression of a transcription factor from the osteoblast differentiation pathway, cbfa1, in mouse was developed [88]. These mice overexpressed cbfa1 after birth, had less active osteoblasts, showed signs of low bone mass and the role of cbfa1 in osteoblastogenesis was elucidated [89]. Another transgenic mouse model was generated using the herpes simplex thymidine kinase genes (HSV-TK) and osteocalcin gene 2 fragment [90]. Osteocalcin is a protein that is expressed during bone formation. In these mice, the expression of HSV-TK in osteoblasts, stop their function and arrested bone formation and is best used to understand the effects of bone resorption when no bone formation occurs [89]. To understand the influence of hypothalamus on bone turnover mainly through the leptin pathway the intracerebroventricular infused mice were generated [89].

Apart from rodent animal models of osteoporosis some large animals like dogs, sheep, goats, and pigs have also been characterized for osteoporosis research. Dogs undergo remodeling after maturity as humans [91] and have Haversian canal system with shorter remodeling cycles, but similar cancellous remodeling cycles [92, 93]. However, there has been a lot of discrepancy in the data obtained from castrated dogs due to various factors including age, number of animals in the study, dietary habits, etc. [94]. Sheep and goats are established models for orthopedic research [95, 96]. Ovariectomized sheep have been used to study osteoporosis [96]. Similarly, ovariectomized goats have also been validated as one of the large animal models to study osteoporosis [95]. However, in ruminants, oral administration of drugs does not give reliable results as estimation of drug doses and clearance rates are difficult to calculate [94]. Pigs have been used in biomedical research as models for several disease [97]. Due to their rapid growth and large size posing a lot of problems, minipigs or micropigs are used as alternatives to study osteoporosis [98]. So far, there is evidence that the spine morphology is similar to humans [99]. However, the regular use of tetracycline on these pigs may pose a problem as

Table 29.3 Animal models for osteoporosis

Animal models	Surgery or genetic manipulations	References
Rat	Ovariectomy	[58, 59]
Mouse	Ovariectomy	[70, 71]
SAMP6	Senescence accelerated mouse	[85]
$OPG^{-/-}$	Osteoprotegrin knockout	[87]
$Cbfa^{-/-}$	Knockout	[88]
HSV-TK	Herpes simplex thymidine kinase	[90]
ICV	Intracerebroventricular infusion	[89]
Dogs	Ovariectomy	[92, 93]
Sheep	Ovariectomy	[96]
Goats	Ovariectomy	[95]
Minipigs	Ovariectomy	[97, 98]

tetracycline binds to bone and may cause problems while assessing bone formation and mineral apposition rates [94].

Overall rodent species like mice and rats are the most popular models recognized. Although naturally they do not undergo menopause, after ovariectomy they show comparable features as in humans—biochemically and morphometrically. Moreover, they are cost-effective and easy to handle both for surgeries as well as for treatment interventions. We have listed the available animal models to study osteoporosis in Table 29.3.

Metabolic Syndrome

Metabolic syndrome (MS) is a term that includes a group of diseases/disorders that increases the risk of cardiovascular diseases. It includes obesity, diabetes and hypertension. Menopause increases the prevalence of MS [100]. One of the major physical changes that occur after menopause is obesity. The body tries to deal with the sudden drop in estrogen by building adipose mass to secrete estrogen. Unfortunately, obesity is a major risk factor for developing type 2 diabetes. However, loss of estrogen decreases insulin sensitivity while normal estrogen levels support pancreatic β cell function by increasing insulin production and protecting the β cells from lipotoxicity, oxidative stress, apoptosis, etc. [101]. With the incidence of obesity and diabetes on the rise, animal models have been developed to study the disorders as well as to test treatment options for the prevention and treatment of these diseases.

As pancreas is the main organ controlling circulating glucose levels in the body, it has been the target initially for animal models. Surgical removal of pancreas [102] or nonsurgical chemical damage induced by toxins such as streptozotocin [103] and alloxan [104] are the most common routes used to induce decrease or loss of normal β cell function. Interestingly, many spontaneously genetic variants among the rodent population also have been isolated and developed into animal models. As for many diseases, many genetically manipulated rodents had also been generated. A few obese rats and mouse have been used in diabetes studies such as fa/fa Zucker rats [105], ob/ob mouse [106], and db/db mouse [107, 108]. As leptin is the protein that is involved with energy metabolism and appetite, these rodents are either leptin resistant (fa/fa Zucker rats and ob/ob mouse) or leptin deficient (db/db mouse). Although fa/fa rats and ob/ob mice do not show hyperglycemia, they develop insulin resistance, while db/db mice develop hyperglycemia, β cell do not keep up with regular insulin production and renal complications [108, 109]. Selective breeding of Wistar rats led to the generation of Goto Kakizaki (GK) rats [110] which develop insulin resistance and decreased insulin secretion as they have decreased islets at birth [111], and they seem to pass these traits to the next generation [112]. Changing the diet of a rat from its natural vegetarian food to lab chow induces obesity, hyperglycemia, and insulin resis-

Table 29.4 Animal models for metabolic disorders

Animal models	Genetic background	Disease expressed	References
Rodents pancreatectomy	Wild type	Diabetes	[102]
Rats (streptozotocin treated)	Wild type	Diabetes	[103]
Rats (alloxan treated)	Wild type	Diabetes	[104]
Zucker fa/fa rats	Leptin resistant	Obesity	[105]
Goto kakizaki (GK)	Selective breeding of Wistar rats	Insulin resistance	[110]
Israeli sand rat	Naturally occurring, diet induced	Obesity, diabetes	[113]
Cohen rats	Selective inbreeding of Cohen rats, diet induced	Diabetes	[115]
Agouti rats and mice	Overexpression of agouti gene	Obesity, diabetes, insulin resistance	[117]
ob/ob mouse	Leptin resistant	Obesity	[106]
db/db mouse	Leptin deficient	Obesity, diabetes	[107, 108]
C57BL/6 mouse	Diet induced	Obesity	[118]
KK	Naturally	Obesity, Insulin resistance	[109, 119]
SHR or kotetsky	Spontaneous obese	Obesity, hypertension	[120, 121]
SHRSP	Spontaneously obese	Obesity, stroke	[120, 122]
WOKW	Inbred Wistar rats	Metabolic syndrome	[123]

tance in the Israeli sand rat (*Psammomy obesus*) [113]. In addition to diabetes, these rats, when fed high-fat diet develop atherosclerosis [114]. Cohen diabetic rats were developed by selective inbreeding of Cohen rats. Two metabolic phenotypes were generated—one strain (CDs) that was sensitive and became highly diabetic when fed high sucrose, low copper diabetogenic diet and the other (CDr) which is resistant and does not develop diabetes even with dietary interventions. The CDs rats showed hyperglycemia and decreased β cell function, and developed nephropathy and retinopathy as well [115]. A spontaneous mutation in the agouti gene resulted in an obese rat which developed diabetes and insulin resistance [116]. Many transgenic mice with mutations in the agouti gene are available now to study obesity induced diabetes [117]. One of the common mouse strains C57Bl/6 can become diabetic with dietary interventions and develop obesity and hypertension [118]. A mouse strain that is naturally obese (KK mouse) also develops islet cell hyperplasia, insulin resistance, and mild hyperglycemia [109, 119]. This mouse model is naturally obese, therefore, may be used to study obesity induced diabetes in humans.

The SHR or Kotetsky rats are spontaneously obese rats and are popular models to study hypertension as they show obesity and hypertension [120, 121]. Some of these rats spontaneously developed hypertension and atherosclerosis in addition to insulin resistance—Stroke prone SHR (SHRSP) strain [120, 122]. A new inbred rat, Wistar Ottawa Karlsburg W (WOKW), a model for MS, develops obesity, hypertension and impaired glucose tolerance [123].

In summary, most available animal models to study MS are spontaneously generated rats (Table 29.4). Many of them show obesity and diabetes as major complications. Jackson Labs has over 50 different genetically altered models for MS related diseases. Only an inbred rat (WOKW rat) seems to develop all three major complications and may be a complete model to study MS.

Conclusions

In the last two decades, many animal models have been developed and characterized with respect to specific diseases. This is also true to diseases related to menopause. With the advancement of molecular technology, there is an explosion of transgenic animals developed with specific gene overexpression or knockouts, enabling to target specific pathways and proteins. Transgenic animals have contributed to the understanding of molecular mechanisms underlying each disease. They also help in connecting the links between pathways as well. For a long time, large and small animals have been used in biomedical research as alternatives to humans because of ethical issues and limitations of using humans as research subjects. Apart from animal models simulating the disease as in humans, there is a need for enough number of animals in each group tested to have statistical significance. Small animals can be used conveniently as they are cost effective and easy to handle when compared to large animals.

So far, transgenic mice have been predominantly used in AD related research. In cardiovascular disease research, however, larger animals are favored, mainly because the vasculature is larger in these animals and are therefore convenient to work with. In osteoporotic research, the ovariectomized rodent model is the favorite animal model and can be picked as "The model" for osteoporotic research, and almost all therapies that are now available have been tested in these models. Metabolic syndrome, being a combination of diseases, has mainly relied on spontaneous variants of rodents for its research. Unfortunately, for studying AD, CVD, and MS, one animal cannot be singled out.

Recently, there have been concerns about the use of animal models in biomedical research which has resulted in strict monitoring measures to reduce any inconvenience and pain that result from these procedures to animals. Considering the fact that humans are highly complex living beings with respect to the different organ systems and the different molecular and physiological mechanisms that is necessary for normal functioning of the body, it is very important to have animal models not only to understand the disease but also to identify and characterize treatment procedures and agents.

Acknowledgement We acknowledge NIH grant AT005232-04.

References

1. Xu H, Gouras GK, Greenfield JP, Vincent B, Naslund J, Mazzarelli L, et al. Estrogen reduces neuronal generation of Alzheimer beta-amyloid peptides. Nat Med. 1998;4:447–51.
2. Schaeffer EL, Figueiro M, Gattaz WF. Insights into Alzheimer disease pathogenesis from studies in transgenic animal models. Clinics. 2011;66 Suppl 1:45–54.
3. Games D, Adams D, Alessandrini R, Barbour R, Berthelette P, Blackwell C, et al. Alzheimer-type neuropathology in transgenic mice overexpressing V717F beta-amyloid precursor protein. Nature. 1995;373:523–7.
4. Chen G, Chen KS, Knox J, Inglis J, Bernard A, Martin SJ, et al. A learning deficit related to age and beta-amyloid plaques in a mouse model of Alzheimer's disease. Nature. 2000;408:975–9.
5. Hsiao K, Chapman P, Nilsen S, Eckman C, Harigaya Y, Younkin S, et al. Correlative memory deficits, Abeta elevation, and amyloid plaques in transgenic mice. Science. 1996;274:99–102.
6. Herzig MC, Winkler DT, Burgermeister P, Pfeifer M, Kohler E, Schmidt SD, et al. Abeta is targeted to the vasculature in a mouse model of hereditary cerebral hemorrhage with amyloidosis. Nat Neurosci. 2004;7:954–60.
7. Holcomb L, Gordon MN, McGowan E, Yu X, Benkovic S, Jantzen P, et al. Accelerated Alzheimer-type phenotype in transgenic mice carrying both mutant amyloid precursor protein and presenilin 1 transgenes. Nat Med. 1998;4:97–100.
8. Chishti MA, Yang DS, Janus C, Phinney AL, Horne P, Pearson J, et al. Early-onset amyloid deposition and cognitive deficits in transgenic mice expressing a double mutant form of amyloid precursor protein 695. J Biol Chem. 2001;276:21562–70.
9. Xu F, Grande AM, Robinson JK, Previti ML, Vasek M, Davis J, et al. Early-onset subicular microvascular amyloid and neuroinflammation correlate with behavioral deficits in vasculotropic mutant amyloid beta-protein precursor transgenic mice. Neuroscience. 2007;146:98–107.
10. Cheng IH, Palop JJ, Esposito LA, Bien-Ly N, Yan F, Mucke L. Aggressive amyloidosis in mice expressing human amyloid peptides with the Arctic mutation. Nat Med. 2004;10:1190–2.
11. Lord A, Kalimo H, Eckman C, Zhang XQ, Lannfelt L, Nilsson LN. The Arctic Alzheimer mutation facilitates early intraneuronal Abeta aggregation and senile plaque formation in transgenic mice. Neurobiol Aging. 2006;27:67–77.
12. Knobloch M, Konietzko U, Krebs DC, Nitsch RM. Intracellular Abeta and cognitive deficits precede beta-amyloid deposition in transgenic arcAbeta mice. Neurobiol Aging. 2007;28:1297–306.
13. Wirths O, Multhaup G, Czech C, Feldmann N, Blanchard V, Tremp G, et al. Intraneuronal APP/A beta trafficking and plaque formation in beta-amyloid precursor protein and presenilin-1 transgenic mice. Brain Pathol. 2002;12:275–86.

14. Rutten BP, Van der Kolk NM, Schafer S, van Zandvoort MA, Bayer TA, Steinbusch HW, et al. Age-related loss of synaptophysin immunoreactive presynaptic boutons within the hippocampus of APP751SL, PS1M146L, and APP751SL/PS1M146L transgenic mice. Am J Pathol. 2005;167:161–73.
15. Casas C, Sergeant N, Itier JM, Blanchard V, Wirths O, van der Kolk N, et al. Massive CA1/2 neuronal loss with intraneuronal and N-terminal truncated Abeta42 accumulation in a novel Alzheimer transgenic model. Am J Pathol. 2004;165:1289–300.
16. Oakley H, Cole SL, Logan S, Maus E, Shao P, Craft J, et al. Intraneuronal beta-amyloid aggregates, neurodegeneration, and neuron loss in transgenic mice with five familial Alzheimer's disease mutations: potential factors in amyloid plaque formation. J Neurosci. 2006;26:10129–40.
17. Ohno M, Cole SL, Yasvoina M, Zhao J, Citron M, Berry R, et al. BACE1 gene deletion prevents neuron loss and memory deficits in 5XFAD APP/PS1 transgenic mice. Neurobiol Dis. 2007;26:134–45.
18. Shin RW, Iwaki T, Kitamoto T, Tateishi J. Hydrated autoclave pretreatment enhances tau immunoreactivity in formalin-fixed normal and Alzheimer's disease brain tissues. Lab Invest. 1991;64:693–702.
19. Oddo S, Caccamo A, Shepherd JD, Murphy MP, Golde TE, Kayed R, et al. Triple-transgenic model of Alzheimer's disease with plaques and tangles: intracellular Abeta and synaptic dysfunction. Neuron. 2003;39:409–21.
20. Billings LM, Oddo S, Green KN, McGaugh JL, LaFerla FM. Intraneuronal Abeta causes the onset of early Alzheimer's disease-related cognitive deficits in transgenic mice. Neuron. 2005;45:675–88.
21. Dierich A, Sairam MR, Monaco L, Fimia GM, Gansmuller A, LeMeur M, et al. Impairing follicle-stimulating hormone (FSH) signaling in vivo: targeted disruption of the FSH receptor leads to aberrant gametogenesis and hormonal imbalance. Proc Natl Acad Sci U S A. 1998;95:13612–7.
22. Tam J, Danilovich N, Nilsson K, Sairam MR, Maysinger D. Chronic estrogen deficiency leads to molecular aberrations related to neurodegenerative changes in follitropin receptor knockout female mice. Neuroscience. 2002;114:493–506.
23. Rumora L, Lovric J, Sairam MR, Maysinger D. Impairments of heat shock protein expression and MAPK translocation in the central nervous system of follitropin receptor knockout mice. Exp Gerontol. 2007;42:619–28.
24. Sairam MR, Wang M, Danilovich N, Javeshghani D, Maysinger D. Early obesity and age-related mimicry of metabolic syndrome in female mice with sex hormonal imbalances. Obesity. 2006;14:1142–54.
25. Baker L, Meldrum KK, Wang M, Sankula R, Vanam R, Raiesdana A, et al. The role of estrogen in cardiovascular disease. J Surg Res. 2003;115:325–44.
26. Daugherty A. Mouse models of atherosclerosis. Am J Med Sci. 2002;323:3–10.
27. Piedrahita JA, Zhang SH, Hagaman JR, Oliver PM, Maeda N. Generation of mice carrying a mutant apolipoprotein E gene inactivated by gene targeting in embryonic stem cells. Proc Natl Acad Sci U S A. 1992;89:4471–5.
28. Coleman R, Hayek T, Keidar S, Aviram M. A mouse model for human atherosclerosis: long-term histopathological study of lesion development in the aortic arch of apolipoprotein E-deficient (E0) mice. Acta Histochem. 2006;108:415–24.
29. Aviram M, Dornfeld L, Rosenblat M, Volkova N, Kaplan M, Coleman R, et al. Pomegranate juice consumption reduces oxidative stress, atherogenic modifications to LDL, and platelet aggregation: studies in humans and in atherosclerotic apolipoprotein E-deficient mice. Am J Clin Nutr. 2000;71:1062–76.
30. Fuhrman B, Rosenblat M, Hayek T, Coleman R, Aviram M. Ginger extract consumption reduces plasma cholesterol, inhibits LDL oxidation and attenuates development of atherosclerosis in atherosclerotic, apolipoprotein E-deficient mice. J Nutr. 2000;130:1124–31.
31. Imaizumi K. Diet and atherosclerosis in apolipoprotein E-deficient mice. Biosci Biotechnol Biochem. 2011;75:1023–35.
32. Nakagami H, Osako MK, Morishita R. New concept of vascular calcification and metabolism. Curr Vasc Pharmacol. 2011;9:124–7.
33. Davis Jr HR, Lowe RS, Neff DR. Effects of ezetimibe on atherosclerosis in preclinical models. Atherosclerosis. 2011;215:266–78.
34. Takahashi S, Sakai J, Fujino T, Hattori H, Zenimaru Y, Suzuki J, et al. The very low-density lipoprotein (VLDL) receptor: characterization and functions as a peripheral lipoprotein receptor. J Atheroscler Thromb. 2004;11:200–8.
35. Stoll G, Bendszus M. Inflammation and atherosclerosis: novel insights into plaque formation and destabilization. Stroke. 2006;37:1923–32.
36. Ohashi R, Mu H, Yao Q, Chen C. Cellular and molecular mechanisms of atherosclerosis with mouse models. Trends Cardiovasc Med. 2004;14:187–90.
37. McNeill E, Channon KM, Greaves DR. Inflammatory cell recruitment in cardiovascular disease: murine models and potential clinical applications. Clin Sci. 2010;118:641–55.
38. Ishibashi S, Brown MS, Goldstein JL, Gerard RD, Hammer RE, Herz J. Hypercholesterolemia in low density lipoprotein receptor knockout mice and its reversal by adenovirus-mediated gene delivery. J Clin Invest. 1993;92:883–93.
39. Leppanen P, Luoma JS, Hofker MH, Havekes LM, Yla-Herttuala S. Characterization of atherosclerotic lesions in apo E3-leiden transgenic mice. Atherosclerosis. 1998;136:147–52.

40. Hofker MH, van Vlijmen BJ, Havekes LM. Transgenic mouse models to study the role of APOE in hyperlipidemia and atherosclerosis. Atherosclerosis. 1998;137:1–11.
41. Zadelaar S, Kleemann R, Verschuren L, De-vries-Van der Weij J, van der Hoorn J, Princen HM, et al. Mouse models for atherosclerosis and pharmaceutical modifiers. Arterioscler Thromb Vasc Biol. 2007;27:1706–21.
42. van der Hoorn JW, Jukema JW, Havekes LM, Lundholm E, Camejo G, Rensen PC, et al. The dual PPARalpha/gamma agonist tesaglitazar blocks progression of pre-existing atherosclerosis in APOE*3Leiden.CETP transgenic mice. Br J Pharmacol. 2009;156:1067–75.
43. Hu P, Zhang D, Swenson L, Chakrabarti G, Abel ED, Litwin SE. Minimally invasive aortic banding in mice: effects of altered cardiomyocyte insulin signaling during pressure overload. Am J Physiol Heart Circ Physiol. 2003;285:H1261–9.
44. Kiss E, Ball NA, Kranias EG, Walsh RA. Differential changes in cardiac phospholamban and sarcoplasmic reticular Ca(2+)-ATPase protein levels. Effects on Ca2+ transport and mechanics in compensated pressure-overload hypertrophy and congestive heart failure. Circ Res. 1995;77:759–64.
45. Stock JH, Reller MD, Sharma S, Pavcnik D, Shiota T, Sahn DJ. Transballoon intravascular ultrasound imaging during balloon angioplasty in animal models with coarctation and branch pulmonary stenosis. Circulation. 1997;95:2354–7.
46. Aikawa M, Sugiyama S, Hill CC, Voglic SJ, Rabkin E, Fukumoto Y, et al. Lipid lowering reduces oxidative stress and endothelial cell activation in rabbit atheroma. Circulation. 2002;106:1390–6.
47. Bustos C, Hernandez-Presa MA, Ortego M, Tunon J, Ortega L, Perez F, et al. HMG-CoA reductase inhibition by atorvastatin reduces neointimal inflammation in a rabbit model of atherosclerosis. J Am Coll Cardiol. 1998;32:2057–64.
48. Largo R, Sanchez-Pernaute O, Marcos ME, Moreno-Rubio J, Aparicio C, Granado R, et al. Chronic arthritis aggravates vascular lesions in rabbits with atherosclerosis: a novel model of atherosclerosis associated with chronic inflammation. Arthritis Rheum. 2008;58:2723–34.
49. Shimizu T, Nakai K, Morimoto Y, Ishihara M, Oishi H, Kikuchi M, et al. Simple rabbit model of vulnerable atherosclerotic plaque. Neurol Med Chir (Tokyo). 2009;49:327–32. discussion 332.
50. Litvak J, Siderides LE, Vineberg AM. The experimental production of coronary artery insufficiency and occlusion. Am Heart J. 1957;53:505–18.
51. Fozzard HA. Validity of myocardial infarction models. Circulation. 1975;52(6 Suppl):III131–46.
52. Xiangdong L, Yuanwu L, Hua Z, Liming R, Qiuyan L, Ning L. Animal models for the atherosclerosis research: a review. Protein Cell. 2011;2:189–201.
53. Nakazawa G, Finn AV, John MC, Kolodgie FD, Virmani R. The significance of preclinical evaluation of sirolimus-, paclitaxel-, and zotarolimus-eluting stents. Am J Cardiol. 2007;100:36M–44.
54. Suzuki Y, Lyons JK, Yeung AC, Ikeno F. The porcine restenosis model using thermal balloon injury: comparison with the model by coronary stenting. J Invasive Cardiol. 2008;20:142–6.
55. Sabbah HN, Stein PD, Kono T, Gheorghiade M, Levine TB, Jafri S, et al. A canine model of chronic heart failure produced by multiple sequential coronary microembolizations. Am J Physiol. 1991;260:H1379–84.
56. Schmitto JD, Ortmann P, Wachter R, Coulibaly M, Sellin C, Popov AF, et al. Chronic heart failure induced by multiple sequential coronary microembolization in sheep. Int J Artif Organs. 2008;31:348–53.
57. Clarkson TB, Mehaffey MH. Coronary heart disease of females: lessons learned from nonhuman primates. Am J Primatol. 2009;71:785–93.
58. Kalu DN, Liu CC, Hardin RR, Hollis BW. The aged rat model of ovarian hormone deficiency bone loss. Endocrinology. 1989;124:7–16.
59. Wronski TJ, Dann LM, Scott KS, Cintron M. Long-term effects of ovariectomy and aging on the rat skeleton. Calcif Tissue Int. 1989;45:360–6.
60. Wronski TJ, Cintron M, Dann LM. Temporal relationship between bone loss and increased bone turnover in ovariectomized rats. Calcif Tissue Int. 1988;43:179–83.
61. Li M, Shen Y, Wronski TJ. Time course of femoral neck osteopenia in ovariectomized rats. Bone. 1997;20:55–61.
62. Wronski TJ, Dann LM, Horner SL. Time course of vertebral osteopenia in ovariectomized rats. Bone. 1989;10:295–301.
63. Danielsen CC, Mosekilde L, Svenstrup B. Cortical bone mass, composition, and mechanical properties in female rats in relation to age, long-term ovariectomy, and estrogen substitution. Calcif Tissue Int. 1993;52:26–33.
64. Yamamoto N, Jee WS, Ma YF. Bone histomorphometric changes in the femoral neck of aging and ovariectomized rats. Anat Rec. 1995;243:175–85.
65. FDA: Guidelines for preclinical and clinical evaluation of agents used for the prevention of treatment of postmenopausal osteoporosis. Division of Metabolism and Endocrine Drug Products. Food and Drug Administration 1994.
66. Banu J, Orhii PB, Okafor MC, Wang L, Kalu DN. Analysis of the effects of growth hormone, exercise and food restriction on cancellous bone in different bone sites in middle-aged female rats. Mech Ageing Dev. 2001;122:849–64.

67. Matsumoto T, Ezawa I, Morita K, Kawanobe Y, Ogata E. Effect of vitamin D metabolites on bone metabolism in a rat model of postmenopausal osteoporosis. J Nutr Sci Vitaminol. 1985;31(Suppl):S61–5.
68. Wronski TJ, Yen CF, Burton KW, Mehta RC, Newman PS, Soltis EE, et al. Skeletal effects of calcitonin in ovariectomized rats. Endocrinology. 1991;129:2246–50.
69. Mosekilde L, Danielsen CC, Sogaard CH, McOsker JE, Wronski TJ. The anabolic effects of parathyroid hormone on cortical bone mass, dimensions and strength–assessed in a sexually mature, ovariectomized rat model. Bone. 1995;16:223–30.
70. Banu J, Bhattacharya A, Rahman M, Kang JX, Fernandes G. Endogenously produced n-3 fatty acids protect against ovariectomy induced bone loss in fat-1 transgenic mice. J Bone Miner Metab. 2010;28:617–26.
71. Banu J, Bhattacharya A, Rahman M, O'Shea M, Fernandes G. Effects of conjugated linoleic acid and exercise on bone mass in young male Balb/C mice. Lipids Health Dis. 2006;5:7.
72. Fernandes G, Bhattacharya A, Rahman M, Zaman K, Banu J. Effects of n-3 fatty acids on autoimmunity and osteoporosis. Front Biosci. 2008;13:4015–20.
73. Kalu DN, Orhii PB. Calcium absorption and bone loss in ovariectomized rats fed varying levels of dietary calcium. Calcif Tissue Int. 1999;65:73–7.
74. Shahnazari M, Martin BR, Legette LL, Lachcik PJ, Welch J, Weaver CM. Diet calcium level but not calcium supplement particle size affects bone density and mechanical properties in ovariectomized rats. J Nutr. 2009;139:1308–14.
75. Banu J, Kalu DN. Site-specific effects of cerivastatin on bone in male Sprague-Dawley rats. Bone. 2004;34:432–42.
76. Rixon RH, Whitfield JF, Gagnon L, Isaacs RJ, Maclean S, Chakravarthy B, et al. Parathyroid hormone fragments may stimulate bone growth in ovariectomized rats by activating adenylyl cyclase. J Bone Miner Res. 1994;9:1179–89.
77. Boyce RW, Wronski TJ, Ebert DC, Stevens ML, Paddock CL, Youngs TA, et al. Direct stereological estimation of three-dimensional connectivity in rat vertebrae: effect of estrogen, etidronate and risedronate following ovariectomy. Bone. 1995;16:209–13.
78. Bryant HU, Glasebrook AL, Yang NN, Sato M. An estrogen receptor basis for raloxifene action in bone. J Steroid Biochem Mol Biol. 1999;69:37–44.
79. Jiu LJ, Morikawa N, Omi N, Ezawa I. The effect of tochu bark on bone metabolism in the rat model with ovariectomized osteoporosis. J Nutr Sci Vitaminol. 1994;40:261–73.
80. Arjmandi BH, Alekel L, Hollis BW, Amin D, Stacewicz-Sapuntzakis M, Guo P, et al. Dietary soybean protein prevents bone loss in an ovariectomized rat model of osteoporosis. J Nutr. 1996;126:161–7.
81. Anderson JJ, Ambrose WW, Garner SC. Biphasic effects of genistein on bone tissue in the ovariectomized, lactating rat model. Proc Soc Exp Biol Med. 1998;217:345–50.
82. Arjmandi BH, Khalil DA, Hollis BW. Ipriflavone, a synthetic phytoestrogen, enhances intestinal calcium transport in vitro. Calcif Tissue Int. 2000;67:225–9.
83. Das AS, Mukherjee M, Mitra C. Evidence for a prospective anti-osteoporosis effect of black tea (Camellia Sinensis) extract in a bilaterally ovariectomized rat model. Asia Pac J Clin Nutr. 2004;13:210–6.
84. Mukherjee M, Das AS, Mitra S, Mitra C. Prevention of bone loss by oil extract of garlic (Allium sativum Linn.) in an ovariectomized rat model of osteoporosis. Phytother Res. 2004;18:389–94.
85. Suda T. Osteoporotic bone changes in SAMP6 are due to a decrease in osteoblast progenitor cells. In: Toshio T, editor. The SAM model of senescence. Amsterdam: Experta Medica; 1994. p. 47–52.
86. Egermann M, Heil P, Tami A, Ito K, Janicki P, Von Rechenberg B, et al. Influence of defective bone marrow osteogenesis on fracture repair in an experimental model of senile osteoporosis. J Orthop Res. 2009;28:798–804.
87. Bucay N, Sarosi I, Dunstan CR, Morony S, Tarpley J, Capparelli C, et al. Osteoprotegerin-deficient mice develop early onset osteoporosis and arterial calcification. Genes Dev. 1998;12:1260–8.
88. Ducy P, Starbuck M, Priemel M, Shen J, Pinero G, Geoffroy V, et al. A Cbfa1-dependent genetic pathway controls bone formation beyond embryonic development. Genes Dev. 1999;13:1025–36.
89. Priemel M, Schilling AF, Haberland M, Pogoda P, Rueger JM, Amling M. Osteopenic mice: animal models of the aging skeleton. J Musculoskelet Neuronal Interact. 2002;2:212–8.
90. Corral DA, Amling M, Priemel M, Loyer E, Fuchs S, Ducy P, et al. Dissociation between bone resorption and bone formation in osteopenic transgenic mice. Proc Natl Acad Sci U S A. 1998;95:13835–40.
91. Fukuda S, Iida H. Effects of orchidectomy on bone metabolism in beagle dogs. J Vet Med Sci. 2000;62:69–73.
92. Martin RK, Albright JP, Jee WS, Taylor GN, Clarke WR. Bone loss in the beagle tibia: influence of age, weight, and sex. Calcif Tissue Int. 1981;33:233–8.
93. Kimmel D. Animal models of osteopenia or osteoporosis. In: Yuchuei H, Freidman RJ, editors. Animal Models in orthopaedic research. Boca Raton, FL, USA: CRC; 1999. p. 280–305.
94. Reinwald S, Burr D. Review of nonprimate, large animal models for osteoporosis research. J Bone Miner Res. 2008;23:1353–68.
95. Leung KS, Siu WS, Cheung NM, Lui PY, Chow DH, James A, et al. Goats as an osteopenic animal model. J Bone Miner Res. 2001;16:2348–55.

96. Zarrinkalam MR, Beard H, Schultz CG, Moore RJ. Validation of the sheep as a large animal model for the study of vertebral osteoporosis. Eur Spine J. 2009;18:244–53.
97. Almond GW. Research applications using pigs. Vet Clin North Am Food Anim Pract. 1996;12:707–16.
98. Mosekilde L, Weisbrode SE, Safron JA, Stills HF, Jankowsky ML, Ebert DC, et al. Calcium-restricted ovariectomized Sinclair S-1 minipigs: an animal model of osteopenia and trabecular plate perforation. Bone. 1993;14:379–82.
99. McLain RF, Yerby SA, Moseley TA. Comparative morphometry of L4 vertebrae: comparison of large animal models for the human lumbar spine. Spine. 2002;27:E200–6.
100. Carr MC. The emergence of the metabolic syndrome with menopause. J Clin Endocrinol Metab. 2003;88:2404–11.
101. Mauvais-Jarvis F. Estrogen and androgen receptors: regulators of fuel homeostasis and emerging targets for diabetes and obesity. Trends Endocrinol Metab. 2011;22:24–33.
102. Bonner-Weir S, Trent DF, Weir GC. Partial pancreatectomy in the rat and subsequent defect in glucose-induced insulin release. J Clin Invest. 1983;71:1544–53.
103. Junod A, Lambert AE, Stauffacher W, Renold AE. Diabetogenic action of streptozotocin: relationship of dose to metabolic response. J Clin Invest. 1969;48(11):2129–39.
104. Lenzen S, Panten U. Alloxan: history and mechanism of action. Diabetologia. 1988;31:337–42.
105. Bray GA. The Zucker-fatty rat: a review. Fed Proc. 1977;36:148–53.
106. Tschop M, Heiman ML. Rodent obesity models: an overview. Exp Clin Endocrinol Diabetes. 2001;109:307–19.
107. Sharma K, McCue P, Dunn SR. Diabetic kidney disease in the db/db mouse. Am J Physiol Renal Physiol. 2003;284:F1138–44.
108. Tesch GH, Lim AK. Recent insights into diabetic renal injury from the db/db mouse model of type 2 diabetic nephropathy. Am J Physiol Renal Physiol. 2011;300:F301–10.
109. Rees DA, Alcolado JC. Animal models of diabetes mellitus. Diabet Med. 2005;22:359–70.
110. Goto Y, Kakizaki M, Masaki N. Production of spontaneous diabetic rats by repetition of selective breeding. Tohoku J Exp Med. 1976;119:85–90.
111. Metz SA, Meredith M, Vadakekalam J, Rabaglia ME, Kowluru A. A defect late in stimulus-secretion coupling impairs insulin secretion in Goto-Kakizaki diabetic rats. Diabetes. 1999;48:1754–62.
112. Gill-Randall R, Adams D, Ollerton RL, Rabaglia ME, Kowluru A. Type 2 diabetes mellitus–genes or intrauterine environment? An embryo transfer paradigm in rats. Diabetologia. 2004;47:1354–9.
113. Ziv E, Shafrir E, Kalman R, Galer S, Bar-On H. Changing pattern of prevalence of insulin resistance in Psammomys obesus, a model of nutritionally induced type 2 diabetes. Metabolism. 1999;48:1549–54.
114. Marquie G, Hadjiisky P, Arnaud O, Duhault J. Development of macroangiopathy in sand rats (Psammomys obesus), an animal model of non-insulin-dependent diabetes mellitus: effect of gliclazide. Am J Med. 1991;90:55S–61.
115. Shafrir E, Ziv E. A useful list of spontaneously arising animal models of obesity and diabetes. Am J Physiol Endocrinol Metab. 2009;296:E1450–2.
116. Klebig ML, Wilkinson JE, Geisler JG, Woychik RP. Ectopic expression of the agouti gene in transgenic mice causes obesity, features of type II diabetes, and yellow fur. Proc Natl Acad Sci U S A. 1995;92:4728–32.
117. Miltenberger RJ, Mynatt RL, Wilkinson JE, Woychik RP. The role of the agouti gene in the yellow obese syndrome. J Nutr. 1997;127:1902S–7.
118. Petro A. The C67BL/6J mouse as model of diet induced type 2 diabtes and obesity. In: Sima AaS E, editor. Animal models of diabetes, a primer. Amsterdam: Harwood Academic; 2001. p. 343–55.
119. Ikeda H. KK mouse. Diabetes Res Clin Pract. 1994;24(Suppl):S313–6.
120. Reaven GM, Chang H, Hoffman BB, Azhar S. Resistance to insulin-stimulated glucose uptake in adipocytes isolated from spontaneously hypertensive rats. Diabetes. 1989;38:1155–60.
121. Kvetnansky R, Rusnak M, Gasperikova D, Jelokova J, Zorad S, Vietor I, et al. Hyperinsulinemia and sympathoadrenal system activity in the rat. Ann N Y Acad Sci. 1997;827:118–34.
122. Yamori Y, Ohtaka M, Horie R, Akiguchi I. Cerebral stroke and myocardial lesions in stroke-prone SHR. Jpn Heart J. 1978;19:609–11.
123. van den Brandt J, Kovacs P, Kloting I. Metabolic features in disease-resistant as well as in spontaneously hypertensive rats and newly established obese Wistar Ottawa Karlsburg inbred rats. Int J Obes Relat Metab Disord. 2000;24:1618–22.

Chapter 30
Phytoestrogen α-Zearalanol in an Animal Model of Menopause

Wen Wang

Key Points

- Estrogen has drawn some serious attention regarding its health benefits.
- The fact that estrogen replacement therapy (ERT) may predispose women to a much higher incidence of breast and endometrial cancers has undoubtedly compromised or jeopardized its clinical application.
- A plant-derived phytoestrogen, α-zearalanol (α-ZAL), has been proposed as a potential replacement for estrogen.
- α-ZAL has shown beneficial effects on blood vessels, osteoporosis, and Alzheimer's disease in animal models of menopause similar with estrogen.
- It has less proliferating effects on uterus and mammary gland compared to estrogen.

Keywords Estrogen replacement therapy • Phytoestrogen • α-Zearalanol • Menopause • Animal model

Abbreviations

ACh	Acetylcholine
AP-1	Activator protein-1
bFGF	Basic fibroblast growth factor
BGP	Bone Gla protein
BMD	Bone mineral density
BMP	Bone morphogenetic proteins
eNOS	Endothelial nitric oxide synthase
EPCs	Endothelial progenitor cells
ET-1	Endothelin-1
17β-E_2	17β-estrodiol
ERT	Estrogen replacement therapy

W. Wang, M.D., Ph.D. (✉)
Department of Pathophysiology, School of Basic Medical Sciences,
Capital Medical University, 10 Xi Tou Tiao, You An Men Wai, Beijing 100069, China
e-mail: wangwen@ccmu.edu.cn;wangwen2102@sina.com

C.J.H. Martin et al. (eds.), *Nutrition and Diet in Menopause*, Nutrition and Health,
DOI 10.1007/978-1-62703-373-2_30, © Springer Science+Business Media New York 2013

ERK	Extracellular signal-regulated kinase
FG	Fibrinogen
Hcy	Homocysteine
HUVECs	Human umbilical vein endothelial cells
HHcy	Hyperhomocysteinemia
H/R	Hypoxia/reoxygenation
LDH	Lactate dehydrogenase
Met	Methionine
NO	Nitric oxide
NOS	Nitric oxide synthase
L-NAME	N-nitro-larginine methylester
Ovx	Ovariectomy
oxLDL	Oxidized low-density lipoprotein
PAI-1	Plasminogen activator inhibitor type 1
PE	Phenylephrine
PT	Prothrombin time
ROS	Reactive oxygen species
TF	Tissue factor
t-PA	Tissue plasminogen activator
VSMCs	Vascular smooth muscle cells
α-ZAL	a-Zearalanol
ZEN	Zearalenone

Introduction

Over the past three decades, the impact of estrogen on the prevention and treatment of atherosclerosis, osteoporosis, Alzheimer's disease, and the aging has drawn some serious attention regarding its health benefits [1, 2]. However, the fact that estrogen replacement therapy (ERT) may predispose women to a much higher incidence of venous thrombosis and breast and endometrial cancers has undoubtedly compromised or jeopardized its clinical application. Although combined estrogen and progesterone therapy may reduce the incidence of endometrial cancer triggered by estrogen mono-therapy, the estrogen-induced increase in the incidence of breast cancer remains elevated despite concurrent progesterone usage [3]. Thus, the search for safe and effective estrogen substitutes becomes a practical issue. Recently, the plant-derived phytoestrogens, which possess some physiological properties of animal-derived estrogen and works as selective estrogen receptor modulator, have been shown to act as potential replacements for estrogen. More than a hundred kinds of phytoestrogen have been identified since the 1950s, with genistein and isoflavone being most common. However, these phytoestrogens also have some negative effects, which cause potential clinical concern [4].

Recently, a plant-derived phytoestrogen, α-zearalanol (α-ZAL), has been proposed as a potential replacement for estrogen [5]. α-Zearalanol, a reductive product of the fungus *Gibberella zeae* (*Fusarium roseum graminearum*) metabolite zearalenone (ZEN), was isolated from culture medium of zearalenone and belongs to the β-resorcylate family (Fig. 30.1). α-ZAL is abundant in plants and vegetables including soybean, wheat, grape, radish, celery, spinach and apple. α-ZAL may facilitate mouse uterine growth and promote weight gain in beef cattle and sheep [6]. Both α-ZAL and its parent compound zearalenone act as universal endogenous hormones for plant growth with α-ZAL being twice as effective as zearalenone, but less toxic [7]. α-ZAL promotes protein synthesis and increases the lean meat ratio of beef cattle and sheep in a manner similar to estrogen. However, little effect on tissue growth was noted for α-ZAL compared with estrogen. α-ZAL is rapidly metabolized in the

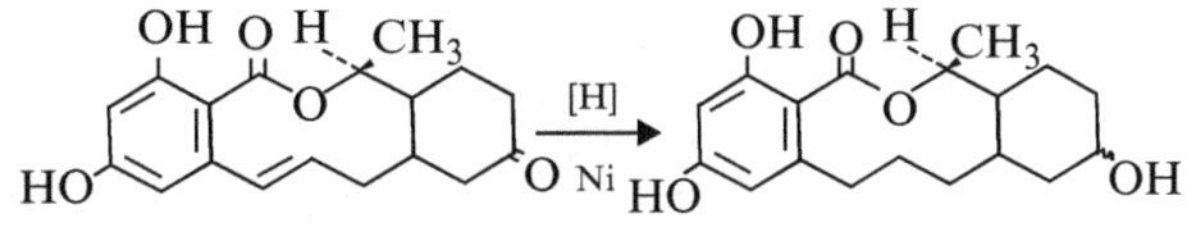

Fig. 30.1 Chemical structures of zearalenone (ZEN) and α-zearalanol (α-ZAL)

body with few residues left in organs such as muscle, heart, liver, pancreas, kidney, and blood. Taking advantage of their estrogen-like properties, both α-ZAL and zearalenone have been used as efficient and safe growth stimulants in diets in animal husbandry. However, little is known of the medical value of these phytoestrogens from clinical studies.

Since 1990s, there are preclinical studies on effects of α-ZAL on proliferating of uterus and mammary gland, blood vessels, osteoporosis, and Alzheimer's disease in animal models of menopause worldwide. What follows are the detailed studies in these fields.

α-ZAL Induces Less Proliferating Effects on Uterus and Mammary Gland Compared to Estrogen

Perhaps the most intriguing and important finding from recent studies was that α-ZAL induced less proliferating effects on uterus and mammary gland compared to estrogen. The uterine enlargement elicited by α-ZAL was only approx 20 % of that associated with equivalent doses of estrogen [8] (Fig. 30.2). The uterus (Fig. 30.3) and mammary gland (Fig. 30.4) displayed little pathological change compared to treatment with 17β-estrodiol (17β-E_2). Although the cellular mechanisms of α-ZAL remain to be elucidated, there is evidence to support that α-ZAL owns the ability to interact with estrogen receptors since α-ZAL has the benzene ring structure resembling 17β-E_2, while its the affinity of binding to the estrogen receptor is estimated to be only one-tenth of that for 17β-E_2. Unlike estrogen, α-ZAL had little effect on normal mouse mammary gland cell proliferation. Deng WH, et al. [9] reported that the effect of α-ZAL on expression of c-myc, c-fos, and epidermal growth factor receptor mRNAs in breast tissues implanted into nude mice was much less than 17β-E_2. They have also studied the effect of α-ZAL on normal human breast [10]. They found that α-ZAL had no significant effect on Bcl-2, proliferating cell nuclear antigen, estrogen receptor, and progesterone receptor expression of mammary epithelial cells in graft specimens, in addition, α-ZAL significantly inhibited the expression of proliferating cell nuclear antigen and facilitated expression of tumor suppressing protein BINI mRNA, suggesting that α-ZAL may have potential protective effect on normal human breast. There was no obvious adverse health effect or mortality during the duration of the α-ZAL treatment. These findings have broadened the research and developmental perspective of α-ZAL.

Benificial Effects of α-ZAL on Blood Vessels

To further evaluate the clinical value of this phytoestrogen, the research groups in Institute of Basic Medical Sciences, Chinese Academy of Medical Sciences & Peking Union Medical College and School of Basic Medical Sciences, Capital Medical University (Beijing, China) have systemically explored the effects of α-ZAL on blood vessels. Their study showed that α-ZAL possessed similar physiological properties of estrogen, such as inhibiting atherogenesis, improving lipid profile, attenuating homocysteine (Hcy)-induced endothelial dysfunction, inhibiting proliferation of smooth muscle cells, inhibiting oxidant stress, inhibiting apoptosis of endothelial cells, improving imbalance of nitric oxide (NO)/endothelin-1(ET-1), improving imbalance of coagulation and fibrinolysis, promoting vascular dilatation, etc.

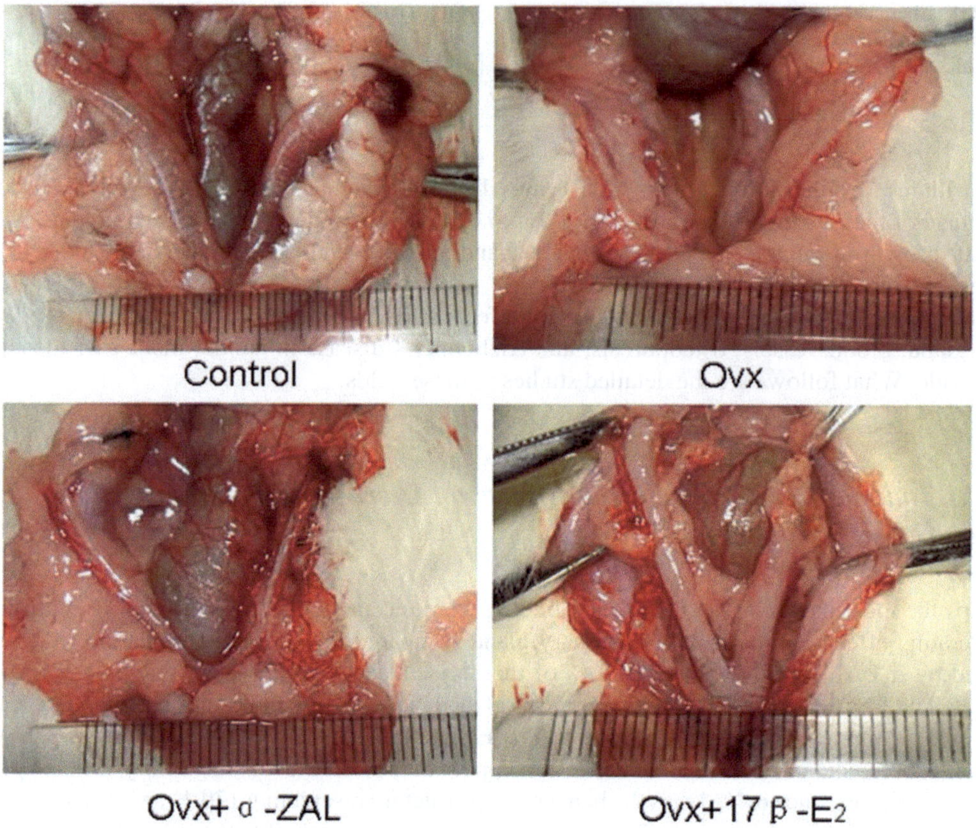

Fig. 30.2 Effects of α-ZAL and 17β-E_2 supplement on uterus growth following bilateral ovariectomy (Ovx) in rats. The size of uterus in Ovx + α-ZAL is greater than that in Ovx, but much smaller than control and Ovx + 17β-E_2. Control: normal rats; Ovx: ovariectomy; Ovx + α-ZAL: supplement with α-ZAL(2.5 mg/kg/d) for 12 weeks after ovariectomy; Ovx + 17β-E_2: supplement with 17β-E_2(2.5 mg/kg/d)for 12 wk after ovariectomy (*Unpublished data of the author*)

α-ZAL Inhibits Atherogenesis and Improves Lipid Profile in Ovariectomized Cholesterol-Fed Rabbits

Dai et al. [11] have tested the effects of α-ZAL on atherosclerosis development in the ovariectomized, cholesterol-fed rabbit model. They found that cholesterol diet-induced atherosclerotic plaque formation was reduced by 50–85 % (plaque area) by α-ZAL treatment, which was as equally effective as 17β-E_2. The plasma lipid total cholesterol, triglycerides low-density lipoprotein-cholesterol (LDL-C), and Apo-protein B (ApoB) declined to various degrees compared to the high cholesterol diet group following α-ZAL treatment. In addition, the level of blood viscosity, plasma viscosity and platelet aggregation rate in α-ZAL treatment group were also significantly decreased compared with nontreatment group, which implying that α-ZAL can improve vascular function both through the adjustment of lipometabolism and hemorheology [12]. These vascular protective effects of α-ZAL were comparable to or greater than those of 17β-E_2. Further mechanistic studies revealed that α-ZAL could reduce vascular smooth muscle cells (VSMCs) proliferation and extracellular Ca^{2+} invasion, and the α-ZAL- elicited protective effects might be related to inhibition of expression of c-myc mRNA and MCP-1 in smooth muscle cells [13].

Xu et al. [14] have evaluated the effect of α-ZAL on oxLDL-induced effect on NO and ET-1 production in human umbilical vein endothelial cells (HUVECs). HUVECs were incubated with

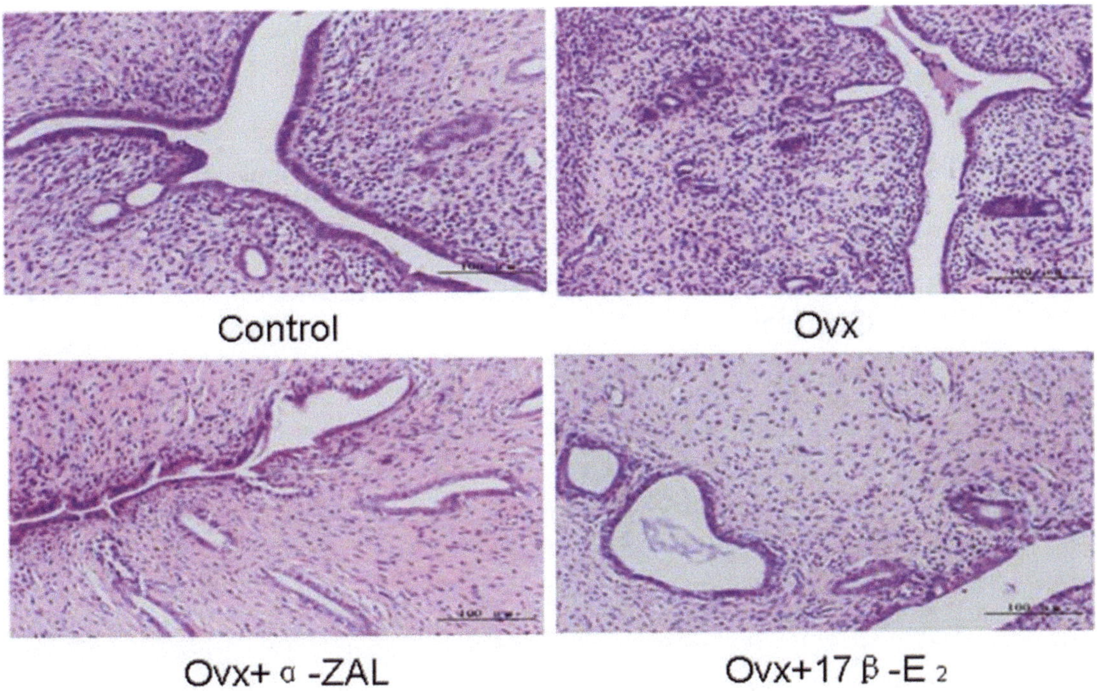

Fig. 30.3 Effects of α-ZAL and 17β-E_2 supplement on histological changes of uterus following bilateral ovariectomy (Ovx) in rats. (H.E. staining, ×20). The uterus in Ovx + α-ZAL group displayed little pathological change compared to Ovx + 17β-E_2 group. Control: normal rats; Ovx: ovariectomy; Ovx + α-ZAL: supplement with α-ZAL(2.5 mg/kg/d) for 12 weeks after ovariectomy; Ovx + 17β-E_2: supplement with 17β-E_2 (2.5 mg/kg/d)for 12 weeks after ovariectomy (*Unpublished data of the author*)

antagonize oxidized low-density lipoprotein (oxLDL, 50 μg/mL) for 24 h in the absence or presence of α-ZAL, 17β-E2 (10–1,000 nM), or the estrogen receptor antagonist ICI182780 (1 μM). Their results indicated that oxLDL significantly reduced NO release and nitric oxide synthase (NOS) activity, and enhanced ET-1 production associated with reduced NOS3 (but not NOS2) expression and enhanced ET-1 mRNA expression. All these oxLDL-induced alterations were significantly attenuated or abolished by co-incubation with α-ZAL or E2, both through an estrogen receptor-dependent mechanism. Either α-ZAL or 17β-E2 or ICI182780 had no direct effect on expression of NOS, ET-1, or NOS activity. These data suggested that the phytoestrogen α-ZAL, like 17β-E2, may effectively antagonize oxLDL-induced decrease of NO and increase of ET-1, which might be protective on endothelial function. Moreover, they examined the effect of α-ZAL on oxLDL-induced extracellular signal-regulated kinase (ERK) phosphorylation, reactive oxygen species (ROS) generation, activation of the transcriptional factor activator protein-1 (AP-1), expression, secretion, and promoter activity of ET-1 in HUVECs [15]. oxLDL (35 μg/mL) significantly enhanced ERK phosphorylation, ROS generation, AP-1 activity, mRNA expression, secretion, and promoter activity of ET-1 in HUVECs, all of which were abrogated by α-ZAL and the antioxidant *N*-acetyl-L-cysteine. Collectively, their data favored the notion that α-ZAL antagonized oxLDL-induced up-regulation of ET-1 gene expression and secretion via suppression of oxLDL-induced ROS accumulation, ERK phosphorylation, and activation of the endothelial transcriptional factor AP-1. It may be therefore speculated that the anti-atherosclerotic property of α-ZAL is mediated through its antioxidant capacity and subsequently, reduction in ET-1 expression via regulation of the redox-sensitive signaling molecules. These findings have shed some lights for the mechanisms responsible for α-ZAL induced endothelial protection and anti-atherosclerotic effects.

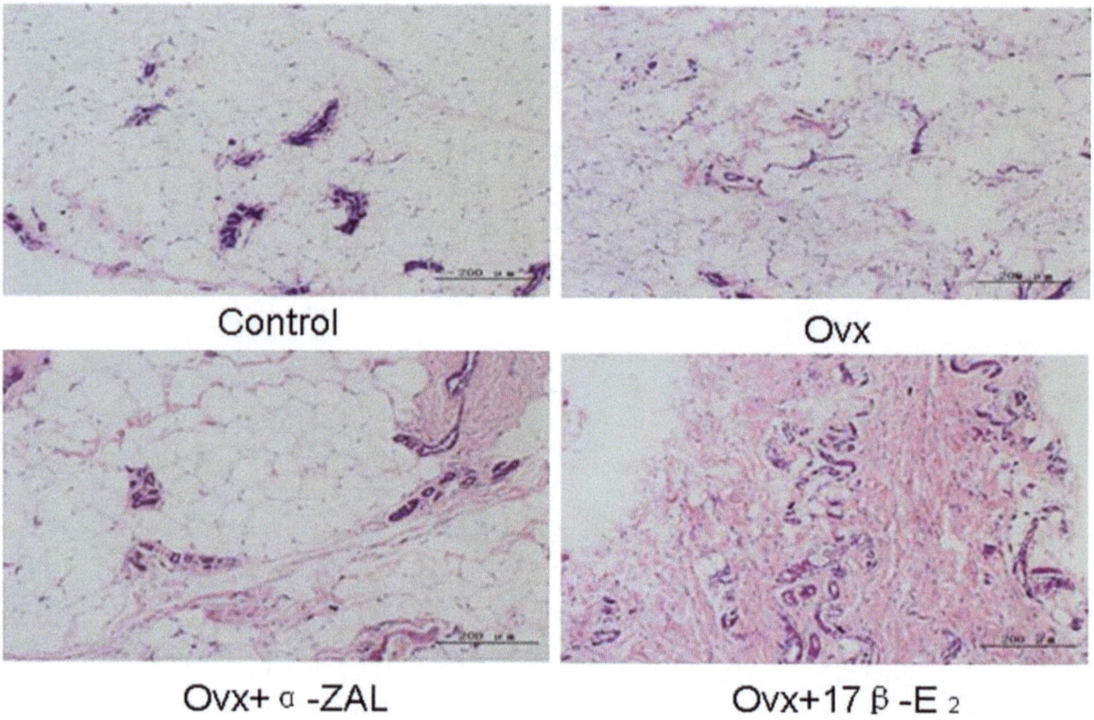

Fig. 30.4 Effects of α-ZAL and 17β-E_2 supplement on histological changes of mammary gland following bilateral ovariectomy (Ovx) in rats. (H.E. staining, ×10). The mammary gland in Ovx + α-ZAL group displayed little pathological change compared to Ovx + 17β-E_2 group. Control: normal rats; Ovx: ovariectomy; Ovx + α-ZAL: supplement with α-ZAL for 12 weeks after ovariectomy; Ovx + 17β-E_2: supplement with 17β-E_2 for 12 weeks after ovariectomy (*Unpublished data of the author*)

α-ZAL Improves Vascular Function in Ovariectomized Hyperhomocysteinemic Rats and Attenuate Homocysteine-Induced Endothelial Dysfunction

Hyperhomocysteinemia (HHcy) is defined as a high plasma homocysteine (Hcy) >15 μmol/L. Clinical studies have showed that up to 40 % of patients diagnosed with early coronary artery, cerebrovascular or peripheral vascular diseases have HHcy. HHcy has been considered to be an independent risk factor for atherosclerosis or even a predictor of cardiovascular diseases. Zhen et al. [16] have investigated the effects of α-ZAL on vascular function in ovariectomized (OVX) hyperhomocysteinemic rats and explore the mechanisms involved primarily. HHcy rat model was induced by diets containing 2.5 % methionine (Met) for 12 wk. They found that supplement of α-ZAL or 17β-E_2 could attenuate the elevation of plasma Hcy and ET-1 levels in variectomized HHcy rats. In rats of *OVX+Met* group, PE elicited significantly greater contraction in a dose-dependent manner in endothelium-intact thoracic aortas rings; ACh elicited significantly less percentage relaxation in variectomized HHcy rats. These effects were significantly attenuated by supplement with α-ZAL or 17β-E_2. Thoracic aortas morphology study also showed severe endothelium injury in ovariectomized HHcy rats, both α-ZAL and 17β-E_2 could attenuate this change. Aortas eNOS expression was decreased in ovariectomized HHcy rats, and supplement with α-ZAL or 17β-E_2 could reverse these changes. These findings demonstrated that α-ZAL could effectively alleviate the impairment of endothelial cells and improve vascular function in ovariectomized HHcy rats by decreasing plasma Hcy and antagonizing decreasing of aortas eNOS expression. This protective effect is somewhat similar with 17β-E_2.

Duan et al. [17] have reported that α-ZAL could attenuate Hcy-induced endothelial dysfunction in vitro similar with 17β-E_2. They found that α-ZAL could antagonize Hcy-induced imbalance of NO/ET-1 and apoptosis in HUVECs. They further explored the mechanisms involved. Their study showed that α-ZAL could inhibit Hcy-induced oxidative stress and ET-1 expression in HUVECs [18]. All above results have suggested the beneficial effect of α-ZAL on Hcy-induced endothelial dysfunction both in vivo and in vitro.

α-ZAL Improves the Imbalance of Coagulation and Fibrinolysis in Ovariectomized Rats and Inhibits the Expression of Tissue Factor in Endothelial Cells

Wang et al. [19] have studied the effect of α-ZAL on coagulation and fibrinolysis in ovariectomized (OVX) rats and compared it with 17β-E_2. After ovariectomy, following the reduce of endogenous estrogen, the rats' blood coagulation activity was increased: prothrombin time (PT) and activity of tissue plasminogen activator(t-PA)were decreased, as well as increased level of fibrinogen (FG), tissue factor (TF), and activity of plasminogen activator inhibitor type 1 (PAI-1). These changes were reversed by 17β-E_2 or α-ZAL replacement. These results suggested that α-ZAL had similar protective effect on improving imbalance of coagulation and fibrinolysis with 17β-E_2 in vivo. TF is a transmembrane glycoprotein that serves as primary initiator of the coagulation cascade by activating factor IX and X, and the presence of circulating TF has been associated with an increased blood thrombogenicity in these diseases. They further explored the effect of α-ZAL on TF expression in HUVECs [20].They found that ZAL could significantly down-regulate the expression of TF protein and mRNA in HUVECs. It is well known that TF gene expression in endothelial cells is mediated by activation of transcription factors, including AP-1 (c-Fos/c-Jun) and NF-κB (c-Rel/p65), and their study showed that ZAL not only decreased c-Jun/AP-1 and NF-κB p65 levels of nuclear extracts, but also inhibited angiotension II-induced activation of them, implying that ZAL decrease TF gene expression in HUVECs maybe through the inhibition of AP-1 and NF-κB [21].

α-ZAL Relaxes Rat Thoracic Aorta Rings In Vitro

Wang et al. [22] have investigated the vasorelaxing effect of α-ZAL on rat thoracic aortas rings and explored the possible mechanisms involved. Intact or endothelium-denuded rat thoracic aortas rings were put in individual organ chamber to observe the endothelium-dependent or independent vasorelaxing effects of α-ZAL. The thoracic aortas rings were pre-contracted with phenylephrine. The results showed that α-ZAL (10^{-10}–10^{-5} M) induced both endothelium-dependent and -independent relaxation of rat thoracic aortas rings. The vasorelaxing effects of α-ZAL were dose dependent whether the endothelium was intact or not. In endothelium-intact aortas rings, α-ZAL induced vasorelaxation might be inhibited by N-nitro-Larginine methylester (L-NAME, NOS inhibitor), methylene blue (guanylate cyclase inhibitor), charybdotoxin (ChTX, Ca^{2+}-activated K^+ channel blocker), glibenclamide (ATP-sensitive K^+ channel blocker), and (−) BayK8644 (L-type Ca^{2+} channel agonist), but not ICI182780(estrogen receptor antagonist). (−) BayK8644 could also inhibit α-ZAL-induced vasorelaxation in endothelium-denuded aortas rings 10^{-7}–10^{-5} M α-ZAL might induce the Phospho-eNOS expression in thoracic aorta tissue, increase the NO level in perfusate and cGMP content in thoracic aorta tissue. Meanwhile, L-NAME might decrease both NO and its downstream cGMP level. Methylene blue might decrease the level of cGMP. These results suggested that α-ZAL might induce a partly endothelium-dependent relaxation of rat thoracic aortas rings. The possible mechanisms involved in this rapid vasorelaxation included activation of eNOS/NO/cGMP pathway, opening of VSMCs ATP-sensitive and Ca^{2+}-activated K^+ channels. Furthermore, this relaxation also appeared to be mediated by both direct and indirect inhibition of voltage-dependent Ca^{2+} channel of VSMCs, while it was not concerned with activation of estrogen receptor.

Protective Effects of α-ZAL on Endothelial Cells from Hypoxia/Reoxygenation Injury

Wang et al. [23] have investigated the effects of α-ZAL on hypoxia/reoxygenation (H/R) injury and mechanism involved in HUVECs. They found that the survival rate (detected by MTT) of HUVECs and the activity of total superoxide dismutase (SOD) were significantly decreased, while the activity of lactate dehydrogenase (LDH) and the level of malondialdehyde were significantly increased after exposed to hypoxia for 3 h and then reoxygenation 1 h (H/R). These changes were reversed by pretreatment with α-ZAL or 17β-E_2 (10^{-9}–10^{-6} mol/L). They also reported that E-selectin, intercellular adhesion molecule-1 (ICAM-1), and vascular cell adhesion molecule-1 (VCAM-1) in supernatant of HUVECs were significantly increased after H (3 h)/R (1 h), and pretreatment with α-ZAL or 17β-E_2 could dose-dependently inhibit the high expression of these cell adhesion molecules induced by H/R injury [24]. These results suggested that α-ZAL could protect HUVECs from H /R injury by inhibiting the oxidative stress or inflammation reaction similar with 17β-E_2.

Protective Effects of α-ZAL on Endothelial Progenitor Cells

In 1997, Asahara et al. [25] first reported the isolation of putative endothelial progenitor cells (EPCs) from human peripheral blood, on the basis of cell surface expression of CD34 and other endothelial markers. Until now, extensive data support the existence of EPCs, their bone marrow origin, and contribution to the formation of new blood vessels in adults. Moreover, the discovery of EPCs had led to the new concept that vasculogenesis and angiogenesis may occur simultaneously in the postnatal life because these cells are able to differentiate when needed into vascular endothelium, through a mechanism recapitulating embryonic vasculogenesis [26, 27]. There are reports that estrogen may have beneficial effects on EPCs' functions, such as migriation, proliferation, differentiation, etc. [28, 29]. Hou et al. [30] have explored the effect of α-ZAL on proliferation of rat EPCs in vitro. They found that α-ZAL could increase EPCs survival rate and cloning formation ability and promoted EPCs proliferation in vitro, and PI3K/Akt inhibitor LY294002 could decrease the proliferation of EPCs. This study implied that α-ZAL could promote proliferation of EPCs in vitro and the PI3K/Akt pathway might be involved in this action.

The Neuroprotective Effects of α-ZAL on Alzheimer's Disease

Alzheimer's disease is a neurodegenerative disorder characterized clinically by progressive dementia and pathologically by intraneuronal neurofibrillary tangles, extracellular deposition of amyloid β peptides (Aβ), and phosphorylation of tau protein. Studies have shown that ERT may reduce the risk of developing Alzheimer's disease in postmenopausal women. Dong et al. [31–33] have explored the neuroprotective effects of α-ZAL on Alzheimer's disease both in vivo and in vitro, and compared this effect with 17β-E_2. They found that treatment with α-ZAL might protect neurons of hippocampus in ovariectomized rats, and α-ZAL could effectively antagonize the β-amyloid induced oxidative damage and apoptosis in cultured rat hippocampal neurons and differentiated PC-12 cells. In all above actions, α-ZAL worked in a manner similar to 17β-E_2. Their results suggested that α-ZAL might be used as a potential substitute of 17β-E_2 in postmenopausal women for Alzheimer's disease prevention.

α-ZAL Reverses Bone Loss Induced by Ovarian Hormone Deficiency in Rats

Osteoporosis is a major widespread metabolic bone disease. The occurrence rate of osteoporosis is increasing internationally as the population ages. The most important mechanism related to osteoporosis is estrogen deficiency. Phytoestrogens, as selective estrogen receptor regulators, might be effective in preventing the postmenopausal osteoporosis caused by estrogen deficiency [34]. Zong et al. [35] have assessed the ability of α-ZAL to prevent bone loss in an ovariectomized rat model of osteoporosis. They reported that α-ZAL at low dose (1 mg/kg) and medium dose (5 mg/kg) could protect the bone against estrogen deficiency similar to 17β-E_2 (0.066 mg/kg) when given once every 3 days for 35 days. The total body bone mineral density (BMD), the expressions of bone morphogenetic proteins (BMP) and basic fibroblast growth factor (bFGF) were up-regulated in the Ovx + α-ZAL groups (1 and 5 mg/kg) compared to the Ovx group, and lower levels of bone Gla protein (BGP), bone alkaline phosphatase, tartrate-resistant acid phosphatase, and tumor necrosis factor α expressions than the Ovx group. This study gave experimental support to administration of α-ZAL to reverses bone loss and prevent osteoporosis after menopausal.

Conclusion

Mounting evidence indicates that zearalenone exists in many plants and vegetables including wheat, cotton, corn, celery, carrot, and beet [36]. As an endogenous sex hormone, zearalenone is believed to play a significant role in herbal development and growth. It is worth mentioning that zearalenone was originally listed as a fungal mycotoxin and used as an index for seed and food contamination because the initial study found animals that consumed spoiled corn (containing zearalenone) displayed feminization and, in pigs, in which estrogen is the pregnancy-recognition signal, zearalenone induces pseudopregnancy [37]. Certain countries considered zearalenone as an exogenous substance for plant contamination and therefore restricted its agricultural applications. As an animal growth promoter, zearalenone has been studied with regard to its effects on organ and gland development [38]. Environmental hormones and their roles in cardiovascular diseases and other postmenopausal symptoms have received special attention over the last 20 years, especially with respect to preventing or reducing cardiovascular morbidity and mortality. As an invironmental hormone, the endogenous zearalenone and its derivative α-ZAL have been the focus of this discussion. As a nonsteroidal estrogen, α-ZAL may lead to hemodynamic alterations, which may display toxicity in the kidney and/or liver. It appears that specific toxicities may be reduced or even reversed by rumen flora in digestive tract of ruminant species, but this is still under debate.

Although a thorough system study on α-ZAL has not been completed yet, worldwide researches in the past 20 years have provided evidence for the beneficial effects of α-ZAL on blood vessels, osteoporosis and Alzheimer's disease in animal models of menopause. In most of these researches, α-ZAL has shown similar effect to 17β-E_2. Although the cellular mechanisms of α-ZAL remain to be elucidated, there is evidence to support that α-ZAL owns the ability to interact with estrogen receptors since α-ZAL has the benzene ring structure resembling 17β-E_2, while its affinity to the estrogen receptor is estimated to be only one-tenth of 17β-E_2. Also in some studies, the protective effect of α-ZAL is not through activation of estrogen receptor, for estrogen receptor antagonist cannot block its action. Thus, the cross-action between α-ZAL and estrogen receptor is worth ongoing effort. Among all these results, the real benefit of α-ZAL might be related to its relatively mild effects on the reproductive organs (e.g., breast and uterus), which means less adverse effects than estrogen. It seems that α-ZAL might be used as a potential alternative for estrogen in postmenopausal women.

To achieve a more rigorous evaluation of α-ZAL, future research should focus on the potential adverse effects of α-ZAL, and compared those to estrogen. The results of these studies will benefit agriculture and animal husbandry, as well as human health. However, clinical efficacy and potential toxicity of α-ZAL in larger trials require further assessment before regarding their use can be established.

Acknowledgments The author would like to thank Prof. Shunling Dai and Dr. Jinhong Duan from Institute of Basic Medical Sciences, Chinese Academy of Medical Sciences & Peking Union Medical College, Beijing, China for their assistance on this article.

References

1. Sullivan JM. Estrogen replacement therapy. Am J Med. 1996;101:4A56S–9. Discussion 59S–60S.
2. Collins P. Clinical cardiovascular studies of hormone replacement therapy. Am J Cardiol. 2002;90:30F–4.
3. Creasman WT. Estrogen and cancer. Gynecol Oncol. 2002;86:1–9.
4. Knight DC, Eden JA. Phytoestrogens—a short review. Maturitas. 1995;22:167–75.
5. Dai SL, Duan JH, Lu Y, Cheng J, Ren J, Deng W, et al. α-Zearalanol, a phytoestrogen for cardiovascular therapy. Endocrine. 2004;25:117–9.
6. Stob M, Boldwin RS, Tuite J. Isolation of an anabolic, uterotrophic compound from corn infected with Gibberella zeae. Nature. 1962;196:1318.
7. Li JL, Zhu TX, Zhang H, Li BR, Deng ZP, Li YS, et al. Studies on zearalenone. Acta Agricul Universitatis Pekinensis. 1980;1:13–28.
8. Wang W, Yang H, Wang HX, Zhang LK. 17β-estradiol and phytoestrogen α-zearalanol on uterus enlarging in ovariectomized rats. J Capit University Med Sci. 2005;26:51–4.
9. Deng WH, Dai SL, Zhang Y, et al. The effects of alpha-zearalanol and estradiol benzoate on expression of c-myc, c-fos and epidermal growth factor receptor mRNAs in breast tissues implanted into nude mice. Gynecol Endocrinol. 2010;26:144–8.
10. Deng WH, Wu YY, Duan JH, Yang L, Wang S, Dai SL. Effects of phytoestrogen α-zearalanol on normal human breast. Acta Acad Med Sin. 2004;26:566–70.
11. Dai SL, Duan JH, Lu Y, Zhang Y, Cheng J, Ren J, et al. Phytoestrogen alpha-zearalanol inhibits atherogenesis and improves lipid profile in ovariectomized cholesterol-fed rabbits. Endocrine. 2004;25:121–9.
12. Zhao XY, Zuo PP, Duan JH, Lu Y, Zhang YH, Cheng JX, et al. Influence of α-zearalanol on lipometabolism and hemorheology in experimental hyperlipidemia rabbits. Chin J Rehabil Theo Pract. 2005;11:924–6.
13. Lu Y, Dai SL, Duan JH, Cheng JX, Zhang YH, Wu XQ, et al. Phytoestrogen α-zearalanol inhibition it against increase of rabbit VSMCs [Ca^{2+}] induced by (−) BayK8644. Chin Phamacol Bull. 2006;22:1147–9.
14. Xu H, Duan J, Dai S, Wu Y, Sun R, Ren J. Phytoestrogen α-zearalanol antagonizes oxidized LDL-induced inhibition of nitric oxide production and stimulation of endothelin-1 release in human umbilical vein endothelial cells. Endocrine. 2004;25:235–45.
15. Xu H, Duan J, Dai S, Wu Y, Sun R, Ren J. α-Zearalanol attenuates oxLDL-induced ET-1 gene expression, ET-1 secretion and redox-sensitive intracellular signaling activation in human umbilical vein endothelial cells. Toxicol Lett. 2008;179:163–8.
16. Zhen PP, Duan JH, Zhao Q, Hou DD, Wang HX, Hong N, et al. Phytoestrogen α-zearalanol improves vascular function in ovariectomized hyperhomocysteinemic rats. Atherosclerosis. 2011;215(2):309–15.
17. Duan J, Xu H, Dai S, Wang X, Wu Y, Zhang Y, et al. Phytoestrogen alpha-zearalanol inhibits homocysteine-induced endothelin-1 expression and oxidative stress in human umbilical vein endothelial cells. Atherosclerosis. 2008;197:549–55.
18. Duan JH, Dai SL, Fang CX, Sun R, Shavali S, Sharma SK, et al. Phytoestrogen alpha-zearalanol antagonizes homocysteine-induced imbalance of nitric oxide/endothelin-1 and apoptosis in human umbilical vein endothelial cells. Cell Biochem Biophys. 2006;45:137–45.
19. Wang W, Zhu GJ, Zu SY. Effects of 17β-estradiol and phytoestrogen α-zearalanol on tissue factor in ovariectomized rats and endothelial cells. Chin J Physiol. 2004;47:67–72.
20. Wang W, Zhu GJ. Comparison between phyoestrogen α-zearalanol and supplementary ectogenesis 17β-estradiol in the effect on coagulation and fibrnolysis in ovariectomized rats. Chin J Clinic Rehabil. 2005;9:195–7.
21. Wang W, Liu W, Zu SY, Zhu GJ. Transcription regulation on tissue factor gene expression in the HUVEC by phytoestrogen α-zearalanol. Basic Clin Med. 2005;25:539–42.
22. Wang W, Jiang DJ, Zhu YF, Liu W, Duan J, Dai S. Relaxing effects of phytoestrogen α-zearalanol on rat thoracic aorta rings in vitro. Chin J Physiol. 2009;52:99–105.
23. Wang W, Qiu XW, Jiang DQ, Zhang LK. Effects of phytoestrogen α-zearalanol on hypoxia/reoxygena tion injury in HUVECs. Chin J Physiol. 2006;22:2110–2.
24. Wang W, Jiang DQ, Qiu XW, Zhu YF, Zhang LK. Influence of a new type of phytoestrogen alpha-zearalanol on the expression of cell adhesion molecule in human umbilical vein endothelial cells following hypoxia/reoxygenation injury. J Clin Rehabili Tis Eng Res. 2007;11:1038–40.
25. Asahara T, Murohara T, Sullivan A, Silver M, van der Zee R, Li T, et al. Isolation of putative progenitor endothelial cells for angiogenesis. Science. 1997;275:964–7.
26. Chade AR, Zhu X, Lavi R, Krier JD, Pislaru S, Simari RD, et al. Endothelial progenitor cells restore renal function in chronic experimental renovascular disease. Circulation. 2009;119:547–57.
27. Wang W, Lang JK, Suzuki G, Canty JM Jr, Cimato T. Statins enhance clonal growth of late outgrowth endothelial progenitors and increase myocardial capillary density in the chronically ischemic heart. PLoS One. 2011;6:e24868.

28. Hamada H, Kim MK, Iwakura A, Ii M, Thorne T, Qin G, et al. Estrogen receptors alpha and beta mediate contribution of bone marrow-derived endothelial progenitor cells to functional recovery after myocardial infarction. Circulation. 2006;114:2261–70.
29. Masuda H, Kalka C, Takahashi T, Yoshida M, Wada M, Kobori M, et al. Estrogen-mediated endothelial progenitor cell biology and kinetics for physiological postnatal vasculogenesis. Circ Res. 2007;101:598–606.
30. Hou DD, Wang W. Phytoestrogen α-zearalanol promotes proliferation of endothelial progenitor cells in vitro. Chin J Microcirc. 2011;21:26–9.
31. Dong YL, Yue Y, Liu FH, Lang SY, Zhang XC, Dai SL, et al. Treatment with phytoestrogen alpha-zearalanol might protect neurons of hippocampus in ovariectomized rats. Endocrine. 2006;30:249–54.
32. Dong YL, Zuo PP, Li Q, Liu FH, Dai SL, Ge QS. Protective effects of phytoestrogen alpha-zearalanol on beta amyloid25-35 induced oxidative damage in cultured rat hippocampal neurons. Endocrine. 2007;32:206–11.
33. Dong YL, Yang N, Liu Y, Li Q, Zuo P. The neuroprotective effects of phytoestrogen α-zearalanol on β-amyloid-induced toxicity in differentiated PC-12 cells. Eur J Pharmacol. 2011;670:392–8.
34. Fanti P, Monier-Faugere MC, Geng Z, Schmidt J, Morris PE, Cohen D, et al. The phytoestrogen genistein reduces bone loss in short-term ovariectomized rats. Osteoporos Int. 1998;8:274–81.
35. Zong SH, Wei B, Xiong CX, Zhao Y, Zeng G, et al. The role of a-zearalanol in reversing bone loss induced by ovarian hormone deficiency in rats. J Bone Miner Metab. 2011. DOI 10.1007/s00774-011-0302-8.
36. Gajecki M. Zearalenone–undesirable substances in feed. Pol J Vet Sci. 2002;5:117–22.
37. Young LG, King GJ. Low concentrations of zearalenone in diets of mature gilts. J Anim Sci. 1986;63:1191–6.
38. Altavilla D, Saitta A, Galeano M, Squadrito G, Marino D, Minutoli L, et al. The phytoestrogen alpha-zearalenol reverses endothelial dysfunction induced by oophorectomy in rats. Lab Invest. 2001;81:125–32.

Chapter 31
Flaxseed and Bone Health in Animal Models of Menopause

Wendy Elizabeth Ward and Lilian U. Thompson

Key Points

- Flaxseed is a widely available food that is often used as a dietary supplement, particularly among postmenopausal women to potentially relieve menopausal symptoms and prevent and/or treat chronic diseases.
- In the ovariectomized rat model of postmenopausal osteoporosis, feeding flaxseed alone does not attenuate the loss of bone mass, structure, and strength that occurs after ovariectomy.
- Combining flaxseed with low or ultralow doses of estrogen attenuates ovariectomy-induced loss of BMD, structure and strength in rats.
- Studies using the athymic nude mouse model, a commonly used model for studying diet and/or drug interventions for breast cancer prevention or treatment, has shown that feeding flaxseed does not impede the effect of soy or its isoflavone genistein or the cancer drug tamoxifen.
- Flaxseed is a healthful food, containing alpha-linolenic acid (ALA), fiber, protein, and many micronutrients and as such may be useful for prevention of chronic diseases other than osteoporosis.

Keywords Alpha-linolenic acid • Bone mineral density • Bone strength • Bone structure • Estrogen • Flaxseed • Lignans • Ovariectomy

Abbreviations

ALA	Alpha-linolenic acid
BMC	Bone mineral content
BMD	Bone mineral density
LV	Lumbar vertebra
SDG	Secoisolariciresinol diglucoside

W.E. Ward, B. Arts & Sci., M.Sc., Ph.D. (✉)
Department of Kinesiology and Center for Bone and Muscle Health, Brock University, 500 Glenridge Avenue, Walker Complex, Room 262, St. Catharines, ON, Canada L2S 3A1
e-mail: wward@brocku.ca

L.U. Thompson, Ph.D.
Faculty of Medicine, Department of Nutritional Sciences, University of Toronto, 150 College Street, FitzGerald Building, Room 316, Toronto, ON, Canada M5S 3E2

C.J.H. Martin et al. (eds.), *Nutrition and Diet in Menopause*, Nutrition and Health,
DOI 10.1007/978-1-62703-373-2_31, © Springer Science+Business Media New York 2013

Introduction

Flaxseed is a commonly consumed dietary supplement, particularly among menopausal and postmenopausal women [1, 2]. The popularity of flaxseed is, in part, due to its relatively high content of omega-3 fatty acid alpha-linolenic acid (ALA) as well as the lignan secoisolariciresinol diglucoside (SDG), which can be metabolized to the mammalian lignans enterodiol and enterolactone. ALA has potential anti-inflammatory properties, whereas the mammalian lignans may have potential hormone-like effects, binding to estrogen receptors or modulating estrogen metabolism depending on the target tissue studied (Fig. 31.1). A decline in endogenous estrogen production that occurs at menopause is often associated with the loss of bone mass and higher risk of fragility fracture. Moreover, lower circulating levels of estrogen is associated with greater T-cell activation that leads to higher levels of proinflammatory cytokines and prostaglandins that stimulate greater production of receptor activator of nuclear factor-κβ that activates osteoclasts [3]. Thus, in theory, both the ALA and lignan components in flaxseed may attenuate the deterioration of bone tissue after menopause.

Studies directly studying the effect of flaxseed intervention on bone health in menopausal/postmenopausal women have reported no direct benefits to bone mineral density (BMD) or on biochemical markers of bone formation or resorption [4–7]. These findings contrast with a study in older adults in which diets that are higher in n-6 to n-3 fatty acids were associated with lower hip BMD [8]. As discussed later in this chapter, effects of flaxseed alone in an animal model—similar to studies in postmenopausal women—demonstrate no beneficial or harmful effect to bone health. However, flaxseed or its lignan or oil component has been shown to modulate the effects of soy or drugs used in prevention or treatment of specific diseases in ovariectomized rodent models.

Ovariectomized Rodent Models for Studying Effects of Flaxseed on Bone Health

This chapter focuses specifically on the effect of flaxseed on bone health in animal models of menopause. Within that context, flaxseed or its bioactives (lignan or oil) have been studied using the ovariectomized rat or mouse model. These studies have used bone strength (peak load) as the primary outcome of interest. Peak load is the maximum force the skeletal site can withstand prior to fracture and is measured using a material testing system, providing a surrogate measure of fracture risk (Fig. 31.2). While the peak load is influenced by many factors, BMD and bone structure at a specific site are two factors that contribute to the strength of a skeletal site (Fig. 31.2). All of the studies to be discussed have measured BMD, and one study measured bone structure to ultimately understand how differences in bone strength have occurred. BMD is a derived measurement—bone mineral content (BMC) is directly measured by dual energy X-ray absorptiometry and expressed as a function of the area of the bone or site measured. BMD strictly represents the amount of mineral present in a bone or at a skeletal site, and because of the complexity of bone tissue and studies that have identified the disparity of BMD measurements and fracture risk, the usefulness of a measurement of BMD in isolation of other outcomes for predicting fracture risk is debated. Bone structure is measured in rodent bones using micro-computed tomography. In the ovariectomized rodent model, the changes in trabecular bone microarchitecture are of particular interest. Among the most common measurements are trabecular number and trabecular separation.

The studies in ovariectomized rats or mice can be grouped into two main research areas (Table 31.1). One area has involved studying whether flaxseed alone or in combination with estrogen replacement therapy preserves bone health in ovariectomized rats. The other area has investigated bone health secondary to outcomes of cancer prevention or treatment in the athymic nude mouse model of human breast cancer.

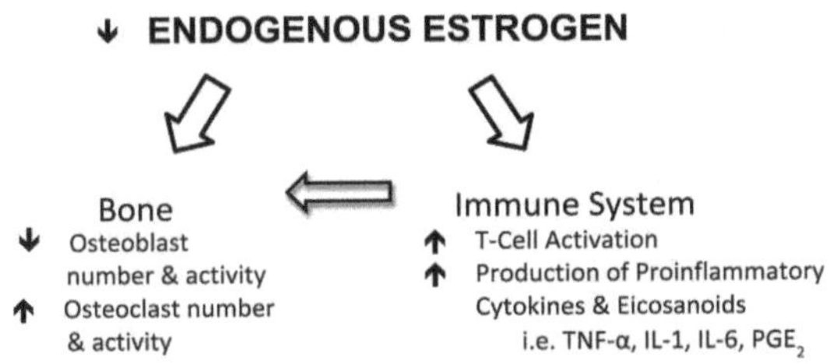

Fig. 31.1 Potential mechanisms by which the lignan and ALA component in flaxseed may modulate bone health. Lignan may have estrogen-like effects with direct effects on bone cell number and activity or indirectly by modulating the immune system. Higher dietary levels of ALA, resulting in a higher dietary ratio of n-3 to n-6 fatty acid that is reflected in bone tissue, may lead to a less inflammatory state within the bone tissue

Fig. 31.2 Approaches used for studying effects of flaxseed on femurs and lumbar spine in ovariectomized rodent models

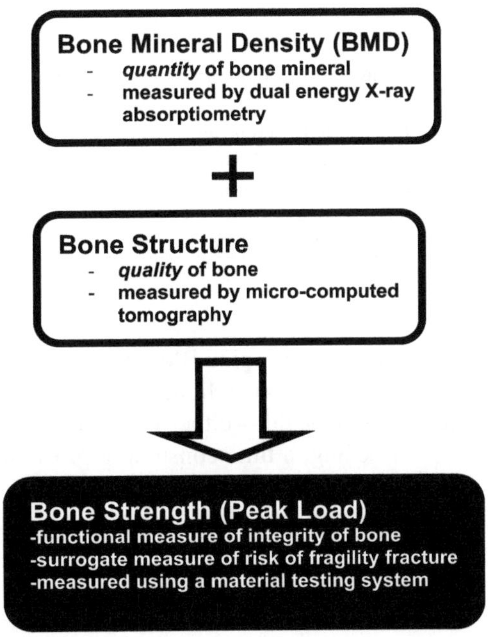

Ovariectomized Rat Model

The ovariectomized rat model can be considered the most commonly used and well-characterized animal model for studying if and how foods or food components attenuate skeletal deterioration that occurs after cessation of endogenous estrogen production. Moreover, the effects of ovariectomy in rats resemble the changes that occur in postmenopausal women: a higher rate of bone turnover and a greater loss of bone at trabecular sites (spine, hip) compared to skeletal sites containing more cortical bone. Ovariectomized rats are also used for testing anti-resorptive or anabolic agents for bone including estrogen, bisphosphonates, parathyroid hormone, calcitonin, or denosumab. A well-documented phenomenon in ovariectomized rats is the hyperphagic state that occurs. Whether the higher food intake and resulting higher body weight itself modulated BMD and strength, had been questioned and thus many studies pair-feed ovariectomized rodents such that they receive an equivalent amount of food as the control rodents. One study in ovariectomized rats has shown that despite the higher food intake and higher body weight in ad libitum-fed compared to pair-fed rats, the effect of ovariectomy

Table 31.1 Summary of the two ovariectomized rodent models in which the effect of flaxseed or its components on bone health have been studied

Intervention	Ovariectomized rodent model	Outcomes measured
Flaxseed alone or in combination with low or ultralow dose estrogen	Sprague–Dawley rats	BMC and BMD of whole femur, whole tibia, and lumbar spine
		Structure of a lumbar vertebra
		Bone strength (peak load) at femur midpoint, femur neck, tibia midpoint and of individual lumbar vertebra
		Lignan distribution in femur, tibia, and lumbar vertebrae
		Fatty acid composition of tibia and lumbar vertebrae
		Serum tartrate resistant acid phosphastase-5β, C-terminal telopeptides of Type 1 collagen, osteocalcin, osteoprotegrin, receptor activator of nuclear factor-κβ
		LV morphology, and tartrate resistant acid phosphatase-5β, osterix, osteocalcin, osteoprotegerin, and receptor activator of nuclear factor-κβ in LV
Flaxseed alone or in combination with soy	Athymic nude mice	BMC and BMD of whole femur and lumbar spine
Enterodiol and enterolactone alone or in combination with genistein		Bone strength (peak load) at femur midpoint, femur neck and of individual lumbar vertebra
Lignan precursor (SDG) and flaxseed oil alone or in combination with tamoxifen		

to femur and lumbar spine BMD and strength were similar [9]. Moreover, the significantly higher fat mass (25 % higher) in ad libitum-fed rats compared to pair-fed rats did not impact any measured outcomes of bone health—either BMD or strength measurements [9]. Findings from this study suggest that pair-feeding, a time-consuming process, of ovariectomized rats is not necessary as food intake does not alter outcomes measured in intact femurs and spine. However, it is important to measure food intake to know the level of intake of the food or food component of interest. The studies using this ovariectomized rat model discussed in this chapter were conducted with similar age rats and for a similar duration (12–14 weeks).

Ovariectomized Athymic Mouse Model

While the ovariectomized mouse model has not been as fully characterized and is not as widely used as the ovariectomized rat model, mice experience a similar loss of bone mineral, changes in bone structure and reduction in bone strength. The ovariectomized mouse model that has been studied extensively with respect to benefits of flaxseed intervention is the athymic nude mouse model. Primary outcomes of these studies have included outcomes of estrogen-dependent breast cancer, and because bone tissue is also sensitive to hormonal changes, secondary outcomes from two studies have included measures of bone health. The nu/nu genetic mutation results in a nonfunctional thymus gland, suppressed T-cell production and, overall, an immunodeficient state that allows human breast cancer cells to be injected without risk of rejection [10]. By removing ovaries at an early age, it is possible to control the level of the estrogen in the mouse, an important consideration when injecting these mice with an estrogen-dependent human breast cancer cell line (i.e., MCF-7 cells).

Flaxseed Intervention: Alone and in Combination with Low or Ultralow Dose Estrogen—At Preventing Loss of Bone Mass and Strength After Ovariectomy in Rats

Flaxseed Alone

Two studies have fed a diet containing 10 % flaxseed by weight (100 g flaxseed per kg of AIN93G diet) to ovariectomized rats for 12 weeks and measured bone quantity and bone strength of lumbar spine and a long bone (femur or tibia or both) [11, 12]. This level of flaxseed represents a realistic level of flaxseed that can be incorporated into the human diet, i.e., 2–5 tbsp or 25–50 g of flaxseed per day. As expected, there was significantly greater incorporation of n-3 fatty acids in LV3 and tibias from these rats. Specifically, ALA was higher and linoleic acid was correspondingly lower among rats fed flaxseed compared to rats not fed flaxseed. Eicosapentaenoic acid was also higher amongst rats fed flaxseed diet. Despite the marked changes in fatty acid composition in the lumbar spine and tibia, deterioration of bone tissue was not attenuated with flaxseed feeding after ovariectomy. BMC, BMD, and peak load measures in lumbar spine and femur were significantly lower than sham-operated controls and similar to rats that were ovariectomized and fed control diet, devoid of flaxseed [11, 12]. While these studies had shown that bone was responsive to changes in fatty acids contributed by flaxseed, whether the lignan component of flaxseed, SDG, with potential hormonal properties, was present in bone tissue had not been determined. A follow-up study using ^{3}H-SDG showed that a very small proportion of the SDG metabolites are incorporated into bone [13], Percentage distribution of ^{3}H-SDG metabolites in bone tissue was relatively low (0.1 %) compared to other hormone sensitive tissues (2.6 % in vagina, 2.3 % in uterus, 1.3 % in mammary tissue) [13]. Of the three skeletal sites measured, vertebra had a higher level of incorporation than long bones (tibia, femur) [13].

Flaxseed in Combination with Low or Ultralow Dose Estrogen

The same two studies [11, 12] described above also included groups in which flaxseed intervention was combined with one of two levels of estrogen that were lower than traditionally used levels of estrogen. The impetus for studying the potential combined effects of flaxseed and estrogen was based on two main aspects: (a) flaxseed is among the most commonly used supplements among menopausal or postmenopausal women, particularly in North America [1, 2]; and (b) findings from the large, multicentered, Women's Health Initiative showing increased risk of cardiovascular disease and invasive breast cancer (but lower fracture rates) prompted consideration of whether lower doses of estrogen therapy could benefit bone health without adverse effects [14]. A review of human studies does suggest that doses of estrogen therapy that are lower than traditional levels such as those used in the Women's Health Initiative can have positive effects on skeletal health, attenuating loss of BMD [14].

The first ovariectomized rat study investigating the combined effect of flaxseed and estrogen used a "low dose" of estrogen (13 μg over 90 days as a slow release subcutaneously placed estrogen pellet) that was titrated to mimic low dose estrogen therapy in women (25 μg transdermal estrogen therapy in postmenopausal women) [11]. The primary objective was to determine whether flaxseed provided additive benefits for estrogen therapy via its bioactive components—ALA and lignans. The greatest benefit of combining flaxseed with low dose estrogen was in peak load of LV2 [11]. Moreover, a higher trabecular number and less trabecular separation of LV5 were observed when flaxseed was combined with low-dose estrogen compared to low dose estrogen alone and these positive effects on LV structure provide an explanation for the higher peak load [15]. Rats receiving flaxseed with low-dose estrogen had similar peak load of LV2, trabecular number and trabecular separation compared to sham-operated control but peak load was not statistically different from low-dose estrogen alone [11, 15]. Similar findings were observed for BMC of LV1-3 [11]. Interestingly, low-dose estrogen alone did not attenuate the loss of BMC and BMD of the lumbar spine induced by ovariectomy but did preserve the strength of LV2—indicating that estrogen was having direct effects on bone structure as opposed to mineral content [11]. Some but not all outcomes measured in long bones (femur, tibia) were altered by ovariectomy, likely due to the greater quantity of cortical bone in comparison to lumbar spine. For outcomes such as whole femur BMD, upper one-third tibia BMC or BMD, or upper one-third femur BMD, none of the interventions attenuated the loss observed with ovariectomy [11].

The second ovariectomized rat study used an ultralow dose of estrogen (7 μg over 90 days as a slow release subcutaneously placed estrogen pellet) that was titrated to mimic ultralow dose estrogen therapy in women (14 μg transdermal estrogen therapy), and the design was identical, except for the dose of estrogen, to the previously discussed study [12]. The rationale for this study was twofold: (a) to determine if flaxseed showed some benefit even when administered with a lower dose of estrogen than previously studied; and (b) to determine if flaxseed might in fact antagonize the effect of such a low dose of estrogen as flaxseed lignan metabolites may modulate estrogen metabolism. Flaxseed feeding was shown to not antagonize the effects of the ultralow dose of estrogen; intervention with either ultralow dose estrogen alone or with flaxseed resulted in similar outcomes [12]. Similar to the study using flaxseed and low-dose estrogen, greatest benefits to bone strength (peak load) were observed in lumbar spine with no benefit to the strength of the femur or tibia [12].

These studies in the ovariectomized rat have shown that flaxseed alone does not attenuate deterioration of bone tissue due to withdrawal of endogenous estrogen but that in combination with low or ultralow dose estrogen, there is a beneficial effect. Arguably, the most important finding is that LV2 is able to withstand a greater compressive force before fracturing. Compression fractures are a common type fragility fracture. Determining the mechanisms by which this effect occurs is ongoing. Rats receiving flaxseed with low dose estrogen have been shown to have lower expression of osteocalcin and higher expression of osteoprotegrin in lumbar vertebra compared to ovariectomized mice fed control diet and that the expression is similar to sham-operated controls [15]. However, the fact that the expression level is not different than low dose estrogen alone suggests that additional mechanisms have not yet been identified [15]. Other outcomes measured in LV that were unchanged included tartrate resistant acid phosphastase-5β, osterix, and receptor activator of nuclear factor-κβ [15].

Flaxseed Intervention: Alone and in Combination with Soy Protein Isolate or Tamoxifen—At Preventing Loss of Bone Mass and Strength After Ovariectomy in the Athymic Nude Mouse Model

The ovariectomized athymic nude mouse model has been used to study the effect of flaxseed or its components in combination with soy or its isoflavones or tamoxifen in breast cancer development and biology. A natural extension of this research has been to investigate these same interventions on other hormone sensitive tissues such as the bone. The intervention studies have fed diets containing 10 % flaxseed by weight or equivalent amounts of SDG or oil present in such diets [16–18].

Flaxseed or Its Lignans in Combination with Soy Protein Isolate or Its Isoflavone Genistein

Flaxseed and soy are commonly used dietary supplements and may be used by breast cancer patients to complement conventional therapies [2]. Moreover, supplements containing bioactive components such as flaxseed lignans (SDG) and soy isoflavones (genistein) are widely used supplements [1]. A study that had previously shown that combined intervention with flaxseed alone and in combination with soy protein isolate—but not soy protein isolate alone—resulted in less tumor growth [19] was followed up with a study to assess effects to other hormone sensitive tissues such as bone [16]. Because soy contains isoflavones with weak estrogenic activity it was possible that the isoflavones could be beneficial to bone health in this model system. Indeed, intervention with soy protein isolate had a positive effect on bone tissue, with a greater effect in femur compared to lumbar spine [16]. Soy protein isolate, unlike flaxseed or the combination of flaxseed and soy protein isolate, resulted in higher whole femur BMC and BMD, and femur midpoint peak load compared to the ovariectomized group fed control diet [16]. Combining with flaxseed attenuated the positive effect of soy protein isolate on whole femur BMD but not peak load at the femur midpoint [16]. Of note is that the athymic mouse responds somewhat differently to ovariectomy due to the fact that T-cell function is suppressed and yet T cell activation is a critical step by which ovariectomy leads to deterioration of bone tissue. This may at least partially explain why LV outcomes are unchanged with interventions. Without a positive control in this study and others it is difficult to assess the effect of ovariectomy at the different skeletal sites. Another interesting finding was that in case of soy protein isolate, tumor volume and whole femur BMD or femur midpoint peak load were positively associated indicating that both the tumors and femur had similar responses to the dietary intervention which was likely estrogenic [16]. Another study investigated the mammalian lignan metabolites of SDG (enterodiol, enterolactone) in combination with the isoflavone genistein [17]. Similar to the effect of soy protein isolate, genistein had an estrogenic effect on femur but not LV, resulting in greater femur BMD [17]. Moreover, as was observed when soy protein isolate and flaxseed were combined, the mammalian lignans did not significantly attenuate the effects of genistein.

Flaxseed in Combination with Tamoxifen

A previous study that used components of flaxseed—SDG or flaxseed oil—alone or in combination with tamoxifen had shown that the components on its own attenuated the growth of breast tumors either in the presence or absence of tamoxifen [20]. Moreover, tamoxifen itself has been shown to result in higher BMD in women as well as other animal studies [21]. Thus, the follow-up study investigating effects on bone health, demonstrated as expected, that tamoxifen had positive effects on femur and LV outcomes (BMC, BMD, and peak load) compared to ovariectomized mice receiving control diet [18]. Unlike tamoxifen alone, neither the SDG or flaxseed oil had positive effects on bone outcomes measured, and as well, when combined with tamoxifen, neither SDG nor flaxseed oil attenuated the positive effect of tamoxifen on bone outcomes [18].

Conclusion

To date, findings from ovariectomy studies suggest that feeding flaxseed or its lignans alone do not attenuate the loss of bone mass, structure, and strength that occurs after ovariectomy. However, there is a benefit to lumbar spine when flaxseed is combined with low dose or ultralow dose estrogen, and the mechanism of action requires further investigation. Using the athymic nude mouse model that has been extensively used to study the protective effects of flaxseed and its lignan or oil as a prevention or treatment strategy for breast cancer, flaxseed subtly attenuates effects of soy or genistein while not modifying the positive effect of tamoxifen. Thus, while flaxseed alone does not modulate bone health this can be viewed as a positive in that there is no negative effect, and in situations in which it has been combined with other foods, food components or drugs it does not overtly interfere with their positive effects to bone. Moreover, flaxseed contains many healthful components and thus incorporating flaxseed into the diet may be beneficial in promoting overall health and preventing other chronic diseases.

References

1. Singh SR, Levine MAH. Natural health product use in Canada: analysis of the national population health survey. Can J Clin Pharmacol. 2006;13:e240–50.
2. Verhoef MJ, Balneaves LG, Boon HS, Vroegindewey A. Reasons for and characteristics associated with complementary and alternative medicine use among adult cancer patients: a systematic review. Integr Cancer Ther. 2005;4:274–86.
3. Pacifici R. Role of T cells in ovariectomy induced bone loss—revisited. J Bone Miner Res. 2012;27:231–9.
4. Brooks JD, Ward WE, Lewis JE, Hilditch J, Nickell L, Wong E, et al. Supplementation with flaxseed alters estrogen metabolism in postmenopausal women to a greater extent than does supplementation with an equal amount of soy. Am J Clin Nutr. 2004;79:318–25.
5. Dodin S, Lemary A, Jacques H, Legare F, Forest JC, Masse B. The effects of flaxseed dietary supplement on lipid profile, bone mineral density, and symptoms in menopausal women: a randomized, double-blind, wheat germ placebo-controlled clinical trial. J Clin Endocrinol Metab. 2005;90:1390–7.
6. Griel AE, Kris-Etherton PM, Hilpert KF, Zhao G, West SG, Corwin RL. An increase in dietary n-3 fatty acids decrease a marker of bone resorption in humans. Nutr J. 2007;6:1–8.
7. Lucas EA, Wild RD, Hammond LJ, Khalil DA, Juma S, Daggy BP, et al. Flaxseed improves lipid profile without altering biomarkers of bone metabolism in postmenopausal women. J Clin Endocrinol Metab. 2002;87:1527–32.
8. Weiss LA, Barrett-Connor E, Von Muhlen D. Ratio of n-6 to n-3 fatty acids and bone mineral density in older adults: the Rancho Bernardo Study. Am J Clin Nutr. 2005;81:934–8.
9. Jiang JM, Sacco SM, Ward WE. Ovariectomy-induced hyperphagia does not modulate bone mineral density or bone strength in rats. J Nutr. 2008;138:2106–10.
10. Kavanaugh CJ, Desai KV, Calvo A, et al. Pre-clinical applications of transgenic mouse mammary cancer models. Transgenic Res. 2002;11:617–33.
11. Sacco SM, Jiang JMY, Reza-Lopez S, Ma DWL, Thompson LU, Ward WE. Flaxseed combined with low-dose estrogen therapy preserves bone tissue in ovariectomized rats. Menopause. 2009;16:545–54.
12. Sacco SM, Jiang JMY, Reza-Lopez S, Ma DWL, Thompson LU, Ward WE. Flaxseed does not antagonize the effect of ultra-low-dose estrogen therapy on bone mineral density and biomechanical bone strength in ovariectomized rats. J Toxicol Environ Health A. 2009;72:1209–16.
13. Sacco SM, Thompson LU, Ganss B, Ward WE. Accessibility of 3H-secoisolariciresinol diglycoside lignan metabolites in skeletal tissue of ovariectomized rats. J Med Food. 2011;14:1208–14.
14. Sacco SM, Ward WE. Revisiting estrogen: efficacy and safety for postmenopausal bone health. J Osteoporos. 2010;708931:8. doi:10.4061/2010/708931.
15. Sacco SM. Flaxseed and lower-dose estrogen: studies on their protective actions and mechanisms in bone using the ovariectomized rat model. Ph.D. Thesis. University of Toronto. 2011.
16. Power KA, Ward WE, Chen JM, Saarinen N, Thompson LU. Flaxseed and soy protein isolate, alone and in combination, differ in their effect on bone mass, biomechanical bone strength, and uterus in ovariectomized nude mice with MCF-7 human breast tumor xenografts. J Toxicol Environ Health A. 2007;70:1088–896.
17. Power KA, Ward WE, Chen JM, Saarinen N, Thompson LU. Genistein alone and in combination with the mammalian lignans enterolactone and enterodiol induce estrogenic effects on bone and uterus in a postmenopausal breast cancer mouse model. Bone. 2006;39:117–24.
18. Chen J, Saggar JK, Ward WE, Thompson LU. Effects of flaxseed lignan and oil on bone health of breast-tumor-bearing mice treated with or without tamoxifen. J Toxicol Environ Health A. 2011;74:756–68.
19. Saarinen NM, Power K, Chen J, Thompson LU. Flaxseed attenuates the tumor growth stimulating effect of soy protein in ovariectomized athymic mice with MCF-7 human breast cancer xenografts. Int J Cancer. 2006;119: 925–31.
20. Saggar JK, Chen J, Corey P, Thompson LU. The effect of secoisolariciresinol diglycoside and flaxseed oil, alone and in combination, on MCF-7 tumor growth and signaling pathways. Nutr Cancer. 2010;62:532–42.
21. Eastell R, Hannon RA, Cuzick J, Dowsett M, Clack G, Adams JE, et al. Effect of an aromatase inhibitor on BMD and bone turnover markers: 2 year results of the Anastrozole, Tamoxifen, alone or in combination (ATAC) trial. J Bone Miner Res. 2006;21:1215–23.

Chapter 32
Flavonoids of Herba Epimedii and Bone Metabolism in Experimental Ovarian Deficiency

Man-Sau Wong and Yan Zhang

Key Points

- Flavonoids of Herba Epimedii could preserve bone health in OVX rodents, including bone histomorphology, micro-structure and bone mass.
- BMP signaling and Wnt signaling pathways are found to be involved in mediating the actions of total flavonoids and icariin in bone cells.
- TF inhibits osteoclast formation by increasing ratio of OPG/RANKL and stimulates bone formation by enhancing Cbfa1 expression.
- Icariin exhibits selective estrogen-like activity, but did not induce uterotrophic effects in vivo.
- Icariin stimulates ERα phosphorylation at Ser118 in a ligand-independent manner without activating ERE-luciferase activity in UMR 106 cells, via the ERα or the ERβ-mediated pathway.

Keywords Bone • Osteoporosis • Herba epimedii • Flavonoid • Icariin • Menopause • Estrogen • Ovariectomy

Abbreviations

Tb.Sp	Trabecular separation
Tb.Th	Trabecular thickness
Tb.N	Trabecular number
SMI	Structure model index
BV/TV	Bone volume/tissue volume
Ct.Th	Cortical thickness

M.-S. Wong, Ph.D. (✉)
Department of Applied Biology and Chemical Technology, The Hong Kong Polytechnic University, Hung Hom, Kowloon, Hong Kong SAR, PRC
e-mail: bcmswong@polyu.edu.hk

Y. Zhang, Ph.D.
University of Shanghai for Science and Technology,
P.O. Box 445, 516# Jungong Road, Yangpu District, Shanghai 200093, China
e-mail: medicineyan@yahoo.com.cn

C.J.H. Martin et al. (eds.), *Nutrition and Diet in Menopause*, Nutrition and Health,
DOI 10.1007/978-1-62703-373-2_32, © Springer Science+Business Media New York 2013

OS/BS	Osteoid surface
MAR	Mineral apposition rate
BFR/BS	Bone formation rate with bone surface as referent
BFR/BV	Bone formation rate with bone volume as referent
BMD	Bone mineral density
SSI	Stress–strain index
OCN	Osteocalcin
BMP	Bone morphogenetic protein
Cbfa1	Core binding factor 1
ER	Estrogen receptor
SAP	Sialoprotein
OPG	Osteoprotegerin
RANKL	Receptor activator of nuclear factor-kB ligand
HRT	Hormone replacement therapy
TCM	Traditional Chinese medicine
TF	Total flavonoids
SRAT	Serum of rats administered TF
ALP	Alkaline phosphatase
BGP	Bone gla protein
ICA	Icariin
EPFs	Epimedium-derived phytoestrogen flavonoids
HEP	Herba epimedii
BM-MSCs	Bone marrow-mesenchymal stem cells
OVX	Ovariectomized
DPD	Deoxypyridinoline
M-CSF	Macrophage colony-stimulating factor
Ca	Calcium

Introduction

Osteoporosis is a metabolic disease of the bone and increases the likelihood of bone fracture. The generalized loss of bone, the development of osteoporosis and the occurrence of fractures increase with age. Whereas bone mineral density (BMD) declines in both men and women with age, women typically start with lower BMD and show an accelerated loss at menopause owing to a decline in estrogen production by ovarian hormone deficiency. It is well known that estrogen deficiency during postmenopause and as a result of ovariectomy leads to acceleration of bone resorption that result in rapid bone loss with a high bone metabolic turnover will increase the risk of the development of osteoporosis in women [1].

Current therapies recommended for postmenopausal osteoporosis treatment include calcitonin, bisphosphonates, raloxifene as well as hormone replacement therapy (HRT). These treatments are viewed as a strategy for the management of climacteric complaints and prevention of osteoporosis. However, recent reports [2] showed that long term use of HRT in postmenopausal women was associated with augmented risks of breast cancer, stroke, and uterine bleeding. At the same time, with the increase in life expectancy of women in both developed and developing countries, the worldwide incidence of postmenopausal osteoporosis are expected to increase dramatically [3]. Thus, there is a strong demand to develop low cost, safe, and effective alternative regimen for management of postmenopausal osteoporosis. Traditional herbal medicine is one of the major candidates that attract the attention of both the afflicted patients as well as the medical professionals.

Use of Traditional Chinese Medicine for Management of Bone Health During Menopause

Traditional Chinese Medicine (TCM) is one of the many different forms of medicine that exist around the globe. Compared to Western Medicine that works with allopathic medicine, TCM follows an entirely different medical system. According to TCM, menopause occurs because we have used up much of our inherited Jing or essence, and at the same time digestive power has decreased so we create less Jing from food. The net loss of Jing results is the creation of a smaller amount of Blood. The available Blood is used to nourish the organs and sinews, with no leftovers to overflow the uterus. The result is the cessation of menses [4].

In Chinese Medicine, menopause reflects our bodies' intelligent conservation of Jing and often results in the classic signs of Kidney Yin Deficiency. Yin is closely related to the feminine hormones such as estrogen and progesterone. Osteoporosis that some women experience at this time would also be related to Yin deficiency and to deficiency of the Kidney in Chinese Medicine [5]. Based on TCM theory, the kidney is responsible for the nourishment of bone, so-called kidney dominates bone, which has been guiding the widely traditional implications of kidney-tonifying herbal medicine for the treatment of fractures and joint diseases for thousands of years in China [2].

Herba epimedii (HEP) is also known as Horny Goat Weed or Yin Yang Huo, and commonly used in traditional Chinese medicine for "strengthening the kidney." It has a proven efficacy in treating cardiovascular diseases and improving sexual and neurological functions [6].

Recent efforts from both Western medical researchers and their Asian and Latin American counterparts focus on the application of Western scientific methods to study the efficacy of traditional medicinal materials. Modern pharmacological studies have indicated that HEP has the efficacy in treating osteoporosis [6]. It is one of the most frequently used herbs in formulas, such as the commercially available formula preparation "Xian-ling-gu-bao" capsule [7], that are prescribed for the treatment of osteoporosis [8]. Its efficacy could be attributed to the bioactive components, flavonoids, contained in HEP. It is well reported that flavonoids, like genistein, daidzein, have bone-preserving functions in postmenopausal women and estrogen-deficient animals [9]. Some of the flavonoids-enriched products, like Novasoy enriched with soy isoflavones [10, 11], have been in market circulation.

Bone loss due to estrogen withdrawal following menopause leads to reduced mechanical strength and ultimately fracture in women. Consequently, in animal study, bilateral ovariectomy serves as an appropriate model for postmenopausal osteoporosis, and the ovariectomized animal models have been widely applied in pathological and pharmacological study on osteoporosis. Additionally, bone cell models, such as osteoblast, osteoclast, and mesenchymal stem cell, are also widely applied for studying the potential molecular mechanism of medical materials on maintaining bone health. The main contents of the following part introduce the effects of HEP on bone metabolism observed in OVX rodents and cell models as summarized in Table 32.1.

Bone Protective Effects of Herba Epimedii Extract

The bone protective effects of HEP have been widely investigated by scientists using in vitro bone cell models and in vivo animal models with modern biological approaches.

The study of the effects of HEP extract on bone properties in experimental model was reported as early as in 1996 by Wu T et al. The study showed that the water extract of HEP worked very well in preventing and minimizing the side effects induced by long-term use of glucocorticoids in rats in which it could antagonize adrenocortical atrophy and osteoporosis associated with glucocorticoid

Table 32.1 Results of HEP flavonoids on bone health in ovariectomized rodents or in bone cells

Study	Treatment	Animal/cell	Major findings
Xie [13], Hong Kong	HEP	OVX rats	Decreased urinary calcium excretion, suppressed serum ALP activity and urinary DPD, increased tibial Tb.Ar and decreased Tb. Sp
Nian [14], China		OVX rats	Prevented the increases in Tb. Sp, moreover, it had remarkable effect on BFR/BV and BFR/BS
Xie [13], Hong Kong		UMR106 cell	Stimulated cell proliferation and increased ALP activity, resulted in a dose-dependent increase in OPG/RANKL mRNA ratio
Jin [15], China		Bone marrow cell from rats	Serum containing HEP, prepared from blood of rats administered orally with HEP extract, decreased the formation of matured osteoclasts induced by RANKL and M-CSF
Chen [17], Hong Kong	Flavonoids	OVX mice	Prevented the deterioration of trabecular bone micro-architecture and suppressed the increase in urinary Ca excretion as well as loss of bone mass and strength at the distal femur, increased renal calcium reabsorption by up-regulating mRNA expression of CaBP-28k and VDR
Zhang [20], China		Human BM-MSCs	The total time needed for osteogenic differentiation of BM-MSCs was significantly shortened by adding total flavonoids
Chen [17], Hong Kong		OVX rodents	Up-regulated mRNA expression of cbfa1, type 1 collagen and osteocalcin of bones
Qian [18], China			Suppressed the osteoclast differentiation by enhancing the ratio of OPG/RANKL in human BM-MSCs [20], in rat osteoblasts [22], and in femur of OVX mice [17], as well as suppressed adipogenic differentiation of bone marrow stromal cells [23]
Chen [17], Peng [23], Hong Kong			
Zhang [20], Liu [22], China			
Nian [29], China	Icariin	OVX rats	Improved BMD and bone strength and prevented the reduction of serum calcium and phosphorus
Mok [30], Hong Kong		OVX mice	Suppressed the loss of bone mass and strength in distal femur
Zhang [31], China		OVX mice	Increased the width and area of trabecular bone and the thickness of cortical bone
Hsieh [37], Taiwan		Primary osteoblast cell cultures	Exerted its osteogenic effects through the induction of BMP-2 and BMP-4 synthesis, subsequently regulating Cbfa1/Runx2, OPG, and RANKL gene expressions
Zhao [38], Japan			

treatment in the animal model [12]. Our study reported in 2005 was the first to employ modern in vitro and in vivo experimental platform to characterize the bone-sparing function of HEP in experimental model of postmenopausal osteoporosis. Four-month-old ovariectomized (OVX) Sprague-Dawley rats were orally administered with HEP extract (110 mg kg^{-1} day^{-1}), 17β-estrogen (2 mg kg^{-1} day^{-1}) or its vehicle for 3 months. We have reported that HEP extract significantly decreased urinary calcium excretion, suppressed serum alkaline phosphatase (ALP) activity and urinary deoxypyridinoline (DPD) level in OVX rats [13].

Histomorphometric analysis (Fig. 32.1) on decalcified bone tissue indicated that HEP extract could prevent ovariectomy-induced bone loss by increasing tibial trabecular bone area and decreasing trabecular separation (Tb. Sp) in rats [13]. Similarly, Nian et al. reported the histological study that the aqueous extract of HEP prevented the increase in Tb. Sp in young OVX rats, and such effect was associated with a remarkable up regulation of bone formation rate both as a reference to bone volume (BFR/BV) and as reference to bone surface (BFR/BS) [14]. However, it is of interest to note that in

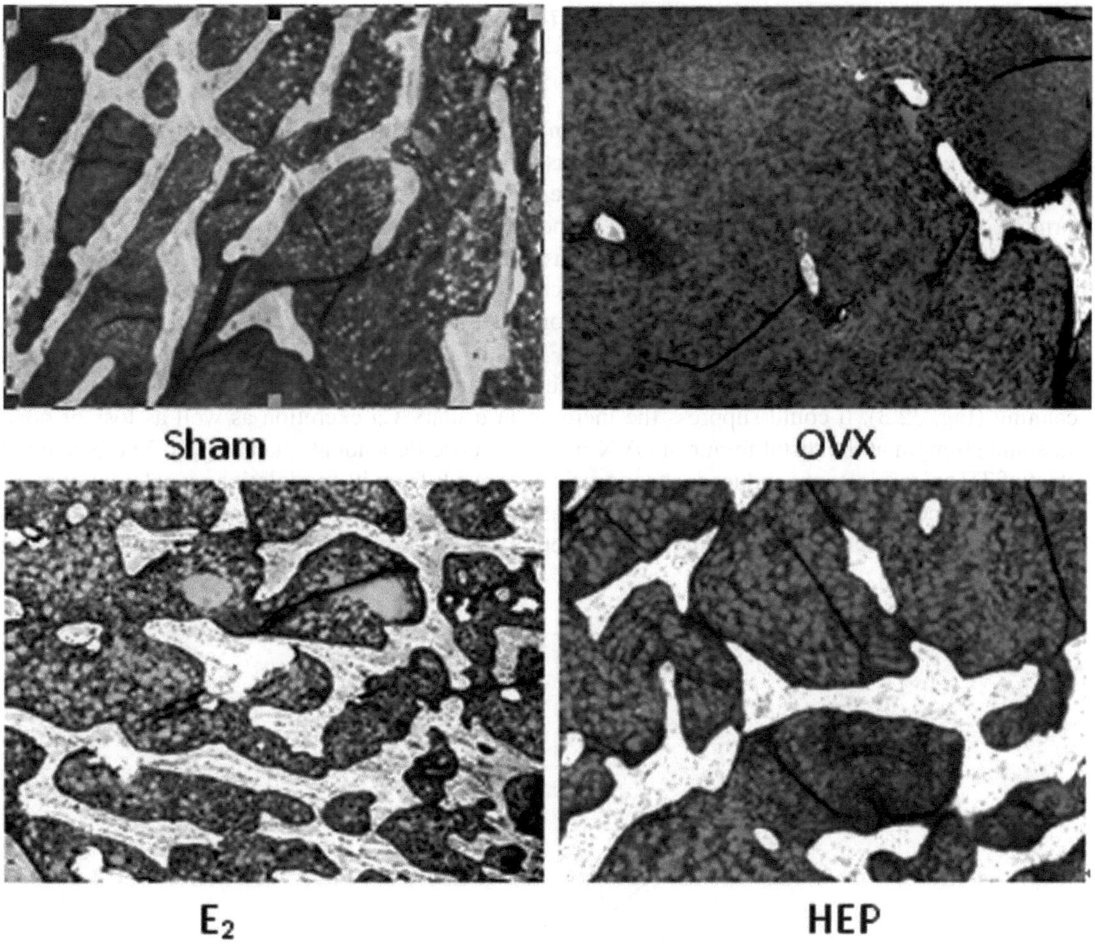

Fig. 32.1 Bone histomorphometric analysis of rat tibia. The images of the metaphyseal trabecular of the sham, OVX, E_2, and HEP groups. The OVX rats were orally administrated with HEP extract (110 mg kg^{-1} day^{-1}), 17-β estradiol (E_2, 2 mg kg^{-1} day^{-1}), or its vehicle for 3 months. Rat tibias were collected, cleaned by removal of adherent tissue, and fixed in chloroform. Upon fixation, diaphyseal segments of the tibias were dehydrated, defatted in acetone followed by ether and then embedded in bioplastic. The blocks were sectioned at a thickness of 5 mm with a Reichert–Jung supercut microtome and digitized using a Leica camera. Sections containing the tibio-fibular junction were coupled to an Olympus AH-2 microscope and were determined using the Leica QW 550 image software (Figure originally published in [13] and permission is granted for reproduction)

both studies HEP extract did not alter trabecular thickness (Tb. Th) and trabecular number (Tb. N) in OVX rats.

Our in vitro study [13] using rat osteoblast-like UMR 106 cells showed that HEP extract significantly stimulated cell proliferation in a dose-dependent manner and increased ALP activity at 200 μg mL^{-1}. It modulated osteoclastogenesis by increasing osteoprotegerin (OPG) mRNA and decreasing receptor activator of NF-κB ligand (RANKL) mRNA expression in UMR 106 cells, resulting in a dose-dependent increase in OPG/RANKL mRNA ratio [13]. The inhibition of HEP on osteoclastogenesis was also demonstrated by the study [15] where serum containing HEP (prepared from blood of rats administered orally with HEP extract) could decrease the formation of mature osteoclasts induced by RANKL and M-CSF. Taken together, HEP treatment can effectively suppress the ovariectomy-induced increase in bone turnover, possibly by both an increase in osteoblastic activities and a decrease in osteoclastogenesis [13].

Bone Protective Effects of Flavonoids, the Major Active Fraction in Herba Epimedii

Flavonoids are class of organic compounds, often naturally occurring and structurally similar to the mammalian estrogens, which many of them act as phytoestrogens in mammals. The consumption of plant-based foods rich in flavonoids and their derivatives may provide an alternative to traditional hormone replacement therapy and has been associated with a reduction in menopausal symptoms, such as hot flashes and vaginal dryness [16]. It has been proven that flavonoids are active component in HEP and have protective effects against ovariectomy-induced bone loss in animal models [17–19]. The major chemical composition of the total flavonoids fraction in HEP is shown in Fig. 32.2.

Our study [17] showed that total flavonoids (TF) isolated from HEP could prevent the deterioration of trabecular bone micro-architecture in OVX mice as determined by the micro-computed tomography scanning (Fig. 32.3). It could suppress the increase in urinary Ca excretion as well as loss of bone mass and strength at the distal femur in OVX mice in a dose-dependent manner [17]. The beneficial effect of TF on ovariectomy-induced osteoporosis may result from its modulation on calcium homeostasis. Our study showed that TF increased renal calcium reabsorption by up-regulating mRNA expression of renal CaBP-28k and vitamin D receptor in OVX mice [17]. Combining with the report

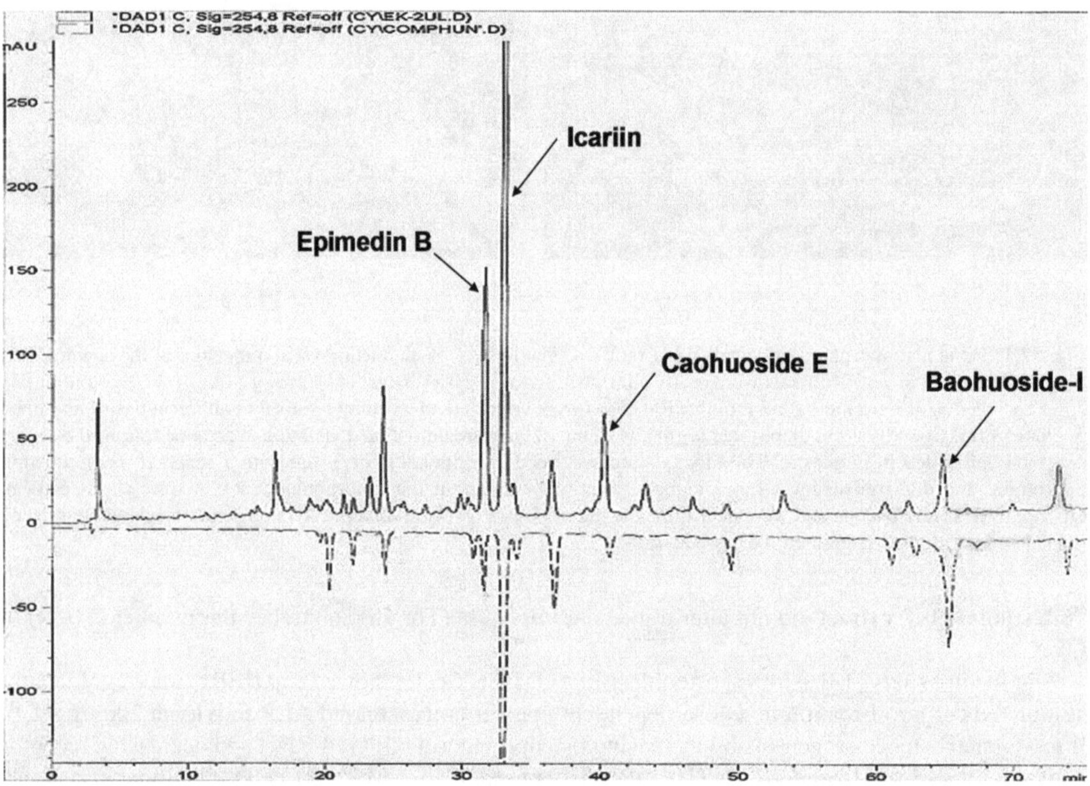

Fig. 32.2 Reverse-phase HPLC for the qualitative analysis of the total flavonoid extract of *Herbal epimidii* (HEP). Icariin, epimedin B, caohuoside E, and baohuoside I are the main active compounds in *Herba epimedii* according to the Chinese Pharmacopoeia. Standard compounds were performed HPLC in the same elution procedure with the total flavonoid extract of HEP. The peaks in the profile of total flavonoids with the same retention time with authentic markers were identified and used for confirmation of the identity of the total flavonoid extract Herba Epimedii (Figure originally published in [17], Cambridge University Press and permission is granted for reproduction)

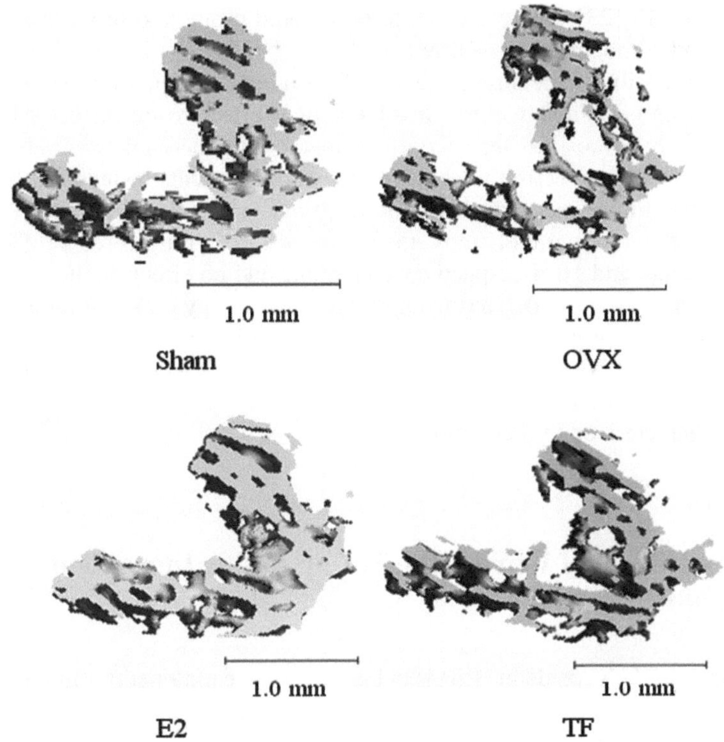

Fig. 32.3 Effects of total flavonoids from HEP on bone microarchitecture at distal femur in ovariectomized mice analyzed by microCT. OVX mice were treated with vehicle (Sham or OVX), 17β-estradiol (E_2, 4 μg $g^{-1}day^{-1}$), or TF (100 μg $g^{-1}day^{-1}$) for 6 weeks. Right femurs from mice were scanned using the microCT system (viva-CT40; Scanco Medical, Bassersdorf, Switzerland) to evaluate microarchitecture in the epiphysis region of the femur end. The scanning position of distal femur was initiated at the distal end of the femur. All scans were done in 21 μm sections to a total of 100 slices per scan. Three-dimensional evaluation was generated by the Scanco compiler in the Virtual Memory System (Figure originally published in [17], Cambridge University Press and permission is granted for reproduction)

of Zhang [19] in which the prevention of osteoporosis in the OVX rat model by TF was found to be independent of an enhancement in intestinal calcium absorption, we can conclude that TF maintains calcium balance in estrogen-deficiency animals is at least in part by increasing renal calcium reabsorption, but not by intestinal calcium absorption.

Recent studies using in vitro model revealed that TF may have direct actions on bone cells. Zhang et al. [20] reported the total time needed for osteogenic differentiation of bone marrow-mesenchymal stem cells (BM-MSCs) was significantly shortened by adding TF. Moreover, TF could increase the expression of Cbfa1 mRNA in the bone of OVX rats in a dose-dependent manner [18]. Cbfa1, a transcription factor specifically expressed in cells of the osteoblast lineage, not only stimulates the differentiation of osteoblast but also serves as a regulator of the major osteoblastic function, i.e., the production of the bone extracellular matrix [21]. It is necessary for osteoblast-specific expression of genes such as osteocalcin, alpha-1 type I collagen (Col), osteopontin, and bone sialoprotein. Studies by our group [17] and others [18] showed that TF administered to OVX rodents stimulated osteocalcin expression and increased the expression of type I collagen mRNA [17] in bones. These findings suggest that TF of HEP might be a bone anabolic agent and Cbfa1 is required for mediating the anabolic effects of TF. In addition, TF was also shown to suppress the osteoclast differentiation by enhancing the ratio of OPG/RANKL in human bone marrow-derived MSCs [20], in rat osteoblasts [22] and in femur of OVX mice [17]. In addition, it was also shown to suppress adipogenic differentiation of bone marrow stromal cells [23]. Therefore, TF of HEP could promote osteogenesis as well as inhibit osteoclastogenesis and adipogenesis concurrently.

Despite the demonstration of the direct effects of TF on bone cells in vitro, study by Wu et al. [24] provided evidence to argue against its direct involvement as effective substance of HEP for treatment of osteoporosis. They hypothesized that certain of metabolites derived from TF and the products induced by these metabolites in serum were the effective components instead. In their study, TF was supplemented into the culture medium of newborn rat calvarial osteoblasts at 0.2, 2, 20, 100, and 200 mg L^{-1}, respectively. In a parallel study, the serum of rats administered TF (SRAT) was added into the medium at 2, 4, 8 and 16 % respectively. TF alone had no effect on the cell proliferation and function expression in osteoblasts derived from rat calvariae at any concentration. In contrast, 2 and 4 % SRAT stimulated cell proliferation and, 4 % SRAT promoted the maturation and function of osteoblast by improving the ALP activity, bone gla protein (BGP) secretion, calcium deposition, and the number of mineralized nodular structures [24]. However, the exact identities of active metabolites in SRAT were not characterized in their study.

Bone Protective Effects of Icariin, the Major Active Ingredient in Herba Epimedii

Icariin, a marker flavonoid glycoside in HEP, is believed to be the major active ingredient that accounts for its bone protective actions. It exists in many species of *Epimedium* plants. Its content in HEP varies among species and sources, and has been reported extensively [6, 25]. The icariin content ranged from 0 to 2.732 % among nine species, in which highest content was found in the *E. pubescens* Maxim, while none was found in *E. leptorrhizum* Stearn [6]. The flavonoid content from 17 species of *Epimedium* was also reported, in which the icariin content ranged from 0 to 14.24 mg g^{-1}. These results show that certain kinds of *Epimedium* plants may serve as better herbal materials as source of flavonoids or icariin for pharmaceutics purposes [6].

Icariin is a prenylated flavonol glycoside with structural formula $C_{33}H_{40}O_{15}$ and molecular weight of 676.67. The chemical structure of icariin is illustrated in Fig. 32.4. Study by Ma et al. [26] suggested that the prenyl group on C-8 of icariin could be the active group that takes part in osteoblastic differentiation and explains for its greater potency in osteogenesis than genistein. The results were in accordance with our in vitro structure–activity study that the prenylation at C-8 could increase the bone-protective effects of genistein on UMR106 cell [27]. These observations were also in agreement with the study by Wong et al. [28] in which they reported that the prenylation at C-8 made icaritin, a metabolite of icariin, a potent phytoestrogen that might exert selective ERα activity using reporter gene system in Hela cells stably expressing ERα or ERβ.

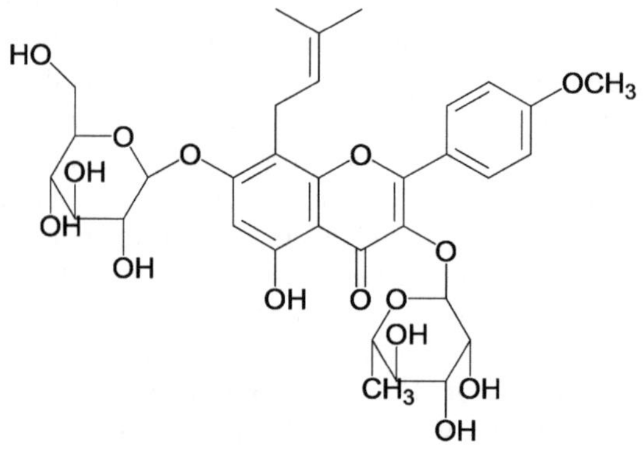

Fig. 32.4 Chemical structure of icariin

To date, only few in vivo studies have been performed to study the effects of icariin on bone health in ovariectomized animals [29–31]. A recent study reported that treatment of OVX rats with icariin could improve BMD and bone strength and prevent the reduction of serum calcium and phosphorus [29]. Our recent study [30] also characterized the in vivo bone protective effects of icariin in which OVX C57BL/6 mice fed with diet containing 0.6 % calcium and 0.65 % phosphorus throughout the course of the study were orally treated with vehicle, 17β-oestradiol (4 μg g^{-1} day^{-1}) or icariin (0.3 mg g^{-1} day^{-1}) for 6 weeks. We found that icariin suppressed the loss of bone mass and strength in distal femur in OVX mice [30]. Study by Zhang et al. [31] also reported that icariin treatment obviously increased the width and area of trabecular bone and the thickness of cortical bone in OVX mice femur based on bone histomorphometric analysis [31], suggesting that icariin can rectify the abnormal metrology index in mice with osteoporosis. Taken together, the in vivo studies revealed that icariin exerted beneficial effects on bone mass, biomechanical strength as well as microstructure of bone in OVX animals.

The beneficial effects of icariin on bone health of OVX animals are, at least in part, due to its regulation on the expression of bone target genes and proteins and its effect on circulating estradiol level. Recent studies showed that icariin increased the mRNA expression ratio of OPG/RANKL in tibia of C57BL/6 mice [30], decreased the protein expression of IL-6 in femur of KM mice following ovariectomy [32]. Studies showed that the serum level of estradiol in icariin-treated rats [29, 33] and mice [34] after ovariectomy was significantly increased compared to OVX model group.

With the demonstration of the estrogen-like bone protective effects of icariin in OVX animals, one should be cautious about the possible side effects of icariin might exert on estrogen-target organs, like uterus. However, based on studies by our group and others neither the wet weight of uterus of OVX rats [33] nor the uterus index of OVX mice [30] were altered upon icariin treatment. These studies suggested that icariin did not induce the uterus hypertrophy and might serve as a potential alternative therapeutic agent for the management of osteoporosis.

Mechanism Study for the Actions of Herba Epimedii and Its Active Constituents in Bone

Although the detailed molecular mechanisms by which the flavonoid components isolated from HEP prevent osteoporosis are not fully understood, several studies have been performed to explore the molecular signaling pathway that might be involved. For instance, Zhang et al. [35, 36] reported that TF enhanced the mRNA expression of BMP-2, BMP-4, Runx2, beta-catenin and cyclinD1 in human bone marrow-derived mesenchymal stem cells. These cellular targets are BMP or Wnt-signaling pathway related regulators, and the osteogenic effects of TF were found to be inhibited by noggin and DKK-1, which are classical inhibitors of BMP and Wnt/beta-catenin signaling pathways, respectively [35, 36]. Similarly, icariin was found to exert its osteogenic effects through the induction of BMP-2 and BMP-4 synthesis in primary osteoblastic culture derived from adult mice, which subsequently lead to the regulation of Cbfa1/Runx2, OPG, and RANKL gene expressions [37, 38]. In addition, the osteogenic effect of icariin was found to be inhibited by the introduction of Smad6 or dominant-negative Runx2, as well as Noggin treatment in primary osteoblastic culture [38]. Thus, both BMP signaling and Wnt/beta-catenin signaling appear to play vital roles in mediating the osteoprotective effects of HEP flavonoids.

In our recently published study, we hypothesized that icariin would act as a phytoestrogens in preventing bone loss induced by estrogen deficiency and promoting osteoblastic functions. We have reported that icariin increased ER-dependent cell proliferation, ALP activity as well as mRNA expression of OPG and the OPG/RANKL ratio in UMR 106 cells. We have also characterized the estrogenic actions of icariin in UMR 106 cells by co-transfection with either ERa or ERb construct as well as

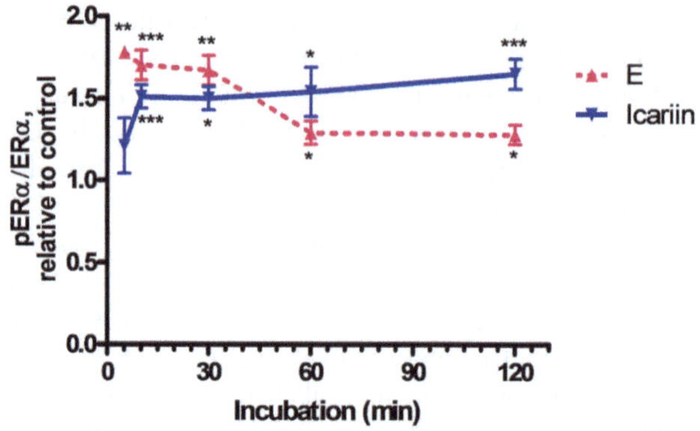

Fig. 32.5 The time course of ER phosphorylation induced by treatment with 10 nM icariin. Cells were treated with vehicle (C), 17β-estradiol (E_2, 10^{-8} M), or icariin (10^{-8} M) for 5 min, 10 min, 30 min, 1 h and 2 h. Proteins extracted from cell lysates were transblotted onto a membrane and probed with anti-phospho-ERα at serine 118 residue (pERα) and anti-ERα (ERα) primary antibodies followed by the corresponding secondary antibodies. Relative intensity of chemiluminescence was measured and phospho-ERα to ERα ratio was calculated. Results were obtained from three independent experiments and expressed as mean ± SEM. *$P<0.05$; **$P<0.01$; ***$P<0.001$ vs. vehicle control (Figure originally published in [30], John Wiley and Sons and permission is granted for reproduction)

estrogen response element (ERE)-luciferase construct. Our results showed that icariin neither activated ERE-luciferase activity in UMR 106 cells via the ERα nor the ERβ-mediated pathway in accordance with the observations of icariin on Hela cells [28]. However, it was found to rapidly increase ERα phosphorylation at Ser118 in UMR 106 cells. As shown in Fig. 32.5, icariin was able to significantly increase the ratio of phosphorylated ERα to ERα expression upon incubation in UMR 106 cells for 10 min ($P<0.001$) and the stimulation was sustained throughout the period of incubation. As serine 118 is the major site for ligand-independent activation of ERa, these results indicated that icariin exerts anabolic effects in bone possibly by activating ER in a ligand-independent manner [30].

Clinical Study Involved the Use of Herba Epimedii for Management of Osteoporosis

As mentioned previously, decoction containing HEP has been prescribed clinically by Chinese medicine practitioners for management of bone diseases with a long history of safe use [39]. Numerous preclinical studies as discussed above involve the use of both in vitro [13, 15] and in vivo [13, 14] models have repeatedly demonstrated its efficacies in improving bone properties using modern experimental approach.

One Singapore research group has systematically examined the estrogenicity of ethanol extracts of taxonomically identified *Epimedium* species prepared under standardized conditions [40]. They established estrogen-responsive bioassay that can measure the pharmacokinetic/pharmacodynamic of estrogen activity in serum [39]. Their results indicated that ethanol extract of HEP exerted estrogenic effects in serum following oral ingestion [28, 39], suggesting its utility for ERT and estrogen-regulated processes such as bone health.

Thus, it is worthwhile to explore its related clinical efficacy using modern approach. An earlier study by Zhao [41] reported that 6 months of HEP extract treatment could improve cancellous bone density and ostealgia in women with osteoporosis as diagnosed by double energy X-ray absorption. A recent study by Zhang et al. [42] performed a 24-month randomized double-blind placebo-controlled clinical trial for evaluating the effect of the *Epimedium*-derived phytoestrogen flavonoids (EPFs) in late postmenopausal women. In this study, subjects were randomized into EPF treatment group ($n=50$; a daily dose of 60 mg Icariin, 15 mg Daidzein, and 3 mg Genistein) or placebo control group ($n=50$) and all participants received 300 mg element calcium daily. The results clearly demonstrated that EPFs exerted beneficial effect on preventing bone loss in late postmenopausal women without resulting in a detectable hyperplasia effect on the endometrium [42].

Conclusions

The effects of HEP total flavonoids (TF) and single flavonoid icariin (ICA) on bone biological parameters and the potential action mechanisms involved in estrogen-deficient animals are summarized in Fig. 32.6. Both TF and ICA could improve bone histomorphology and micro-structure as well as increase bone mass in OVX rodents. BMP signaling (up-regulate BMP-2, BMP-4, and Cbfa1) and Wnt (up-regulate beta-catenin and cyclin D1) signaling pathways are found to be involved in mediating the actions of TF and ICA in bone cells. Moreover, TF inhibits osteoclast formation by increasing ratio of OPG/RANKL and stimulates bone formation by enhancing Cbfa1 expression which in turn triggers the expression of osteocalcin, collagen and bone sialoprotein in osteoblastic cells. ICA exhibited selective estrogen-like activity by increasing serum estradiol level of OVX animals, but did not induce uterotrophic effects in vivo. In addition, ICA stimulates ERα phosphorylation at Ser118 in a ligand-independent manner without activating ERE-luciferase activity in UMR 106 cells, via the ERα or the ERβ-mediated pathway.

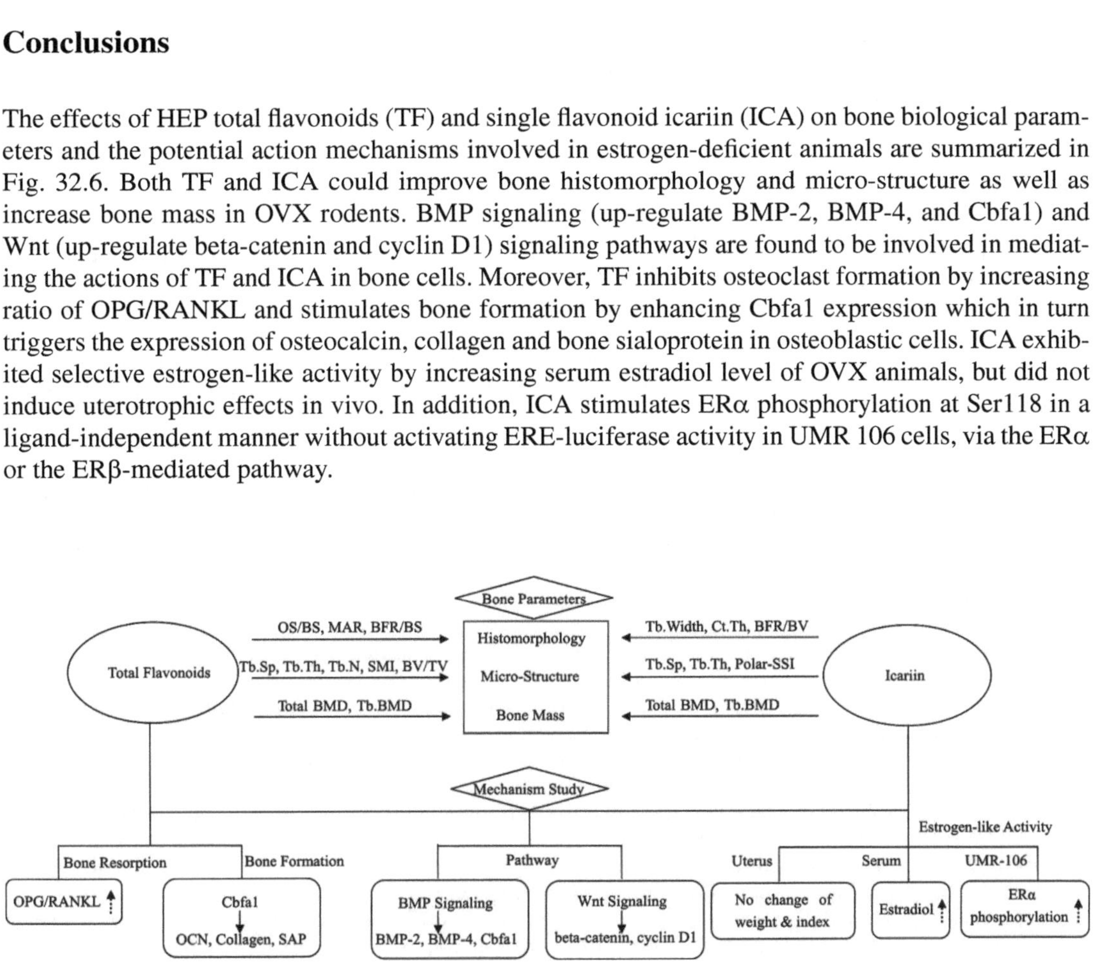

Fig. 32.6 Summary of the effects of HEP total flavonoids (TF) and single flavonoid icariin (ICA) on bone parameters and the potential mechanisms involved in estrogen-deficient animals. Both TF [17, 23] and ICA [29–31] could improve bone histomorphology and micro-structure as well as increase bone mass in ovariectomized (OVX) rodents. The sharing molecular pathways for TF and ICA are BMP (up-regulate BMP-2, BMP-4, and Cbfa1) and Wnt (up-regulate beta-catenin and cyclin D1) signaling [35–38]. Additionally, TF inhibited osteoclast-involved bone resorption by increasing ratio of OPG/RANKL [17, 20, 22] and stimulated osteoblast-involved bone formation by enhancing Cbfa1 expression which secondarily induces expression of OCN, collagen, and SAP [17, 18]. ICA exhibited selective estrogen-like activity by increasing serum estradiol level [29, 33, 34] and ERα phosphorylation at Ser118 [30], but it did not induce uterus hypertrophy of OVX animals [30, 33]. *Tb.Sp* trabecular separation, *Tb.Th* trabecular thickness, *Tb.N* trabecular number, *SMI* structure model index, *BV/TV* bone volume/tissue volume, *Ct.Th* cortical thickness, *OS/BS* osteoid surface, *MAR* mineral apposition rate, *BFR/BS* bone formation rate with bone surface as referent, *BFR/BV* bone formation rate with bone volume as referent, *BMD* bone mineral density, *SSI* stress–strain index, *OCN* osteocalcin, *BMP* bone morphogenetic protein, *Cbfa1* core binding factor 1, *ER* estrogen receptor, *SAP* sialoprotein, *OPG* osteoprotegerin, *RANKL* receptor activator of nuclear factor-κB ligand

Future work will be needed to evaluate the clinical efficacy of flavonoids of HEP as an alternative regimen for the management of bone health in ageing people with high risk of bone loss, especially in postmenopausal women. Simultaneously, the herbal quality standard for Herba Epimedii from different sources should be established according to the content of active flavonoids or single compound. It is hope that with the demonstration of clinical efficacy and safety of the use of HEP as well as the improvement of quality of the herbal material, HEP will be accepted internationally as an alternative regimen for management of osteoporosis.

Acknowledgments This work was partially supported by Hong Kong Scholars Program (XJ2011022) and China Postdoctoral Science Foundation funded project (2012M511115) for Yan Zhang.

References

1. Pie JE, Park JH, Park YH, et al. Effect of genistein on the expression of bone metabolism genes in ovariectomized mice using a cDNA microarray. J Nutr Biochem. 2006;17:157–64.
2. Stevenson JC. Prevention of osteoporosis: one step forward, two steps back. Menopause Int. 2011;17:137–41.
3. Reginster JY, Burlet N. Osteoporosis: a still increasing prevalence. Bone. 2006;38(Suppl):4S–9.
4. Kastner J. Chinese nutrition therapy: dietetics in traditional Chinese medicine. 2nd ed. Stuttgart: Georg Thieme; 2009.
5. Zhang Y, Wong MS, Wu CF. Anti-osteoporotic effects of medicinal herbs and their mechanisms of action. Asian J Trad Med. 2006;1:105–11.
6. Sze SC, Tong Y, Ng TB, Cheng CL, Cheung HP. Herba epimedii: anti-oxidative properties and its medical implications. Molecules. 2010;15:7861–70.
7. Guan XY, Li HF, Yang WZ, et al. HPLC-DAD-MS(n) analysis and HPLC quantitation of chemical constituents in Xian-ling-gu-bao capsules. J Pharm Biomed Anal. 2011;55:923–33.
8. Sun Y, Lee SM, Wong YM, et al. Dosing effects of an antiosteoporosis herbal formula—a preclinical investigation using a rat model. Phytother Res. 2008;22:267–73.
9. Zhang Y, Chen WF, Lai WP, Wong MS. Soy isoflavones and their bone protective effects. Inflammopharmacology. 2008;16:213–5.
10. Jones G, Dwyer T, Hynes K, et al. A randomized controlled trial of phytoestrogen supplementation, growth and bone turnover in adolescent males. Eur J Clin Nutr. 2003;57:324–7.
11. Zhang Y, Li Q, Wan HY, Helferich WG, Wong MS. Genistein and a soy extract differentially affect three-dimensional bone parameters and bone-specific gene expression in ovariectomized mice. J Nutr. 2009;139:2230–6.
12. Wu T, Cui L, Zhang Z, et al. Experimental study on antagonizing action of Herba epimedii on side effects induced by glucocorticoids. China J Chin Mater Med. 1996;21:748–51.
13. Xie F, Wu CF, Lai WP, et al. The osteoprotective effect of Herba epimedii (HEP) extract in vivo and in vitro. Evid Based Complement Alternat Med. 2005;2:353–61.
14. Nian H, Xu LL, Ma MH, et al. Prevention of bone loss by aqueous extract of Epimedii sagittatum in an ovariectomized rat model of osteoporosis. J Chin Integra Med. 2006;4:628–33.
15. Jin L, Yang YQ, Wang S. Herba epimedii effect on osteoclast formation induced by RANKL and M-CSF and on the expression of FN. J Huazhong Norm Univ Nat Sci. 2009;43:640–64.
16. Levis S, Strickman-Stein N, Ganjei-Azar P, et al. Soy isoflavones in the prevention of menopausal bone loss and menopausal symptoms: a randomized, double-blind trial. Arch Intern Med. 2011;171:1363–9.
17. Chen WF, Mok SK, Wang XL, et al. Total flavonoid fraction of the Herba epimedii extract suppresses urinary calcium excretion and improves bone properties in ovariectomised mice. Br J Nutr. 2011;105:180–9.
18. Qian G, Zhang X, Lu L, et al. Regulation of Cbfa1 expression by total flavonoids of Herba epimedii. Endocr J. 2006;53:87–94.
19. Zhang G, Qin L, Hung WY, et al. Flavonoids derived from herbal Epimedium Brevicornum Maxim prevent OVX-induced osteoporosis in rats independent of its enhancement in intestinal calcium absorption. Bone. 2006;38:818–25.
20. Zhang JF, Li G, Meng CL, et al. Total flavonoids of Herba epimedii improves osteogenesis and inhibits osteoclastogenesis of human mesenchymal stem cells. Phytomedicine. 2009;16:521–9.
21. Zhang Y, Dong XL, Leung PC, Wong MS. Differential mRNA expression profiles in proximal tibia of aged rats in response to ovariectomy and low Ca diet. Bone. 2009;44:46–52.
22. Liu Y, Zang H, Zhang H, Chen J. Effect of Herba Epimedii Flavone on expression of OPG and RANKL in rat osteoblasts. J Chin Med Mater. 2005;28:1076–8.

23. Peng S, Zhang G, He Y, et al. Epimedium-derived flavonoids promote osteoblastogenesis and suppress adipogenesis in bone marrow stromal cells while exerting an anabolic effect on osteoporotic bone. Bone. 2009;45:534–44.
24. Wu MS, Zhao SZ, Li E, Bai X, Hao XH. Effect of total flavonoids of *Epimedium sagittatum* and its metabolites on osteoblast proliferation and function expression. Chin Pharmacol Bull. 2009;25:613–6.
25. Zhou ZZ, Luo JG, Guo BL, Kong LY. Analysis of bioactive flavonoids and resources research of main Herba epimedii species from different origins. J China Pharm Univ. 2010;41:146–50.
26. Ma HP, Ming LG, Ge BF, et al. Icariin is more potent than genistein in promoting osteoblast differentiation and mineralization in vitro. J Cell Biochem. 2011;112:916–23.
27. Zhang Y, Li XL, Yao XS, Wong MS. Osteogenic activities of genistein derivatives were influenced by the presence of prenyl group at ring A. Arch Pharm Res. 2008;31:1534–9.
28. Wong SP, Shen P, Lee L, Li J, Yong EL. Pharmacokinetics of prenylflavonoids and correlations with the dynamics of estrogen action in sera following ingestion of a standardized Epimedium extract. J Pharm Biomed Anal. 2009;50:216–23.
29. Nian H, Ma MH, Nian SS, Xu LL. Antiosteoporotic activity of icariin in ovariectomized rats. Phytomedicine. 2009;16:320–6.
30. Mok SK, Chen WF, Lai WP, et al. Icariin protects against bone loss induced by oestrogen deficiency and activates oestrogen receptor-dependent osteoblastic functions in UMR 106 cells. Br J Pharmacol. 2010;159:939–49.
31. Zhang JJ, Wen Y, Zhang GL, Xiao J. Analysis of the effects of icariin on the mice with osteoporosis through index of histomorphometry of bone. Guizhou Med J. 2010;34:404–5.
32. Wen Y, Zhang JJ, Chen XM, Ren GY, Zhang GL. Effects of icariin of examining the expression level of interleukin-6 in mice models of experimental osteoporosis. Guizhou Med J. 2010;34:781–3.
33. Wu MS, Zhao SZ, Ren LZ, Wang R, Bai X. Effects of icariin on expression of the estrogen receptor beta mRNA of bone and different hypothalamic nuclei in ovariectomy rats. Chin Pharmacol Bull. 2011;27:29–33.
34. Wu JS, Zhang Y, Wen Y, Zhang JJ. Effects of icariin on serum estradiol of ovariectomized mice. Guizhou Med J. 2010;34:79–80.
35. Zhang JF, Li G, Chan CY, et al. Flavonoids of Herba epimedii regulate osteogenesis of human mesenchymal stem cells through BMP and Wnt/beta-catenin signaling pathway. Mol Cell Endocrinol. 2010;314:70–4.
36. Zhang JF, Xie WD, Zhang YO, et al. WNT/beta-catenin signaling involved in the osteogenesis of human MSCs induced by flavonoids of Herba epimedii. Prog Modern Biomed. 2010;10:1006–8.
37. Hsieh TP, Sheu SY, Sun JS, Chen MH, Liu MH. Icariin isolated from *Epimedium pubescens* regulates osteoblasts anabolism through BMP-2, SMAD4, and Cbfa1 expression. Phytomedicine. 2010;17:414–23.
38. Zhao J, Ohba S, Shinkai M, Chung UI, Nagamune T. Icariin induces osteogenic differentiation in vitro in a BMP- and Runx2-dependent manner. Biochem Biophys Res Commun. 2008;369:444–8.
39. Yap SP, Shen P, Li J, Lee LS, Yong EL. Molecular and pharmacodynamic properties of estrogenic extracts from the traditional Chinese medicinal herb Epimedium. J Ethnopharmacol. 2007;113:218–24.
40. Shen P, Guo BL, Gong Y, et al. Taxonomic, genetic, chemical and estrogenic characteristics of Epimedium species. Phytochemistry. 2007;68:1448–58.
41. Zhao LN. Clinical evaluation of Herba epimedii on osteoporosis. Modern J Integra Chin Trad West Med. 2003;12:922–3.
42. Zhang G, Qin L, Shi Y. Epimedium-derived phytoestrogen flavonoids exert beneficial effect on preventing bone loss in late postmenopausal women: a 24-month randomized, double-blind and placebo-controlled trial. J Bone Miner Res. 2007;22:1072–9.

Chapter 33
Dietary Plant Maslinic Acid in Ovariectomy Model of Menopause

Jian Luo and Mingyao Liu

Key Points

- The relationship between menopause and skeletal health
- The animal model of menopause and its use in research
- The background of maslinic acid (including sources of maslinic acid), and pharmacological research into maslinic acid
- The effects of maslinic acid on the ovariectomy mouse model
- Maslinic acid's potential toxicity in animal model

Keywords Maslinic acid • Animal model of menopause • Ovariectomy • Diet • Skeletal health

Abbreviations

BMD	Bone mineral density
BMM	Bone marrow macrophage
RANKL	Receptor activator of nuclear factor kappa B ligand
RANK	Receptor activator of nuclear factor kappa B
OPG	Osteoprotegerin
IL	Interleukin
GM-CSF	Granulocyte-macrophage colony-stimulating factor
M-CSF	Macrophage colony-stimulating factor
PGE_2	Prostaglandin-E_2
TNFa	Tumor necrosis factor a
TGFb	Transforming growth factor b
VCD	4-Vinylcyclohexene diepoxide
GnRH	Gonadotropin-releasing hormone
LH	Luteinizing hormone
FSH	Follicle-stimulating hormone

J. Luo, Ph.D. (✉) • M. Liu, Ph.D.
The Institute of Biomedical Sciences, East China Normal University,
500 Dongchuan Road, Shanghai 200241, P.R. China
e-mail: jluo@bio.ecnu.edu.cn; mliu@ibt.tamhsc.edu

C.J.H. Martin et al. (eds.), *Nutrition and Diet in Menopause*, Nutrition and Health,
DOI 10.1007/978-1-62703-373-2_33, © Springer Science+Business Media New York 2013

HIV	Human immunodeficiency virus
AIDS	Acquired immunodeficiency syndrome
WHO	World Health Organization
GLT-1	Glial glutamate transporter
NF-kB	Nuclear factor-kappa B
MAPK	Mitogen-activated protein kinase
GP	Glycogen phosphorylase
SHR	Spontaneously hypertensive rats
MMP	Matrix metallopeptidase
CTR	Calcitonin receptor
OVX	Ovariectomy

Introduction

Ovarian hormones shape women's health throughout their lives, especially with respect to bone mass. Menopause occurs when ovarian follicles become depleted, usually during women's late 40s or early 50s. The transition from reproductive to nonreproductive status is the result of minor reductions in female hormonal production by the ovaries. After the reproductive system, the skeleton is the system that is most affected by menopause. The main reason for menopause-induced osteoporosis is estrogen deficiency accompanied by production of proinflammatory cytokines, such as TNFa and RANKL, all of which cause excess bone resorption. Maslinic acid, a pentacyclic triterpene acid, is present in many dietary plants, especially in olive fruit skins and hawthorn. The dietary compound has attracted much interest because of its proven pharmacologic safety and its many biological activities, such anti-inflammatory, antiviral, antioxidant, and anti-diabetogenic activities and anti-colon cancer and anti-astrocytoma properties. In this report, we focus on maslinic acid in animal models of menopause and introduce the relationship between menopause and skeletal health in an animal model of menopause.

Menopause and the Skeleton

During an organism's lifetime, bone homeostasis strikes a balance between bone formation by osteoblasts and bone resorption by osteoclasts [1]. Normally, bone formation predominates before the age of 30 years, which causes rapid increases in bone mineral density (BMD) during adolescence and early adulthood. After the age of 30, bone resorption exceeds bone formation, resulting in losses in bone mass [2]. In women, age-related bone loss starts earlier than men because of menopause. Menopause-induced bone loss in women can be divided into two phases: an initial accelerated phase that occurs at the time of menopause and continues for 5–8 years and a prolonged, slower phase that lasts until death. During the initial accelerated phase, bone formation and bone resorption biochemical marker levels can be increased by 45 % and 90 %, respectively [3]. These results indicate that imbalances in bone formation and bone resorption lead to bone loss and rapid decreases in BMD. In particular, a loss of 20–30 % in the cancellous bone and 5–10 % in cortical bone occurs during the initial accelerated phase. The prolonged, slower phase continues throughout senescence. The predominant characteristic of this phase is easy fractures of the hip, pelvis, humerus, and tibia.

The mechanisms by which menopause induces bone loss are diverse. The well accepted theory is that a deficiency of hormonal factors produced by healthy ovaries. Among these hormonal factors, estrogen is the most important to bone loss. Estrogen modulates the central signaling RANKL/OPG/

RANK pathway in osteoclastogenesis by regulating OPG and RANK expression [2]. Estrogen deficiency during menopause leads to decreased expression of OPG and increased expression of RANK. Osteoclastogenesis and bone resorption become highly activated. In addition to RANKL signaling, proinflammatory cytokines, such as tumor necrosis factor a (TNF-a), interleukins 1 and 6 (IL-1, IL-6), granulocyte-macrophage colony-stimulating factor (GM-CSF), macrophage colony-stimulating factor (M-CSF), and prostaglandin-E_2 (PGE_2), become increased in the bones of estrogen-deficient individuals. All of the cytokines can interact with RANKL pathway and then induce bone resorption. For example, IL-1 and TNF-a increase expression of RANKL, whereas PGE_2 increases expression of RANKL and decreases expression of OPG. Estrogen also increases the production of transforming growth factor beta (TGF-beta) in bone marrow, which suppresses bone resorption by inhibiting osteoclast activity. Conversely, estrogen deficiency suppresses TGF-beta production and induces bone resorption. In addition, estrogen can directly block osteoclast differentiation by inhibiting the activity of RANNL-mediated Jun NH2-terminal kinase in osteoclast [4]. Taken all together, estrogen suppresses osteoclast activity by modulation of several mechanisms and deficiency of estrogen results in excess osteoclast activity and bone resorption through modulation of several mechanisms.

Animal Model of Menopause

Rodents comprise the most extensively used animal models of menopause. These include the intact aging model, chemically induced model, and ovariectomy model. Animal model studies can further our understanding of ovary-related diseases in perimenopausal and postmenopausal women. In the intact aging model, female rodents experience natural hormonal fluctuations that occur in middle age, which is similar to women's menopause. However, the retention of ovarian tissue and a substantial transitional period makes the hormonal milieu in rodents quite different from human menopause [5]. Recently, a chemically induced rodent model of menopause has been developed using the occupational chemical, 4-vinylcyclohexene diepoxide (VCD) [5]. In this model, VCD is injected into mice daily to selectively deplete small ovarian preantral follicles by acceleration of the natural process of atresia (apoptosis) through follicle-specific pathways. However, this model usually takes a long time to establish and highly costly [6]. Currently, the most common method is bilateral ovariectomy, which can be used in the study of osteoporosis and in drug discovery [7–9]. US Food and Drug Administration (FDA) guidelines dictate that the ovariectomized rat model is necessary for the testing of any preventive or treatment strategy for osteoporosis [10]. The features of ovariectomy-induced bone loss mimic menopause-induced changes in human bones [7, 11]. As in the initial accelerated phase in humans, bone mass decreases dramatically immediately after ovariectomy as bone resorption exceeds bone formation [11]. When bone resorption and formation become balanced again, bone remodeling finds a new steady state. This is consistent with the prolonged, slower phase in human menopause. In mature, ovariectomized rats, statistically significant bone loss starts in the proximal tibial metaphysis after 14 days, in the lumbar vertebrae after 60 days, and in the femoral neck after 30 days [12]. It finally reaches a steady state in the proximal tibial metaphysis after 90 days and in the lumbar vertebrae and femoral neck after 270 days [12, 13]. In contrast, ovariectomy does not lead to bone loss in the epiphysis of long bones, in the distal tibial metaphysis, or in the caudal vertebrae [14–17]. Though the ovariectomized animal model is well established in menopause research, it has two very visible disadvantages. First, almost all menopausal women retain their ovaries and experience a gradual rather than precipitous reduction of hormone secretion [11]. In this way, ovariectomized animal cannot model natural, transitional menopause [18]. Second, in addition to estrogens, certain other hormones play important roles in menopause such as LH, FSH, and gonadotropin-releasing hormone (GnRH), but these are fully abrogated in ovariectomized animals [11, 19].

Sources of Maslinic Acid

Maslinic acid, a pentacyclic triterpene acid, is present in significant amounts in dietary plants. It is especially abundant in certain plants, such as olive, hawthorn, jujube, and wood avens [1]. It accounts for 80 % of the wax in olive skins. These dietary plants also have been safely used for centuries in traditional Chinese medicine and Indian Ayurvedic for the treatment of various ailments, to aid digestion, to enhance immunity, to promote blood circulation, and to dispel blood stasis. As a chemical compound, maslinic acid can be obtained from two sources. First, it can be isolated from plants such as olive oil. In virgin olive oils, the concentration of maslinic acid averages 20–98 mg/kg, and it can reach 212–356 mg/kg in high-quality olive oil. The highest concentrations can be found in crude olive pomace oils (212–1,485 mg/kg). The other method is semi-synthesis from the cheaper commercially available oleanic acid [20].

Maslinic Acid and Existing Pharmacological Research

In modern pharmacological research, maslinic acid has attracted a great deal of interest in multiple biological activities. It has been proven that maslinic acid can induce cancer apoptosis in melanoma, Raji, colon cancer, adenoid cystic carcinoma, breast cancer, pancreatic cancer, liver cancer, and astrocytoma [21]. Another antitumor agent, tumor necrosis factor alpha (TNFa) markedly potentiates apoptosis-inducing activity of maslinic acid [22]. It also has anti-angiogenic activity during tumor growth [23]. Studies of potential molecular mechanisms of maslinic acid have indicated that it induces cell apoptosis by targeting topoisomerase I to suppress DNA synthesis and target the NF-kB signaling pathway to inhibit cell survival. Oxidation reactions can produce free radicals, which cause cell damage and cell death, and finally induce human diseases such as neurodegenerative diseases, coronary heart disease, and aging [24, 25]. Maslinic acid has been found to significantly inhibit the lipopolysaccharide (LPS)-induced nitric oxide, suppress the production of IL-6 and TNFa, and reduce the generation of hydrogen peroxide in LPS-stimulated murine macrophages [26, 27]. These reports suggest a potential biopharmaceutical application of maslinic acid in the prevention of oxidative stress and proinflammatory cytokine production. Human immunodeficiency virus (HIV) causes acquired immunodeficiency syndrome (AIDS). The serine protease is very important for the release of the virus release, it has been reported that maslinic acid could suppress the activity of the serine-protease and prevent the spread of the HIV by 80 % [28]. Similar results were obtained in antibacterial experiments. Maslinic acid was found to strongly affect antimicrobial activity against gram-positive bacteria and yeasts, including *S. aureus*, *S. agalacticae*, and *C. albicans*, but not against gram-negative organisms [29]. Resistance to antimicrobial is common. The World Health Organization (WHO) has suggested that researchers should develop novel-style antibacterial drugs. The antiviral and antibacterial properties of maslinic acid indicate its potential against resistant microbes. Maslinic acid also has antiparasitic activity [30]. ICR mice were infected with *P. yoelii* (malaria) and treated with maslinic acid (40 mg/kg) daily. The survival rate of the infected mice increased from 20 % to 80 % when treated with maslinic acid, and the maturation of the parasite was delayed from day 3 to day 7, which led to synchronization of the intraerythrocytic cycle and accumulation of schizonts by day 6 [30, 31]. All these experiments suggest that maslinic acid can function as a parasitostatic agent in vivo. Diabetes is a group of metabolic diseases caused by insufficient insulin production or an inability of cells to respond to the insulin [32]. Diabetes can be separated into three groups (type-1, type-2, and gestational diabetes) depending on the pathogenesis [33]. Recently, maslinic acid has been found to reduce blood glucose activity in a mouse model of type-2 diabetes [34, 35]. Daily administration of maslinic acid at dosages of 10 mg/kg or 30 mg/kg every day for 2 weeks showed a significant reduction in the blood glucose levels in the type-2 diabetes KK-A(y) mice, suggesting that maslinic acid might reduce blood glucose levels partially through reducing insulin resistance [34, 35]. In the insulin pathway, inactivation of glycogen phosphorylase (GP) was found to mimic insulin stimulation of hepatic glycogen synthesis. It's been reported that maslinic acid could inhibit the activity of muscle glycogen phosphorylase A (GPA), which may be the mechanism by which maslinic acid affects diabetes [34, 35]. Diabetes and hyperglycemia can increase the risk of many human diseases, including changes in vision, cardiovascular disease, and cerebral ischemic injury. It has been reported that maslinic acid can also affect focal cerebral ischemia in hyperglycemic rats. Treatment with maslinic acid increases the expression of the glial glutamate transporter (GLT-1) by inhibiting NF-kB signaling [35, 36]. In this way, maslinic acid can modulate hyperglycemia, thereby preventing the exacerbation of brain lesions [35, 36]. Persistent hypertension can cause a number of severe human diseases, such as stroke, myocardial infarction, heart failure, and arterial aneurysm [37]. The induction of vasorelaxation is one therapeutic technique used in clinical settings. In isolated aorta from spontaneously hypertensive rats (SHR), maslinic acid was found to induce dose-dependent vasorelaxation, suggesting that maslinic acid elicits vasorelaxation in hypertensive rats [38].

Effect of Maslinic Acid on Mouse Model of Menopause

To determine whether maslinic acid has any effect on menopause-induced bone loss, we employed an ovariectomy mouse model. Ovariectomy dramatically induces the bone loss in 2–3 months in mouse. However, administration of maslinic acid prevents ovariectomy-induced bone loss, as indicated by histomorphometric analysis. Histomorphometric parameters, including bone value/total value (BV/TV), trabecular space (Tb.Sp), and trabecular number (Tb.N), all of which are indicative of bone mass, were recovered when ovariectomy mice were treated with maslinic acid (Fig. 33.1). Bone mass is regulated by both osteoblast and osteoclast cells. To determine which cells maslinic acid affects, we first performed an osteoblast differentiation assay and bone nodule formation assay in vitro. Maslinic acid was found to have little effect on osteogenesis, suggesting that maslinic acid does not affect osteoblast cells. Maslinic acid was found to inhibit osteoclastogenesis in a dose-dependent manner in two standard in vitro mouse osteoclast differentiation models, mouse bone morrow monocyte differentiation model and mouse osteoclast precursor cell line RAW264.7 cell differentiation model (Fig. 33.2). Similar results were obtained in an actin-ring formation assay. The osteoclast actin-ring is a prerequisite for osteoclast bone resorption and it is the most obvious characteristic of mature osteoclasts during osteoclastogenesis [1]. The size and number of actin-ring structures were significantly decreased when the cells were treated with maslinic acid (Fig. 33.3). An osteoclast function assay on dentin slices also showed that maslinic acid suppresses resorption lacunae and pit formation caused by mature osteoclasts. To further confirm that maslinic acid inhibits osteoclastogenesis, the osteoclastic parameters were examined in an ovariectomy mouse model. As expected, the osteoclast surface/bone surface (OcS/BS), osteoclast number/bone surface (N.Oc/BS), and eroded surface/bone surface (ES/BS) were also recovered in ovariectomy mice treated with maslinic acid (Fig. 33.4). Serum protein levels of TRACP 5b reflects osteoclast activity in vivo, and the results of an examination of the serum protein level of TRACP 5b also confirmed that TRACP 5b levels were higher in OVX mice than in sham-operated control mice, but maslinic acid treatment significantly decreased the TRACP 5b level induced by OVX (Fig. 33.5). Taken together, all the in vivo and in vitro evidence indicates that administration of maslinic acid can prevent ovariectomy-induced bone loss by suppressing osteoclast activity. These results suggest that dietary plants, which are abundant in maslinic acid, can be useful for the skeletal health of menopausal women.

To determine the mechanism underlying the action of maslinic acid in osteoclasts, we found that maslinic acid suppresses IkBa phosphorylation and degradation; blocks NF-kB/p65 phosphorylation, nuclear translocation, and DNA-binding activity; and abrogates the expression of the NF-kB luciferase

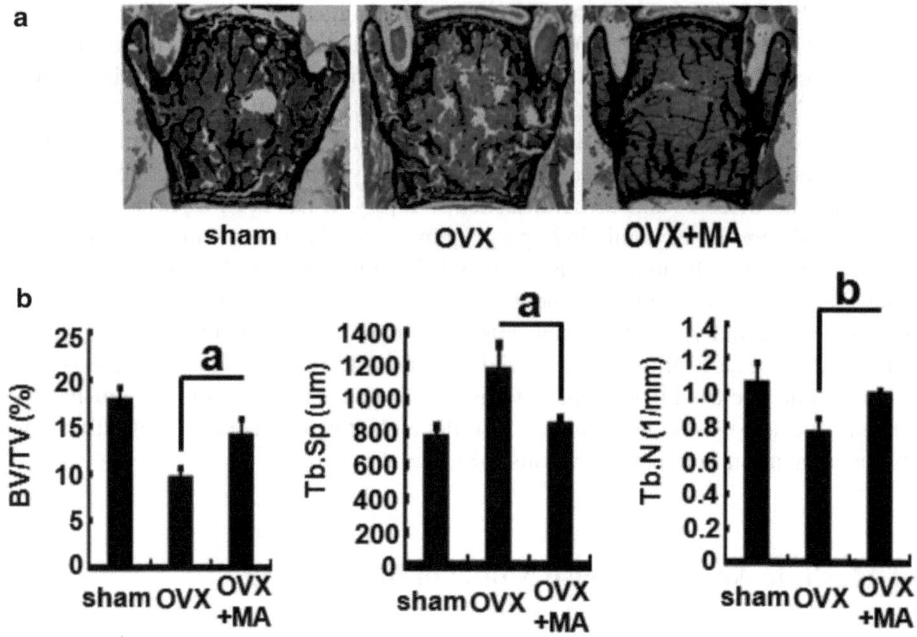

Fig. 33.1 Maslinic acid prevents ovariectomy-induced bone loss. (**a**) Representative von Kossa stained sections of lumbar vertebrae from sham, OVX mice, and OVX+MA mice. (**b**) The bone mass related parameters including bone value/total value (BV/TV), trabecular space (Tb.Sp), and trabecular number (Tb.N) were analyzed by OsteoMeasure Analysis System. The histograms showed the mean+SEM of six sets of analysis of parameters from sham, OVX mice, and OVX+MA mice (Reproduced from J Bone Miner Res. 2011;26:644–56 with permission of the American Society for Bone and Mineral Research)

reporter gene. Maslinic acid inhibits phosphorylation of MAPKs (p38, JNK, and ERK), as indicated by Western blot analysis and AP-1 luciferase reporter gene expression. This suggests that maslinic acid can inhibit RANKL-induced activation of NF-kB and MAPK signaling pathways. In this way, it can decrease the downstream expression of the NFATc1 osteoclastogenesis-related marker genes, including *TRACP*, *MMP-9*, *c-Src*, *CTR*, and *cathepsin K*.

In summary, maslinic acid has been shown to suppress osteoclastogenesis and mediate osteoclast activity in vitro and in vivo. Its inhibitory effects have been found to occur through the suppression of NF-kB and MAPK/AP-1 activation and the expression of NFATc1. These findings suggest that maslinic acid could be a suitable agent in the treatment of osteoclast-related diseases, such as osteoporosis, and that dietary plans rich in maslinic acid may be helpful for osteoclast-related conditions, such as menopausal osteoporosis.

Toxicity of Maslinic Acid

As the standard of living increases, people need to be more careful to eat green and organic foods. Maslinic acid is abundant in lots of green dietary plant, such as olives, hawthorn, jujube, and wood avens. Olive oil, which is abundant in maslinic acid, has been characteristic of the cuisine of the Mediterranean Basin for millennia. Epidemiological studies have suggested that olive oil has protective effects against oxidants and certain malignant tumors. This has also been proven of maslinic acid

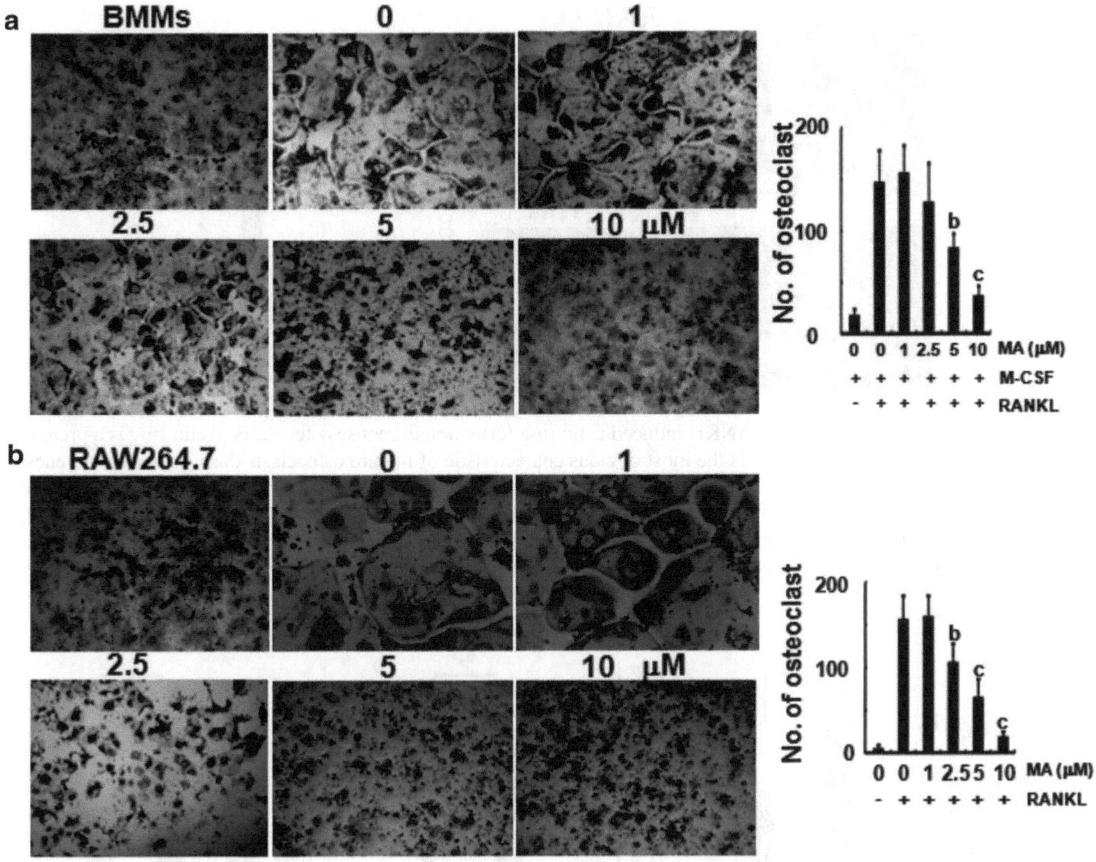

Fig. 33.2 Maslinic acid inhibits osteoclast differentiation in BMMs and RAW264.7. BMMs and RAW264.7 osteoclast differentiation models are two standard in vitro osteoclast differentiation models. BMM precursors with RANKL and M-CSF treatment and mouse osteoclast precursor cell line RAW264.7 cells with RANKL treatment can be differentiated into mature osteoclasts. (**a**) MA inhibits RANKL-induced mouse BMMs differentiation. *Left*, photographs of cells (original magnification, X100). *Right*, TRAP-positive multinucleated (>5 nuclei) osteoclasts were counted. *Column*, means of three experiments carried out in triplicate; *bar*, SD; $^{b}P<0.01$, $^{c}P<0.001$ versus RANKL plus M-CSF. (**b**) MA inhibits RANKL-induced RAW264.7 cell differentiation. *Left*, photographs of cells (original magnification, X100). *Right*, TRAP-positive multinucleated (>3 nuclei) osteoclasts were counted. *Column*, means of three experiments carried out in triplicate; *bar*, SD; $^{b}P<0.01$, $^{c}p<0.001$ versus RANKL alone (Reproduced from J Bone Miner Res. 2011;26:644–56 with permission of the American Society for Bone and Mineral Research)

[22]. Hawthorn (thorn apple) is native to temperate regions of the northern hemisphere in Europe, Asia, and North America. The traditional Mexican Christmas punch contains cooked hawthorn fruit. Hawthorn fruits are also used to make many kinds of traditional snacks in Iran, China, Korea, United States, and Canada. It is reasonable to speculate that maslinic acid is at most minimally toxic. Research has revealed its pharmacological safety in human mononuclear cells, malaria-infected mice (40 mg/kg), diabetic mice (30 mg/kg), tumor-bearing mice (50 mg/kg), and fish (rainbow trout) (250 mg/kg), even at high doses [39]. To evaluate the toxicity of maslinic acid in the models of menopause, the ovariectomy mice were subcutaneously injected with 10 mg/kg every 2 days for more than 3 months, and body weight was recorded every day [1]. The results showed that maslinic acid had little effect on the body weight of the ovariectomy mice (Fig. 33.6). This suggests that this compound is only minimally toxic to these ovariectomy mice.

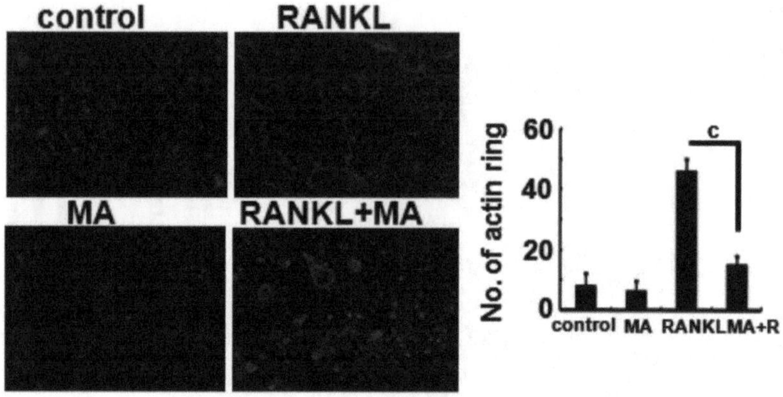

Fig. 33.3 Maslinic acid suppresses RANKL-induced actin ring formation in mouse osteoclasts. Actin-ring is a prerequisite for osteoclast bone resorption and is the most obvious characteristic of mature osteoclasts during osteoclastogenesis. BMMs cells (2×104 cells) were incubated with or without RANKL (50 ng/ml) in the presence of M-CSF (50 ng/ml), followed by treatment with or without 5 μM MA. Cells were fixed and stained for F-actin (*top*). Osteoclasts with actin-rings were counted (*bottom*). *Column*, means of three experiments carried out in triplicate; *bar*, SD; [c]$P<0.001$ (Reproduced from J Bone Miner Res. 2011;26: 644–56 with permission of the American Society for Bone and Mineral Research)

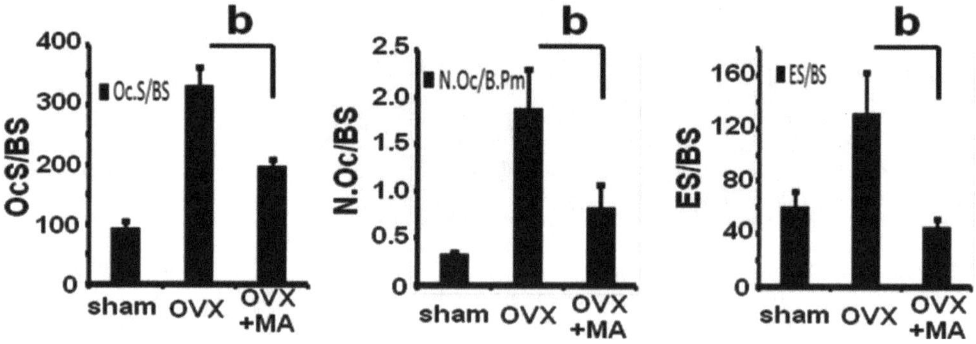

Fig. 33.4 Administration of maslinic acid inhibits osteoclastic parameters in ovariectomy mouse model. Sham, OVX, and OVX+MA mouse lumbers were sectioned and stained for the osteoclast activity. Osteoclast related parameters were analyzed by the OsteoMeasure Analysis System. The parameters including osteoclast surface/bone surface (OcS/BS), osteoclast number/bone surface (N.Oc/BS), and eroded surface/bone surface (ES/BS) were dramatically more common in OVX mice than in sham-operated controls. These parameters in MA-treated OVX mice were significantly lower than in OVX mice ([b]$P<0.01$, $n=6$) (Reproduced from J Bone Miner Res. 2011;26:644–56 with permission of the American Society for Bone and Mineral Research)

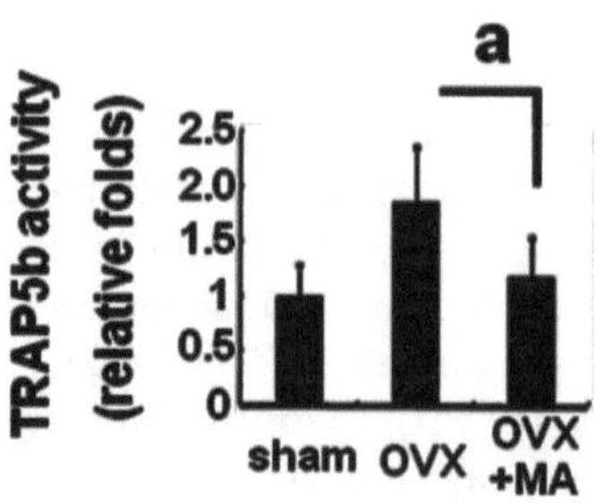

Fig. 33.5 Administration of maslinic acid inhibits serum osteoclast biomarker in ovariectomy mouse model. The serum TRACP 5b reflects osteoclast activity in vivo. The serum TRAP5b level was higher in OVX mice than in sham-operated mice, while MA treatment significantly decreased the TRAP5b levels induced by ovariectomy ([a]$P<0.001$, $n=6$) (Reproduced from J Bone Miner Res. 2011;26:644–56 with permission of the American Society for Bone and Mineral Research)

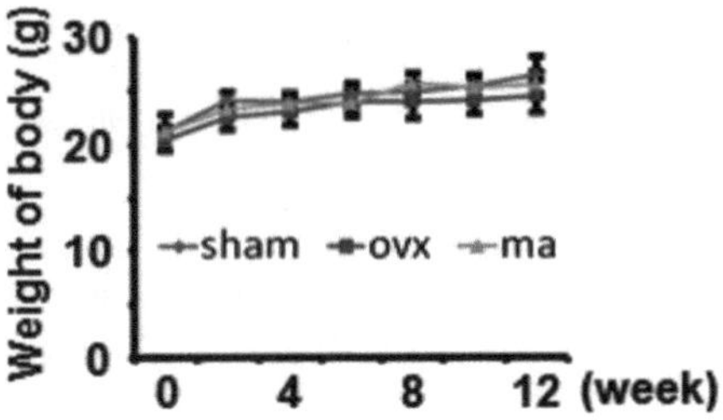

Fig. 33.6 Maslinic acid has little effect on mouse body weight in ovariectomy mouse model. Eight-week-old C57BL/6 female mice were treated with vehicle (OVX) or with 10 mg/kg MA every 2 days (OVX+MA) for 90 days. Body weight was recorded every week ($n=6$) (Reproduced from J Bone Miner Res. 2011;26: 644–56 with permission of the American Society for Bone and Mineral Research)

Conclusion

Maslinic acid is abundant in many green dietary plants and plant foods, including olive oil, hawthorn, and jujube. This suggests that maslinic acid is only minimally toxic. Maslinic acid has a specific inhibitory effect on osteoclastogenesis and mediates osteoclast activities in vitro and in vivo, but not in osteoblasts. In an ovariectomized mouse model, the administration of maslinic acid significantly prevents ovariectomy-induced bone loss over 2–3 months. This suggests that, maslinic acid may be a potential agent in the treatment of menopause-induced osteoporosis.

References

1. Li C, Yang Z, Li Z, Ma Y, Zhang L, Zheng C, et al. Maslinic acid suppresses osteoclastogenesis and prevents ovariectomy-induced bone loss by regulating RANKL-mediated NF-kappaB and MAPK signaling pathways. J Bone Miner Res. 2011;26(3):644–56.
2. Mirza FS, Prestwood KM. Bone health and aging: implications for menopause. Endocrinol Metab Clin North Am. 2004;33(4):741–59.
3. Garnero P, Sornay-Rendu E, Chapuy MC, Delmas PD. Increased bone turnover in late postmenopausal women is a major determinant of osteoporosis. J Bone Miner Res. 1996;11(3):337–49.
4. Riggs BL, Khosla S, Melton 3rd LJ. Sex steroids and the construction and conservation of the adult skeleton. Endocr Rev. 2002;23(3):279–302.
5. Van Kempen TA, Milner TA, Waters EM. Accelerated ovarian failure: a novel, chemically induced animal model of menopause. Brain Res. 2011;1379:176–87.
6. Wright LE, Christian PJ, Rivera Z, Van Alstine WG, Funk JL, Bouxsein ML, et al. Comparison of skeletal effects of ovariectomy versus chemically induced ovarian failure in mice. J Bone Miner Res. 2008;23(8):1296–303.
7. Jee WS, Yao W. Overview: animal models of osteopenia and osteoporosis. J Musculoskelet Neuronal Interact. 2001;1(3):193–207.
8. Lo JC, Burnett-Bowie SA, Finkelstein JS. Bone and the perimenopause. Obstet Gynecol Clin North Am. 2011;38(3):503–17.
9. Gass M, Dawson-Hughes B. Preventing osteoporosis-related fractures: an overview. Am J Med. 2006;119(4 Suppl 1):S3–11.
10. Thompson DD, Simmons HA, Pirie CM, Ke HZ. FDA guidelines and animal models for osteoporosis. Bone. 1995;17(4 Suppl):125S–33.
11. Lelovas PP, Xanthos TT, Thoma SE, Lyritis GP, Dontas IA. The laboratory rat as an animal model for osteoporosis research. Comp Med. 2008;58(5):424–30.
12. Li M, Shen Y, Wronski TJ. Time course of femoral neck osteopenia in ovariectomized rats. Bone. 1997;20(1):55–61.
13. Wronski TJ, Dann LM, Horner SL. Time course of vertebral osteopenia in ovariectomized rats. Bone. 1989;10(4):295–301.

14. Li XJ, Jee WS. Adaptation of diaphyseal structure to aging and decreased mechanical loading in the adult rat: a densitometric and histomorphometric study. Anat Rec. 1991;229(3):291–7.
15. Li M, Shen Y, Qi H, Wronski TJ. Comparative study of skeletal response to estrogen depletion at red and yellow marrow sites in rats. Anat Rec. 1996;245(3):472–80.
16. Ma YF, Ke HZ, Jee WS. Prostaglandin E2 adds bone to a cancellous bone site with a closed growth plate and low bone turnover in ovariectomized rats. Bone. 1994;15(2):137–46.
17. Miller SC, Bowman BM, Miller MA, Bagi CM. Calcium absorption and osseous organ-, tissue-, and envelope-specific changes following ovariectomy in rats. Bone. 1991;12(6):439–46.
18. Gallagher JC. Effect of early menopause on bone mineral density and fractures. Menopause. 2007;14(3 Pt 2):567–71.
19. Sniekers YH, Weinans H, Bierma-Zeinstra SM, van Leeuwen JP, van Osch GJ. Animal models for osteoarthritis: the effect of ovariectomy and estrogen treatment—a systematic approach. Osteoarthritis Cartilage. 2008;16(5):533–41.
20. Wen X, Zhang P, Liu J, Zhang L, Wu X, Ni P, et al. Pentacyclic triterpenes. Part 2: Synthesis and biological evaluation of maslinic acid derivatives as glycogen phosphorylase inhibitors. Bioorg Med Chem Lett. 2006;16(3): 722–6.
21. Martin R, Carvalho J, Ibeas E, Hernandez M, Ruiz-Gutierrez V, Nieto ML. Acidic triterpenes compromise growth and survival of astrocytoma cell lines by regulating reactive oxygen species accumulation. Cancer Res. 2007;67(8):3741–51.
22. Li C, Yang Z, Zhai C, Qiu W, Li D, Yi Z, et al. Maslinic acid potentiates the anti-tumor activity of tumor necrosis factor alpha by inhibiting NF-kappaB signaling pathway. Mol Cancer. 2010;9:73.
23. Lin CC, Huang CY, Mong MC, Chan CY, Yin MC. Antiangiogenic potential of three triterpenic acids in human liver cancer cells. J Agric Food Chem. 2011;59(2):755–62.
24. Elahi MM, Kong YX, Matata BM. Oxidative stress as a mediator of cardiovascular disease. Oxid Med Cell Longev. 2009;2(5):259–69.
25. Napolitano A, Manini P, d'Ischia M. Oxidation chemistry of catecholamines and neuronal degeneration: an update. Curr Med Chem. 2011;18(12):1832–45.
26. Marquez Martin A, de la Puerta Vazquez R, Fernandez-Arche A, Ruiz-Gutierrez V. Supressive effect of maslinic acid from pomace olive oil on oxidative stress and cytokine production in stimulated murine macrophages. Free Radic Res. 2006;40(3):295–302.
27. Marquez-Martin A, De La Puerta R, Fernandez-Arche A, Ruiz-Gutierrez V, Yaqoob P. Modulation of cytokine secretion by pentacyclic triterpenes from olive pomace oil in human mononuclear cells. Cytokine. 2006;36(5–6):211–7.
28. Xu HX, Zeng FQ, Wan M, Sim KY. Anti-HIV triterpene acids from Geum japonicum. J Nat Prod. 1996;59(7):643–5.
29. Braca A, Morelli I, Mendez J, Battinelli L, Braghiroli L, Mazzanti G. Antimicrobial triterpenoids from Licania heteromorpha. Planta Med. 2000;66(8):768–9.
30. Moneriz C, Marin-Garcia P, Bautista JM, Diez A, Puyet A. Parasitostatic effect of maslinic acid. II. Survival increase and immune protection in lethal Plasmodium yoelii-infected mice. Malar J. 2011;10:103.
31. Moneriz C, Mestres J, Bautista JM, Diez A, Puyet A. Multi-targeted activity of maslinic acid as an antimalarial natural compound. FEBS J. 2011;278(16):2951–61.
32. Chan L, Terashima T, Urabe H, Lin F, Kojima H. Pathogenesis of diabetic neuropathy: bad to the bone. Ann N Y Acad Sci. 2011;1240:70–6.
33. Bikman BT, Summers SA. Ceramides as modulators of cellular and whole-body metabolism. J Clin Invest. 2011;121(11):4222–30.
34. Liu J, Sun H, Duan W, Mu D, Zhang L. Maslinic acid reduces blood glucose in KK-Ay mice. Biol Pharm Bull. 2007;30(11):2075–8.
35. Guan T, Qian Y, Tang X, Huang M, Huang L, Li Y, et al. Maslinic acid, a natural inhibitor of glycogen phosphorylase, reduces cerebral ischemic injury in hyperglycemic rats by GLT-1 up-regulation. J Neurosci Res. 2011;89(11):1829–39.
36. Qian Y, Guan T, Tang X, Huang L, Huang M, Li Y, et al. Maslinic acid, a natural triterpenoid compound from Olea europaea, protects cortical neurons against oxygen-glucose deprivation-induced injury. Eur J Pharmacol. 2011;670(1):148–53.
37. Doggrell SA, Brown L. Rat models of hypertension, cardiac hypertrophy and failure. Cardiovasc Res. 1998;39(1):89–105.
38. Dongmo AB, Azebaze AG, Donfack FM, Dimo T, Nkeng-Efouet PA, Devkota KP, et al. Pentacyclic triterpenoids and ceramide mediate the vasorelaxant activity of Vitex cienkowskii via involvement of NO/cGMP pathway in isolated rat aortic rings. J Ethnopharmacol. 2011;133(1):204–12.
39. Fernandez-Navarro M, Peragon J, Amores V, De La Higuera M, Lupianez JA. Maslinic acid added to the diet increases growth and protein-turnover rates in the white muscle of rainbow trout (Oncorhynchus mykiss). Comp Biochem Physiol C Toxicol Pharmacol. 2008;147(2):158–67.

Chapter 34
Interlinking Diet, Nutrition, Menopause and Recommended Resources

Roshanna Rajendram, Rajkumar Rajendram, Vinood B. Patel, and Victor R. Preedy

Key Points

- Women are increasingly seeking non-drug alternatives to hormone replacement therapy.
- Proven and putative alternatives to the medical management of menopause include lifestyle changes (physical activity, healthy diet, not smoking), food supplements, and herbal medicines.
- Prescription medicines also offer other modes of treatment.
- There is thus a wide range of treatment regimens for menopause. For example, food fortification with vitamins and minerals may help to ameliorate some of the symptoms of menopause.
- This chapter lists the most up-to-date resources on the regulatory bodies, journals, books, professional bodies and Web sites that are relevant to an evidence-based approach to not only food fortification for women during menopause but also other forms of treatment.
- These resources effectively interlink diet, nutrition, and menopause to further advance the alleviation of symptoms and to enhance our understanding of a complex life stage.

Keywords Menopause • Diet quality • Nutrition • Evidence • Resources • Books • Journals • Regulatory bodies • Professional societies

R. Rajendram, B.Sc. (hons) (✉)
School of Medical and Dental Sciences, University of Birmingham,
Edgbaston, Birmingham, West Midlands B15 2TT, UK
e-mail: rxr744@bham.ac.uk

R. Rajendram, A.K.C., B.Sc. (hons), M.B.B.S. (dist), M.R.C.P. (UK), F.R.C.A.
Departments of General Medicine and Intensive Care, John Radcliffe Hospital,
Oxford, Oxfordshire OX3 9DU, UK

Diabetes and Nutritional Sciences Research Division, School of Medicine, King's College London,
Franklin-Wilkins Building, 150 Stamford Street, London SE1 8WA, UK
e-mail: rajkumarrajendram@doctors.org.uk

V.B. Patel, B.Sc. (Hons), Ph.D.
Department of Biomedical Sciences, School of Life Sciences,
University of Westminster, London, UK
e-mail: vinoodpatel@yahoo.co.uk

V.R. Preedy, Ph.D.
Diabetes and Nutritional Sciences, School of Medicine, King's College London,
Franklin Wilkins Buildings, 150 Stamford Street, London SE1 9NU, UK
e-mail: victor.preedy@kcl.ac.uk

C.J.H. Martin et al. (eds.), *Nutrition and Diet in Menopause*, Nutrition and Health,
DOI 10.1007/978-1-62703-373-2_34, © Springer Science+Business Media New York 2013

Introduction

Over the last decade, the controversy surrounding hormone replacement therapy has changed the management of menopause dramatically [1]. Data from surveys suggest that when women choose a therapy to treat menopausal symptoms safety is the most important issue. This is followed by efficacy, duration of action, onset of symptom relief and risk of side-effects. Cost is far less important to women than efficacy [1].

Women increasingly want non-drug options. Proven alternatives to the medical management of menopause include lifestyle changes (physical activity, healthy diet, not smoking), food supplements and herbal medicines [1].

Potential solutions to improving the diet of menopausal women include promotion of dietary change (requiring education, advice and incentives), dietary supplementation, and fortification of food. Educational interventions are, in theory, the ideal solution. However, changing dietary habits on the population level is challenging [2]. To take a single example, experience with the management of iron deficiency anaemia at the level of the general population suggests that dietary change may have poor efficacy, at least in the short term [3]. Dietary supplementation is a rapid and cost-effective solution for individuals at risk of deficiency that also limits overdose in those with adequate dietary intake. However, supplements may have adverse side effects and compliance may be poor.

Food fortification is another potential solution. This involves enrichment of food with nutrients to greater concentrations than those naturally present [4]. The use of food fortification as a public health intervention for nutritional deficiencies has increased recently. Food fortification has a wider and more sustained impact than supplementation. Although not without limitations, food fortification is an important intervention to treat micronutrient malnutrition. Such fortification can potentially have a beneficial effect on the diet quality of menopausal women and may help to ameliorate some of the symptoms of menopause.

However, for the treatment of menopause food fortification alone is unlikely to be sufficient for most women. A combination of food fortification with the promotion of dietary change with or without dietary supplements is likely to be more helpful and could reduce the reliance on medical management of menopause. Understanding the psychological and physiological changes in menopause *per se* may also be beneficial for women and their health practitioners. Examples and applications of treatment regimens such as food fortification in menopause can be found in this book and also via the recommended resources in the tables below.

This chapter provides recommendations for additional reading about the role of nutrition, diet (including food fortification) in menopause. Sources include professional bodies which regulate the food fortification industry (Table 34.1), and also journals (Table 34.2), books (Table 34.3), professional societies (Table 34.4) and Web sites (Table 34.5) which provide invaluable information about this subject.

Table 34.1 Important professional bodies which regulate food fortification

Regulatory body	Web address
European Food Safety Authority	http://www.efsa.europa.eu/
Food Standards Australia New Zealand	http://www.foodstandards.gov.au/consumerinformation/fortification/
US Food and Drug Administration	http://www.fda.gov

Table 34.2 Journals which publish research about menopause and/or diet and nutrition

Journal name	Web address
American Journal of Obstetrics and Gynaecology	http://www.ajog.org/
British Journal of Nutrition	http://journals.cambridge.org/action/displayJournal?jid=BJN
International Journal of Cancer	http://onlinelibrary.wiley.com/journal/10.1002/(ISSN)1097-0215
Magnesium Research	http://www.magnesiumresearch.com/index.phtml
Menopause	http://www.menopause.org/journals/m/m_index.aspx
Menopause International	http://mi.rsmjournals.com
Molecular and Cellular Endocrinology	http://www.journals.elsevier.com/molecular-and-cellular-endocrinology/
Obstetrics and Gynaecology	http://journals.lww.com/greenjournal/pages/default.aspx
Przegl d Menopauzalny	http://www.termedia.pl/Czasopisma/Przeglad_Menopauzalny
Public Health Nutrition	http://journals.cambridge.org/action/displayJournal?jid=PHN
The American Journal of Clinical Nutrition	http://onlinelibrary.wiley.com/journal/10.1111/(ISSN)1365-2796
The Japan Society for Menopause and Women's Health	http://www.jmwh.jp/index.html
The Journal of Internal Medicine	http://www.wiley.com
The Journal of Nutrition	http://jn.nutrition.org/
The Lancet	http://www.thelancet.com
The New England Journal of Medicine	http://www.nejm.org

Table 34.3 Books and other publications concerning menopause and/or diet and nutrition

Book title	Authors or editors	Publisher	Date	City and country
Animal models of diabetes	E. Shafrir	CRC Press	2007	Florida, USA
Animal models in cardiovascular research	DR. Gross	Springer	2009	London, UK
Chinese nutrition therapy: dietetics in traditional Chinese medicine	J. Kastner	Thieme	2009	New York, USA
Diagnostyka i terapia wieku menopauzalnego	T. Perty ski (Editor)	Wydawnictwo medyczne Urban & Partner	2004	Wrocław, Poland
Focus on homocysteine and the vitamins involved in its metabolism	C. Bolander-Gouaille	Springer	2002	Paris, France
Handbook of animal models in Alzheimer's disease	G. Casadesus	IOS Press	2011	Washington, USA
Management of the perimenopause. Practical pathways in obstetrics and gynecology	JH. Liu, MLS Gass (Editors)	McGraw-Hill Medical Publishing Division	2006	New York, USA
Managing the monstrous feminine. Regulating the reproductive body	JM. Ussher	Routledge	2006	London, UK
Menopause and culture	GE. Berger	Pluto Press	1999	London, UK
Nutritional epidemiology of breast cancer	AL. Ronco, ED. Stéfani	Springer	2011	Amsterdam, the Netherlands
The ageing skeleton	CJ. Rosen, J. Glowacki, JP. Bilezjkian	Academic Press	1999	Sandiego, USA

Table 34.4 Professional Societies which provide information about menopause and/or diet and nutrition

Society Name	Web address
American Society for Bone and Mineral Research	http://www.asbmr.org/Default.aspx
Asociación Española para el Estudio de la Menopausia	http://www.aeem.es/
Institute of Medicine	http://www.iom.edu/Reports/2010/Dietary-Reference-Intakes-for-Calcium-and-Vitamin-D.aspx
International Menopause Society	http://www.imsociety.org/
International Osteoporosis Foundation	http://www.iofbonehealth.org/
Linus Pauling Institute	http://lpi.oregonstate.edu/infocenter/
National Osteoporosis Foundation	http://www.nof.org/aboutosteoporosis/prevention/calcium
Polskie Towarzystwo Menopauzy i Andropauzy	http://www.3gin.am.lublin.pl/PTMA.htm
Senologic International Society	http://www.sisbreast.org
The British Menopausal Society	http://www.thebms.org.uk/index.php
The National Academies Press	http://www.nap.edu/topics.php?topic=287
The North American Menopause Society	http://www.menopause.org/
Vitamin D council	http://www.vitamindcouncil.org

Table 34.5 Relevant resources on the Web concerning micronutrient deficiency, disease or risk factors in menopause

Name	Web address
Centres for disease control and prevention: nutrition for everyone	http://www.cdc.gov/nutrition/everyone/basics/vitamins/calcium.html
European Parliament and Council. Regulation on nutrition and health claims made on foods; 2006	http://ec.europa.eu/food/food/labellingnutrition/claims/index_en.htm
Magnesium online library	http://www.mgwater.com/index.shtml
Mayo clinic: osteoporosis	http://www.mayoclinic.com/health/osteoporosis/DS00128
Medline plus: menopause	http://www.nlm.nih.gov/medlineplus/menopause.html
Medline plus: osteoporosis	http://www.nlm.nih.gov/medlineplus/osteoporosis.html
National Institute of Health: osteoporosis and related bone diseases national resource centre	http://www.niams.nih.gov/Health_Info/Bone/default.asp
Nutra ingredients	http://www.nutraingredients.com/Regulation
Portal dojrzałej kobiety (Web site with information on menopause and ageing and nutrition)	http://www.menopauza.pl
US department of Health and Human services: women's health	http://www.womenshealth.gov/menopause/
World Health Organization & Food and Agriculture Organization of the United Nations. Guidelines on food fortification with micronutrients; 2006	http://www.who.int/nutrition/publications/guide_food_fortification_micronutrients.pdf

Acknowledgements We would like to thank the following authors (in alphabetical order) for contributing to this list of resources: J Aloia, SS Avinash, J Banu, E Bielawska-Batorowicz, LM Chiechi, R D'Anna, HR Franke, B Haliloglu, I Kiyoshi, C Larroy, G Paradisi, A Ronco, RJ Schwen, W Wang, Dr M-S Wong and IZ Zubrzycki.

References

1. Johnston J. Managing the menopause: practical choices faced in primary care. Climacteric. 2011;14 Suppl 2Suppl 2:8–12.
2. Fletcher RJ, Bell IP, Lambert JP. Public health aspects of food fortification: a question of balance. Proc Nutr Soc. 2004;63:605–14.
3. Huch R, Schaefer R. Iron deficiency and iron deficiency anemia: a pocket atlas special. Stuttgart, Germany: Georg Thieme Verlag; 2006. p. 35.
4. Fortification of food with micronutrients: the role and position of FAO. www.ceecis.org/iodine/01_global/01_pl/01_01_other_fao.pdf. Accessed 15 Oct 2011

Index

C.J.H. Martin et al. (eds.), *Nutrition and Diet in Menopause*, Nutrition and Health,
DOI 10.1007/978-1-62703-373-2, © Springer Science+Business Media New York 2013

D

E

MIX
Papier aus verantwortungsvollen Quellen
Paper from responsible sources
FSC® C105338

If you have any concerns about our products,
you can contact us on
ProductSafety@springernature.com

In case Publisher is established outside the EU,
the EU authorized representative is:
Springer Nature Customer Service Center GmbH
Europaplatz 3, 69115 Heidelberg, Germany

Printed by Libri Plureos GmbH
in Hamburg, Germany